*The American Medical
Women's Association*

The Women's
Complete
Wellness Book

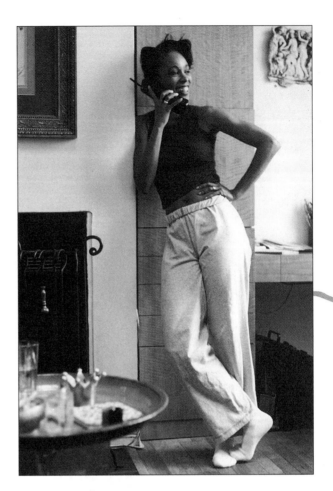

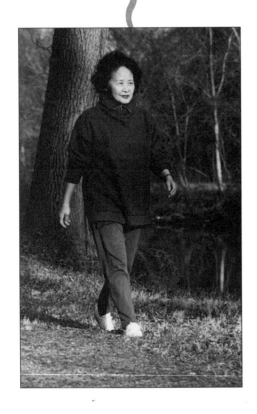

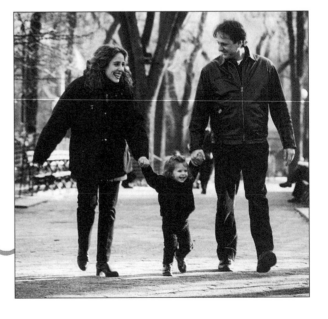

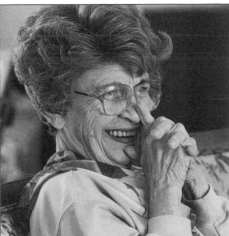
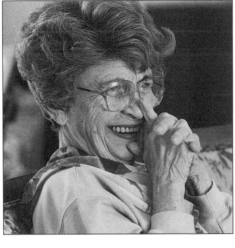
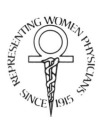

The American Medical Women's Association

The Women's *Complete* Wellness Book

Debra R. Judelson, M.D., F.A.C.C., F.A.C.P.

  Medical Director, Women's Heart Institute

  Senior Partner, Cardiovascular Medical Group of
    Southern California

  1996–97 President, American Medical Women's
    Association

Diana L. Dell, M.D., F.A.C.O.G.

  Assistant Professor, Duke University Medical Center,
    Department of Obstetrics & Gynecology

  Senior Resident, University of North Carolina—
    Chapel Hill, Department of Psychiatry

  1994–95 President, American Medical Women's
    Association

PRODUCED BY THE PHILIP LIEF GROUP

St. Martin's Griffin ≋ New York

This book provides comprehensive information relating to women's health issues, but should not be used as a substitute for medical advice. The reader should consult a physician for individual medical problems.

THE WOMEN'S COMPLETE WELLNESS BOOK. Copyright © 1998 by The Philip Lief Group, Inc., and The American Medical Women's Association. All rights reserved. Printed in the United States of America. No part of this book may be used or reproduced in any manner whatsoever without written permission except in the case of brief quotations embodied in critical articles or reviews. For information, address St. Martin's Press, 175 Fifth Avenue, New York, N.Y. 10010.

Produced by The Phillip Lief Group

Photographs by David Kelly Crow
Illustrations by Precision Graphics

ISBN 0-312-25472-5

First published in the United States by Golden Books Publishing Co., Inc.

First St. Martin's Griffin Edition: March 2000

10 9 8 7 6 5 4 3 2 1

Table of Contents

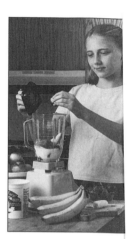

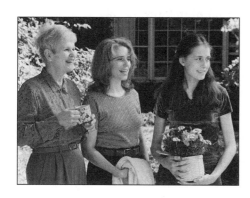

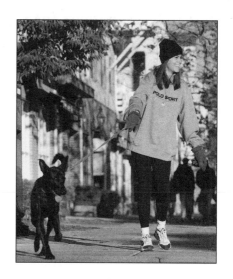

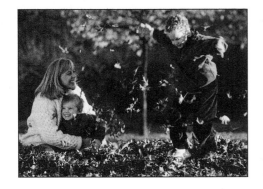

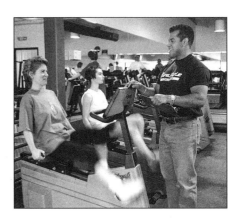

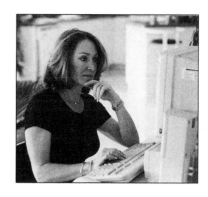

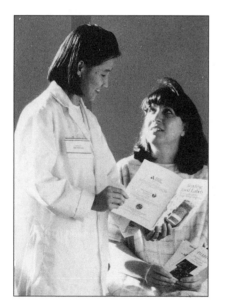

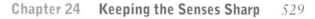

Acknowledgments

I am grateful for the work of the researchers, experts, physicians, and organizations that constantly expand our knowledge in women's health, and for the women's health movement, which has raised our awareness about the issues important to women and their families. These contributions, the pioneering efforts of the American Medical Women's Association, and the support of our membership have made this book possible.

I appreciate, thank, and dedicate my efforts to:
my family, who encouraged me and forgave me the time I spent on this project;
my parents, who inspired me to have limitless goals and ambitions; and
my patients, who taught me that being well in both mind and body is what health is all about.

Debra M. Judelson, M.D.

~~~~~~~~

I am grateful to the American Medical Women's Association for fueling the women's health movement in this country. And I am deeply honored by the efforts of Eileen McGrath, J.D., AMWA's executive director, for her enduring support of women physicians and the special care they bring to the patients they serve.

Diana L. Dell, M.D.

Introduction

Modern medical science has traditionally been more focused on the diagnosis and treatment of disease than with its prevention, screening, and early detection. As "miracle cures" for common illnesses were developed through scientific research, the average woman began to feel less responsibility for taking the basic steps to prevent illness—engaging in regular exercise, eating a variety of healthy foods, and avoiding dangerous substances. Further, as medical information became more complex and difficult to understand, many women lost sight of their health risk factors. Others were unaware of obvious symptoms of illness or put off their own medical appointments because they were too busy caring for other family members or concerns. *The Women's Complete Wellness Book* offers women a path back to a practical approach to good health and the reassurance that wellness is very much within every woman's reach and control.

Wellness can be defined for each woman as *her own ideal degree of good health.* Achieving wellness, then, presents a different challenge for every woman. Genetic factors, the environment, stress, age, existing medical conditions, and attitudes toward health and health care combine to form the degree of wellness a woman can expect to achieve. Active wellness requires that a woman take responsibility for learning about her body and about the internal and external factors that influence her health. In this process, she also learns about taking steps to avoid negative influences and foster positive ones. According to this definition, a woman with arthritis is well if she has learned as much as she can about her condition and has successfully reduced her joint pain and preserved her mobility in spite of her arthritis. She may, in fact, claim a higher degree of wellness than a woman without arthritis who does nothing to minimize her potential health risks.

Women can lead the movement toward the basic principles of wellness. Those who embark on a wellness program designed to prevent disease—rather than waiting passively for illness to strike and then depending on their health care system to choose the right treatment for them—find this experience enormously empowering. The primary mission of *The Women's Complete Wellness Book* is to help women take control of every aspect of their health and begin living the quality life that good health provides and every woman deserves.

All the information a woman needs to achieve her optimal health and maintain wellness is contained in the pages of this book. Most recommendations in health books are based primarily on studies of the health concerns of men and assume that women's concerns are the same. Traditional health books usually limit their discussions to symptoms and treatments rather than prevention and an overall health outlook. *The Women's Complete Wellness Book,* on the other hand, bases its information as much as possible on the study of women, embraces a broad spectrum of topics focused on wellness, and addresses many issues that typical health books and encyclopedias skim over or avoid altogether.

Part I, "The Goal Is Wellness," presents an overview of the health issues most relevant to women today. Readers learn how to assess their own genetic and environmental risk factors using a family medical history and personal health risk assessment. An important discussion of health care plans and doctors reminds every woman that although she controls her own wellness, she is never alone in her efforts to achieve optimal health. She will, in the course of her life, work with a variety of medical practitioners and needs to feel comfortable communicating with them. The important decisions a woman makes about her health care providers and her health insurance plan can either facilitate or impede her goal of optimal health. Women who have a strong understanding of the principles of wellness feel empowered to partner with doctors and health plans that they can depend upon to help them live well throughout their lives.

Part II, "Checking Up for Total Wellness," provides a thorough, detailed discussion about routine care and the health concerns that arise most often in each life stage. The importance of proactive, routine care from birth to old age is emphasized, including up-to-date information on when to schedule checkups and vaccinations. Part II helps each reader construct a lifetime wellness plan for herself.

Part III, "A Healthy Lifestyle," offers sound guidelines for making sensible lifestyle choices. Easy-to-understand explanations of the role of good nutrition, regular exercise, and adequate rest and relaxation in preventing disease and living a quality life are presented in an engaging, compelling fashion.

Part III also examines the fundamentals of a healthy lifestyle that are not typically covered in other health books—mental health concerns, injury and accident prevention, sexuality, relationships and communication, violence prevention, family planning, pregnancy, and menopause. These are issues of particular importance to women. Relationships, for example, can be destructive and even dangerous, or they can provide the joy and intimacy necessary for ideal good health. Examining relationships in this light can allow women to renew their commitment to making relationships as healthy and constructive as possible. A woman's mental and emotional life, long considered only peripheral to good health, can actually work for or against her on her road to wellness. Concerns about the violence all women fear and many women face every day has a dramatic impact on both emotional and physical well-being. These "non-disease" topics are as essential to the prevention of injury and preservation of health as are the knowledge and discussion of such topics as cancer and infectious disease.

Part IV, "Maintaining the Balance of Wellness," illuminates the inner workings of a woman's body—the complex systems that operate together to keep us well. A basic knowledge of how these systems function can help women better understand the behaviors and lifestyle choices that cause imbalances leading to illness, infection, or disease. Part IV begins with a discussion of the cardiovascular system and how to lower your risk of heart disease—the number one killer of women in the United States. Also included are chapters that focus on reducing your risk of cancer (including an explanation of the major cancers that strike women), protecting your body from infection, lowering your risk of metabolic disease, keeping your senses sharp, and strengthening your bones and muscles. As with all other topics in this book, the focus is on understanding disease prevention and maintaining healthy systems in every life stage.

Achieving wellness does not require a sudden or complete overhaul of daily activities. Wellness is a process and a state of mind that requires only a few moments of attention each day. The clear and concise information we have gathered for *The Women's Complete Wellness Book* will help every woman tailor her own program to meet her specific needs and goals for her optimal health. We dedicate this book to your wellness and the wellness of those you care for!

Debra R. Judelson
M.D., F.A.C.C., F.A.C.P.

Diana L. Dell
M.D., F.A.C.O.G.

PART I

The Goal Is Wellness

With all that women do in the course of a day, most do not take the time to stop and think, "I feel well today; I am healthy." Only when a fever—or something more worrisome, such as blurred vision or a lump in the breast—occurs do most women turn their attention to their health.

The wellness approach to health encourages you to learn all you can about your body and your personal health while you are well. It then directs you to take the necessary steps to keep yourself well throughout your life. At issue is not just good health, but self-awareness, self-direction, and self-control. The wellness approach empowers you to take charge of your own health and well-being so that you can become a partner with your doctor in maintaining your good health, not just as a patient trying to regain it.

In order to understand the goal of wellness, it is important to first discover what helps women stay well—and what makes them sick. Chapter 1 looks at women's health in the United States today and identifies some of the greatest threats to good health. You may be surprised to find, for example, that cardiovascular disease, not breast cancer, is the leading cause of death for women. Learning this essential fact—and many others—is likely to convince you to say to yourself, "I am well now, but what can I do to avoid falling victim to cardiovascular disease or some other serious condition?"

Your wellness program begins with you evaluating your current health status and determining the particular risks you face as an individual, based upon your family medical history and your lifestyle. By exploring your past, you can learn a great deal about your health future. Chapter 2 offers an in-depth look at the most common health conditions and their risk factors. The chapter includes a family medical history and health risk assessment form that you can fill out and analyze with your doctor's help. By taking a look at what risk factors may threaten your wellness in the future, you can begin now to improve your chances of remaining healthy.

Central to the success of your wellness program is choosing the right doctor to work with you. Routine examinations show your health status now and keep your health profile up-to-date, providing both you and your doctor opportunities to develop a realistic plan for optimum health. Chapter 3 helps you navigate the health care system and make well-informed choices about health insurance and health care providers. When you establish a positive, trusting relationship with a doctor while you are well, you can count on her knowledge of your particular health profile to help you prevent illness and to give the most effective treatment if you do become ill.

If you are a healthy woman in the United States, you hold the power to improve your chances of living into your seventies or eighties. Part I of this book illustrates that with the gift of a long life comes the responsibility to ensure that your *quality* of life remains high, as well.

A **Dynamic** **Approach** *for a* **Longer,** **Healthier Life**

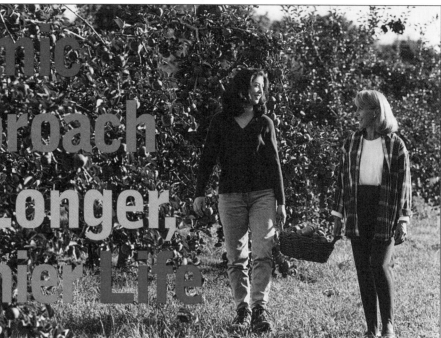

Women are recognizing the importance of taking a proactive role in their own wellness. That is, they are learning not to wait until they are ill to seek medical help and advice. Nor are women depending solely on their doctors and health care providers to tell them what they need to know about staying well. Rather they are actively seeking information that helps them optimize their well-being while they prevent the illnesses that compromised the health of women in earlier generations.

Most women have traditionally thought of health and health care in "either/or" terms: either they were sick and needed help to get better or they were not sick and could ignore health care. But as the new century approaches, this view of health and health care services is changing. Women and their health care professionals are beginning to assess health along a continuum of wellness. Instead of asking, "Am I sick?" more women are now asking, "How well am I?" and "How well can I be?"

Wellness means feeling and being as healthy as you can possibly be. The way to achieve wellness is to optimize your physical and emotional conditions: to lead a healthy lifestyle by eating well, getting adequate rest and exercise, reaching and maintaining your optimal weight, managing stress, avoiding cigarettes and drugs, investigating your family history and risks for disease, and preventing accidents and violence. For many women, wellness also means keeping a chronic health problem under control—whether it is a minor one, such as an allergy, or a more serious condition, such as diabetes or high blood pressure.

Studies show that the medical and personal costs of staying healthy are far less in the long run than the costs of dealing with and treating preventable illness and disease after they have taken root. Thinking of health in terms of wellness not only helps reduce risks for disease, it also prompts us to detect problems *before* they become so far advanced that they cannot be treated or cured without costly and complicated efforts.

Adopting a philosophy of wellness makes sense for every woman, since women now fill many more roles than they did in decades past. They are wives and mothers, but they are also breadwinners, money-managers, and educators for their families. Furthermore, they frequently are called upon to be the health care "specialists" in their homes, with responsibility not just for their own health, but for the health of their entire families, from newborns to aging parents. With all their other responsibilities, it is essential for women not to let personal and family wellness fall through the cracks. Promoting healthy habits at home and choosing a health care system and health care providers will always be among their most important roles.

Facts *About* Women
and Their Health

In the United States, the average life expectancy at birth for females is 75.7 years. However, given the absence of disease or accidental death, women can expect to live an average of 79 years. This age is dramatically higher than women's life expectancy in 1900, when the average woman lived only to age 48.

A longer life, of course, does not necessarily mean a better life. The quality of your life, especially in old age, depends to a great extent on the quality of your health. The way to ensure that those extra years are productive and satisfying is to begin taking responsibility for your own wellness now, whether you are a young woman just beginning to think about health issues or a woman who is past retirement age.

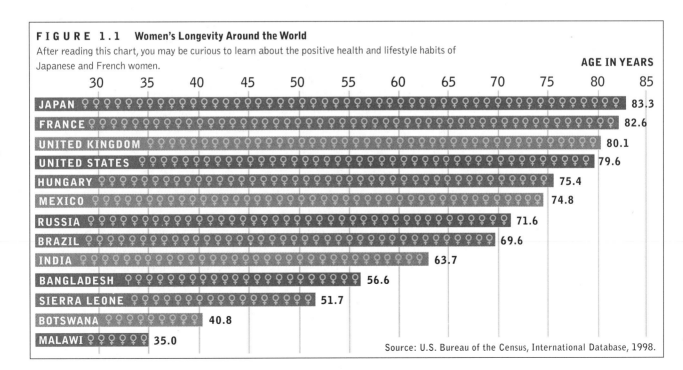

FIGURE 1.1   Women's Longevity Around the World

After reading this chart, you may be curious to learn about the positive health and lifestyle habits of Japanese and French women.

Source: U.S. Bureau of the Census, International Database, 1998.

Managing Life Stresses

Stress has always been a fact of every woman's life. The responsibilities of caring for aging parents, young children, husbands, and/or ailing siblings have typically fallen to women. Today, new kinds of stress are taking their toll on women in addition to the traditional ones.

Women today are handling some of the same life problems that were once the domain of men. The number of women who work for wages outside the home has increased dramatically in the last few decades. At the same time, however, household maintenance and primary childcare remain largely the responsibility of women. The demographic shift that places women in the workplace has brought them more financial security and economic power, but these assets have come with a cost. Women are statistically more at risk today for stress-related illnesses than they have ever been before.

Balancing Work, Family, and Wellness

For many women, working outside the home or managing a business from a home office adds burdens to their lives as they try to juggle the obligations that come with both a career and a family. The issue is time—or rather lack of it. An eight-hour work day combined with six to ten hours of "second-shift" work—cleaning, helping kids with their studies, preparing meals and filling lunch boxes, arranging for extra-curricular activities for children, not to mention attending to the emotional needs of children, husbands, and friends—adds up to a "time crunch" that makes it difficult for women to tend to their own health needs until they realize that something is wrong.

Heart disease is the leading cause of death in women, and since 1989, statistics show that more women than men in the United States die of this disease. This relatively recent phenomenon has become a kind of barometer indicating that many women are not aware of their risk, do not receive adequate diagnostic and screening care, and do not pay close enough attention to the symptoms of serious disease. The increase in incidence of heart disease further reveals that women's responsibilities are growing, stress levels are rising, and spare time for heart-healthy activities is shrinking.

Many women feel driven to "do it all" without realizing the toll on their health such an unrealistic goal takes. Single mothers have the extra burden of family responsibilities in addition to their careers. Women without children often focus more on their careers, volunteer work, expanding educational goals, and keeping up with extended families as they neglect their personal health needs. At-home wives and mothers immerse themselves in their spouse's and children's needs, volunteer work, and, again, the needs of the extended family. Women who choose a career and a family fill every minute of every day trying to be successful in both those realms. When "doing it all" means sacrificing good health, or when women find they just cannot make the time to practice a healthy lifestyle, exercise, and see their doctor for wellness checks, then it might be time to learn to do less. In other words, if being successful at all you do for your own sake and for the sake of others is important to you, then one of the most important things you can do is preserve your health so that you can continue to be successful for a long time.

Wellness: *A New Perspective* on Health

Unlike traditional health care, which focuses on treating and curing disease, wellness promotes the techniques of maintaining good health and offers sound advice for resolving problems when they do arise. Besides improving the quality of your life, the major benefit of the wellness approach is that it makes you less dependent on your doctors and health care providers by giving you the primary responsibility for your own health and well-being.

The first step in taking charge of your own health is to know yourself. This means assessing the risk factors for illness that are unique to you—those that run in your family or are present because of where you work, where you live, and *how* you live—your lifestyle. (Chapter 2 discusses this topic in detail.) If you find you are at risk for particular disorders, you can take positive steps to reduce the chances you will contract those diseases. Another important step is to develop a positive, cooperative relationship with your doctor by scheduling routine screening tests and examinations, with emphasis on your higher risk concerns. Such examinations give you an opportunity to speak with the doctor about your overall health; they reassure you that your wellness program is working for you; and they help detect illnesses before they pose serious threats to your health.

Detecting Problems Early

Early detection is an essential component of preventive health care. The most important tools used to detect health problems early are routine assessments and screening.

Routine Assessment. An estimated one-third of American women are at risk for health problems that have not been detected but that can be treated. This is one of the most compelling reasons for routine examinations by your doctor. It is recommended that you have at least one routine assessment each year or so, during which your doctor can direct her attention to a complete physical examination and any other evaluations or procedures warranted by your particular health profile, rather than focusing on an acute illness. (Part II of this book discusses all the routine assessments recommended at each stage of a woman's life.)

During routine visits, your doctor can also gather information to determine whether you should receive special tests. For example, during a routine visit to your gynecologist, she will do breast and pelvic examinations. If any abnormalities or changes from the last visit are seen, you may be referred for further tests.

Some women who know they are at risk avoid scheduling routine assessments because, they say, they are afraid they will find out that something is wrong. This is an understandable fear. But facing fears, even to find out a problem exists, is easier than being constantly afraid. Routine examinations yield high gains in terms of long-term good health, and they give you and your doctor a chance to talk over any topics of concern that may have arisen since the last visit. When you are seeing your doctor regularly, she can more easily keep track of your health history. In fact, there are many benefits of developing a closer working relationship with your health care provider.

wellness **tip**

Regular checkups are key to good health, even if you have no signs of problems. Routine examinations are advised for women of all ages. Try making your appointments for routine visits well in advance— near your birthday, for example. Make them a priority so you will not be tempted to cancel or reschedule them.

Screening. Screenings are defined as procedures or tests that are done in the absence of any signs or symptoms of disease. Screening may be done for a number of reasons. Some screening tests, such as the Pap smear for cervical cancer, are recommended for adult women of all ages, regardless of their health history. Other tests, such as a mammogram to detect breast cancer or a sigmoidoscopy or colonoscopy to detect rectal and colon cancer, are done on a regular basis starting at a certain age. This is because the risk of these cancers rises with age. But other screening tests may be done only if a woman has a family history of a particular health problem, which automatically increases her own risk.

Screening, such as with blood tests, is also a way of identifying health conditions that need closer monitoring. It is recommended that women who have high cholesterol, for example, have regular tests to measure complete lipid levels so that problems can be monitored—and treated—early. Treating high cholesterol by changing your lifestyle or using medication as needed is much easier and much less costly (both personally and financially) than undergoing heart surgery for a blocked artery or living with the effects of a stroke.

It is impractical to use every screening test on every person every time. Continuing studies of the natural history of disease (called epidemiology) helps medical experts make recommendations for who should be screened for what and when.

Wellness and the Quality of Life

When you take steps, such as improving your eating habits, to help prevent disease, you also begin to feel good on a daily basis, thus improving the quality of your life. Exercise, another component of wellness, is a proven "stress-buster." It not only tones your muscles, facilitating ease of movement and reducing the risk of injury and heart disease, it also releases endorphins, the "feel good" substances that are believed to help control the body's reaction to pain and tension. All these benefits boost self-esteem and lead to a sense of well-being, which greatly enhances your enjoyment of life.

Following the basics of good health—nutrition, exercise, and stress management—is easier than you think and helps you get more enjoyment out of life.

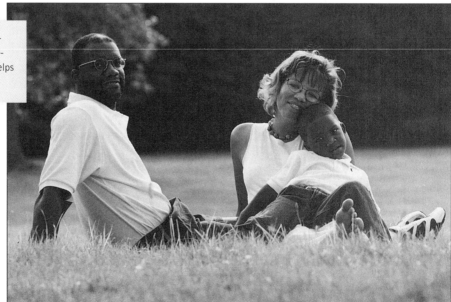

The Dollars and Health Sense of Preventive Medicine

Preventive care saves money as well as lives. Screening procedures and efforts to change behaviors that affect health can prevent and control diseases that cost a great deal to treat. For example:

- Programs that help pregnant women quit smoking can save over $6 for each dollar spent.
- Each dollar spent on teaching diabetics how to manage the disease saves $2 to $3 in hospital costs.
- For every dollar spent on educating schoolchildren about drug use and safe sex, $14 is saved in avoided health care costs for drug abuse treatment, unintended pregnancy, and sexually transmitted diseases (STDs).

Overcoming Barriers to Wellness

Although the outlook on health care is changing toward more preventive care, many women still lack information about the benefits of a wellness approach to health. An estimated 40 percent of American women do not take the simple steps that can help them stay well throughout their lives. In 1991, 42 percent of adult white women did not have a routine physical in the prior year, 44 percent of women over age 40 did not have a screening mammogram in the past two years, and 44 percent did not have a Pap smear. These routine tests are designed to detect disease in the early stages. That could save thousands of lives—and dollars—each year.

One reason so many women do not receive adequate routine health care is that their doctors are unaware that women's health needs are different from men's, and so they have not advised women appropriately. Further, women are often dissatisfied with their health care relationship—25 percent of women feel "talked down to" by their physician, and 17 percent reported being told that their health problems were "all in their head," according to a 1993 survey conducted by the Commission on Women's Health at Columbia University. Until recently, most health research has focused on male patients, and researchers have assumed that their conclusions apply equally well to both sexes. This assumption is being challenged, however, as more researchers and doctors are learning about the specific health issues women face and how women's bodies react to illness and disease.

Women as health care consumers, however, are only slowly becoming aware that there is health information available just for them, and that finding that information can keep them healthy longer. In addition, the health care system is starting to recognize the need to educate female patients and to make its information available to all patients.

Other factors that limit women's access to the wellness approach to health include poverty and illiteracy. Studies show that women with low incomes are less likely to seek routine preventive care services. Many neighborhoods and rural areas do not have convenient centers for preventive care, and even if they are available, many women cannot afford to use them.

Finally, even when a woman does have access to preventive care services, her everyday responsibilities and pressures may keep her from taking advantage of them. As stated earlier, many women feel pressed for time to do all of the things they need to do for their careers and their families. Going to the doctor when they do not feel ill seems like a low priority for many.

Common Barriers to Breast Cancer Screening

Several studies have identified the most common reasons women do not use health services to screen for breast cancer:

- **Cost.** Many women cite cost as the reason they do not use early detection programs. Many are not aware of the availability of low-cost programs.
- **Time Constraints.** Women feel their day is already more than full. Making time for preventive health care is not a typical priority.
- **Lack of Physician Referral.** Studies have shown that women are more likely to be screened if their physician advises it.
- **Fear of Results.** Women do not want to find that they have cancer.
- **Transportation.** Because many women lack a way to get to a screening center, the location of screening facilities is important.
- **Communication Barriers.** Communication styles and methods sometimes do not accommodate the needs of the women seeking services. This is especially true for illiterate women and women whose first language is not English.
- **Lack of Childcare.** Many women need help to arrange childcare in order to be able to use screening.

Some of these barriers to preventive health care are not within our control—but many are. Wellness takes a surprisingly small amount of time. The busiest of women can substitute healthy snacks for junk food, can park farther from the store or office entrance, can walk for twenty minutes a day, and can schedule an hour for a wellness checkup during each year. We can work together to improve health care for all women by being aware of legislation that affects women, by participating in political discussions, and by encouraging members of Congress to put the topic high on their agendas. Finally, we can educate ourselves. The information we need is available. Keeping this book at your bedside table, for example, and reading sections for only a few minutes a night will raise your awareness of the importance of wellness and give you practical tools to use in meeting your health needs.

Major *Health Risks* to Women

The health risks women face vary according to age, economic status, ethnic background, and educational background. Young women, for example, are less likely to contract diseases that are not prevalent in their families, but are more likely to die from accidents, such as motor vehicle accidents, and suicide than are older women. As women age, heart disease and cancer pose greater risks to their health. Older women are also much more likely than younger women to develop osteoporosis, a disease that weakens bone tissue and can lead to injury and disability.

Among African American women, the rates of deaths from breast cancer, AIDS, and hypertension are higher than for white women, who have a higher

TABLE 1.1

Leading Causes of Death in American Women in 1995

Rank	Cause	Number	Number of deaths per 100,000 women
1	Heart diseases	360,161	275.8
2	Cancer (including breast cancer)	245,740	188.2
3	Stroke	87,124	66.7
4	Lung diseases (other than cancer)	41,473	31.8
5	Pneumonia and influenza	40,254	30.8
6	Accidents and injuries	28,915	22.1
7	Diabetes mellitus	28,395	21.7
8	Kidney diseases	11,346	8.7
9	Septicemia	11,140	8.5
10	Atherosclerosis	10,503	8.0
	All other causes	188,226	144.1

Source: National Center for Health Statistics, 1996.

risk of death from smoking-related lung diseases, like emphysema. Poor women are more likely to wait before seeing a doctor, even if symptoms of a serious disease are present. They are also more at risk for diseases that are caused by—or made worse by—poor nutrition. Women who are poorly educated also tend to delay visiting a doctor, and avoid screening and diagnostic testing because they are less aware of the options available to them. For these reasons, society has much to gain by making wellness information available to all women, through various means.

Advances in medical research for women have revealed several major health risks women face going into the twenty-first century. In order to take advantage of this research, read the general descriptions below, consider whether you are at risk for these diseases, and then learn as much as you can by referring to more detailed sections throughout this book. It has been said that good health is everything, and you have everything to gain with the wellness approach to your health.

Heart Disease

Of the approximately one million women who died in 1995 from all causes, more than one-third of them died from heart diseases (see Table 1.1). Since the early 1900s, heart disease—and specifically coronary artery or coronary heart disease (CHD)—has been the leading cause of death in both women and men in the United States. CHD is caused by a buildup of fatty deposits in the inner walls of the major blood vessels (arteries) that lead to the heart. This buildup can partly or completely block the flow of blood to the heart. When an artery becomes totally blocked, a heart attack or stroke can result.

Although the mortality rate from CHD has been declining since the 1970s, this drop has been greater in men than in women. Men's rate of death from CHD fell by 30 percent between 1979 and 1993, but women's fell by only 23 percent. Consider these statistics:

- In 1993, about one-third of all deaths in the United States were due to CHD.
- An estimated 70 million Americans have some form of heart disease.
- As many as 150,000 people every year have fatal heart attacks from CHD.

Risks for Heart Disease. Until the 1990s, men had higher rates of CHD than women at all age groups. They still have more risk factors for CHD. However, as larger numbers of women smoke and pursue lifelong careers outside the home, their stress levels and risks are also rising.

From the late 1970s to the mid-1990s, the gap between men's and women's rates of death from CHD gradually narrowed as men's rate decreased and women's increased. By 1994, the two rates were nearly identical: 284 of every 100,000 men and 278 of every 100,000 women died from heart disease in that year. Now, CHD is the leading cause of death in American women of nearly all races. The exception is Asian/Pacific Islander women, for whom it is the second leading cause of death (after cancer). The disease occurs in more than twice as many African American women as white women. The risk is lower in American Indian, Asian, and Hispanic women than in white women.

The risk of CHD increases as women age, with an acceleration as women become postmenopausal and lose the natural protective effects of the hormone estrogen. The risk for women aged 55 and over is ten times higher than for those

wellness
warning

Smoking and excessive drinking are the leading causes of health problems for white women, while sedentary lifestyle and obesity are the leading causes for African American and Hispanic women. A sedentary lifestyle poses the biggest health threat to Asian women. White women and more educated women suffer from more alcohol-related health problems than other women, especially when drinking starts early in life.

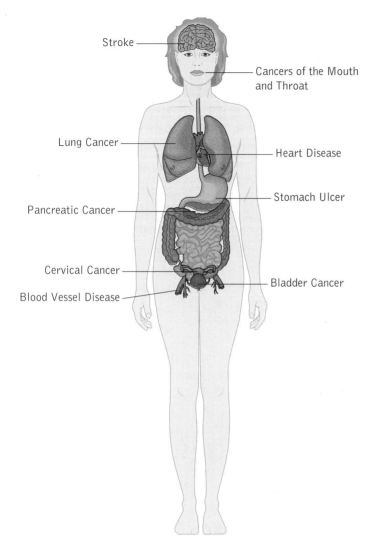

Stroke

Cancers of the Mouth and Throat

Lung Cancer

Heart Disease

Stomach Ulcer

Pancreatic Cancer

Cervical Cancer

Bladder Cancer

Blood Vessel Disease

FIGURE 1.2

The Health Threats of Smoking

Smoking has negative effects on many areas of the body, but even if you have been smoking for many years, you can reduce your risk of developing certain conditions and diseases by quitting now.

aged 35 to 54 years. About one out of every nine women aged 45 to 64 has some type of heart disease; after age 65, this rate increases to one in three.

The Framingham Study. In 1948, a coalition of researchers began to study a group of women and men over their lifetimes in order to see how many developed heart disease and what factors placed them at risk. Called the Framingham Heart Study (after the Massachusetts town in which it is based), the research is ongoing today and has enrolled four generations of women and men.

One of the findings of the Framingham study has been that women appear to develop CHD about ten years later in life than men do. It has also showed that, although more men than women get CHD, after age 65 this gap begins to narrow.

The Framingham study has yielded valuable information about risk factors for CHD. Its most clear-cut conclusions have been that people who eat foods high in fat and cholesterol, who do not engage in regular physical activities or get enough exercise, and who smoke cigarettes are at increased risk for heart disease.

The Framingham study misled researchers for years because it looked at males and females in the same manner. Now, more sophisticated tests have revealed that women's cardiac risk does not follow the male pattern; specifically, that chest pain is not an accurate marker for risk in women as it is for men. Another significant difference is that those women in the study who had heart attacks suffered more complications, had higher mortality, and had more repeat heart attacks than men.

Smoking-Related Illnesses

A great deal of research has focused on the risks of tobacco use, especially cigarette smoking. Studies show that smoking is linked to lung cancer, high blood pressure, heart disease, and stroke. Yet despite the wealth of knowledge about the hazards, many women—more than one-fifth of those over age 18—continue to smoke. The number of smokers is highest among women aged 25 to 34. This statistic is troubling, since these are the prime childbearing years, and smoking is known to increase the risk of miscarriage and other pregnancy problems.

Using tobacco increases a woman's risk for chronic health problems and early death:

- Nearly one-third of all deaths from cancer are linked to tobacco use.
  - ➤ About 62,000 women die from lung cancer each year. These deaths are largely due to smoking.

> ➤ In addition to lung cancer, smoking is a major risk factor for cancers of the cervix, mouth, throat, kidney, bladder, and possibly breast.

- The risks of heart attack and stroke are greatly increased in women who smoke. These risks are actually increased more in younger than in older women.
  - ➤ An estimated 34,000 women die each year from heart attacks that are thought to be linked to smoking.
  - ➤ About 8,000 women die from strokes linked to smoking each year.
- Smoking damages the health of a woman and her baby during and after pregnancy:
  - ➤ Up to one-fifth of women smoke during their pregnancies. These women run a higher than average risk of miscarriage, stillbirth, premature birth, and infant death.
  - ➤ Smoking during pregnancy is a major cause of low birth weight in infants.
  - ➤ Research suggests that babies born to mothers who smoke during or after their pregnancies are more likely to die from SIDS (sudden infant death syndrome).

Breast Cancer

Breast cancer is second only to lung cancer as a cause of cancer deaths in women. A number of factors increase a woman's risk for breast cancer:

- **Aging.** The risk of breast cancer increases with age; the highest rates are seen in women in their mid to late 70s.
- **Family history of breast cancer.** Having a first-degree relative (mother, sister, or daughter) with breast cancer increases the risk. Less risk is associated with second-degree relatives (aunt or grandmother).
- **Previous breast cancer.** Women who have had breast cancer, even if it was treated successfully, are more likely to get it again.
- **Previous non-cancer breast problems.** Benign breast disease, such as fibro-cystic changes, increases the risk of breast cancer.
- **Older age at first childbirth.** Women who never have children or who delay childbirth until their late 30s or early 40s are at an increased risk for breast cancer.

The good news is that a woman's chances of surviving breast cancer are very high—up to 97 percent—when it is caught before it has spread to other sites in the body. The best way to detect breast cancer at an early stage is to examine your breasts monthly, have regular checkups with your gynecologist, and receive mammograms *at least* every other year after age 40. Breast cancer screening with mammograms is the most effective way to detect breast cancer in its earliest, most treatable stage. Mammograms detect cancer an average of 1.7 years before the woman can feel a lump herself. It can also locate tumors that are too small to be felt during a breast examination. Screening mammograms and proper treatment have been shown to reduce the risk of death from breast cancer by 30 percent for women aged 50 to 69 years.

AIDS and HIV

AIDS, or acquired immunodeficiency syndrome, has claimed nearly one-quarter of a million lives in the United States since the disease was first recognized in the early 1980s. Although AIDS rates have always been higher in men than in

wellness **tip**

Quitting smoking isn't easy, but it is always possible. Smoking-cessation programs, counseling, and methods, such as nicotine gum or patches, can help. The basic principles behind quitting for good are given in Chapter 13.

women, more than 10,000 women are found to have the disease each year. Between 1988 and 1996, almost 50,000 American women died of AIDS. It is the fourth leading cause of death in women 25 to 44 years of age.

AIDS is caused by a virus called HIV (human immunodeficiency virus) that attacks the body's immune system, making it vulnerable to life-threatening diseases. HIV is mainly spread through contact with an infected person's blood, body secretions, or semen. Babies can become infected before birth if the mother has HIV.

Since the disease was first identified, more than twice as many African American as white women have died from AIDS. In 1995 alone, AIDS caused more than 4,000 deaths among African American women, almost 40 percent more than in white women. The disease is slightly less common in Hispanic women than in white women. American Indian and Asian women have relatively low rates of AIDS.

When AIDS was first identified, most women who were found to have the disease had become infected through the use of intravenous drugs. Today, however, heterosexual contact is the leading cause of AIDS among all women. But intravenous drug use remains a major cause of AIDS in women. Most women who are infected during sexual intercourse get the disease because their male partners are intravenous drug users.

Sexually transmitted HIV infection causes more cases of AIDS in women in their 20s than in older women. Because AIDS can take years to develop after a person is exposed to the virus, it is thought that these women were infected in their teens.

Women of all ages and races can reduce their risk of HIV and AIDS by having monogamous relationships in which both partners agree not to have sex with anyone else, and by always using latex condoms during sex. Women who use intravenous drugs can lower their risk by getting into a drug treatment program and by not sharing needles with others.

Chronic Diseases

Long-term health problems are major causes of disability in women, especially older women. These include chronic conditions, which can be treated but not completely cured. Many women have more than one chronic disease. Among women aged 65 to 85, 31 percent have one chronic disease, 27 percent have two, 24 percent have 3 or more, and 18 percent have no chronic diseases. Women with chronic diseases must learn to manage them in order to stay healthy and to make life as comfortable and active as possible. In this endeavor, a good relationship with her doctor is crucial for a woman.

Most people think of chronic illness as inevitable for women as they age. But the truth is that most chronic conditions can be prevented, delayed, or successfully treated. However, because women live an average of seven years longer than men (the U.S. Bureau of the Census estimates that there are some 25,000 women over the age of 100 in the United States!), they are particularly prone to chronic health problems.

Arthritis. A painful and sometimes disabling disease of the joints, arthritis affects almost 40 million people in the United States. More than half—23 million—are women. As both women and men age, the number who develop arthritis rises until about age 65. After that age, the rate levels off among men but continues to rise among women. More than half of women over 65 have arthritis. African American women are especially prone to disability due to arthritis.

The most common forms of arthritis are osteoarthritis and rheumatoid arthritis. In osteoarthritis, the tissue in the joints begins to break down, causing pain and stiffness. This type of arthritis is by far the most common. About half of all cases of arthritis in women, and three-fourths of all cases in both sexes, are osteoarthritis. Rheumatoid arthritis affects fewer women but is much more severe. It is thought that rheumatoid arthritis is caused by a problem with the immune system, causing it to "backfire" and attack healthy tissue in the joints.

The presence of arthritis restricts a woman's movements and places limits on her ability to enjoy life fully. When the disease becomes severe, a woman may be unable to exercise or work and may have pain much of the time. Arthritis can be treated but is never completely cured. Treatment is aimed at reducing pain, stiffness, and swelling in order to allow a woman to remain as active as possible. Disabling arthritis is a major cause of dependency as women age.

More research is needed to find out what causes arthritis. Some risk factors are known to be linked to the disease. Women who are obese and have an inactive lifestyle, for example, are at high risk for arthritis. As is true of so many health problems, women can reduce their risk of arthritis by eating well and exercising regularly.

Osteoporosis. About one-fifth of American women have osteoporosis, a disease in which bone density is reduced. The disease affects many more women than men, most likely because it is linked to the lower bone density developed by women in childhood and the increased bone mineral loss caused by reduced estrogen levels after menopause. The risk of osteoporosis increases dramatically after age 50, and more than 90 percent of women have developed the disease by age 80. In fact, complications of

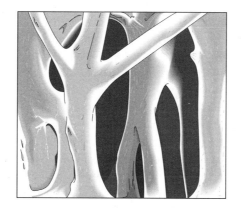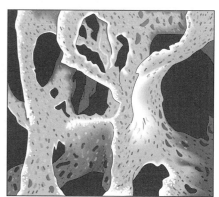

FIGURE 1.3 Osteoporosis and Bone Health
By the time they reach 80, more than 90 percent of women have developed osteoporosis, a condition characterized by decreased bone density. On the left is dense, healthy bone; on the right is bone affected by osteoporosis.

osteoporosis cause death in 2.4 percent of postmenopausal women, about the same mortality rate as postmenopausal breast cancer. It is more common in white women of slender build and in women who smoke.

Severe osteoporosis can lead to fractures and to malformations of the spinal column, causing a hump in the shoulders and shortened stature. Women can prevent or delay the onset of this disease by engaging in weight-bearing exercises, such as jogging, walking with weights, or low-impact aerobics. Many doctors also advise women to build up their calcium "bank" throughout their young adult years by eating more foods with natural sources of calcium (such as low-fat dairy products) or by taking calcium supplements. Yet 61 percent of women over 45 are not familiar with osteoporosis, and 79 percent of women aged 18 to 44 (and 58 percent of women over 65) do not get an adequate amount of calcium.

wellness **tip**

The National Domestic
Violence Hotline,
800-799-SAFE
(800-799-7233), is a
toll-free, 24-hour number
that you can call any time
you feel threatened by an
abuser. Trained personnel
are always available to
help you take action to
protect yourself and your
children.

Special tests to screen for the early signs of osteoporosis can detect changes in bone density. Doctors sometimes suggest these tests for women who are at high risk for osteoporosis because treatment to reverse this disease _is_ available.

Diabetes. It is estimated that more than 4 million American women currently have diabetes. This is a disease in which a hormone called insulin, which normally regulates the body's level of glucose (blood sugar), does not carry out its function properly. The disease is among the ten leading causes of death in all women. Among African American women, the rate of diabetes is higher than in women of other races: in 1995, it was the fourth leading cause of death in African American women. Diabetes is an increased risk for Native American and Hispanic women as well.

Even if controlled, diabetes can cause serious health problems:

- **Heart disease** is 2 to 4 times more common in people with diabetes.
- **Stroke** is 2.5 times more common in people with diabetes.
- **High blood pressure** is present in 60 to 65 percent of people with diabetes.
- **Blindness** in people aged 20 to 74 is caused most often by diabetes, especially poorly controlled diabetes.

Diabetes can also lead to kidney problems, nerve disease, and circulatory problems that require amputation of a lower limb. It can also cause serious complications during pregnancy. Sometimes the disease occurs for the first time during pregnancy, when it is called gestational diabetes. It may or may not subside after the pregnancy.

Treatment for diabetes focuses on controlling blood glucose levels using exercise, diet, and oral medication. In more severe cases, insulin injections may be needed.

Women can lower their risk of diabetes by exercising, eating well, and maintaining a healthy weight. Diabetes in one pregnancy increases the risk of the disease recurring in the next pregnancy. It is recommended that women who have had gestational diabetes be screened for blood glucose levels during subsequent pregnancies.

Violence

Violence at the hands of male partners is a part of life for 1.8 million American women each year. It is estimated that up to 22 percent of married women experience violence from their husbands each year. As many as 30 percent of women treated in emergency rooms have injuries or symptoms related to physical abuse.

Variously called domestic violence, family violence, and partner or intimate violence, physical abuse from a woman's husband or boyfriend cuts across all lines of race, ethnicity, and age. Pregnancy is no buffer against the problem: up to 20 percent of women have experienced violence during their pregnancies. Some studies indicate that violence from a woman's partner actually begins or increases when she is pregnant.

Why women who are battered stay with their partners is one of the most complex questions within the women's health arena. A fundamental aspect of any abusive relationship is the victim's lack of self-confidence and self-esteem, as well as fear of the abuser. The problem seems to be affected by both the man's and the woman's family histories. Research has shown that children growing up in violent households are more likely to have abusive relationships themselves—

the boys are more likely to become abusers, and the girls are more likely to become victims. In this way, family violence can continue through generations.

Fear and shame prevent many battered women from reporting the crimes, and as a result it is generally accepted that the rate of domestic violence is much higher than the estimates indicate.

Mental Illness

Nearly one-half of American women develop symptoms of a mental health problem at some point between the ages of 15 and 54. Women are far more likely than men to suffer from anxiety and depression, the two most common mental problems among American adults. Some researchers link the high rate of depression among women to domestic violence, sexual abuse (occurring during childhood), feelings of inadequacy in balancing home and work responsibilities, and/or poverty.

Both anxiety and depression can be treated in most people with counseling, medication, or a combination of both. Women can lower their risk of these problems by using stress management techniques and getting professional help.

Anxiety. A group of disorders known as anxiety disorders includes phobias, panic disorder, and posttraumatic stress disorder. About 30 percent of women and about 19 percent of men experience an anxiety disorder at some point in their lives.

Depression. Depression, the second most common mental disorder in Americans, occurs in about 17 percent of all adults. More women (21 percent) than men (13 percent), however, are afflicted with major depression at some point in their lives.

Depression is a major cause of impaired physical, social, and work-related functioning in adult women. It also increases the risk of suicide. Recognition and treatment of the problem are needed to prevent depression from becoming a chronic problem in a woman's life.

Women's Health: *The* Search *for* Answers

At all levels of health care policy and research, women's health is coming under increasing scrutiny. Because of heightened efforts to learn more, exciting projects are in progress at national and local levels. Numerous programs are under way to advance the cause of women's health and to make information on preventive care available to all women.

Healthy People 2000

In 1990, the U.S. Public Health Service sought to bring together government, professional, and citizen-based organizations to set goals for the nation's health by the start of the next century. Named "Healthy People 2000," this project has taken shape as a national prevention initiative to improve the health of all Americans.

wellness
warning

Because the known risk factors for anxiety and depression are of special concern for so many women, it is important to be informed about the early warning signs of these problems. See Chapter 12 for a description of risk factors, and if you feel you need help, by all means seek it.

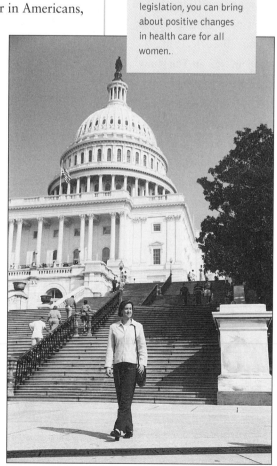

By taking an active interest in health legislation, you can bring about positive changes in health care for all women.

Joining the Women's Health Initiative

The Women's Health Initiative is a large clinical trial that has benefitted from the investment of scientific expertise and adequate funding. Women of all ages, but particularly those between the ages of 50 and 79 years old, are being sought as volunteers for research in 40 universities and hospitals all over the United States. Activities will range from answering questionnaires to participating in studies that examine the effects of aging on women. The study will follow the progress of 164,500 volunteers for up to 12 years. You can find out more about joining this important effort by contacting the Women's Health Initiative at 800-54-WOMEN (800-549-6636).

Following are its three major goals:

- To increase the span of healthy life
- To reduce inequalities in access to and quality of health care
- To provide access to preventive care

To achieve these goals, 22 major arenas were targeted for improvements in health status, risk reduction, and service delivery. One arena is the health of American women. Special efforts are underway to identify the missing links in current research on women's health and to increase the numbers of women enrolled in clinical studies.

The Women's Health Initiative

The National Institutes of Health established the Women's Health Initiative (WHI) in 1991 to explore the most common causes of death, disability, and impaired functioning in women past the age of menopause. One of the largest preventive studies in the United States, WHI is a 15-year, multi-million-dollar research effort focusing on heart disease, cancer, osteoporosis, and Alzheimer's disease in older women. Under the project, numerous clinical studies are being carried out across the nation to identify risk factors for these problems and to explore promising new approaches to prevent them, including the role of lifestyle, diet, and hormone replacement.

What *You* Can **Do**

There are many things you can do to help improve your health and health care options for you and all women:

- Identify your risk factors for diseases and disorders, and then work with your physician to make decisions about lifestyle and intervention that can minimize those risks.
- Schedule regular checkups with your doctor.
- Recognize that good nutrition, appropriate exercise, and adequate rest can improve your energy level and your quality of life.
- Find ways to manage stress and other triggers for both physical and mental illness. Limit your use of alcohol and drugs, learn good communication skills, take a proactive stance against violence, and utilize your accident-prevention skills.
- Protect yourself from sexually transmitted diseases.
- Read the health news in magazines and newspapers.
- Keep up with legislation that relates to women's health, and voice your opinion to your local lawmakers as well as your senators and congressmen.
- Consider volunteering to participate in a research study. Research is done to answer important health questions. By participating in clinical research, you can become a key component in the health recommendations that women will follow for decades to come.

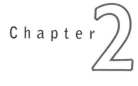

Family History *and* Lifestyle Assessment

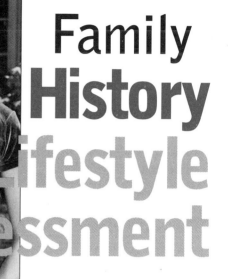

If you were to interview a hundred women about their health, their lifestyles, and the health of their families, you could find out which women are most likely to develop certain diseases by determining each woman's risk factors—the conditions in her life that indicate susceptibility to disease. Risk factors might be genetic. That is, genes carrying the potential for increased susceptibility to disease might be passed down through generations within one family. Risk factors might also be environmental, depending on where and with whom a woman lives and works. Risk factors might be based on lifestyle choices that increase the likelihood of disease. Often, risk for disease is based on a combination of genetics, environmental conditions, and lifestyle choices, all of which can cause a disease or condition to develop.

The first step in the wellness approach to health is to learn all you can about your own risk factors. Women are understandably reluctant to examine the possible health risks they live with, fearing that the knowledge will only add more anxiety to their lives. But risk assessment is a constructive, positive, "know your enemy" approach to wellness.

Learning all you can about the potential health risks you face is an important step in adopting a wellness approach to your health and longevity. Taking the time to learn about your risk factors and how to avoid dangerous situations may reduce the likelihood that you will face serious illness or injury.

Having a risk factor for a particular disorder does not mean you will definitely contract the disease. Just about everybody has at least one or two risk factors for disease. It does mean, however, that you are more *likely* to contract the disorder than someone who does not have the same risk factor, especially if you allow environmental or lifestyle choices to work against you. Acknowledging

preview

▶ **Family History**

▶ **Environmental Factors and Lifestyle Choices**

▶ **Early Detection**

▶ **Common Health Conditions and Their Risk Factors**

▶ **What You Can Do**

this greater probability is your absolute best defense against getting sick and your best chance for an early diagnosis and cure if you do get sick.

For example, you have a friend who dislikes going to the gynecologist. She is 30 years old, has no gynecological problems, and has no history of health problems in her family. So she just does not go. And she brags about it. You don't particularly like going to the gynecologist, either; but you learned some time ago that your grandmother died of cervical cancer at age 35, and your aunt is fighting the disease now. Consequently you never miss your annual appointment for an examination. If you had not acknowledged the genetic risk factors in your family, you might have been influenced by your friend to avoid the gynecologist's office until symptoms of a problem prompted a visit, rather than taking advantage of early detection options with checkups. If you develop cervical cancer, having routine checkups and screenings will increase the chances of an early diagnosis when a cure is still possible.

It is best to examine your risk factors for disease during your twenties, but it is never too late to improve your odds of living a long, healthy life. Begin by filling out the Family Medical History and Health Risk Assessment Form (Figures 2.1 and 2.2) to the extent that you can. Then show them to your physician and ask for her help in completing them. Your doctor can then counsel you in terms of lifestyle choices that might help reduce the probability of illness. She can also help you decide when screening and testing should begin. Finally, your doctor can recommend vaccinations, medications, dietary supplements, food choices, and other preventative therapies if they are appropriate.

This chapter describes how you can determine your personal risk factors for the most common diseases and begin taking steps to address them. Using the information in this chapter, you can go to the doctor with a clear idea of what questions to ask and what to expect so that the partnership between you and your physician can be most beneficial to your long-term health.

Family *History*

Certain diseases are strongly linked to risk factors passed down through families, so the easiest way to tell whether you may have inherited a risk factor is to complete a family health history. Examples of the most likely inherited diseases include diabetes, early heart disease, and some types of cancer.

A family medical history lists members of your family, including deceased relatives, and notes each person's specific health problems, the age the problem occurred, as well as their cause of death, if deceased. A completed history can show trends of diseases that run in your family. It can even predict at what age you may be susceptible to those diseases.

For a family medical history to be most effective, it should include both your immediate family (parents, brothers, sisters, and your own children) and your extended family (grandparents, and aunts and uncles who share one-fourth of your genes). Remember to include only blood relatives and make sure to include both sides of the family. Only serious diseases, medical conditions, and causes of death, if applicable, need to be mentioned in the history. If you doubt whether an

FIGURE 2.1
Family Medical History

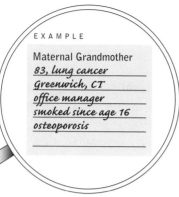

EXAMPLE

Maternal Grandmother
83, lung cancer
Greenwich, CT
office manager
smoked since age 16
osteoporosis

Take an important first step in planning your wellness program by filling in the chart and discussing it with your doctor. For each relative, note age and cause of death (if applicable), birthplace and occupation, and any applicable health problems (from the list below). Add any necessary details, e.g. if cancer or allergies, state type. Also note if any blood relations had medical problems at a young or early age (below the age of 40 years). Add lines if necessary to include as much pertinent information as possible.

Maternal Grandmother	Maternal Grandfather	Paternal Grandmother	Paternal Grandfather

Aunts	Uncles	Aunts	Uncles

Mother	Father

Sibling	Sibling	Sibling

Examples of Health Problems	Cancer	Hearing disorder	Mental disorder	Respiratory system
Alcoholism	Diabetes	Heart disease or	Nerves/Muscles	Stroke
Allergies	Digestive system	disorder	Osteoporosis or	Tuberculosis
Arthritis	Drug sensitivities	High blood pressure	other bone	Urinary problem
Blood/Circulation	Glaucoma or other	Kidney disorder	disorder	Major surgery
	eye disorder	Liver disorder	Reproductive system	Other

FIGURE 2.2
Health Risk Assessment Form

Date: _____

Name: Last _____
       First _____
       Middle _____

Personal Medical History

1. How do you rate your current health? (circle one)
   Excellent   Good   Fair   Poor

2. What is your main medical problem?
   _____
   _____

3. Are there other medical problems of concern?
   _____

4. What medications are you on?
   _____

5. What operations have you had? (give date if known)
   Include tonsillectomy, appendectomy, hernia repair,
   gynecological procedures, plastic surgery, or major surgery.
   _____
   _____

6. What hospitalizations have you had for nonsurgical
   illnesses?_____
   _____

7. What other major illnesses have you had?
   _____

8. What medications are you allergic to? (give reaction
   if known) _____

9. What other foods or items are you allergic to?
   _____

Weight

1. What do you regard as your ideal weight?
   _____ pounds

2. Are you at that weight, underweight, or overweight?
   _____

3. What health problems do you attribute to weight?
   _____

4. What contributes to problems in your weight? (Travel,
   snacks, business lunches, lack of exercise,
   pregnancy, etc.)_____

5. Are you trying to lose weight now? Y   N
   If yes, how? _____

Cholesterol/lipid level

1. Have you had your cholesterol/lipids checked? Y   N
   Were they elevated? _____

2. Do you know your most recent results for HDL/LDL/
   Triglyceride? (circle one) Specify: _____

3. Are you on a diet to limit your fat intake to lower
   your cholesterol/lipids? Y   N

4. Do you take vitamins (niacin or others) or medication for your cholesterol/lipids? Y   N Specify?
   _____

5. Do you have any health problems related to your
   cholesterol/lipids? _____
   _____

Diet

1. Is your diet usually healthy? Y   N

2. Is your intake of fat or cholesterol low/moderate/high?
   (circle one)
   Do you limit your intake of fat? Y   N
   Cholesterol? Y   N

3. How many eggs do you use a week? _____

4. How much milk do you drink daily? _____
   Is it whole, skim, 1%, or 2%? _____

5. Do you limit your intake of salt, meat, or other items?
   Y   N

6. How many caffeinated beverages (coffee, tea, cola)
   do you drink a day? _____
   What side effects do you have from caffeinated beverages?_____

7. Do you drink wine, beer, or hard liquor? Y   N
   If yes, how often? (circle one)
   Rarely   Once or twice a week   Daily

8. Do you have any health problems from alcohol use?
   _____

9. Do you take vitamin C? Y   N
   Vitamin E? Y   N
   Calcium? Y   N
   Other supplements (including multivitamins)?_____

CONTINUED NEXT PAGE

Stress

1. Do you sleep well at night? Y N
   How many hours do you get nightly? _____
2. Do you handle and control the stress in your life?
   Y N
3. How many hours do you drive a day _____
4. Is your work a source of excess stress for you? Y N
5. Do you consider yourself compulsive, easily upset, or
   frequently depressed? _____
6. Were you ever the victim of violence or abuse, either
   physical or emotional? Y N
   If yes, are you at risk now? Y N
   What problems do you have that are related to this?
   _____

HIV Profile

1. Have you ever been tested for HIV? Y N
   Results _____ When _____
2. Have you ever used intravenous drugs? Y N
3. Have you ever had a blood transfusion? Y N
4. Have you been sexually active? Y N
   If yes, have you had sex with men, women, or both?
   _____
5. Have you had sexual relations with men who have sex
   with men? Y N Don't know
6. Do you use latex condoms during intercourse?
   Y N
   Each and every time? Y N
7. Have you ever been treated for sexually transmitted
   diseases? Y N
   Have you had venereal warts? Y N
   Genital herpes? Y N

Exercise

1. How often do you exercise? (circle one)
   Never   Rarely   Once or twice a month
   Once or twice a week   Almost daily
2. What is the average amount of time that you exercise?
   _____
3. Is your exercise formal or informal? _____
4. Which activities do you participate in? (circle any)
   Aerobics, Jogging, Bicycling, Swimming, Tennis, Golf,
   Treadmill, Weight machines, Stairmaster, Walking,
   Free weights, Gardening, Other _____
5. What symptoms, if any, do you have when you exercise?
   _____

Smoking

1. Do you currently smoke cigarettes? Y N
   If yes, how many a day? _____
   How many years have you smoked? _____
2. If you don't smoke now, have you smoked in the past?
   Y N
   If yes, how many a day? _____
   How many years did you smoke? _____
   When did you quit? _____
3. Have you ever smoked a pipe or cigar? Y N
   Do you still smoke? Y N
   If yes, how much? _____
4. Have you chewed tobacco? Y N
   For how long? _____
   Do you still use it? Y N
5. Are you exposed to secondhand smoke? Y N

Health Habits

1. Do you wear a seat belt/shoulder harness every time
   you ride in a car? Y N
2. Do you ever ride in a car when the driver (including
   yourself) has been drinking? Y N
3. When was your last complete physical examination?
   _____
4. Are your immunizations up-to-date for:
   tetanus/diptheria? Y N   Influenza? Y N
5. Do you do a monthly breast self-exam? Y N
   Have you had a mammogram? Y N
   If yes, what were the results and when was it done?
   _____
6. When was your last Pap smear? _____
   Have you ever had an abnormal Pap smear? Y N
   If yes, what treatment did you receive? _____
7. Have you ever had a stress test? Y N
   If yes, results? _____
8. Have you ever had a sigmoidoscopy or colonoscopy?
   Y N
   If yes, reason and results? _____
9. Do you use any over-the-counter medications?
   Y N
   Which medications, and for what? _____
   _____

Source: Adapted from the Health Risk Assessment Form used by the Cardiovascular Medical Group of Southern California, Beverly Hills, CA. Debra R. Judelson, MD, Medical Director, © 1997.

wellness **tip**

If you have one or more relatives who contracted a serious disease while still young, it is more likely that you are at risk for that disease. Alert your doctor.

illness is significant enough to consider, go ahead and record the health problem, and let your physician assess its importance.

Some people are able to research their family health histories with just a few quick telephone calls to relatives. In other cases, it may not be so easy. Family members are sometimes reluctant to talk about certain conditions that may be embarrassing or uncomfortable to discuss, such as mental retardation, depression, or multiple miscarriages. In other cases, the information may not be available because relatives just don't know details or are deceased.

While not every relative has to be included on the history, it is helpful to have as much information as possible. In the case of relatives who withhold information, sometimes a tactful explanation of the purpose of the family history is helpful. If you have relatives who died and no one knows the circumstances, you may wish to contact family doctors, who will often reveal pertinent medical information in such cases. Or you may wish to check with the state health department, which keeps death records, to determine whether death was caused by a serious disease.

If you are an adopted member of your family, it is just as important to gather information about your blood relatives. Many adoption agencies can release health information, or if you know your birth parents, you can ask them.

Once you have completed your family health history, you can look for patterns. For example, diseases that affect two or more relatives should raise a concern. Diseases that strike at a young age (thirties, forties, or fifties rather than eighties) also should be examined closely. Most experts on inherited diseases recommend that screening for these diseases start a decade or more before the earliest family member was diagnosed. Many inherited diseases declare themselves at an earlier age with each generation.

While some patterns may be obvious to you, others are less obvious. That is why it is important to share your family history with your physician. Physicians can apply their knowledge and experience to your particular history and evaluate it more thoroughly than you can. For example, your doctor may have information about your particular ethnic group's susceptibility to certain diseases that will shed light on trends in your family's health history. Also, your doctor may know about the clustering of certain medical conditions and screen more thoroughly for those in areas for which you have increased risk.

Once you and your physician identify your health risks, you can take appropriate precautions. For example, if you are at risk for premenopausal breast cancer, your physician may send you for early screening and a mammogram instead of waiting until the usual age for such evaluations. It is also important to update your family history whenever anyone dies or is diagnosed with serious illness.

Environmental Factors *and*
Lifestyle **Choices**

Genes are not the only risk factors that should be considered in a health assessment. Most health problems seem to result from the combination of a genetic predisposition to particular disorders, environmental factors that trigger those diseases, and lifestyle choices. Environmental factors include some variables that

Preventive Surgery Could Stop Disease Before It Starts

Suppose your family medical history reveals that you are at very high risk for ovarian cancer. Would you consider having your ovaries removed to prevent the disease from occurring in your body?

That question poses a dilemma for many women at risk for this and other diseases. In the above example, removing the ovaries would virtually eliminate the possibility of ovarian cancer, but it would also bring on early menopause, which is associated with other problems, like osteoporosis and heart disease.

Many doctors and patients are reluctant to remove healthy ovaries or other organs and tissue when there is no disease present. Yet when clear trends emerge within their families, more and more women are discussing the option with their doctors.

Similar considerations arise among women who have developed breast cancer. Since they are at increased risk for developing cancer in the other breast, some women request removal of their healthy breast to decrease the cancer risk, even though this is not the standard of care for breast cancer treatment.

Doctors warn, however, that preventive surgery (also called prophylactic surgery) gives women a false sense of security. An operation that removes healthy organs and tissues does not guarantee against disease. Breast cancer can develop in tissue surrounding the breast, which is not removed during surgery. So even with both breasts removed, women who have had breast cancer must continue screening and consider treatment options to reduce the chance of recurrence elsewhere in the body.

Following are questions that are important to ask your doctor if you believe you might be a candidate for preventive surgery:

- What are the chances of my developing the disease without surgery? After prophylactic surgery?
- What are the potential complications of the surgery?
- Will surgery make me susceptible to other diseases or disorders?
- What follow-up will be necessary on my part?
- What is the cost of the surgery? Is it covered under my health insurance?
- Is the prophylactic surgery recommended, experimental, or discouraged in my situation?

It is vital that you do not make a quick decision, especially during the period when you are recovering from the news that you are at risk for a disease. Take time to gather information, think through all your options, and be sure you have the support of friends and family.

---

are not entirely within your control. If the work you do exposes you to potentially harmful chemicals, for example, you need to be sure that your employer is doing everything possible to minimize your exposure, but you might not be able to eliminate it altogether without changing your job or profession.

Air pollution is a fact of life for many women, and most are not in a position to move away from the neighborhood or city in which they live. Women who live with people who smoke or who work in health care facilities where they are exposed to disease can take certain precautions, but some risk is inevitable in such situations. When outside influences are beyond your control, it is best to take them into consideration when you assess your total risk profile and do what you can to minimize risk in other areas.

Unlike environmental factors, lifestyle choices are almost entirely within the control of the average woman. Even women who are at risk for disease from genetic causes can maximize good health both by avoiding risky behaviors and by making healthy choices in terms of diet and exercise. While some women underestimate the impact of lifestyle choices, many experts believe these choices have a profound effect on health. If you can change your lifestyle to eliminate or curb unhealthy habits, you can do a lot to keep yourself well and reduce your risk, even if a disease is prevalent in your family.

Your doctor can help you develop a plan for a healthy lifestyle that is tailored to your particular set of risk factors. But any healthy lifestyle begins with the following choices:

- Observe a diet low in fat and high in fruits and vegetables.
- Abstain from smoking, excessive drinking, and drugs.
- Practice safer sex.
- Maintain a normal body weight.
- Exercise regularly.
- Get adequate rest.
- Monitor and reduce your stress level.

Choosing healthy alternatives such as these will improve the quality of your life now while decreasing your risk of disease both now and later in life. By modifying how you live, you can overcome the threat of disease and live a long, healthy life. Part III of this book closely examines all the elements of a healthy lifestyle.

Early *Detection*

Decades ago, people died from diseases because they were unaware that they were affected, had no treatment options, such as for infectious diseases, or did not seek out treatment when available. Today, however, advances in technology allow us to investigate problems and uncover diseases before they progress beyond the point where treatment is possible. Yet many people still remain at risk for premature death because they do not make use of tests that can detect early signs of a health problem. Instead, they seek care only when serious symptoms develop.

Early detection of disease offers the best chance for a favorable prognosis. It is especially crucial for certain illnesses that begin early in life but do not produce symptoms until much later, such as heart disease and cancer in some families. Early detection involves regular monitoring for diseases associated with personal risk factors. Results of these tests will alert you to potential concerns and allow you to get immediate treatment if needed.

If you discover you are at risk for certain disorders, it is important for you to be assertive and remind doctors of your family tendencies toward certain diseases. Ask your doctor to include as part of your medical record her recommendations for regular screenings for these conditions. Then, be diligent about getting those tests and checkups. It just may save your life.

Common Health Conditions *and* Their Risk Factors

While every woman's risk profile is different, this section details some common health conditions and their risk factors. The list offers information for only the most common health problems. Therefore, if your risk profile includes other less common diseases or disorders, contact your doctor, health care provider, or

Doctor and Patient: A Partnership in Care

It used to be that a doctor's recommendation was taken as gospel. After all, she went to medical school. Yet, more and more patients today are questioning their doctors. While they do not know more about medicine, they do know their own bodies and risks—and they know what they want. This may, for example, include avoiding surgery if medication can provide similar results. Questioning your doctor does not mean that you no longer trust her. It just means that you need all of the pertinent information in order to participate in the decision-making process.

In fact, questioning your doctor helps make your health care a partnership, where each party brings special expertise to the discussion. Even if you decide to follow your doctor's advice after all, you will be actively involved in the process of maintaining your good health.

If you think it might be uncomfortable to question your doctor, here are some tips that may help. Try them with your current physician. If your physician is not receptive to your taking an active role, you may want to consider changing doctors to one who is easier to talk with. Active participation in medical decision-making for yourself and your family is not an unreasonable request—it is the best way to optimize health. Doctor-patient communication is also discussed in Chapter 3.

- **Do your homework.** Research your health problem or questions so you will be able to talk about them intelligently.

- **Write down your questions.** Do this in order of most to least, important. This will ensure you will not forget anything and will allow the initial focus to be on your most important questions. Also, limited time would not delay your more urgent questions.

- **Pose your questions politely and respectfully.** Do not put the doctor on the defensive with questions like "You are not planning to do that, are you?" Instead, ask, "Why do you think that is best for me?"

- **Schedule extra time when you make your appointment.** Then, the doctor will have enough time to spend with you. If that is not possible because of other patients' needs, be willing to book a second appointment a few days later to talk further.

- **Talk to the doctor in her office and not in the examination room, if possible.** Many patients (and doctors) feel more comfortable if you are not undressed and wearing a paper gown. Whether talking in the office or the examination room, everyone communicates better with clothes on!

- **Consider bringing a tape recorder or taking notes.** This will help you remember your conversation and any specific advice, instructions, or recommendations. You might also ask the doctor to write down details or provide handouts. Many doctors have answers to commonly asked questions already prepared as a handout.

- **Consider bringing along a family member or friend.** They may be able to add another viewpoint to the discussion and pick up on things the doctor said that you did not notice.

- **Keep track of the answers you receive.** While your doctor may be pleased that you asked certain questions, she can be understandably frustrated if you ask the same questions at each visit or have not read the handouts or information she gave you at the last visit.

agencies, such as the American Heart Association or the Lupus Foundation of America, to obtain information on those conditions so you can take appropriate action. You can find more information about each of the diseases below in other sections of this book (check the table of contents and index).

Iron-Deficiency Anemia

Red blood cells carry oxygen to all parts of your body, providing the ingredients necessary to energize your body. You need iron to produce these red blood cells. When you do not have enough iron, your body does not produce enough red blood cells and therefore does not get enough oxygen. This condition is called iron-deficiency anemia. Severe iron-deficiency anemia can temporarily weaken

A diet rich in dark green, leafy vegetables—such as spinach and kale—can help prevent iron-deficiency anemia.

you, decrease your endurance, and impair your brain function—especially memory and logic—and so can affect your daily life. The good news is that the condition is both preventable and correctable with iron supplements and changes in diet.

Women are prone to iron-deficiency anemia because it is often caused by the loss of blood during the menstrual period. As the body tries to regenerate lost blood, more iron is needed than many women consume in their everyday diets. If you do not eat enough iron-rich foods or take an iron supplement, you may encounter an iron deficiency at some point in your life. If the deficiency is serious enough, you will contract iron-deficiency anemia.

In addition to blood loss during menstruation, anemia has other possible causes, which are less common. If you do not consume enough vitamin B_{12}, you can contract a rarer form of anemia called pernicious anemia. This type of anemia is found among vegetarians who do not take B_{12} supplements or eat at least some meat products, and it affects women with conditions restricting their ability to absorb B_{12} (such as those with autoimmune diseases or low stomach acid). Women on long-term acid suppression medication may become B_{12}-deficient and anemic as well.

Though symptoms of B_{12} deficiency are different for each woman, most experience one or more of the following: tingling of extremities, weakness, fatigue, lack of energy, decreased memory, shortness of breath, paleness, decreased endurance during exercise, rapid pulse, loss of appetite, and a need for more sleep than usual. B_{12} deficiency and resulting anemia are conditions that evolve over several months or years, with symptoms appearing gradually and intensifying.

Are You at Risk for Iron-Deficiency Anemia? Any woman with a heavy menstrual period lasting seven to ten days or longer is at risk for iron-deficiency anemia. In fact, about ten percent of American women of childbearing age are iron-deficient and about three percent have iron-deficiency anemia. African American women tend to be at greater risk because they are more likely to have benign fibroid tumors that cause heavy menstrual bleeding. Pregnant women also are at greater risk because the fetus draws iron from them, which has to be replaced.

Detecting Anemia. Iron-deficiency anemia is usually detected with blood tests that measure the hemoglobin concentration and iron levels in your blood. B_{12}-deficiency anemia is also detected by blood testing—a specific test that measures your body's B_{12} level. Both kinds of anemia may be completely asymptomatic until very severe, which is why physical examination without blood testing may not detect your anemia.

Cardiovascular Disease

Cardiovascular disease—or heart disease—is the number one killer of women in the United States. Yet it often goes undiagnosed and untreated in women until the disease has progressed to dangerous stages.

Heart disease is diagnosed when an examination reveals an abnormality in the heart or in the blood vessels supplying it. The common abnormalities are degenerative conditions that occur as we age (more often appearing after menopause in women), called coronary artery disease (CAD). In CAD, the arteries have become narrowed or blocked with fatty tissue deposits, preventing efficient blood circulation. Heart disease can also be caused by birth defects, hypertension (high blood pressure), and by some infectious diseases, such as rheumatic fever.

Classic symptoms of heart disease depend upon the cause but often include shortness of breath, fatigue, weakness or faintness, swelling of the abdomen, legs, and ankles, chest discomfort, or a rapid or irregular heartbeat.

Are You at Risk for Cardiovascular Disease? Risk for cardiovascular disease has many components. Untreated high blood pressure increases the risk of developing CAD, having a heart attack, or experiencing congestive heart failure. High total cholesterol (over 240 mg/dl) almost doubles your chances of contracting heart disease, and more than one in five American women fall within this category. Cigarette smokers are more than twice as likely to experience a heart attack as nonsmokers and are two to four times as likely to die from it. Even smoking a few cigarettes increases your risk. If you are postmenopausal, or if you experienced an early or surgical menopause, you also are at greater risk for CAD. If you are an African American woman, you are twice as likely to die from a heart attack as women of other ethnicities. And if you have a family history of early heart disease, you are at increased risk.

Detecting Cardiovascular Disease. Heart disease can be initially detected through a careful history and examination by your doctor. The diagnosis can be confirmed through a physical examination and evaluation that includes blood tests measuring lipids and cholesterol, stress tests that evaluate the impact of blood vessel narrowing, or using imaging techniques that view blood flow to the heart. Doctors may employ other diagnostic or screening measures to determine the presence or extent of disease. These include an electrocardiograph (EKG), an echocardiogram, or x-rays of the heart, lungs, and blood vessels. An EKG measures the electrical impulses of the heart. An echocardiogram provides a picture of the structure and function of the heart using sound waves. X-ray techniques usually involve injecting dye into specific blood vessels, and are more invasive than an EKG or echocardiogram. Some doctors utilize "rapid CT" (a modified version of the CAT scan that gathers images very quickly) to screen for CAD. Since this technique shows calcification of coronary arteries less commonly found in women than men, it is less reliable as a screening technique for CAD in women.

Lung Cancer

Lung cancer affects more men than women, but at the same time it is the leading cause of cancer death among women in the United States. Women are catching up with men in cases of lung cancer because the number of women who smoke is increasing. Approximately 80 to 85 percent of all lung cancers are directly linked to cigarette smoking.

Women who do not smoke are unlikely to develop primary lung cancer, but a tumor in the lung might be the first sign that cancer has developed elsewhere and is spreading. Recent studies have concluded that secondhand smoke exposure causes lung disease among people who do not smoke.

Lung cancer is also linked to environmental factors, especially exposure to asbestos. It is important that women who work around known carcinogens, such as asbestos, take every precaution to protect themselves against breathing contaminated air. If you live in a house built before 1970, you should have the house inspected for asbestos, which was used as insulation for ceilings, floors, and pipes. Asbestos removal requires an expert and is quite expensive. However, it is essential to have the work done if risk of exposure is present, to protect your health as well as the health of your family. The combination of asbestos exposure and smoking is more deadly than either exposure is alone.

Are You at Risk for Lung Cancer? You are at risk of developing lung cancer if:

- You smoke.
- You work around industrial carcinogens, such as radon gas, asbestos, and radiation.
- Your home exposes you to asbestos or radon.

Detecting Lung Cancer. Your physician would suspect the possible presence of lung cancer if you complain of a nagging cough that brings up blood, chest pain with coughing, or an unexplained loss of appetite and weight. A chest x-ray might reveal a tumor, and computerized axial tomography (CAT scan) or magnetic resonance imaging (MRI) would be required to determine the extent of the tumor. It is recommended that women over 40 have baseline x-rays against which future x-rays can be compared. Smokers or people with a family history of lung cancer not related to cigarette smoking should be screened earlier with chest x-rays to detect the disease before it causes symptoms or spreads.

Breast Cancer

Breast cancer is the second leading cause of premature death among women who have cancer. It is estimated that one in nine women will develop breast cancer in the United States if they live to 85 years of age. However, only 1 in 25 women will die of it. Because the prevalence of breast cancer is growing, checking for the disease must be a regular part of every woman's health regime. The disease is often treatable in its early stages, and most early-stage tumors of the breast are noticed first by women themselves.

Are You at Risk for Breast Cancer? Recent research on breast cancer indicates clear risk factors. Some research results, however, are controversial. For example, one study linked the risk of breast cancer with a high-fat diet, and a few years later a second study contradicted the evidence of the first. Even the prolonged use of postmenopausal hormone replacement therapy has conflicting results in studies, though most researchers do believe it slightly increases risk. The list below represents confirmed high-risk indicators. If you fall into any one of these categories, you should talk to your physician about early detection and possible early intervention. However, most women who develop breast cancer do not have an identifiable risk factor; so all women need to be screened.

FIGURE 2.3   **Breast Self-Examination**

Conduct a monthly self-examination, after your menstrual period, to check for signs of breast cancer.

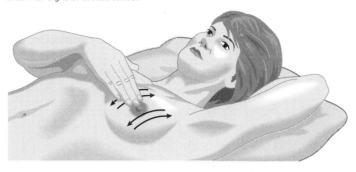

STEP 1 Standing in front of a mirror, place your hands on your hips and look for any changes in the size or shape of your breasts, puckering, dimpling, or changes in skin texture. Gently squeeze each nipple and look for any discharge.

STEP 2 Lying down, place a towel or flat pillow under your right shoulder and your left hand above your head. (You can also do the self-exam in the shower.) Use the finger pads of your right hand to gently touch every area of your left breast, feeling for unusual lumps or thickening. You can use a spiral pattern, moving your hand from the outer portion of your breast to the nipple, or you can move your hand up and down from one side of the breast to the other. Repeat this check with your left hand on your right breast.

STEP 3 Standing, rest your arm on a firm surface and examine the underarm area. Use the same circular motion you used when lying on your back. Also check your collarbone and neck area for any lumps or thickening.

You are at increased risk for breast cancer if you:

- Have a mother or a sister who has had breast cancer, especially before menopause.
- Have never had children, or began having children after age 30.
- Did not breastfeed your children.
- Are more than 40 percent over your ideal body weight.
- Had a late menopause.

Detecting Breast Cancer. The most effective way to detect breast cancer is with a combination of a monthly breast examination and regular mammography screening. It is easiest for you to conduct the breast examination yourself (Figure 2.3). On your next visit to your general doctor or gynecologist, ask her to examine your breasts thoroughly, to point out to you any lumps or thick spots that are not a cause for concern, and to instruct you in breast self-examination. It is good to have the doctor's input in the beginning, as most women find lumps or bumps that are simply glands or benign cysts. Your doctor can help you distinguish between these naturally occurring lumps and those that might indicate the presence of a tumor.

If you are under the age of 40 and are not at high risk for breast cancer, a doctor should examine your breasts at least once every three years. When you are over the age of 40, you should have an examination every year. It is recommended that you get a baseline mammogram soon after turning 40, then every year or two. After age 50, it is a good idea to have a mammogram every year. Of course, if you are in a high-risk group for breast cancer, you should consult your doctor and set up a regular schedule for screening as soon as you determine your risk factors.

Varicella (Chickenpox)

You are probably familiar with chickenpox. A common childhood illness, it erupts as red patches with clear blisters that can itch as they heal. The varicella-zoster virus, which causes chickenpox, also causes another disease called shingles, which is a slightly more severe form of the disease.

When chickenpox occurs in children, it is relatively mild. However, when it occurs in adults, the disease can be severe. While only five percent of the cases of chickenpox (from 1990 to 1994) occurred in adults, more than half of the deaths from chickenpox resulted when adults who were infected with varicella contracted varicella pneumonia.

Adults who have never had chickenpox can reduce their likelihood of serious complications from the disease by receiving the chickenpox vaccine.

Are You at Risk for Chickenpox? People most at risk for complications from the varicella virus are teenagers and women who have neither had chickenpox nor been vaccinated. In addition, health care workers, teachers, and women who work in health facilities, schools, or day care facilities are at risk if they have not had the disease or the vaccination.

The relatively new chickenpox vaccination is 70 to 90 percent effective against the disease. If you are at risk for the disease, getting two doses of the vaccine should protect you from infection. If you are pregnant, avoid the vaccine for now. Because it is made from a live virus, there is a small chance that the virus could be passed to your baby during the pregnancy.

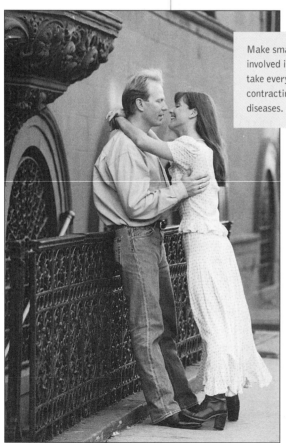

Make smart decisions about becoming involved in a physical relationship and take every possible precaution against contracting sexually transmitted diseases.

Detecting Varicella. Detection of chickenpox is usually easy because of the distinctive symptoms of the disease. You can confirm the presence of the disease with a doctor's visit. Tests are also available to determine whether or not you have had the varicella virus in the past. If you have had chickenpox once you will not get it again.

Sexually Transmitted Diseases

One in four people in the United States will eventually contract at least one sexually transmitted disease (STD). These diseases are particularly dangerous to women because if left untreated, STDs can result in pelvic inflammatory disease, a serious infection that causes pelvic pain and, in the worst cases, infertility.

While there are a variety of STDs, some common ones include gonorrhea, chlamydia, syphilis, herpes, and HIV. (HIV is discussed in a separate section later in this chapter.) Each disease is caused by contact with a specific microorganism that is usually passed between sexual partners in an exchange of body fluids. STDs also can be transmitted from mother to child during pregnancy. Infection in babies can be severe, causing death in about 40 percent of the cases. (A full discussion of STDs appears in Chapter 22.)

One reason STDs are dangerous is that they often present few or no symptoms, especially in women. Many women are not alerted to the fact that they have an STD until they encounter difficulty getting pregnant or have symptoms of pelvic inflammatory disease, which is difficult to cure. Symptoms that have been present initially sometimes disappear for years, or decades, giving a woman no cause for alarm. For example, some women who have syphilis may initially see or feel sores in and around their genitals or throat. These disappear, but the disease does not. In later stages syphilis can adversely affect vital systems throughout the body and eventually cause damage to the brain, nervous system, and heart. The importance of prevention and screening cannot be overemphasized. Herpes, for example, another serious STD, is contagious *before* sores appear and can be spread by genital or oral exposure.

Are You at Risk for STDs? Since symptoms are not reliable in identifying STDs, it is especially important to determine what your risk factors are. The best defense against these dangerous and debilitating diseases is an excellent offense. That is, it is important to take every possible precaution against contracting STDs. While not being sexually active is the obvious solution, it is not practical or realistic for most of us. A mutually monogamous sexual relationship, where both you and your partner have absolutely no other sexual partners, is powerful protection against STDs, provided you both enter the relationship disease-free. If you recognize even *one* of the risk factors below as having ever applied to you, do not hesitate to confide in a doctor, who will test you for specific STDs based on your risk factors. If you have one or more of the higher risk behaviors (those in the list followed by an asterisk), it is best to be honest with your physician so that you can be screened more often and rechecked after treatment.

You are at risk for sexually transmitted diseases if you:

- Have more than one sexual partner at the same time now, or have had more than one in the past.
- Have a partner who has ever had a partner other than you.
- Do not use a condom during sexual intercourse, or use them infrequently.*
- Have a condition affecting your cervix (for example, a cervix that bleeds easily when examined).
- Have had at least two sexual partners in the last year.
- Have had a STD before.
- Have sexual partner(s) with STDs, such as syphilis, or have sores that can transmit the herpes virus, a discharge, or a history of these symptoms.*
- Have traded sex for money or drugs.*
- Use drugs intravenously.*

*higher-risk behaviors

Detecting Sexually Transmitted Diseases. While symptoms may not appear, detection is often straightforward. Results often can be found with a blood test or sophisticated culture. The blood test measures antibodies present in your system

wellness
warning

The most common "silent" sexually transmitted disease is chlamydia. It can and should be checked for, even in sexually active women with no symptoms, because early treatment can be effective in preventing pelvic inflammatory disease and preserving fertility. Make sure your doctor talks with you about chlamydia screening each year when you have your annual examination.

to fight the disease. Culture samples are scrapings or secretions taken from areas thought to be infected, such as the cervix or rectum. A laboratory technician examines samples for the organisms that cause STDs.

Hepatitis

Hepatitis is an inflammation of the liver caused by virus, drugs, toxic chemicals, and/or alcohol. It is diagnosed by blood tests that show elevated liver enzymes, reflecting how much liver damage has occurred. While the liver is often able to repair itself, repeated exposure can cause severe damage (called cirrhosis) and even liver failure. Avoiding exposure to toxic drugs and chemicals and limiting alcohol use can dramatically reduce your risk. However, some forms of hepatitis are infectious; the most common forms of infectious hepatitis are viral.

There are five known types of viral hepatitis, called hepatitis A to E, but the first three are the most common. Hepatitis A is caused by consuming food or water contaminated with the hepatitis A virus. This is the most common form of hepatitis and one with which Americans are most familiar. Formerly called infectious hepatitis, hepatitis A is seen frequently among children in developing countries or areas with bad sanitation, and among U.S. adults and children who visit those areas. Hepatitis A rarely causes severe liver damage. A vaccine is now available and should be used by travelers and those exposed to others with the virus.

Hepatitis B is the most serious form of hepatitis. Spread through contact with body fluids and blood, hepatitis B is much more contagious than HIV, the virus that causes AIDS. That is because the hepatitis B virus can live outside the body for up to a week. People can acquire the virus from using toothbrushes, nail files, ear-piercing instruments, surgical instruments, or blood products that have been contaminated with the virus. However, the hepatitis B virus is most commonly transmitted through sexual contact and intravenous drug use.

Though serious, hepatitis B is preventable. A vaccine, available since the mid-1980s, can protect you from becoming ill as well as prevent you from passing the virus to someone else. However, the majority of people in the United States have not received the vaccine and remain at risk for the disease. Increased use of this vaccine is encouraged, especially among young adults and intravenous drug users.

Like hepatitis B, hepatitis C is spread through contact with body fluids and blood. Unlike hepatitis B, it is not preventable through a vaccine at this time. This type of hepatitis is most commonly transmitted through blood transfusions, but sexual contact with an infected person can also lead to the disease.

Are You at Risk for Hepatitis? Depending on the type of viral hepatitis, risk factors vary. Hepatitis A risk factors are distinct, while hepatitis B and C share similar risk factors.

You are at risk for hepatitis A if you:

- Are Native American and/or Native Alaskan.
- Travel to developing areas with poor sanitation, such as Mexico, the Middle East, Central and South America, Africa, India, and Pakistan.
- Are a resident of a long-term care facility.

- Engage in high-risk sexual behavior, with multiple partners and without condom protection.
- Are an intravenous drug user.
- Work in a health care, laboratory, or childcare setting.
- Are a member of the military.

You are at risk for hepatitis B and hepatitis C if you:

- Are an intravenous drug user.
- Travel to developing countries.
- Engage in high-risk sexual behavior, with multiple partners and without condom protection.
- Work in a health care or laboratory setting, or in a mortuary.
- Have received blood products.
- Are a transplant or dialysis patient.
- Get frequent manicures or tattoos in establishments where the instruments are not sterilized after each use.

Detecting Hepatitis. A blood test is the only way the presence of this disease can be confirmed, although a doctor may suspect the problem based on your history or an examination. The source of a hepatitis A infection (such as eating at a restaurant) can sometimes be traced. If a restaurant is the suspected source, it is especially important to immediately alert health authorities.

HIV

HIV (human immunodeficiency virus) is the virus that causes AIDS (acquired immunodeficiency syndrome). Because it destroys cells in the immune system, HIV weakens the body's defense against disease. It is transferred through direct contact with blood or body fluids, such as through intravenous needles or sexual intercourse. Infected mothers also can pass HIV to their babies in the womb, during birth, or during breastfeeding.

More and more women are becoming infected by HIV. The World Health Organization (WHO) estimates that more than 13 million women will have been infected by the year 2000.

Experts think that women may be more susceptible than men to HIV for several reasons. Women have a larger mucosal surface exposed during sexual intercourse, increasing their ability to become infected during a sexual encounter. Semen typically contains higher concentrations of HIV than do vaginal secretions, making sexual activity with male partners riskier.

Are You at Risk for HIV? As serious as HIV is, it is preventable. If you think you are at risk, your best defense is to change your lifestyle to minimize the potential for contracting HIV. (See Chapter 22 for a full discussion of preventing HIV.) You are at risk for HIV if you:

- Engage in high-risk sexual behavior, such as intercourse with more than one partner, or do not use condom protection each and every time you have intercourse.

wellness **tip**

Health officials now recommend that all expectant mothers be screened for hepatitis B and that all newborns be immunized against the disease. Consult your obstetrician or health provider for more information. Many experts recommend that the hepatitis B vaccination be part of every child's standard immunization schedule.

wellness **tip**

During flu and cold season, keep your fingers and hands away from your face. This helps prevent a virus from entering your mucous membranes. If you must touch any part of your face, wash your hands thoroughly first, then do not touch anything else before you touch your face. If you have personal contact with others, including shaking hands, wash your hands as soon as possible.

- Are an intravenous drug user.
- Had a blood transfusion between 1975 and 1985. (During this time, blood was not routinely checked for the presence of HIV antibodies.)
- Are the child (under age 18, living at home) of a mother at risk for HIV.

Detecting HIV. Because the HIV infection often produces no symptoms initially, the only way you can know you are infected is to be tested for it. If you have any reason to think you might be infected, get tested as soon as possible, both to learn what life-enhancing treatments are available and to avoid spreading the virus to others. There are a variety of tests available that check blood or body fluids for the presence of antibodies fighting the virus. However, tests may not show the presence of HIV until six months after initial infection.

You can choose to be tested in a doctor's office, laboratory, or at home with a mail-in kit. Whether the test is performed at home or in a health care setting, positive results are usually communicated in person or on the telephone by a professional counselor.

Having a negative result does not guarantee that you do not have HIV in your body, especially if tested shortly after exposure to the virus. It only means that the virus has not been detected. If you find out that you were exposed to someone who is HIV-positive, ask your doctor to perform the more sophisticated tests now available, which can show evidence of the virus earlier than the standard HIV test. Make sure you are retested if the results are negative, and use condoms during sexual activity. HIV is most contagious in the early weeks of the disease, often before the standard tests are positive.

Influenza

Influenza, better known as the flu, is not often thought of as a serious or deadly disease. Yet it is the cause of death for 10,000 to 20,000 Americans annually—mostly among newborns, the elderly, or the chronically ill. Among healthier people, influenza is responsible for workers missing millions of sick days each year.

Like the common cold, the flu is a respiratory infection caused by viruses. The flu virus can linger in the air for up to three hours, making it easy to catch. However, the flu is more serious than a cold, affecting multiple organ systems.

Are You at Risk for Influenza? Anyone interacting with people on a daily basis is at risk for influenza. Typically, cases of influenza appear most often during the winter months (December through March) when people spend time in close quarters inside warm buildings. In many cases, frequent hand washing can help reduce your risk.

There are several strains of the flu virus, including influenza A, B, and C. Each flu season, a vaccine is made up for the most popular strains. In the past, the vaccine was recommended for older women, women with respiratory ailments, and others who have one or more of the risk factors below. However, many health experts consider the disease serious and recommend the vaccine for all adults, primarily because of the loss of work days for those who become ill and the highly contagious nature of the disease. If you do not receive a vaccination, influenza A is the only strain that later can be treated with an anti-viral medication, like amantadine or rimantadine.

Is It a Cold or the Flu?

The flu is like a cold—so much so that patients and even doctors sometimes misdiagnose it. Following is a breakdown of the specific symptoms for the flu and for the common cold. While these diseases do share symptoms, you will notice they vary in their severity.

SYMPTOMS	THE FLU	COMMON COLD
aches/pains	severe	slight
fatigue/weakness	severe	slight
extreme exhaustion	yes	never
headaches	yes	rarely
high fever	yes	rarely
stuffy nose	sometimes	yes
sneezing	sometimes	yes
sore throat	sometimes	yes
chest discomfort	yes	yes
cough	yes	yes
serious congestion	rarely	sometimes

If you are unsure whether you have a cold or the flu, treat yourself as if you have the flu. Get plenty of bed rest, drink plenty of fluids, call your doctor if your temperature exceeds 101°F or symptoms become severe.

There is no truth to the phrase, "Feed a cold, starve a fever." However, most people do best with symptomatic treatment—rest, fluids, and taking decongestants for stuffy noses, antihistamines for sneezing and runny noses, and acetominophine or aspirin for body aches, fever, and throat pain. (Avoid giving aspirin to children and teenagers because of the rare risk of Reye's syndrome.) Most people with the common cold feel well enough to continue usual activities but should avoid exposing others to the cold virus if possible. Those with the flu should rest in bed to give their body a chance to fight the virus.

You are especially at risk for the flu if you:

- Live in a long-term care facility.
- Have a chronic medical condition, such as heart–lung disease, diabetes, cystic fibrosis, certain blood disorders (hemoglobinopathies), or kidney disease.
- Have chronic respiratory problems, such as asthma.
- Have a weak immune system.
- Are over age 65.
- Work in a health facility or medical office, laboratory, childcare setting, or school.
- Are a family member, coworker, or are close to someone with influenza.

Detecting Influenza. Since flu symptoms are typical and treatment is limited, you usually do not need a doctor's examination to confirm the diagnosis or treat yourself. In fact, going to the doctor's office may expose others to the virus and so may be discouraged in many cases. However, if you experience severe or unusual symptoms, or have chronic respiratory disease or a weakened immune system, consult your doctor immediately. Occasionally, other serious diseases mimic flu symptoms, or your flu may turn into life-threatening pneumonia.

If you have just started to experience flu symptoms during an influenza A epidemic, call your doctor promptly about the use of antiviral medication. While not for everyone, this medication can shorten the duration and reduce the intensity of your flu symptoms, if caused by influenza A. Since there is no way your doctor can diagnose influenza A in time for treatment to be helpful, during an epidemic the medication is usually offered at the onset of flu symptoms.

Measles, Mumps, and Rubella

Measles, mumps, and rubella are a trio of infections caused by viruses—often grouped together because the vaccines to prevent them are given together. These diseases usually affect children, as they are highly contagious and can be easily spread from person to person in settings such as schools. Some of these infections also can be passed from a pregnant woman to her fetus with harmful results, including birth defects and miscarriage.

Measles is a disease characterized by a red rash. The virus infects the respiratory tract, often invading it initially through the nose and throat through tiny, airborne droplets. The disease lasts for about two weeks.

Mumps is caused by a virus that attacks glandular and nervous tissue, including the salivary glands. Symptoms include fever, pain in front of the ears, and swelling of the salivary glands. In some cases, patients may experience vomiting, headaches, and a stiff neck, or even temporary swelling of the brain and spinal cord. Less frequently, the pancreas, ovaries, breasts, or thyroid gland may be affected. In men, the testes can be affected. In most cases, mumps patients recover with no lasting effects. In some cases, however, more serious complications occur, such as permanent deafness or loss of fertility.

Rubella, also called German measles, is a milder form of measles during the course of which the lymph glands become tender and enlarged. Soon, a rash of small pink spots appears on the face and neck and spreads within 24 hours to the rest of the body. Both the rash and fever disappear within a day or two. The real danger is contracting the disease during pregnancy, because it can lead to miscarriages and birth defects.

Are You at Risk for Measles, Mumps, or Rubella? If you have had the measles, mumps, or rubella vaccinations, or if you have contracted these diseases, you are not at risk for getting them. (In rare instances, the vaccine may not have been 100 percent effective so the disease can still occur unless you received two doses. Your doctor can test your susceptibility, especially to rubella, if you are considering future pregnancies.) All three diseases are more dangerous in adults than in children, so if you believe you may be at risk, get the proper vaccinations.

You are at risk for measles, mumps, and rubella if:

- You were born after 1956 and you have not had the diseases and have not had the vaccinations.
- You have not had two shots of the vaccines.
- Laboratory tests show you are at risk.

Disease in the Environment?

While experts agree that lifestyle choices definitely influence health, there is a controversy over whether environmental pollutants have a similar effect. Some scientists believe that when numbers of women who live in the same geographic area experience repeated miscarriages and/or have children with birth defects, for example, the cause must be linked to toxic elements in their local shared environment. They believe that public awareness reduces exposure and prevents further cases.

Critics argue that there is no direct causal link between environmental factors and disease. They attribute the rise in statistics on disease to better detection and reporting methods. According to them, there was a similar number of cases (or even more) decades before, but the medical community did not have the tools to diagnose them correctly or did not report them vigilantly.

Some environmental pollutants have been proven to be linked to disease, including air pollution, pesticides, certain chemicals in cosmetics, industrial waste, and even certain types of plastics. All of these materials are man-made. Experts say natural toxic materials—which are just as potent—have been around for millions of years, allowing humans to build up a resistance to them, which is why they do not seem to cause clusters of illness.

While scientists around the world continue to study this controversy, women concerned about environmental causes of disease in their area should contact the local health authorities and environmental groups for information.

- You spend time where a lot of other teens and young adults do (such as at a high school or college, or in the military).

Detecting Mumps, Measles, and Rubella. A doctor's visit is usually necessary to confirm the presence of measles, mumps, and rubella. Laboratory tests can show whether you have been infected with these viruses in the past, and another test in two to three weeks can confirm a recent infection. (Tests are usually not needed if you have doctor's records or family records confirming prior infection.) If you use your obstetrician/gynecologist as your primary care physician, or if your family practitioner has an obstetrical practice, talk to the doctor *before* going into the office—in order to keep you out of contact with pregnant women.

Tuberculosis

Tuberculosis (TB) is an infection caused by an organism called *Mycobacterium tuberculosis*. It primarily affects the lungs, causing a chronic cough, exhaustion, weakness, loss of appetite, and fever. It can then spread from the lungs to other parts of the body. If untreated, tuberculosis can be fatal, especially for older people, babies, and those with weakened immune systems.

While TB virtually disappeared as a health threat in developed countries from the 1940s to the 1980s, it has reemerged as a killer. New strains of TB have proven impervious to the antibiotics that have controlled it in the past, and the AIDS epidemic has created a whole new population with increased susceptibility to TB.

Transmission of TB occurs as it is passed through the air in droplets when someone coughs, sneezes, sings, or laughs. Yet you can get tuberculosis and not have active TB, meaning you will have no signs of the disease. In many people's bodies, the TB infection is kept under control, and it never becomes active.

Are You at Risk for Tuberculosis? While anyone exposed to people in a confined space may be affected by TB, you are at particular risk if you are:

- Native American and/or Native Alaskan.
- Living in a long-term care facility.
- Living in crowded or unsanitary conditions.
- Infected with HIV.
- Infected with a chronic illness that lowers your resistance.
- An intravenous drug user.
- A user of cortisone or immunosuppressive drugs.
- A health care or laboratory worker.
- An alcoholic.

Detecting Tuberculosis. The first step in diagnosing TB is usually a tuberculin skin test. This is done regularly for students in public schools and employees in health care facilities. If positive, the test may indicate tuberculosis, but it does not mean the disease is active or that there is any danger of it becoming so. In people under the age of 35, treatment after a positive skin test is recommended to reduce the likelihood of the disease becoming active when you are older and have a lower resistance.

A chest x-ray can confirm the diagnosis of active tuberculosis. It can show signs of active lung infection, which, along with a doctor's examination, patient symptoms, and laboratory testing, can indicate the need for treatment. In addition, samples of sputum from your lungs can be analyzed for TB bacteria, to see if you are spreading the disease to others. However, such tests may take four to six weeks to get results, as TB bacteria grow very slowly. Therefore, treatment may be started before results are back in people with abnormal chest x-rays and symptoms suggestive of active TB.

What *You* Can **Do**

We have listed only the most common health conditions and their risk factors and those that pose particular problems for women. Of course, each woman is different, and you are likely to have risk factors mentioned in this book as well as others. The most important thing is to become aware of your personal risks for disease.

Remember, it is never too late to improve your odds of living a long, healthy life. Once you determine your risk profile, you can make lifestyle changes to overcome your risk factors:

- Start and maintain a family medical history to determine your personal risk factors for disease. (See Figure 2.1 at the beginning of this chapter for a worksheet that helps you assess your risk factors.)
- Share your family history chart with your physician. Identify the diseases and disorders for which you may be at risk.
- Check with your doctor on lifestyle changes you can make to reduce those risk factors from developing into disease, and begin to incorporate those changes into your and your family's daily routines.
- Take the necessary preventive measures, such as vaccinations and screening tests, to maintain your good health status.
- Schedule regular checkups with your doctor to keep a close watch on your health.

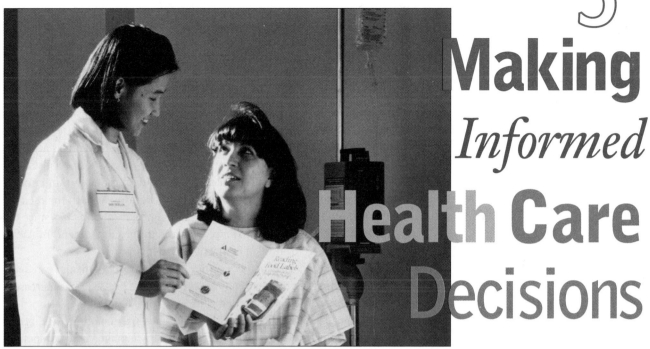

Making *Informed* Health Care Decisions

The health care system in the United States is undergoing a dynamic change. In response to escalating costs, new systems for the delivery of care have emerged with the hope of focusing on preventive care—wellness—in addition to treatment. Never before have so many options been available. The choices are numerous, the decisions are complex, and the costs for health insurance can still be high. Women today must be savvy consumers as they choose health care for themselves and their families. As the health care system continues to evolve and change, it is important for women to be actively involved in learning about their options and in making decisions.

Health Care Cost

Traditionally, payment for health care in the United States has been provided in a system in which payers—usually employers or the government—paid all or most of the premiums, individuals went to the licensed medical practitioner of their choice, an insurance company paid its share of the bill, and the patient was responsible for any uncovered balance. Those who did not have health care benefits at work or were not eligible for government programs, such as Medicaid, Medicare, or a Veterans Affairs hospital, either paid for an individual health insurance policy themselves or chose not to have health insurance coverage at all.

As the cost of health care and insurance coverage has risen, employers and the government have become less willing to cover the mounting costs. Consequently, more Americans than ever either have no health insurance or are absorbing the bulk of the costs for these services out of their own pockets. During 1994, about 10.5 million Americans relied on self-paid individual health insurance as their only source of health care coverage. In 1996, 41 million Americans—most of them working families without employer-provided insurance—were uninsured primarily because they could not afford individual insurance or had a preexisting condition that prevented them from obtaining insurance coverage.

Since the 1980s, it has become apparent that the many "miracle" drugs and high-tech options were saving life and limb but were also very expensive. Insurance providers began exploring ways to contain spiraling costs. "Managed care" emerged as the solution. This system is actually designed to manage cost. It channels access to care through a primary care physician, limiting unnecessary access to specialists, and places restrictions on the type of care that can be provided under certain circumstances. Despite the criticism that managed care has generated in both the medical and consumer communities, it has grown significantly in the United States since the 1980s, primarily due to its lower cost to employers and to the government. By 1996, some 125 million people were enrolled in managed care plans.

With the growth of managed care, concerns about its impact on health care have also grown with resulting government vigilance. Legislative pressure has increased, and numerous issues are being examined. For example, federal legislation now requires that coverage be allowed for longer hospital stays after childbirth and breast cancer surgery, overriding previously set, shorter limits by managed care companies. Additional mandates on coverage will no doubt be forthcoming as consumers and legislators strive to protect health care benefits in the face of cost-cutting restrictions.

As another cost-cutting measure, employers began requiring their employees to contribute more to their health insurance premiums, making health coverage less comprehensive, and introducing higher deductibles and copayments (deductibles and copayments will be discussed later in the chapter). Some employers stopped offering health insurance altogether. The Commonwealth Fund, a nonprofit organization that monitors health issues, forecasts that more and more employers will choose this route in the future.

Health care reform measures have been introduced in state and federal legislatures, but the prospects of a complete restructuring of the industry seem unlikely in the foreseeable future. Meanwhile, an increasing number of individuals cannot afford basic coverage and do not qualify for assistance from the government. Women and children are disproportionately affected by a lack of insurance. Women often work in areas in which insurance is not provided, such as service industries,

Preexisting Conditions

A preexisting condition is a diagnosed medical condition that you had before you joined a health plan or tried to take out health insurance. Such a condition may be excluded from coverage, or you may have to wait for a period of time before coverage becomes effective. When considering health coverage it is important to be alert for such exclusions. If you have a preexisting condition and are changing plans, obtain new health care coverage before your current coverage expires. Some insurance companies may waive the waiting period if you join them while you are still in another plan. Do not try to hide a diagnosed preexisting condition; medical records can be found to document it. The insurance plan may not cover the problem when the time comes to treat it or may even demand a refund if it is discovered after the treatment.

and do not earn enough to pay for private insurance. Lack of health care exerts a high cost economically and in human suffering for both the individual and society.

Types *of* Health Care **Plans**

Factors to consider in choosing a health care plan can be overwhelming. There are any number of reasons why you may be confronting this decision:

- You are just starting a job and have to select a plan.
- You are given the opportunity to change your plan at work.
- You are trying to find private (individual) health care coverage on your own.

In other cases, you may have to switch plans for involuntary reasons. Many employers change the plans they are offering because of dissatisfaction with a plan, in order to control internal costs, or because of corporate budgetary constraints. Switching to a new health plan may also require you to find new health care providers. When you are given a choice of plans, it is important to know the types of plans available, costs, coverage benefits, and limitations. You will want to have as much information as possible to make the most of your health care dollars.

There are two main types of plans available: fee-for-service and managed care. Fee-for-service may present more out-of-pocket costs to the member but offers a wider range of options for choosing doctors and services. Managed care may be more economical but typically limits members' choices of physicians and services. Traditional fee-for-service coverage has become less available as managed care becomes the dominant offering in a cost-conscious economy. Managed care plans tend to cover more preventive care services than fee-for-service plans. Some health insurance plans offer dental and eye care either as a part of the basic plan or at an additional cost.

When given a choice of health care options, such as from an employer, consider these questions:

- Do I want to be able to use my present doctor or any other doctor I wish?
- Do I wish to have direct access to a wide range of specialists?
- Do I prefer to use a female health care provider or women's health center?
- Do I want to be able to use any hospital I choose?
- Am I willing to pay more in premiums, deductibles, and copayments to ensure the provider choices I want?
- Are my time and convenience worth more than cost savings?
- Do I have a particular health condition or concern which may have better coverage with a particular plan?

Fee-for-Service Health Care

If you answered yes to any of the preceding questions, your choice leads to what is known as a fee-for-service, or indemnity, arrangement. Fee-for-service plans provide a full range of medical benefits, including doctors' visits and outpatient and inpatient hospital stays.

Dental and Eye Care Insurance

Dental care insurance is often available as an optional feature (sometimes called a "rider") in a fee-for-service or managed care insurance plan. It also may be obtained from a managed care plan that has been organized specifically to provide dental services on a prepaid basis. The degree of coverage varies considerably among plans, and it is important to pay close attention to services, deductibles, and copayments.

Many fee-for-service and managed care insurance plans cover the medical aspects of eye care, and some subsidize the cost of vision correction. If your plan has provisions for eye care, it will probably include periodic exams and treatment of such medical problems as glaucoma and cataracts, but may not pay for any or all of the cost of eye glasses or contact lenses. To receive eye care under a managed care plan you may need to be referred to an eye care facility by your primary care physician.

With a fee-for-service plan, you choose your doctor and hospital. When you visit either one, you pay the provider directly and submit a claim to your insurance company for reimbursement. Sometimes the provider is willing to bill the insurance company directly and you are responsible for any uncovered balance. Most doctors, hospitals, and other health care providers accept this type of insurance. Your out-of-pocket costs may be higher than in a managed care plan. You may need to pay a deductible before costs are reimbursed by your insurance company.

According to a U.S. Bureau of Labor Statistics study, plans of medium and large employers in 1993 had annual deductibles between $100 and $300 and total out-of-pocket expenses of no more than $1,500 for most employees. In the individual market, deductibles are more commonly between $250 and $2,500 and out-of-pocket maximums start at $1,200 but can exceed $6,000 annually.

Even fee-for-service plans have some degree of managed care since they can require you to get approval from the insurance company before you can be electively admitted to a hospital or surgical center (a process called precertification or preauthorization). Your doctor's proposed treatment may also have to undergo a medical review by the insurance company in a process called utilization review. Some plans cover annual physicals while others may not cover routine examinations without a specific diagnosis.

The main difference between a fee-for-service plan and a managed care plan is that in a fee-for-service plan you are free to see any doctor or specialist you or your physician wishes, as often as you wish, and the insurance company will pay its agreed portion of the bills. Personal choice of providers and locations for tests and hospitalization are the paramount factors in deciding to use a fee-for-service plan. Another benefit is that physicians have the flexibility to order tests and treatments at the time and location most convenient to you. This flexibility can be very important if you have limited time off from work. Even so, it may be wise to check with your primary doctor to get recommendations before seeing a specialist to avoid duplication or conflicting treatments so your care can be coordinated.

Managed Health Care

Managed care organizations arose from a concern about the rising costs of providing unrestricted medical care and, consequently, the cost of insurance premiums. It was thought that total health care costs could be controlled (or "managed") if plan members were provided with low cost preventive care and screening services to detect diseases in the early stages when they are more easily and successfully treated. Additionally, having a primary care physician (also known as the PCP) coordinate all aspects of an individual's health care would allow the PCP to treat common problems without referral to specialists. This restriction on a patient's ability to go to a more expensive specialist on her own, without preapproval (or "referral") from the PCP, would reduce or delay "unnecessary" specialist visits. The managed care plan would further control costs by negotiating discounted fees with health care providers, who accept the lower fees in return for the promise of a large number of patients or the ability to continue seeing patients whose plans have changed. This multi-faceted approach was a well-intentioned effort to reduce health care costs while implementing preventive health care measures. Unfortunately, it has not worked well. Patient and employer/payee dissatisfaction has been high, and managed care organizations

Most Common Concerns About Managed Care Plans

Managed care plans have supporters and critics. If you are unfamiliar with managed care plans or are being offered a managed care plan at work, think about the following concerns:

- **Access.** How easy is it to get an appointment? How long do you have to wait in the waiting room? Can you talk with your doctor or the doctor's assistant on the telephone or by E mail? What do you do when an emergency or an urgent issue occurs? What must you do if you and your doctor decide you need to see a specialist? Where do you go for tests?
- **Continuity of care.** Will you see the same health care provider—whether it is a doctor, nurse, or therapist—whenever you need care?
- **Coordination.** If you see a primary care doctor and one or more specialists, how will your care be coordinated so that no information falls through the cracks?
- **Flexibility.** Can you switch doctors in the plan if you are unhappy with your first choice? How can you get a second opinion? What happens if you disagree with the plan's decision not to cover certain services? What is the appeal process that they follow?

Source: National Committee for Quality Assurance

have realized that there is often a rapid turnover in plans—so that providing preventative services has not been in their economic best interest. The plans have given employers "predictable" costs, without predictably saving them money.

Critics of Managed Care. Critics of managed care argue that these plans have not provided preventive care, they have not actually improved the state of health care in this country, and overall health care costs have not been reduced. Studies show that costs have only been reduced for employers.

Other criticisms of managed care relate to the referral process primary care physicians are required to use to refer patients to specialists. Different plans use different processes to approve or authorize a referral, so it is not often the sole decision of the PCP. Some managed care plans have a payment structure that penalizes doctors who refer patients to specialists. Other experts criticize the so-called "gag rule," in which doctors are prohibited from discussing with patients certain treatments that are not covered by the plan. There are also concerns that patients might not receive adequate medical care in situations where groups of doctors receive a preset fee per patient per year, called a capitated fee, in exchange for providing all medical care allowed by the plan. If the fee is too low to cover the cost of medically necessary services (such as vaccinations for infants) or if certain patients require considerably more care than others, the groups essentially make less money and may be forced to curtail services or go out of business.

The "Gatekeeper" Primary Care Provider. In a managed care plan your health care provider is your primary care physician, whom you select from a group of participating doctors. That doctor will usually be a family physician, internist, or obstetrician/gynecologist. If the physician is not an obstetrician/gynecologist, you will generally be allowed to see one without first going through your PCP (known

Glossary of Health Care Coverage Terms

Here are some definitions that will help you navigate through health care terminology:

CAPITATED FEE: A fee paid to a health care provider for medical services on a per person rather than a per procedure basis. Under the system of capitation, a managed care plan pays each of its participating doctors a fixed fee per month for every member of the plan for whom the doctor is responsible, regardless of how much or how little care the member receives from the doctor.

CLINICAL PRACTICE GUIDELINES: Carefully developed criteria used for diagnosing and treating specific medical conditions. These guidelines are based on clinical literature and expert consensus. They provide guidelines to help a health plan administrator evaluate appropriateness and medical necessity for care.

COINSURANCE PAYMENT: A percentage amount a patient is required to pay toward a covered benefit. Usual coinsurance payments are 10 to 20 percent of total payments. Some patients have a second insurance policy that covers the coinsurance payment. Most insurance policies have a maximum coinsurance payment that the individual or family is required to pay each year.

COPAYMENT: A preset amount, such as $5, $10, or $20, that the patient pays each time she goes to a doctor's office and receives a service covered by the plan.

DEDUCTIBLE: A preset amount the patient must pay each year before the insurer will begin paying for services. This feature is common to indemnity plans (see fee-for-service). A typical deductible is $200 or $250 annually per individual or family member. Some deductibles apply when out-of-plan physicians or services are used.

FEE-FOR-SERVICE: A way of paying for medical care in which a doctor charges a fee for each service provided and an insurance company pays all or part of the fee. There may be a copayment, coinsurance payment, and/or an annual deductible for the patient. Also called an indemnity plan.

FORMULARY: A list of drugs for which a managed care plan will pay, usually chosen because the drugs are "cost effective."

HMO: Health maintenance organization. A federally defined health plan using a defined group of physicians and facilities that provide care in return for a preset monthly payment.

IPA: Independent practice association. A federally defined network of health care providers that contracts as a single entity with employers and/or insurers to provide comprehensive health care for a preset monthly payment.

MANAGED CARE PLAN: An umbrella term for many types of health plans that provide health care in return for reduced or preset monthly payments and coordinate care through a defined network of physicians and hospitals. These include HMOs, PPOs, and some other insurance plans.

PPO: Preferred provider organization. A health plan that restricts fully covered care to a defined group of physicians and hospitals and pays physicians on a discounted fee-for-service basis.

PRECERTIFICATION: Advance approval required by an insurance plan for admission to a hospital or certain procedures.

as self-referral or direct access) for routine gynecological care, and in some plans and states, for any gynecological problems.

Your primary care physician is sometimes referred to as a "gatekeeper," because she is the doctor who "opens the gate," or requests authorization for referrals, to most specialty care (other than routine obstetrician/gynecologist care). Referrals are also required for many tests or procedures performed in the doctor's office or hospital. Most managed care plans have a reviewer (often a nurse or physician) who authorizes referrals based on information the PCP provides and a panel of physicians who decide on questionable situations.

Managed Care Plans. Managed care plans come in several varieties. They include preferred provider organizations (PPOs) and health maintenance organizations

(HMOs); there is also a new hybrid of PPOs and HMOs called a point-of-service (POS) plan. These plans differ in the degree of risk that the providers assume, the degree of preventive care provided, the selection of doctors and specialists, the cost of their coverage, the extent of pretreatment authorization, the restrictions they place on you as to how and where your care is provided, and the degree to which out-of-plan care is covered.

Preferred Provider Organization (PPO). A PPO is a group that represents doctors and hospitals who have agreed to see patients at a discounted fee that has been negotiated with an insurance plan. If the plan member goes outside that group for medical services, she has to pay the difference between the fee permitted by the PPO and the amount charged by the doctor visited. In general, PPOs are selected by people who are willing to pay more of their health care costs in order to be able to have freedom of choice in which doctors they see. There are no claim forms to fill out when a plan member uses a doctor on the list of preferred providers; if the plan member uses a doctor who is not on the list, she will need to complete certain forms for each visit and pay more out of pocket.

Health Maintenance Organization (HMO). An outstanding HMO offers a wide range of doctors and hospitalization benefits. It also offers an assortment of covered preventive care features, such as periodic physical examinations, mammography and Pap smear screenings, immunizations, smoking cessation workshops, nutrition and exercise training, and general health education. An HMO pays doctors and hospitals a fixed amount to provide services to its members. Doctors are either members of a staff or group that usually contracts exclusively with the HMO, or are members of an IPA or network that contracts with the HMO on a nonexclusive basis.

HMO members are required to choose a group or IPA affiliated with the HMO, usually designating a particular physician as their PCP. The PCP provides most of the routine medical care and coordinates additional services. Visits to specialists, special tests, and elective surgery require an approved referral from the plan member's primary care doctor. Life-threatening emergency care is always covered, but nonemergency care, even in an emergency room, may require authorization.

An HMO is one of the most economical types of plans because of the restrictions outlined above. In addition to an annual premium (all or part of which may be paid by your employer), you may need to pay a nominal copayment at each doctor visit. There are no claim forms to complete. However, visits to physicians other than your PCP, nonauthorized tests or specialist visits, out-of-area non-life-threatening emergency care, and particular services (cosmetic surgery, for example) may not be covered. You may need to come back to the physician several times and get x-rays or laboratory tests elsewhere. You should consider the restrictions and minor delays in determining the true cost of HMO coverage for you and your family.

Point-of-Service (POS) Plan. POS plans are hybrids of HMOs and PPOs. Like PPOs and HMOS, they offer plan members a network of participating providers. If a plan member uses an in-network provider, she usually pays a copayment at

wellness **tip**

According to the American Association of Health Plans, some 81 percent of managed care plans offer women the choice of an obstetrician/gynecologist as their primary care provider or allow them to see one for routine care without going through their primary care physician.

wellness **tip**

The "gatekeeper" concept and the authorization procedure have raised concerns about access to care. For instance, your primary care physician (PCP) may not agree with a treatment that you think you should have or the plan may not authorize a referral or procedure that your PCP requests. All plans, however, are required to have a process for grievance and dispute settlement, a feature you should examine before deciding on a managed care plan. Any time you disagree with a decision, you should request an appeal, either from your PCP or from the plan.

Sources of Information About Health Care Plans

- Contact your benefits department at work or check with your union.
- Read the benefits contract from each plan you are considering, sometimes called a subscriber agreement or certificate of coverage. Make sure you understand the contract of the plan you choose.
- Get an information packet from the plans you are considering, including member handbook, newsletter, health promotion literature, and annual report. Find out whether the plans you are considering publish an annual HEDIS—Health Plan Employer Data and Information Set—report, which provides data about the plan and compares its performance to regional and national standards.
- Attend information meetings conducted by the plan.
- Call the plan's member services department with questions.
- Talk with coworkers who have used the plan and ask about any problems they may have encountered.
- Get information about the National Committee for Quality Assurance (NCQA) report card, which shows how a managed care plan rates in such areas as doctor qualification, prevention, quality management, and member satisfaction.
- Contact your state insurance counseling office.
- Ask your state and county medical boards and associations about particular doctors from the plan.

the time of service, similar to an HMO. POS plans also allow plan members to go to any out-of-network providers and get unauthorized tests done, although the plan member is then subject to a deductible and a varying percentage of fees once the deductible has been met. Claim forms are required when plan members use an out-of-network provider. This plan offers more flexibility in choosing physicians and hospitals and protects those who work or travel away from their PCP, while limiting costs for usual medical care.

Sources of Health Care *Coverage*

If your employer or your spouse's employer provides health care coverage, you are one of the fortunate majority of Americans. Otherwise, you must search the individual insurance market for a policy that provides coverage you can afford.

Employer-Sponsored Health Insurance

Typically, if an employer offers coverage, the employer will pay 80 to 100 percent of the premiums for an unmarried employee's coverage and about 70 to 100 percent for family coverage. Most employers offer only one or two plans from which to choose and often limit the type of insurance options offered, such as HMO. Employees may also choose to supplement their employer's plan with an individual plan in order to expand coverage. If you are thinking about using your spouse's plan, a major consideration is what would happen to your coverage if your spouse loses that job or retires. You will want to know when open enrollment occurs for your employer's insurance plan so as not to miss an opportunity to sign up or change your coverage.

The Individual Insurance Market

Affordability is usually the main concern for people seeking to obtain individual, or private, health care coverage, since the individual pays the entire premium and out-of-pocket costs. If you think the chance of your needing medical care is minimal but you want coverage in case of an accident or catastrophic illness (called major medical coverage), you may wish to choose a plan that offers a high deductible or copayment but a low premium. Some women, regardless of their health status, may only be able to afford insurance with this very high cost-sharing structure. For those with few anticipated health costs, this coverage may be much less expensive, as you pay out of pocket for the few services you need and save the difference that you do not spend on more expensive premiums. If you expect ongoing medical care, consider paying higher premiums with a lower deductible and coinsurance limit so that you can meet your deductible and coinsurance limit early in your care and become eligible for fully covered benefits. Sources of information about individual plans include:

- **Insurance agents or brokers.** Refer to your telephone company's Yellow Pages or other directories, and contact those professional agents or brokers who deal with well-known insurance companies.
- **Advertisements.** Watch for advertisements on TV, on the radio, and in newspapers to see which insurance companies and managed care organizations focus their sales on the individual market in your area.
- **Health care advocacy groups.** Contact those in your community.
- **Blue Cross/Blue Shield.** Contact your local Blue Cross/Blue Shield organization, particularly if you have a preexisting condition that you believe may keep you from getting adequate coverage through other sources; the Blue Cross/Blue Shield organizations are the insurers of last resort in several states.
- **Your personal physician or local hospital.** Ask what plans patients have that they are pleased with. The local county medical association often has listings and referrals available.
- **A group-sponsored health care plan.** Join this plan, sometimes called a small group plan.

   Here are some ideas for locating such a group:

- Ask friends and relatives.
- Talk to other people who do the same kind of work you do. Many professional and trade organizations offer their members health care coverage.
- Discuss the matter with your religious leader, who may know of a group.
- If you are a student or college alumnus, check with your school.
- If you are a temporary employment agency employee, check with the agency through which you receive your assignments.
- If you are a farmer, contact your farm cooperative.
- If you are 50 years old or over, contact the American Association of Retired

---

Typical Coverage by a Managed Care Plan

Managed care plans vary in the types of services and procedures they cover. A typical plan covers:

- **Doctor visits.**
- **Routine tests.**
- **Inpatient and outpatient hospital care.**
- **Preventive measures, such as physical examinations, breast and cervical screenings, and immunizations.**

Some benefits are more likely to be "optional" with greater expense incurred:

- **Cost of prescription medications**
- **Eye care**
- **Dental care**
- **Nutrition and exercise training**
- **Weight maintenance programs**
- **Smoking cessation workshops**
- **General health education**

wellness **tip**

Check with your personnel director and health care insurance provider when there is a major change in your life. Life changes—marriage, having a child, losing a dependent, retirement (especially if you have dependents), divorce, or a death in the family—can expand or reduce your coverage needs. Timely notification of changes is critical to making sure you and your family are properly covered.

Persons (AARP) and find out whether their health plans have been extended to your state. If so, this could be an attractive option, and joining AARP is quite inexpensive.
- Consider joining other special interest or professional organizations that provide sponsored group coverage.
- Contact your state's or county's health care or insurance group for information on programs available in your area.

Government Health Programs

Medicare is a federal government-sponsored health care plan for retired people at least 65 years old and for younger people with end-stage renal disease or other disabilities certified by the Social Security Administration. Medicare has a Part A and a Part B. Part A covers inpatient hospital medical costs and is available at no cost to the participant. Part B covers 80 percent of doctors' costs and various outpatient costs, for which the participant or a third party has to pay a monthly premium.

Even though you may have Parts A and B there will still be some costs that are not paid, such as deductibles, coinsurance, and most medications. For these you can purchase supplemental insurance, known as Medigap, which is available at several levels differentiated by the degree of extra coverage and cost. Medigap insurance is now coordinated with Medicare benefits to avoid duplicate coverage. Medicare has some limits regarding length of coverage, so if you have significant medical problems, additional coverage should be considered.

You will be notified by the Social Security Administration of your eligibility for Medicare coverage and given instructions at least three months before you reach age 65. For more information call the Medicare hot line: 800-638-6833.

Do not wait until age 65 to learn as much as you can about Medicare. It is a good idea to study eligibility and benefits carefully—explore what is covered and what is not—so you can create an adequate savings plan for retirement early in your adult life. For example, for you to qualify for Medicare Part A at no cost, you must be eligible for Social Security benefits. Otherwise, you will have to pay a fee for Part A. That could mean a fee for Part A, a fee for Part B, and a fee for an optional Medigap policy of your choice.

Medicaid is a government-sponsored health care plan for people with medical needs but very low income and savings levels, regardless of their age. Medicaid often serves as a Medigap insurance for Medicare patients with limited funds and may cover most of Part B, deductibles, and coinsurance. It will also cover long-term custodial or nonmedically necessary nursing home care. Specifications vary from state to state so call your state Medicaid office for information about your area.

Some veterans are eligible for medical treatment at Veterans Affairs hospitals and medical facilities. Benefits can be quite comprehensive for qualified veterans. Contact the Veteran Administration for more information.

Other Health-Related Insurance Policies

Other policies, known as limited-benefit plans, are generally used to supplement other health plans and should not be considered comprehensive health plans.

Short-Term Major Medical Insurance. Some insurance companies offer short-term major medical insurance policies. These policies are made available to individuals who are between jobs and without health coverage.

FIGURE 3.1
Health Plan Checklist

This checklist is designed to help you evaluate a health plan regardless of whether you have only one plan from which to choose or whether you are comparing plans. Before using the checklist you may want to read the plan's certificate of coverage (the legal document that describes the responsibilities of the plan and the member) and member handbook, which will explain all the coverages, what is not covered (exclusions), and many other details.

If you have access to only one plan, going through the checklist will help you better understand the plan and help you identify areas where you need to obtain more information either from your employer's benefits department or directly from the plan's member services group. If you are comparing plans, fill out a checklist for each plan and then decide which one works best for you.

General Considerations

1. Does the plan cover:

   Mental health services?   Dental care?
   Substance abuse treatment? Vision care?
   Physical therapy?   Cosmetic surgery?
   Occupational therapy?   Oral surgery?
   Reconstructive surgery?

2. Are you satisfied with the plan's grievance procedure?

3. If you will be participating in this plan as a dependent, do you understand what happens to your health care coverage by this plan if you were no longer a dependent?

4. Is there a maximum dollar amount of services you can use each year, for a particular disease, or during a lifetime?

5. Does your plan allow you to use another doctor, emergency room, or HMO while you are traveling in the United States?

6. Does the plan provide coverage while traveling in a foreign country?

About the Doctors

1. Does the plan offer you the choice of an obstetrician/gynecologist as your primary care provider or permit you to see one without referral?

2. Can you expect to receive an appointment with your primary care physician within an acceptable time?

3. Are the doctors located near your home or office?

4. Can you see your doctor during evening or weekend hours?

5. Will you be able to see the same doctor at each scheduled visit?

6. Will the plan allow you to see a doctor outside the plan?

7. Is there an additional cost to you to see a doctor outside the plan? What is the extra cost to do this?

8. How easy is it to change your doctor?

9. Are there any limitations in regard to being referred to a specialist by your primary care physician? Is preauthorization necessary? How long can it take?

10. Are a large majority of the plan's doctors board certified? Is your doctor certified?

11. Does the plan review the doctors' credentials (current licenses, liability claims, felony convictions, disciplinary actions, etc.) every two years?

12. Does the plan review each doctor's performance annually?

13. Do the doctors use "clinical practice guidelines" as part of their efforts to provide high-quality health care?

Disease Prevention and Health Education

1. Are any of the following prevention programs available in the plan?

   Well-woman visits   Cervical screening
   Breast screening   Diabetes screening
   Cholesterol screening   Occupational coun-
   Exercise counseling   seling to prevent
   Weight maintenance   repetitive motion
     counseling   injury (carpal tun-
   Smoking cessation   nel syndrome, for
   Nutrition counseling   example)

CONTINUED NEXT PAGE

2. Does the plan offer counseling and support groups to help patients adjust to the effect an illness has on life at home or work?
3. Does the plan teach a member how to self-manage a chronic illness (diabetes, for example)?
4. Does the plan provide referrals to home health care, Meals-on-Wheels, senior centers, and other community services?

The Child Rearing Years

1. Does the plan provide family planning services?
2. Does the plan cover infertility diagnosis and treatment?
3. Does the plan include full pregnancy-related services as soon as you enroll?
4. Does the plan have a hot line for expectant mothers and does it include a postpartum period?
5. Does the plan cover pregnancy termination services?
6. Will the plan permit you to use a doctor who specializes in children's health care?
7. Will the plan permit you to use a hospital that specializes in the care of children?
8. Does the plan allow regular well-baby visits?
9. Will your children be covered while away at school?

Preexisting Conditions

1. Does the plan cover all or any preexisting conditions as soon as you enroll? What is the waiting period?
2. Is there a time limit in covering certain conditions? For example, if you have had a breast biopsy that was benign, will the plan cover another biopsy in the future?

Drugs and Durable Medical Equipment

1. Are prescription drugs covered by this plan?
2. Is there a procedure for using a drug that is not on the formulary?
3. Are the pharmacies where you can get prescriptions filled convenient for you?
4. Are durable medical equipment (wheelchairs, hospital beds, crutches, canes, walkers, etc.), implants, and prosthetic and orthopedic devices covered by the plan?

The Emergency Room

1. Are you required to obtain advance approval to visit an emergency room for a life-threatening problem?
2. Are you required to obtain advance approval to use an emergency room for a non-life-threatening problem?
3. Is it a simple procedure to obtain approval to use emergency room services?
4. Will there be a time when the plan will not pay for an emergency room visit?
5. Do you have to use a special facility for non-life-threatening emergencies?

Surgery

1. Can you choose your surgeon and anesthesiologist?
2. Will the plan provide you with a list of surgical procedures that are serious enough to allow a hospital stay?
3. Will the plan provide you with a list of surgical procedures that are performed on an outpatient basis?
4. Are there any of the above procedures you would prefer not to have performed on an outpatient basis?

Single-Disease Insurance. This type of insurance is available and pays you only if you get an illness or disease covered by the policy (cancer, for example). These are not comprehensive health plans, and most experts do not consider them a good way to spend your health care money.

Hospital Indemnity Plans. These plans pay a fixed amount for hospital and medical expenses each day you are in a hospital. The policy amount is paid to you and not to the hospital and usually is a limited, fixed reimbursement for hospital or medical-surgical expenses.

Long-Term Disability Insurance. This type of insurance provides protection against loss of income due to an accident or sickness. Even though you may be offered this type of coverage through your employer, you may wish to reevaluate whether it is adequate. Ideally, it is best to have coverage to age 65 when Medicare takes over. In some cases benefits may be combined with Social Security benefits for disability and must fulfill their criteria. If you are buying this coverage on an individual basis, insist on guaranteed renewability.

Long-Term Care Coverage. This type of coverage, not to be confused with long-term disability coverage, provides a wide array of services to help compensate for a chronic condition or illness that limits your ability to perform activities essential to daily living, not complex medical care. These activities can range from helping a frail, elderly person dress, eat, and use the bathroom to skills training and medication management for a mentally ill person to technical and nursing care for a ventilator-dependent child.

Financial *Considerations*

A key point in judging any plan is its cost: How will your plan be paid for? What is the best value for your money? The plan's certificate of coverage will show copayments, deductibles, and coinsurance. The premium amounts can be obtained from your employer's benefits department or from the group to which you belong or from your private insurance carrier. Take time to carefully assess the cost of any plan you are considering. If you have access to only one plan, going through this exercise will help you better understand the provisions of your plan. If you are comparing plans, it will help you decide which is the best plan for you based on cost. Remember, however, that cost is not the sole determining factor in selecting a health plan. Other considerations are your individual health care needs as well as those of your family, convenience, travel, plan restrictions, savings, and your tax status. The checklist that appears in Figure 3.1 on pages 49–50 can also help you assess all the variables.

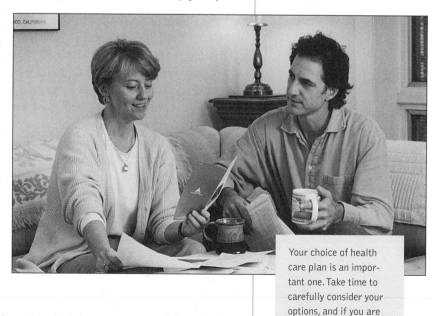

Your choice of health care plan is an important one. Take time to carefully consider your options, and if you are married, discuss them with your spouse.

Income Tax Deductions

Women who are self-employed should keep in mind that a portion of their health insurance costs is tax deductible. For the 1997 tax year, 40 percent of such costs is deductible; by 2006, the amount is scheduled to gradually rise to 80 percent. Also, out-of-pocket health care costs in excess of 7.5 percent of your adjusted gross income can be deducted if you itemize your expenses. Consult your tax adviser for details.

wellness **tip**

Some states have set up insurance pools for high-risk individuals or have made other forms of insurance available to accommodate people or employers who are unable to obtain health care insurance. Contact your state insurance counseling office for local information.

Medical Savings Accounts

The Health Insurance Portability and Accountability Act of 1996 (the Kassebaum-Kennedy Bill) authorized the creation of 750,000 tax-exempt medical savings accounts (MSAs) beginning in 1997. After four years, Congress will determine whether to extend that figure or expand the coverage.

An MSA can be set up only by someone who is self-employed or who works in a small business (50 or fewer employees). Similar to the popular individual retirement accounts (IRAs), contributions to MSAs can be deducted from income when calculating federal income taxes. To participate, people must have health insurance policies with high annual deductibles; the act says "high deductible" means $1,500 to $2,250 for a single person and $3,000 to $4,500 for a family. The requirement for a high deductible is intended to make the policy premium more affordable without removing the responsibility for usual health care costs from the individual. The intent is that personal responsibility will make consumers more cost conscious in choosing health care services that they truly want and need.

The cost of services is paid out of the MSA. If you set up an MSA, you can deduct from your taxable income up to 65 percent of your annual deductible if you are single or 75 percent if you have a family. Interest earned on the money in an MSA is not taxable. As the money saved in an MSA accumulates, it can be used in years when you have additional health care costs.

Example: If you have a family and your health insurance policy premium (paid by you or your employer or both) has an annual deductible of $3,000:

1. You can pay into your MSA up to 75 percent of the $3,000, or $2,250 per year.
2. You can deduct the $2,250 from your taxable income for the year.
3. Since your deductible is $3,000, payment by the insurance company will kick in once you pay $3,000 out of your own pocket. You have probably noticed that you only put in $2,250, but that is only for the year you set up the MSA; hopefully you will not have to spend any of that, and in the second year you will have accumulated $4,500 plus earnings. If you have to spend up to your deductible at that point, you should have around $1,500 left over for future health care costs.

If you are a small-business owner or are self-employed, you can get information about setting up an MSA from the Employers Council on Flexible Compensation in Washington, D.C., at 202-659-4300. In the future, investment firms, insurance companies, and other organizations will offer MSA plans.

Legislation Supporting Women

In addition to establishing medical savings accounts, the Health Insurance Portability and Accountability Act of 1996 provides several reforms that make it easier for women and their families to get and keep comprehensive health insurance:

- An uninsured woman applying for group coverage cannot be refused coverage for herself or her family (or be charged a higher premium) because of a past or present medical problem. Neither can she or her family be refused such coverage if she changes from one health plan to a new group plan.

- A woman who loses her job and continues group coverage under COBRA must be covered for a newborn or adopted child under COBRA without waiting for the group's open enrollment plan.
- A woman applying for group coverage may not be discriminated against because she is a victim of domestic violence.

For a complete list of examples, send a stamped, self-addressed envelope to the Women's Legal Defense Fund, 1875 Connecticut Avenue, N.W., Washington, DC 20009, and ask for the fact sheet titled "What the New Health Insurance Reform Law Means for Women and Their Families."

Choosing *Your*
Health Care Providers

Your primary care physician, specialist doctors, and other health care professionals are important people in your life. When selecting them, consider their training, credentials, experience, and how well you think you will be able to relate to them.

Levels of Medical Care

There are three levels of medical care. The components and complexity of care provided depend on individual needs, the health care organization, and insurance coverage:

- **Primary Care.** The first contact you have with a health care provider can take place in a doctor's office, an emergency room, or a walk-in clinic. Primary care is obtained on the patient's own initiative, that is, no referral is needed.
- **Secondary Care.** This level of care is provided by a physician who specializes in a particular field of medicine, such as ophthalmology, psychiatry, or dermatology. If you are a member of a managed care plan, you generally will need an authorized referral to see a specialist; fee-for-service patients do not usually need a referral and can go directly to any specialist.
- **Tertiary Care.** This level of care consists of such complex procedures as heart surgery, organ transplants, and brain surgery, all requiring extensive training and advanced equipment and facilities. Sophisticated diagnostic tests are also included in tertiary care; examples of such tests are magnetic resonance imaging (MRI) and computerized axial tomography (CAT scan). A doctor's authorized referral is needed for tertiary care and preauthorization may also be needed.

Primary Care Physicians. According to the American Medical Association, "primary care consists of the provision of a broad range of personal medical care (preventive, diagnostic, curative, counseling, and rehabilitative) in a manner that is accessible, comprehensive, and coordinated by a licensed M.D. or D.O. Care may be provided to an age-specific or gender-specific group of patients, as long as the care of the individual patient meets the above criteria." It is recommended that every woman choose a primary doctor to coordinate and oversee all her health care needs. It is best to choose a doctor early in adult life rather than after a medical problem arises. Your PCP provides preventive care and is familiar with all aspects of

COBRA

When you leave a group health insurance plan you may be able to continue coverage on an individual basis. A federal law (the Consolidated Omnibus Budget Reconciliation Act—known as COBRA) states that if your employer has 20 or more employees and you leave the employer's group plan, you must be offered the option of purchasing the same coverage. You can do this for 18 months and at no more than 102 percent of the total cost of the coverage. Note that "total" means what you and your employer combined were paying.

Some states have similar laws applying to coverage by employers of fewer than 20 people. Several states also require carriers to allow group members to convert their policies to comparable individual coverage.

These conversion privileges are expensive and are generally higher than you would pay if you obtained new individual coverage. However, you may find one of them to be an option if you leave your job and do not intend to start a new job immediately or if you have a preexisting medical condition.

FIGURE 3.2
Choosing a Primary Care Physician
An important decision every woman needs to make is whether to have an obstetrician/gynecologist, family physician, or internist as her primary care physician.

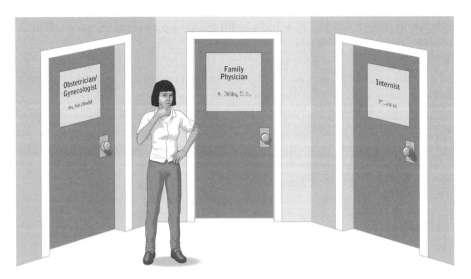

your health care needs, lifestyle, and family history. Your PCP keeps a complete medical history of all aspects of your health, including all prescriptions you take or that have ever been prescribed, tests that have been administered and their results, and factors in your work or personal life that may affect your health.

Your PCP can be a family physician, internist, or obstetrician/gynecologist. Both family physicians and internists provide a full range of health care. Some women prefer to see doctors of osteopathy, who use both conventional medicine and manipulation of the muscles and bones to prevent or treat illness. Some women choose an obstetrician/gynecologist as their PCP during their reproductive years and continue care if the physician has had extra training to do this; for their postmenopausal years, women often choose an internist or family physician as their PCP, choosing an internist if they develop any significant health conditions or concerns that require ongoing monitoring or treatment.

In certain cases, a woman's primary care physician is called a principal care physician. In such cases, patients with chronic health problems regularly see a subspecialist of internal medicine rather than a family physician, internist, or obstetrician/gynecologist. For example, a woman with chronic heart problems would regularly visit her cardiologist (acting as her principal care physician), instead of going to a primary care physician.

The doctor you choose as your PCP should be someone with whom you feel comfortable and are able to communicate. Your doctor should be able to explain the components of the office visit, discuss any health problems, encourage your questions, and answer them fully in terms you can understand. A 1997 study published in *The Journal of the American Medical Association* found that patients want to be personally connected to their PCP and specialists. Good two-way communication fosters this process and helps build the doctor-patient relationship.

Specialists. When you need the care of a specialist, work closely with your PCP in the selection process. Be sure you understand why a specialist is required and any financial responsibility you may assume. The specialist may diagnose and recommend a treatment and will typically do so in consultation with your PCP. Evaluate your specialist in the same way you did your PCP (that is, make sure you learn her training, experience, and the hospitals where she has patient-admission privileges). Ask questions so you fully understand all the information provided. If you wish to get a second opinion on the diagnosis or treatment plan of a specialist, discuss the matter with your PCP. Also, clarify whether the primary care responsibility will shift to the specialist during the course of a particular treatment.

Many specialties have subspecialties in which a doctor may pursue additional training. For example, the pediatric specialty has some 15 subspecialties ranging from pediatric cardiology to pediatric urology; internal medicine subspecialties include cardiology, gastroenterology, endocrinology, pulmonology, rheumatology, and neurology. The American Board of Medical Specialties recognizes the following list of medical specialties:

- Allergy and immunology (treatment of allergies, asthma, and allergic skin problems)
- Anesthesiology (administration of anesthetic agents [pain relief] and monitoring of patients during surgery and invasive procedures)
- Colon and rectal surgery (evaluation and treatment of conditions of the intestinal tract, colon, rectum, and anal canal)
- Dermatology (evaluation and treatment of conditions of the skin, mouth, genitalia, hair, and nails)
- Emergency medicine (acute evaluation and treatment of urgent health problems in a hospital based setting)
- Family practice (total health oversight, treatment of general health problems, including minor surgery, of all ages of patients and their family members)
- Internal medicine (total health oversight, diagnosis, and nonsurgical medical treatment of adult health conditions, from general to complex) Many subspecialties of internal medicine use procedures that are sophisticated and curative, such as cardiology (heart) or gastroenterology (stomach and intestines).
- Medical genetics (diagnosis and counseling of inherited diseases)
- Neurological surgery (evaluation and surgical treatment of conditions of the brain, spinal cord, and nervous system)
- Neurology (disorders of the brain and peripheral nervous system)
- Nuclear medicine (diagnostic testing using radioactive substances, treatment of thyroid disease and tumors with radioactive substances, and radiation exposure)
- Obstetrics and gynecology (treatment of female reproductive organs; pregnancy, labor and delivery, hormone therapy)
- Ophthalmology (treatment of the eyes)
- Orthopedic surgery (surgery on the limbs, spine, and related parts)
- Otolaryngology (treatment of the ears, nose, and throat)
- Pathology (microscopic examination of tissue, cells, and body fluids to diagnose diseases)
- Pediatrics (childhood, preadolescent medicine)
- Physical medicine and rehabilitation (treatment of disease and injury by such means as manipulation, massage, exercise)
- Plastic surgery (reconstructive and cosmetic surgery)
- Preventive medicine (disease prevention)
- Psychiatry (treatment of mental illness)

- Radiology (diagnosis of disease and conditions through use of x-ray testing)
- Surgery (treatment of diseases, injuries, and deformities through operative procedures)
- Thoracic surgery (surgery on the heart, lungs, and chest)
- Urology (treatment of the male genitals; urinary tract and bladder in men and women)

Other Members of the Health Care Team. Any number of allied health professionals may provide care for you in a doctor's, eye doctor's, or dentist's office. Following are several examples of professionals who may make up your health care team:

- **Dental hygienists** clean your teeth, take dental x-rays, show you how to floss and brush your teeth, and provide related dental care under the supervision of a dentist.
- **Emergency medical technicians** provide immediate care in emergency situations; they usually reach the emergency site by ambulance.
- **Home health aides** provide personal care services to sick and disabled individuals who are homebound.
- **Licensed practical nurses** have graduated from an accredited school of nursing and are licensed to provide basic nursing care under the supervision of a registered nurse or a doctor.
- **Medical technologists** perform the laboratory tests your doctor orders.
- **Nurse midwives** have completed nursing training with additional specialized training in normal childbirth. They do not use obstetric forceps, perform cesarean deliveries, or treat high-risk pregnancy patients. Their philosophy of care considers pregnancy to be a natural state and not a medical condition. They also provide many other services, such as prenatal care, advice on diet and exercise, and follow-up care for the mother. Nurse midwives can perform gynecologic checkups, breast examinations, and Pap tests, and can provide birth control advice.
- **Nurse practitioners** are registered nurses who have received special training in preventive care and in diagnosing and treating routine or minor ailments under the supervision of a doctor.
- **Occupational therapists** assist individuals who are recovering from a mental or physical disability, perhaps due to an accident. Working under the direction of a physician, they devise therapeutic activities to strengthen their patients' motor and nervous systems and psychological outlook and help patients learn or relearn skills for daily living and/or basic employment.
- **Opticians** make and fit eyeglasses and contact lenses in accordance with the prescriptions of ophthalmologists and optometrists.
- **Optometrists** examine your eyes, using special instruments, for defects in vision and eye disorders in order to prescribe glasses, contact lenses, or other corrective measures.
- **Osteopaths** are physicians who use conventional medicine and a system of manipulation of the muscles and bones to promote structural integrity that could restore or preserve health.
- **Paramedics** provide care in emergency situations. Paramedics are more highly trained that emergency medical technicians, who can also administer emergency care.

- **Pharmacists,** also known as druggists, dispense medicine in accordance with your doctor's prescription. They check for drug interactions and can often give advice on medication use.
- **Physical therapists,** working under the direction of a physician, treat individuals with a disability, disease, or injury by means of heat and cold treatment, therapeutic exercise, and massage. The objective of physical therapy is to speed rehabilitation and prevent deformity.
- **Physician assistants** work under the supervision of a doctor and are trained to perform many basic clinical evaluations and procedures traditionally performed by the doctor.
- **Podiatrists** diagnose and treat diseases, injuries, and abnormalities of the feet. They are the only health care practitioners other than physicians who can independently prescribe drugs and perform surgery to treat their patients.
- **Psychologists** specialize in the study of human behavior and mental health. They provide psychological therapy, counseling, and testing.
- **Radiologic technicians** take and develop x-rays under the direction of a physician.
- **Registered dietitians** provide dietetic and nutritional advice to help their patients achieve and maintain good health.
- **Registered nurses** have graduated from a state-approved school of nursing, have passed the professional nursing state board examination, and have been granted a license to practice within a given state.
- **Social workers** provide social services, such as assistance with financial problems and living arrangements, to people in need or under physical or mental duress who are unable to handle such matters on their own.
- **Speech pathologists and audiologists** measure hearing ability and evaluate and treat speech disorders and swallowing disorders.

Doctor Training and Certification

Doctors go through many years of formal training and, in order to maintain their licenses, are required to participate in continuing medical education (CME) seminars and courses for the length of their careers. The level of training of a doctor is related to the degree of specialization. Your state may require that doctors complete training leading to a minimum number of CME credits in order to maintain a medical license in the state.

Getting a Medical Degree. To become a doctor one must complete a course of instruction at a medical school or college of osteopathy, which usually takes four years. The doctor then takes a state licensing examination, which, if successfully completed, along with one year of postgraduate training (the internship) leads to a license to practice medicine in a particular state.

Residency. After medical school most doctors enter postgraduate training—or residency—in a particular area of interest. The residency takes three to seven years. After the first year, the doctor is fully licensed in the state. During this training period the doctor is actually practicing medicine, although under the supervision of more experienced doctors.

Alternative Medical Practitioners

The federal Office of Alternative Medicine classifies alternative therapies seven ways:

1. Diet, nutrition, and lifestyle changes
2. Mind/body control (biofeedback, yoga)
3. Alternative systems of medical practices (acupuncture, homeopathic medicine, Ayurveda)
4. Manual healing (chiropractic medicine, aromatherapy, acupressure)
5. Pharmacologic and biologic treatments (chelation therapy, metabolic therapy)
6. Bioelectromagnetic applications (electroacupuncture, blue light treatment)
7. Herbal medicine

You may obtain these therapies from licensed physicians or specialized practitioners who may or may not be medical doctors. Note that very few of these practices have had their effectiveness tested in clinical studies. This federal office was established to try to increase studies of treatments likely to be effective.

Board Certification. To measure competence after a residency program, doctors may take an exam to qualify as "board certified" in that specialty. Each accredited specialty has a board that certifies doctors' competency in that field. When a doctor becomes board certified, you can feel comfortable that the doctor has completed an approved residency program under proper supervision and now has demonstrated knowledge of the specialty by passing an exam. The exam may be written or oral or both. Applicants also may need to present a list of conditions they have treated to show the extent of their experience.

After board certification in a specialty field, a doctor may opt for additional training called a "fellowship" and take an exam for board certification in that subspecialty. For example, a doctor may be board certified in obstetrics and gynecology and its subspecialty of maternal and fetal medicine. "Board eligible" is used to describe a physician who has completed the required training and is still in the process of getting certification. In obstetrics and gynecology, for example, the doctor cannot take the second part of the exam (orals) until at least her third year of practice.

Recertification. Some of the specialty governing boards have established requirements for board recertification, usually every seven to ten years. Since recertification is a fairly recent undertaking, some boards have not set up requirements, and other boards do not require doctors to recertify if they were originally board certified before a certain cutoff date.

Not all doctors are board certified, but that does not mean they are not competent in their field. They may have just completed their residency, may be studying for the exam, may not have passed the exam the first time and are studying to try again, or for some other reason have chosen not to seek certification. In choosing a physician, however, it may be helpful to know the doctor's certification status.

The Doctor's Track Record

In addition to education, training, and certification, the doctor's experience can help guide your choices. Find answers to these questions:

- How long has the doctor been practicing medicine in general and the specialty in particular?
- How long has it been since the doctor completed medical school and residency?
- Does the doctor serve on the faculty of a medical school, have patient-admission privileges at a teaching hospital, or teach students or residents in their office?

You may run into a situation in which you are evaluating an older doctor who has years of experience but no board certification or a young doctor who has just completed residency and passed board exams but has considerably less experience than an older doctor. Do not hesitate to ask questions in order to make informed decisions.

The Public Citizen Health Research Group in Washington, D.C., has published a list of doctors in each state who have been sued for malpractice or had some other action taken against them. For a copy of your state's *Questionable Doctors* call 202-588-1000. The cost is $19. If your doctor is on the list, call and ask for an explanation before jumping to conclusions.

Communicating *Effectively*
with **Your** Doctor

It is important that you have a high comfort level in dealing with your doctor. Above all, it is important that you feel comfortable discussing your health care and feel that the doctor understands you and is willing to communicate fully with you. You should not feel rushed or brushed off by the doctor during a visit. You should feel your doctor is taking adequate time and paying full attention to you during your visits. You should not feel judged or talked down to by your doctor. Be wary of a doctor who will not discuss serious issues because "they may worry you." Your doctor should be able to explain medical conditions and procedures in terms you can understand.

Many factors can contribute to your comfort level, and they do not have to be based on personal rapport. For example, you may be more comfortable with a female doctor, a doctor of your own ethnic or religious group, one near your own age, or one who shares your views on philosophical, social, or cultural issues. If English is not your first language, your first requirement may be that the doctor speak your native language fluently.

The Take Time to Talk Advisory Council

The Take Time to Talk Advisory Council is made up of representatives from the nation's largest and most important health care associations for women—including the American Medical Women's Association, the American College of Obstetricians and Gynecologists, the American Academy of Nurse Practitioners, and the American Academy of Family Physicians. On December 2, 1997, the Council endorsed the proclamation printed below to kick off a series of patient and physician education efforts nationwide to address the nature and scope of barriers to positive, effective communication between health care providers and patients. (These efforts also include a formal survey, the results of which are summarized in the sidebar on this page.) The proclamation supports the Council's belief that the health care professional-patient relationship is the most vital component in the continuing health of every American.

The Take Time to Talk Proclamation

To achieve the highest level of health for each individual, every American—patients and providers—must be an active participant in the health care conversation.

As patients, we must speak freely, truthfully, and in confidence to our physician, nurse practitioner, physician assistant, or other health care provider about any issue which we feel may affect our physical, mental or spiritual health, even if some personal issues may be embarrassing or painful to discuss.

As health care providers, we must go beyond the technical expectations of our professions to nurture those under our care. We must listen respectfully and thoughtfully to our patients and fully explore their health concerns and needs, even if we are pressed for time.

Specifically, patients are urged to:

Doctor, Can We Talk?

A 1997 survey of primary care physicians and adults 18 years of age and older found these barriers to effective patient-physician communication:

Reluctance to talk. 93% of physicians agreed that serious medical problems could be averted if patients were more willing to talk about them; 68% reported serious difficulties treating patients who are hesitant or embarrassed to talk about their health problems.

Time barriers. 67% of physicians said that not being able to spend enough time with patients is a serious problem. 17% of patients said they avoided talking to a doctor about a health problem because the doctor seemed rushed or too distracted.

Other findings. 61% of doctors felt that medical school did not prepare them well for physician-patient communication. Physicians also felt that lack of health care education and knowledge among patients is a communication barrier.

Source: Take Time to Talk Advisory Council, chaired by C. Everett Koop, M.D., ScD. Survey conducted by Louis Harris and Associates, Inc.

- Take time to seek medical care and counsel on a regular basis, even if only to talk over questions.
- Inform their primary health care provider of any and all changes in their health status.
- Promptly attend to personal medical issues—even those which may seem frightening or that may be embarrassing or difficult to talk about.
- Make the most of their medical office visits. Prepare in advance. Make a list of issues and questions to discuss. Then, listen carefully and ask questions to make sure you understand the advice.

In turn, providers are urged to:

- Take time to listen to each patient.
- Allow patients to tell their story so that you fully understand their medical concerns and their expectations for treatment.
- Respond without judgment, criticism, or condemnation and with sensitivity to medical issues that may seem frightening to the patient or that may be embarrassing or difficult to talk about.
- Ensure that your advice is understood. Explain the issue carefully and don't leave the subject until you believe the patient understands.
- Be understanding. Remember that bad news or an unfavorable diagnosis renders many patients unable to hear what else you might say.

Finding a Doctor Who's Right for You

Many times doctors are chosen on the basis of recommendations of friends, relatives, and coworkers. This is generally not the best way unless you make it clear what you are looking for in a doctor; a doctor your friend likes may not be right for you.

If you are selecting a doctor in an HMO you may be limited to the doctors under contract with the plan. Even though the plan will probably indicate its doctors are all well-qualified, it is still wise to do some checking.

Following are some sources of information about doctors:

- Your current doctor, nurse practitioner, or physician assistant
- Local medical societies
- Local hospitals
- Local referral agencies
- A managed care plan's member services department
- The American Medical Association's physician database (http://www.ama-assn.org)
- "Dentists Information Bureaus" (in the Yellow Pages of your telephone directory or call 1-800-DENTIST, which has data on dentists in some 28 states)
- The American Board of Medical Specialties
- Your state medical board

In addition, the "Physicians and Surgeons Information Bureaus" section of the Yellow Pages of your telephone directory is a good place to start, especially if you live in a sizeable city. You will find locator services and hospitals that have special departments to help you find a doctor based on the requirements you give them.

FIGURE 3.3

The Prepared Patient's Checklist

Photocopy and fill out this checklist before each doctor visit.

Things to Bring

☐ Insurance card

☐ Social Security number

☐ Address and phone number of your appointment, where to park, money for parking

Things to Ask

What do I want to talk about?

_____

_____

_____

What are my symptoms?

_____

_____

_____

When did this all start?

_____

_____

_____

What was I doing then, or what had I just finished doing?

_____

_____

_____

If it hurts, what kind of pain do I feel?

_____

_____

_____

Where does it hurt?

_____

_____

_____

When does it hurt?

_____

_____

_____

What makes it better or worse?

_____

_____

_____

Have I ever had anything like this before? When?

_____

_____

_____

What prescription medicines have I taken in the last month?

_____

_____

_____

What over-the-counter drugs am I taking?

_____

_____

_____

What natural or alternative medicines or therapies am I using?

_____

_____

_____

What health care providers am I seeing regularly or have I seen in the last two months?

_____

_____

_____

What did I see each for?

_____

_____

_____

What did each recommend?

_____

_____

_____

What do I expect to happen from this visit today?

_____

_____

_____

What other questions do I have?

_____

_____

_____

Source: Take Time to Talk Advisory Council, chaired by C. Everett Koop, M.D., ScD. For further information, call 800-931-3321.

Smart Choices

You can feel assured you have found the right doctor when:

- **The doctor does not accept telephone calls during a consultation.**
- **The doctor treats you like a responsible, intelligent person.**
- **The doctor listens to you, does not interrupt when you describe symptoms, and encourages you to air your concerns about treatment.**
- **The doctor is well-informed about preventive health measures, such as nutrition, exercise, and the use of screening tests.**
- **The doctor discusses with you the pros and cons of medical procedures and therapies and explains the implications of test results.**
- **The doctor is an excellent source of knowledge and makes you feel cared for.**

Source: "Health Care's Front Line: Primary Care Physicians." Health Pages. http://www.thehealthpages.com/ar-pcpdr.htm (October 13, 1997).

Health *Care* Settings

Health care can be provided in a variety of settings. Your choice of settings will be determined by your health insurance plan as well as where your physician has patient-admission privileges. Having a preference for a certain setting or hospital could affect your choice of physician also.

Private Practices

A private practice physician can provide medical care as a solo practitioner (one doctor who practices alone) or as a member of a group practice (doctors who work out of, and share financial responsibility for, the same office suite or facility). A group can be doctors in the same specialty (for example, pediatricians) or it can be made up of doctors in several specialties.

Private practice physicians see private patients who are either covered by a fee-for-service health insurance policy or are paying for their own health care. They may also take managed care patients under an agreement with one or more managed care plans. Some have certain laboratory and diagnostic services available whereas others refer their patients elsewhere for these services.

Hospitals

It is recommended that your choice of a hospital be made on the basis of quality and convenience. A hospital that offers a variety of services and experience with complex procedures is preferred over one that is more limited. The selection of a hospital often depends on where the physician has patient-admission privileges and with which health care facility a managed care organization has an agreement. Take these factors into consideration when selecting a physician and a health care plan.

Hospitals go through a process of accreditation through the Joint Commission on Accreditation of Healthcare Organizations. This organization establishes criteria for care and evaluates the quality of staff and equipment. It is also becoming increasingly involved in a facility's success at treating patients.

Community or General Hospitals. The most common type of hospital in the United States is the community or general hospital. These hospitals vary in size and can be a nonprofit or for-profit entity. In general, the larger the hospital, the wider the range of services, since it can afford a larger contingent of highly qualified specialists and sophisticated technology and equipment. Community hospitals are generally thought to provide a more usual or primary level of care. Many hospitals have units that specialize in intensive care, coronary care, neonatal intensive care, or critical care. Larger hospitals are more likely to have all of these units.

Specialty Hospitals. Some hospitals specialize in treating a particular kind of patient or illness. There are hospitals that specialize in the treatment of women and children, patients needing physical rehabilitation, as well as certain diseases, such as cancer. Some hospitals specialize in certain treatments by using medical contractors who assume responsibility for patients undergoing those treatments. The hospital does not have to provide treatment staff and equipment that may be used only occasionally or at less than full capacity.

Teaching Hospitals. Teaching hospitals are usually associated with university medical schools. They are the clinical training arm of the medical school. These hospitals have at least one postgraduate program approved for specialty training. Most of the staff teaches in the medical school and/or performs medical research. Since teaching hospitals provide all levels of care, from primary to tertiary, you can expect excellent technical resources and doctors who are highly qualified and up-to-date on medical developments. You may also receive care from physicians in training. Make sure doctors identify their role and find out who the most senior physician is that is responsible for your care. If any care questions arise, you may request that the senior physician speak with you directly regarding your care. Often, the multiple physicians providing care in the teaching setting have the potential to improve and personalize the care you would otherwise have received.

Emergency Care. Most hospitals have emergency rooms, but they may not be open 24 hours a day or be staffed by a doctor around the clock. Therefore, if you live in a community without a full-service emergency room, determine in advance where you would want to be taken in the event of an emergency that requires those services.

In recent years, many people, especially in large cities, use the emergency room as a primary care facility for any kind of ailment. This can be very expensive and may not be covered by your health plan. If you have a true emergency, however, you should go immediately to an emergency room. They cannot legally refuse to treat you if you have a real emergency; ability to pay is not a basis for turning you away in a true emergency. However, be aware that minor problems are treated at a much higher price in emergency rooms, and it is much more costly to go there for routine care. Most managed care plans will question payment for routine care in an emergency room.

Walk-in Care Centers

So-called walk-in centers operate as urgent care facilities, especially when a hospital emergency room is far away. Many are open 24 hours a day and provide care when your primary care physician's office is closed. Costs tend to be higher than what your doctor would charge but lower than a traditional emergency room. If you do not live near a hospital emergency room, you may want to familiarize yourself with the doctors and services of your local walk-in care centers before you actually need to take advantage of such care.

Some managed care programs do not cover care of non-life-threatening conditions in an emergency room and stipulate that such care be provided in a designated walk-in center. It is a good idea to locate these centers in advance and to be familiar with the criteria for the cost of care to be reimbursed. Emergency room care that is not covered by your health plan can be very expensive for you.

Ambulatory Surgical Centers

Ambulatory surgical centers are used for surgery that is often performed under local anesthesia, with the patient going home the same day. A surgical center can be independent or associated with a hospital. Costs may be lower than if performed in a regular hospital. If possible, it is recommended that you use an accred-

wellness **tip**

To check on accreditation of hospitals and other types of health care facilities mentioned in this section, contact the Joint Commission on Accreditation of Healthcare Organizations at 708-916-5800.

ited ambulatory care center. Research the costs before choosing an ambulatory care center; privately owned facilities may have very high prices. By asking for the complete fee for the facility, staff, anesthesia, and pre- and postoperative care, you can decide if you should have your procedure there or at another facility.

Community Health Clinics

Community health clinics primarily provide ambulatory care in rural areas and inner-city neighborhoods where medical care is scarce and there are many individuals without health insurance or primary care doctors. In addition to providing primary health care, these clinics promote public health in cooperation with community schools, churches, and social service groups. To locate such a clinic, call your health department or look in the Yellow Pages of your telephone directory.

Women's Centers

Women's centers provide programs and services of interest to women: educational programs, libraries, counseling, screening, as well as diagnosis and treatment of health conditions. A women's center can be a clinic or a group of programs associated with a hospital. In addition to primary care, services can include obstetrics, reproductive care, and mental health services—all in one facility staffed by physicians and other health care providers. Please note that not all women's centers are staffed by female physicians.

Health Care Concerns While Traveling

Most health plans have provisions for obtaining care when you are away from home. Obtaining care while traveling is easier with some plans than others, however, and it pays to do some research in advance so you will be prepared. Those who have special health concerns may wish to check out any risks to which they may be exposed while traveling. You should seek information from a doctor skilled in travel related health concerns at least two months before traveling to places with poor sanitation or to exotic places.

Travel in the United States. If you have fee-for-service health coverage and you need to see a doctor while traveling, you can choose any available local doctor. When traveling outside your managed care plan's coverage area, you will have to comply with your plan's requirement for out-of-area medical attention. Most plans require you to call for advance approval of your visit to a doctor. After-the-fact approval is needed for a legitimate visit to an emergency room. It is a good idea to take with you information on how to contact your plan should it be necessary, including your plan identification card and extra copies of the card.

Some HMOs allow members to use a national network of HMOs while traveling in the United States when diagnosis and treatment of a condition cannot wait until you return home. Call 800-223-0654 (American Association of Health Plans) to find out whether there is a participating plan in the area you are visiting.

Travel Abroad. While planning a foreign trip, it is a good idea to discuss health care needs and facilities with your travel consultant and seek medical advice at least two months before your travel to deal with pretravel needs. If your health care policy covers you regardless of where you are, there should be no reason to purchase special health care insurance for the trip. If your policy does not cover you while you are abroad, you may wish to consider obtaining special trip insurance to cover injury or illness incurred while on your trip.

If you are a Medicare participant, you may be eligible for limited benefits only in Mexico and Canada and none elsewhere. You will thus need to rely on your Medigap coverage or special trip coverage.

Check with your usual physician, a travel-specialist physician consultant, or the Centers for Disease Control and Prevention about health risks in the areas you will be visiting. Get a list of English-speaking physicians there in case you need them, and be sure you have received all the necessary vaccinations and pretrip medications. It is a good idea to avoid places where health risks exist if you are, or could be, pregnant or have significant health problems.

Advance *Directives*

It is important to consider in advance how you would like your health care administered if you become too ill to make your own decisions. Advance directives include two important documents: a living will and a durable power of attorney for health care. Neither of these documents goes into effect if you are able to represent yourself when a decision has to be made regarding medical treatment.

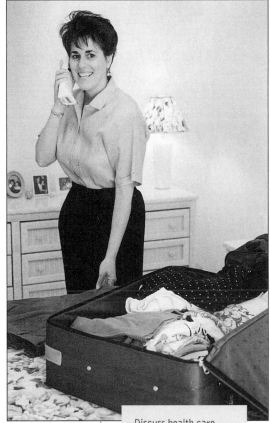

Discuss health care needs and facilities with your travel agent and primary care physician before leaving for a trip overseas.

Many people wait to create these documents in their later years. Unfortunately, accidents frequently lead to situations where patients cannot speak for themselves. Some state laws permit spouses or families to make medical decisions in such cases, but others make no provision for patients who have no living will or a durable power of attorney.

The Living Will

A living will is a legal document that informs doctors, relatives, and friends how you wish your health care to be administered if you become terminally ill or permanently unconscious. In it you can state any extraordinary measures you would like taken, and you can state those you would not like taken. For example, if an accident or illness leaves you unable to survive without artificial breathing equipment, and you are likely to remain unconscious for the rest of your life, your living will can relieve your family of the decision whether to remove the equipment. Other items discussed in a living will may include feeding tubes, surgery, medication, and use of cardiopulmonary resuscitation (CPR) to reestablish a normal heartbeat (those who do not wish to be resuscitated may issue a DNR—do not resuscitate—order in their living will). See Figure 3.4 for an example of a living will.

Durable Power of Attorney

The durable power of attorney document designates a relative or close friend to make health care decisions for you if you become incapacitated or declared

FIGURE 3.4   SAMPLE

Living Will and Health Care Surrogate

Florida Living Will

Declaration made this _____ day of _____ ,
19_____. I, _____ ,
willfully and voluntarily make known my desire that my
dying not be artificially prolonged under the circumstances
set forth below, and I do hereby declare:

If at any time I have a terminal condition and if my
attending or treating physician and another consulting
physician have determined that there is no medical probability of my recovery from such condition, I direct that life-prolonging procedures be withheld or withdrawn when the
application of such procedures would serve only to prolong
artificially the process of dying, and that I be permitted to
die naturally with only the administration of medication or
the performance of any medical procedure deemed necessary to provide me with comfort care or to alleviate pain.

It is my intention that this declaration be honored by my
family and physician as the final expression of my legal right
to refuse medical or surgical treatment and to accept the
consequences for such refusal.

In the event that I have been determined to be unable to
provide express and informed consent regarding the withholding, withdrawal, or continuation of life-prolonging procedures, I wish to designate, as my surrogate to carry out
the provisions of this declaration:

Name:_____
Address: _____
_____ Zip Code: _____
Phone: _____

I wish to designate the following person as my alternate
surrogate, to carry out the provisions of this declaration should
my surrogate be unwilling or unable to act on my behalf:

Name:_____
Address: _____
_____ Zip Code: _____
Phone: _____

Additional instructions (optional):

I understand the full import of this declaration, and I am emotionally and mentally competent to make this declaration.

Signed: _____

Witness 1:
   Signed:_____
   Address:_____

Witness 2:
   Signed:_____
   Address:_____

Florida Designation of Health Care Surrogate

Name: _____
        (Last)   (First)   (Middle Initial)

In the event that I have been determined to be incapaci-
tated to provide informed consent for medical treatment
and surgical and diagnostic procedures, I wish to designate
as my surrogate for health care decisions:
Name:_____
Address: _____
_____ Zip Code: _____
Phone: _____

If my surrogate is unwilling or unable to perform his
duties, I wish to designate as my alternate surrogate:
Name:_____
Address: _____
_____ Zip Code: _____
Phone: _____

I fully understand that this designation will permit my
designee to make health care decisions and to provide, withhold, or withdraw consent on my behalf; to apply for public
benefits to defray the cost of health care; and to authorize
my admission to or transfer from a health care facility.

Additional instructions (optional):

I further affirm that this designation is not being made as
a condition of treatment or admission to a health care facility. I will notify and send a copy of this document to the following persons other than my surrogate, so they may know
who my surrogate is:

Name:_____
Address: _____

Name:_____
Address: _____

Signed: _____
Date: _____

Witness 1:
   Signed: _____
   Address: _____

Witness 2:
   Signed: _____
   Address: _____

Reprinted with permission from Choice in Dying, 1035 30th Street, NW,
Washington, DC 20007, 800-989-9455. Note: Living wills and health surrogate forms are state-specific. Choice in Dying strongly advises using documents specific to the state in which one resides.

incompetent, whether or not death is imminent. For example, you might not be able to understand information being given to you by medical professionals or be able to consent to proposed treatments. Your designee can act on your behalf by deciding to give consent or to refuse it. Make certain your designee understands your wishes completely and agrees to comply with those wishes.

Considerations Before Completing Advance Directives

Before completing advance directive forms, devote some time to thinking about your wishes and then discuss them with your partner, family, and close friends. In the case of the power of attorney, it is important to discuss your plans with the person you wish to designate as your spokesperson. That person must agree to being designated and must understand fully how you wish your health care to be handled under as many types of situations as you can anticipate. Discuss with your primary care physician the way you would like end-of-life situations handled and make sure she knows who you have designated to speak for you.

Each state has its own requirements covering living wills and power of attorney forms. If you maintain more than one residence, you will want to make sure you use the correct form for each state in which you live. Once the forms are prepared properly, give signed copies to all your doctors and immediate family members or to a close relative or friend. It is also wise to carry a copy of each in your purse and keep copies in places where they are certain to be found when needed.

If you are admitted to a health care facility without these completed forms, the facility is required to inform you of your rights under state laws to make a living will or durable power of attorney. Waiting until this stressful period arrives does not allow you much time to think about your desires or talk to the person whom you would like to designate. As with most aspects of health care, you are more likely to get what you want by planning in advance.

If you are the primary caregiver of a child or elderly parent, a living will and durable power of attorney are also helpful in ensuring that your wishes are carried out regarding a new guardian.

What *You* Can Do

Today's health care consumer is faced with many decisions about health care. The costs are high, not only for insurance but also for paying for care without it. It pays to be an active, informed consumer:

- Know what your health insurance policy covers and does not cover.
- Do not let your health insurance policy lapse before you have a replacement policy.
- Select your doctor before you need one.
- Develop a close professional relationship with your doctor and other health care providers.
- Become familiar with health care facilities in your area that meet your needs.
- Prepare a living will and durable power of attorney and speak with your family and close friends about your preferences for treatment.

wellness **tip**

For a nominal fee you can obtain a copy of your state's living will and durable power of attorney forms (with instructions). Call 800-989-9455 (Choice in Dying, a Washington, DC, nonprofit organization). If you live in more than one state, be sure to ask for each state's forms. For an additional fee you can file a copy of your documents with that organization and, in return, receive a wallet-sized card that tells where your forms are maintained in case that information is needed.

PART II

Checking Up for Total Wellness:
Routine Examinations
Throughout a Woman's Life Stages

One of the most effective tools a woman has to help her stay well and detect the early warning signs of disease is the periodic health checkup, also known as the well-woman examination.

Many women think to go to the doctor only when they are ill, but that may be too late. At a periodic health examination, a woman can learn how to recognize the warning signs that represent risks to her health. These routine examinations include health advice and services tailored to the woman's stage in life. This information helps her identify any needed care and to make lifestyle changes that will help her stay as healthy as possible. In addition, during routine examinations a woman's doctor can detect disease in its very early stages, treat it more easily, and, in some cases, prevent the progression of the disease or condition.

Many women think of the well-woman examination as an annual checkup (or a full physical), but a woman's doctor may deem it necessary to perform only a partial examination or one or two basic tests at each periodic health examination. Some women may need to see a doctor annually, whereas others may need a well-woman examination less frequently. The frequency of the examination and what is performed each time are tailored to the needs of a woman based on her age, medical history, general health, and the presence or absence of risk factors.

A complete well-woman examination includes care in three areas:

1. Screening
2. Counseling
3. Immunizations

Part II of this book focuses on how these three elements of the periodic health examination can help a woman stay well during all the stages of her life. (The keys to a healthy lifestyle are described in Part III.)

Part II reflects the findings and recommendations of the U.S. Preventive Services Task Force, which was founded in 1984 to study what types of health care made the greatest difference in keeping people well. The task force, which was made up of a diverse group of health care specialists from many fields, examined hundreds of articles in medical journals and books, debated the merits of different kinds of care, and listened to the opinions of hundreds of experts. In order for members of the task force to recommend a specific type of health care, they had to agree that it met the following conditions:

- It was effective in preventing illness or detecting it early.
- It was cost-effective.
- Overall, the benefits of receiving the care outweighed the risks it might carry.

The results of the task force's research was published in 1996 as the *Guide to Clinical Preventive Services, Second Edition.*

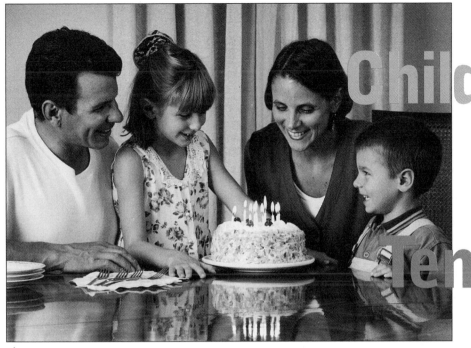

Chapter 4

Childhood: Birth *to* Ten Years

At no time in life do people grow and change as rapidly as in childhood. Over their first ten years, children pass a predictable series of milestones in their physical, cognitive, social, and emotional development. Well-baby and well-child physician checkups are necessary to make sure children are developing physically, mentally, and emotionally within average time frames, and to detect and treat any health problems early.

Infants and young toddlers cannot speak to describe how they feel, and even young children who can talk typically do not have the verbal skills and vocabulary to describe physical symptoms. That is why it is recommended that you establish a relationship between your child and one doctor who can get to know your child and keep track of patterns in her development.

Your relationship with your child's doctor is important, too. As you get to know your child's physician, you can ask questions about your child's health and get reassurance about all areas of her development including social, emotional, and cognitive development. Such a relationship will save a great deal of unnecessary worry on your part, since you can feel sure that the doctor knows your child well enough to spot problems before they become serious, and that she will communicate the problems to you clearly. Suggestions for how to develop a strong doctor-parent-child relationship are given at the end of this chapter.

A quick survey of almost any pediatrician's waiting room reveals that, while fathers accompany their children to the doctor's office more often than in the past, it is still typically the mother who attends. It is always a good idea for both parents to get to know the doctor, however, since well-child visits help the parents learn important strategies for:

- Helping newborns learn to sleep through the night and older infants and toddlers learn to adopt a predictable nap and meal schedule.
- Keeping children safe.
- Encouraging good eating and hygiene habits.

This chapter describes what to expect during wellness checkups for children up to ten years old and outlines key concerns for parents during these early years. It also offers information and tips to help mothers and fathers keep their children healthy. The routine and preventive care described here is designed for the parents of children who are not ill as a way of ensuring continued good health throughout the child's life.

The Periodic Health Examination

Although adults too benefit from regular checkups with the doctor, for children, such checkups are *absolutely essential*. Preventive services for children are usually performed during special, prescheduled visits called well-baby and well-child visits. Visits are more frequent when a baby is young and then are spaced farther apart as the child grows older.

A child's first wellness examination takes place in the minutes after she is born, when those attending the birth give her a general physical examination. During this time, the internal and external organs are checked and vital signs are assessed. As the child grows, wellness visits are usually recommended at the following ages:

- 2 weeks
- 1 month
- 2 months
- 4 months
- 6 months
- 9 months
- 12 months
- 15 months

- 18 months
- 24 months
- 3 years
- 4 years
- 5 years
- 6 years
- 8 years
- 10 years

During these visits, the doctor offers three basic services: screening, counseling, and immunization (see box).

Screening

Screening gives the doctor a baseline against which to compare future developments in your child's health. Each time you take your child to the pediatrician, she will compare current data to data from previous visits and provide you with a clear picture of your child's progress and the state of her health. Screening also detects potential health risks before they develop into illness. Following are screening tests you can expect when you take your child to the doctor.

Height and Weight. Measuring height and weight provides important benchmarks to assess a child's physical growth and development. Her changing height

Periodic Health Examination

The following health services are performed at each regularly scheduled well-child visit unless a specific age is mentioned.

Screening. The doctor uses these measurements and tests to look for signs of health risks in well children:

- Height and weight
- Blood pressure
- Vision and hearing examination
- Hemoglobin test (at birth)
- Phenylalanine level (at birth)
- Thyroid test (at birth)

Counseling. Depending on the age of your child, the doctor will review information about your role in keeping your children well:

- Preventing injuries
- Providing a well-balanced diet and encouraging children to enjoy being physically active
- Monitoring the quality of your child's environment
- Taking appropriate actions to prevent substance use
- Fostering good dental health habits

Immunizations. The immunizations listed here are recommended for all healthy children. See Table 4.1 on page 82 for a typical immunization schedule:

- Diphtheria–tetanus–pertussis (DTP)
- Poliovirus
- Measles–mumps–rubella (MMR)
- *H. influenzae* type b (Hib)
- Hepatitis B
- Varicella

wellness **tip**

In between well-baby and well-child visits, jot down questions that you want to ask at the next visit. Bring your list with you, and also bring a pad to write down the answers. If you get into a lengthy discussion or if your doctor provides a lengthy answer, taking notes can help you remember details.

indicates how her bones are developing. Her weight indicates whether she is eating well. A baby who fails to gain weight, or loses weight in the first year of life, might be diagnosed as "failure-to-thrive," and steps will be taken to learn the source of the problem. On the other hand, if a young child is gaining too much weight, the pediatrician can counsel parents about what is a reasonable diet to help that child reach and maintain a healthy weight.

Starting with the first well-baby visit, a child's height and weight are typically plotted on a growth chart that shows how her growth compares with that of other children her age (Figure 4.1 on page 72). Measurements are expressed in percentiles. For example, a male toddler who weighs 27 pounds at age 15 months is in the 75th percentile for weight (meaning that 75 percent of male toddlers his age

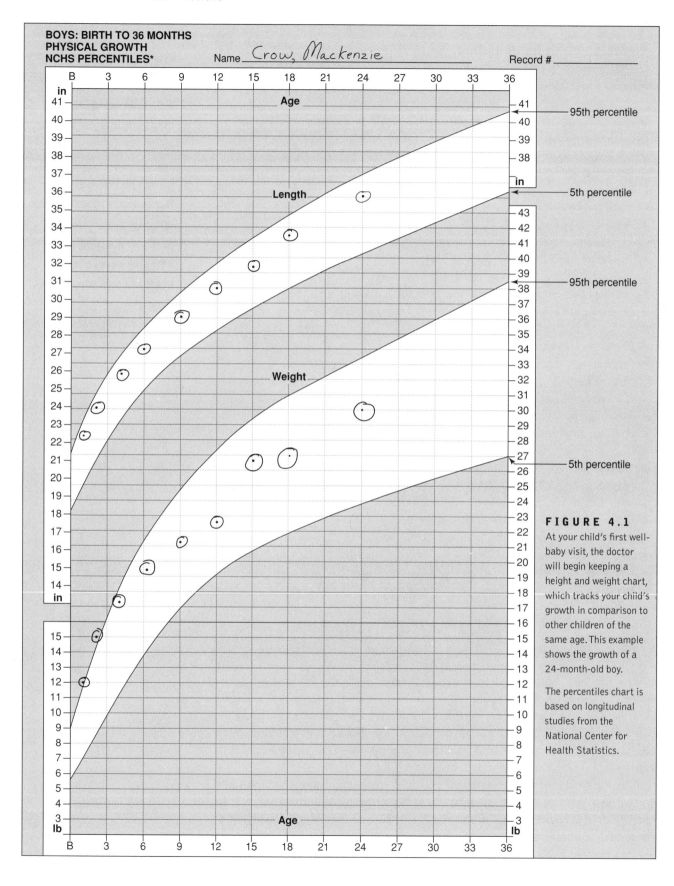

FIGURE 4.1

At your child's first well-baby visit, the doctor will begin keeping a height and weight chart, which tracks your child's growth in comparison to other children of the same age. This example shows the growth of a 24-month-old boy.

The percentiles chart is based on longitudinal studies from the National Center for Health Statistics.

are lighter than he is). If he is 32 inches long, he is in the 75th percentile for height (meaning that 75 percent of male toddlers his age are smaller than he is).

Most doctors do not become concerned about a child's growth unless she is significantly off the percentile scale in either direction. Infants who are large at birth or gain a great deal of weight in the weeks following birth typically slow down their growth by age one, and smaller infants typically "catch up" in a similar time frame.

Blood Pressure. High blood pressure can occur even in children. Because high blood pressure runs in some families, children born to parents with high blood pressure should be observed to see if they have the problem as well. It is thought that children who have high blood pressure are more likely to have high blood pressure as adults. It also increases the risk of other health problems later in life, such as diabetes and heart disease.

High blood pressure in children is often caused by an illness. For example, some types of kidney disease cause high blood pressure. Regular screening, therefore, is very important. Taking early action to lower blood pressure can help prevent problems in later years. If your child's blood pressure is high, the doctor will explore the cause for it and will counsel you on ways to lower the blood pressure.

Vision and Hearing Checkups. The typical newborn can focus on an object only when it is 8 to 14 inches away. During well-baby visits, the doctor will check your infant's eyes by moving an object in an arc to see if the child can follow it. She will also ask you what you have observed in terms of your child's visual alertness. At about three months, an infant will begin to follow the arc. Informal eye checks are a routine part of well-baby visits during the first three years.

Starting at about two years of age, every child should receive an annual eye examination by an eye care specialist. An ophthalmologist can determine whether the child has any eye diseases or vision problems. As many as one in ten preschool children have vision problems that go unnoticed without testing. Tests in young children include screening for amblyopia and strabismus. Ambylopia is commonly called "lazy eye." One eye weakens, and the other eye works harder as a result to compensate for the weakened eye. Strabismus occurs when the eyes cannot focus together well.

Although difficulty in focusing the eyes is common in newborns, within a few weeks infants should be able to move their eyes together. It is important to detect both amblyopia and strabismus early. The earlier these vision problems are detected, the more easily they can be treated. Both can result in permanent vision difficulties or vision loss if untreated.

Nearly all elementary schools test students' vision. Poor vision may also be detected if a child has trouble reading or seeing the blackboard at school. If your child's school provides annual vision testing, you may not have to take her to an eye doctor. However, if your child needs corrective lenses or if she is diagnosed with an eye disorder, you will need to see an ophthalmologist.

During the first few well-baby visits, the doctor will usually asks the parents if the baby responds to their voices and turns toward loud or sudden noises. A child's ability to respond to sounds in each ear can be determined very early. Sometimes it is necessary to test with special equipment to determine mild or

wellness **tip**

Research has shown that until about five months of age, infants respond more actively to black and white patterns than to color. Look for a black and white mobile (most are made of printed cardboard or stuffed fabric shapes) to hang over your baby's crib. A nice feature is an adjustable hanger that raises the height of the mobile from your baby's face as her field of vision lengthens.

uneven hearing problems. Well-baby and well-child visits also include checking the ears with an otoscope to make sure color, fluid, and movement of the ear drum are normal. The otoscope detects any sign of ear infections, which should always be treated as early as possible to prevent hearing loss.

Hemoglobin Test. This blood test, often performed at birth, detects the type of hemoglobin in an infant's blood. Hemoglobin is a protein in red blood cells that carries oxygen in the blood. Some abnormal types of hemoglobin cause conditions called hemoglobinopathies, which are illnesses passed from parent to child. One such illness is sickle cell disease, which usually occurs in people of African descent, and another is Tay-Sachs disease, which occurs mostly in Jewish people of European descent. People from other ethnic groups who should be on the alert for hemoglobinopathies are those whose ancestors are from the Caribbean, Latin America, the Mediterranean region, the Middle East, and Southeast Asia.

Since hemoglobinopathies are inherited, if one child is affected, others may be as well. Genetic counseling and testing are available to parents to help them understand the risk of the disease in themselves and their children. Early hemoglobin testing can allow affected children to begin early interventional medical care. Although hemoglobinopathies cannot be cured, special care can ease symptoms and prevent complications.

Phenylalanine Test. This test (called the PKU test) detects the amount of phenylalanine, a naturally occurring amino acid, in an infant's blood. Infants are tested within seven days after birth. The result of the test may be inaccurate in infants tested earlier than 24 hours after birth because phenylalanine is present only after an infant has had a few feedings. People who have the disease phenylketonuria (PKU) are unable to digest phenylalanine. This inherited illness, in which higher-than-normal levels of phenylalanine circulate in the blood, is referred to as an inborn error of metabolism. PKU occurs in about one in every 14,000 births. Untreated PKU can result in mental retardation and neurologic problems.

Children found to have high levels of phenylalanine are prescribed special diets low in this substance. If the diet is maintained, the harmful effects of PKU can be minimized. It is especially important for pregnant women with PKU to maintain the appropriate diet because high levels of phenylalanine can harm the fetus.

Tests for T_4 and TSH. Both T_4 and TSH are hormones made by the thyroid gland. Tests that show the levels of these hormones in the blood indicate thyroid function. If the thyroid is overactive and produces high levels of hormones, hyperthyroidism occurs. If the thyroid is underactive and produces low levels of hormones, hypothyroidism occurs.

The level of thyroid hormones in infants' blood is tested in the first week of life. In the United States, T_4 is usually checked first; if it is too low, then TSH is checked. (TSH is a hormone made by the pituitary gland that stimulates thyroid gland function.) If TSH is higher than normal, the infant has hypothyroidism. Untreated hypothyroid infants have stunted growth and are usually mentally handicapped. If hypothyroidism is detected and treated early, though, infants show few effects of the condition. It occurs in about one in every 4,000 births.

Counseling

During regular checkups, your child's doctor can explain what you can do at home to keep your child well. The reason this counseling is so important is that accidents that occur in the home and motor vehicle injuries are among the leading causes of death in children from birth to ten years. First-time parents especially cannot anticipate the numerous ways small children can get in harm's way, and a doctor's advice may save a life. In addition to counseling you about safety issues, the doctor will offer advice on your child's diet, physical activity, dental health, and overall healthy lifestyle.

Injury Prevention. Injuries are the fourth leading cause of death among children, followed by automobile accidents. There are many steps parents can take to keep their children safe in the car, during outside play, and in the home.

Car Travel and Air Bags. In many countries of the world, the law requires that children ride in the back seat of cars until they are 13 years old. The back seat is considered safest for children because they are protected on all four sides by the bulk of the car. If possible, place your child's car seat in the center of the back seat (facing toward the back until your infant weighs 20 pounds and can sit up well). Make sure the shoulder straps and the strap in between the legs fit snugly but not too tightly. For infants, place a rolled receiving blanket or small towel around the head for extra padding and to hold the head in place. Specially-proportioned cushion inserts are also available for this purpose.

If your car is equipped with a passenger-side air bag, you have another compelling reason to put your child in the back seat at all times. The air bags currently in use are designed for adults. The force of the inflating bag has caused death or serious harm to a number of children sitting in the front seat. Infants in car seats are especially vulnerable. Until safer air bags become available, the rear seat remains the safest location in a car for all children.

Bicycle Safety. Hospital emergency room personnel see numerous children every month who have had accidents while riding bicycles. It is essential to teach children to avoid riding near traffic and to wear a helmet while riding. Look for the ANSI (American National Standards Institute) or SNELL (Snell Memorial Foundation) marking on a helmet, indicating that it has been professionally tested and has met or exceeded safety standards. If your child has learned to ride a bicycle, review with her the "rules of the road" for bike riders: always ride on the right side of the road, signal when turning, ride defensively, never assume drivers in cars can see you. It is a good idea to ride with your child on her first several outings to be sure she understands the rules and can handle her bike well enough to travel on the roadway.

Fire and Burn Prevention. Fires and burns are leading causes of accidental death and injury in children, but they are often avoidable. Install smoke detectors on each level of home, especially near bedrooms. Make a point to test detectors regularly during the year to make sure they are working properly. Purchase flame-retardant sleepwear for your children. Teach children not to play with matches

Infants at Risk

Both a child's family history and her environment may pose risks to her health. These risks can be observed by and/or discussed with the doctor during routine visits and may require special tests or care. The following factors indicate infants at risk for health problems.

Infants who:

- **Are preterm or low birth weight**
- **Are from low-income families or families who have recently emigrated from developing countries**
- **Have mothers at risk for HIV**
- **Are exposed to tuberculosis through family members or other contacts**
- **Are taken to developing countries in which certain diseases are prevalent**
- **Live with their mother in an institution**
- **Have chronic medical conditions**
- **Are exposed to lead in their home or community**
- **Live in a town with inadequate water fluoridation**
- **Have a family history of skin cancer or who have fair skin, eyes, and hair**

wellness tip

If you have an air bag in the front passenger seat of your car, put your child in the back seat at all times. If your child must ride in the passenger seat, be sure she is properly restrained by a car seat or safety belt. Move the seat as far back as possible from the panel that contains the air bag.

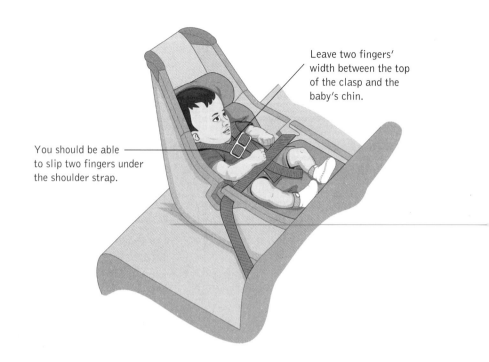

Leave two fingers' width between the top of the clasp and the baby's chin.

You should be able to slip two fingers under the shoulder strap.

FIGURE 4.2 Car Seat Safety

Before traveling, be sure to secure your child's car seat in the center of the back seat. The car seat should face toward the rear until the child weighs 20 pounds and can sit up well.

and to stay away from hot surfaces. Never leave a crawling infant or toddler alone near a hot oven, woodstove, kerosene heater, or fireplace, or where there are candles burning. Put protective barriers over fireplaces and stove dials. To avoid accidental scalding from hot water, set hot water heaters to a temperature no higher than 120 to 130°F.

Preventing Falls. Falls are another hazard that can easily be prevented by taking some basic precautions. Too often, parents think their child is too young to be at risk of a fall and so do not take preventive action. However, children make developmental leaps in their motor skills almost overnight. One day your toddler may be able to climb up on a chair and reach the window, whereas the day before she was not. Place guards on windows and gates at the top and bottom of stairs. Dress your child carefully, avoiding pants legs that are too long, pajamas with "feet" that are too long, or socks and slippers without rubberized gripping. Never leave a young child or infant unattended, especially in a baby walker. Walkers are not safe for use around stairs. Families with pools need to be especially cautious. A fence around the pool will help prevent a toddler from falling into the pool. You must also be alert to the risk of drowning if your neighbors have pools. As soon as they are capable of understanding, make sure your children know that they should never enter or play near water without an adult present.

Preventing Accidental Overdose or Poisoning. Anything that could be harmful to children is best stored safely out of reach. Purchase over-the-counter and prescription medications in childproof containers and store them away from children—in a locked cabinet or drawer, if possible. Toxic substances, such as cleaning supplies, must be kept locked up and out of children's reach. When possible, buy non-toxic alternatives. Keep products in their original containers—do not put them in containers that have been used to hold food.

If a child ingests a poisonous substance, call the local poison control number. Do not assume that the best response is to induce vomiting, since some poisons, especially corrosives, cause more harm when vomiting is induced. Keep syrup of ipecac on hand, but do not administer it until you are directed to do so by the poison control center.

To avoid accidents and poisoning, anticipate your child's physical developmental changes and prepare your home ahead of time. At each well-baby and well-child visit, ask your doctor what developmental milestones are upcoming and what actions you can take to prevent accidents and injuries.

Gun Safety. Guns are hazardous in any home but particularly in homes with children. Half of all gun owners keep their weapons in an unlocked area. According to the Educational Fund to End Handgun Violence, in 1991, 1,441 unintentional shooting fatalities occurred, 551 of them involving children aged 19 or younger.

While it is recommended that guns not be kept in the home, parents who do choose to keep them are strongly advised to store them locked and unloaded, and to teach their children that guns are not toys and that they must never touch them. (See Chapter 14 for a detailed discussion of gun safety in the home.) If you learn that your children's friends have guns in their homes, discuss the situation with the parents and ask them to lock the guns away. Children are much more likely to explore and tamper with "forbidden" items when they are with other children than when they are alone.

Preventing SIDS. Sudden infant death syndrome, or SIDS, is the third leading cause of death in young children. The risk is typically described as 2 in 1,000. As its name suggests, SIDS victims die in their sleep for no apparent reason. Recent studies have concluded that infants who sleep on their stomachs are more likely to die of SIDS than those who are placed on their backs to sleep. These studies contradict a long-standing belief that babies placed on their backs are at risk of choking if they "spit up" while lying in that position. It now seems that babies are capable of avoiding choking on their own and that the risk of SIDS is much greater than the risk of choking. If you are worried about the back of the baby's

CPR Training

When accidents happen, parents and day care providers who are trained in cardiopulmonary resuscitation (CPR) can start lifesaving measures right away. The American Red Cross offers CPR classes, including those teaching techniques designed for babies and young children. Some ob/gyn practices offer infant CPR classes to their patients. Older children may be encouraged to learn CPR and first aid as well, perhaps through instruction offered by a scouting, YWCA, or YMCA program.

head becoming flat, you can place her head to the side or lay the baby on her side, supported by a blanket.

The factors that increase a baby's risk for SIDS are not known, but some experts believe the following factors may increase risk:

- If the baby once survived a life-threatening event during which she stopped breathing, turned blue, or required resuscitation
- If she has had episodes of apnea in which she stopped breathing for 20 seconds or less
- If she was a low birth weight or premature baby
- If she was born to a mother who lacked adequate prenatal care
- If she was born to a mother who smoked during the pregnancy

Diet and Exercise. Just as with adults, diet and exercise are the keys to wellness for children. But a child's nutritional and physical needs are not the same as those of an adult. Following are tips to help you understand the differences.

Diet. An infant's best first diet is breast milk alone. It naturally provides not only the right amounts of nutrients (at the right temperature) but also offers some protection against infection. Breast milk provides iron, which is required to prevent anemia. If a mother chooses not to breastfeed her infant, or weans her infant before six months, formula fortified with iron also gives children the nutrients they need to grow, but it does not provide the immune system protection. (See Chapter 18 for a more detailed discussion of breastfeeding.) Once solid foods are introduced, iron-fortified cereal (a typical "first food") can help ensure that a child gets enough iron.

A Healthy Weight for a Healthy Child

Up to 25 percent of American children weigh too much. Being overweight carries the same health risks for children as it does for adults. Overweight children often grow up to be overweight adults.

Keeping children at a healthy weight requires that you provide a well-balanced diet and help them get regular exercise. The most effective way to help children develop good eating habits is to set guidelines for the whole family, including the adults. Have your child help you choose recipes, shop for food, and prepare meals and snacks. Look for children's books (fiction or nonfiction) that discuss healthy eating or outdoor activities. Encourage a love of and respect for nature (children who love nature generally enjoy spending time outdoors). Engage in active play and outdoor recreational activities with your child on a regular basis.

Avoid giving your children fatty, salty, and sugary foods. A child who never develops a taste for these foods is less likely to eat them regularly as an adult. Give your children healthy snacks. Fruit is a good choice because it tastes sweet, is low-calorie, full of fiber, and helps prevent tooth decay. Pack lunch boxes so that children have good food to eat while at school. Make sure your day care provider knows your family policy on sweets and fatty foods. Good caregivers will cheerfully accommodate these requests.

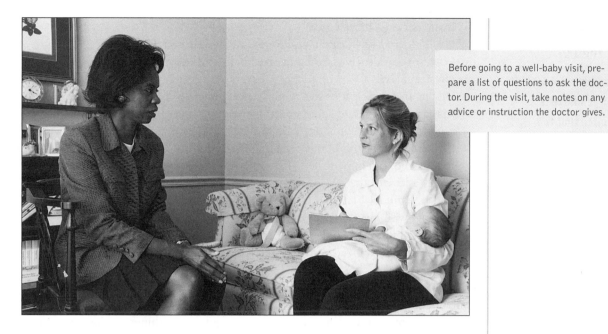

Before going to a well-baby visit, prepare a list of questions to ask the doctor. During the visit, take notes on any advice or instruction the doctor gives.

Some parents mistakenly think that feeding their young children low-fat food and dairy products prevents them from becoming overweight. It is important to realize that young children need some fat in their diets for proper growth. For this reason, whole-fat dairy products are advised for children under the age of two (including cow's milk, which is usually introduced between 9 and 12 months). After age two, your child can eat low-fat dairy products, but at no time should a child be given an extremely low-fat diet. After age two, about 30 percent of a child's daily calories can come from fat.

Once children begin solid foods, parents are wise to begin immediately structuring their meals and snacks around the basic rules of a healthful diet. Though children do have individual tastes—and some children will never like certain foods—it seems that the earlier in a child's life a certain food is offered, the more likely a child will continue to enjoy it later. (Certain foods, including shellfish, berries, peanuts, raw honey, and egg whites, should not be introduced until age one to avoid the development of allergies and serious, even fatal, reactions because of the baby's unsophisticated digestive and immune systems.) Include a variety of nutrient-dense foods and adequate amounts of grains, fruits, and vegetables. These foods are good sources of vitamins and minerals as well as dietary fiber, which helps prevent some cancers. (See Chapter 8 for more information on eating for wellness.)

Exercise. Young children in this country do not get enough exercise. Toddlers generally enjoy active play, which helps them grow and develop. But after the toddler years, many young children need encouragement to participate in active play. They may be shy or lack the social skills to join a group. They may simply watch too much television (including videos) or spend too much time in front of the computer. If your child leans toward passive or inactive play, find ways to encourage her:

Turn Off the TV

Physicians, nutritionists, and child psychologists generally agree that too much TV creates sedentary, unimaginative children and the commercials encourage materialism and eating high-fat, salty, and sugary foods. Try to avoid using the TV as a babysitter. Limit viewing, and encourage your children to play outdoors, weather permitting, for a set period of time each day, such as the hour before dinner.

- Invite her on a bicycle ride.
- Play hide-and-seek, catch, and follow-the-leader with her.
- Look for toys, such as different-sized balls and tricycles, that encourage physical play.
- Design an obstacle course in your backyard, and ask her to help you build it.
- Make sure your child spends part of every day outside, weather permitting (it is good to ask potential day care providers if they schedule this).
- If your child is shy, ask your pediatrician about ways to help her learn to make friends and join in play.
- Foster a love of the outdoors—take your children on nature walks.
- Be a role model—let your children see that you value physical activity, such as jogging, walking, or aerobic dance.
- As your children get older, encourage them to stay active—in free play and games or in organized activities and sports.

Environment. You are responsible for monitoring the quality of the environment surrounding your child. You do not always have control over the air and water quality in your immediate vicinity, but there are many things over which you do have control. It is a good idea to have your water tested for lead and other contaminants, especially if you live in an older house with lead pipes. Lead is known to cause diminished brain function in children. If you have well water, it is also important to check the water quality frequently. Another dangerous source of lead is from paint that peels off the walls in older buildings and is ingested by crawling infants and toddlers, who explore their world by putting everything they find into their mouth.

Tobacco smoke poses another environmental hazard to children's health. Secondhand smoke has been proven to be dangerous, increasing the risk of SIDS and, later, the risk of lung cancer and heart disease. Being exposed to secondhand smoke increases a child's risk for infections, such as tonsillitis and respiratory, ear, bacterial, and viral infections. It also worsens asthma in children who have the condition. Parents who smoke are advised to quit, both for their benefit and that of their children. If you do continue to smoke after your children are born, smoke outdoors or in a room where your children do not spend time. Avoid smoking in the car when your child is with you.

It is a good idea to begin telling children at a young age about the dangers of smoking and advising them not to start. Today, most individuals who smoke began during high school or earlier; many of them have parents or older brothers or sisters who smoke. Starting smoking early is linked to a more severe addiction to nicotine later in life.

Controlled Substances. It is never too early to begin talking to your children about the dangers of alcohol and drug use. Reports of children being offered these substances in elementary and middle school by peers and older children are growing. Your pediatrician may be able to give you tips on broaching these sensitive subjects with your children. Remember, too, that parents are role models for their children and should use alcohol moderately, if at all, avoid tobacco and street drugs completely, and use prescription drugs only as intended.

Curbing a Sweet Tooth

Research shows that you can teach your baby not to crave sweets, or at least increase the chance that she won't. A baby's tongue is like a clean slate at birth. Refrain from giving her all forms of refined sugar, including maple sugar, brown sugar, and corn syrup, during the first and second years. Instead, offer foods such as plain cottage cheese, plain yogurt, unsweetened applesauce, as well as pureed fresh ripe fruits, such as peaches, bananas, and pears and steamed and pureed fresh vegetables (fruits can be mixed with cottage cheese or yogurt, vegetables with cottage cheese). If you use jarred baby foods, make sure they contain no sugar, corn syrup, or other "natural" sweeteners. The longer you hold off on products with refined sugar the better. Explain your rationale to relatives and caregivers, too, so they support your efforts.

wellness **tip**

Kids may find brushing and flossing more enjoyable with toothpaste and brushes made especially for them. Flavored dental floss may help, as well. If you find that your children brush too quickly, set an egg timer for two minutes and tell them they need to brush until the time is up.

Dental Health. Caring for a child's teeth is an important part of overall wellness. The major dental problem for children is cavities. By the age of three, 60 percent of children have at least one cavity. Even primary teeth need protection from cavities. If they are lost to tooth decay, and the permanent tooth does not emerge soon afterward, the other primary teeth can move to fill the gap, causing irregular growth in the permanent teeth.

Your pediatrician will tell you that dental care begins early by preventing "baby bottle tooth decay." Putting an infant to bed with a bottle is not recommended. When milk, formula, or juice remains in a child's mouth all night, tooth decay usually results. Some parents leave a bottle with their babies thinking they are easing their way into sleep. But once children get attached to the routine, it can be hard to stop.

Regular dental hygiene can begin as soon as a child's first teeth appear. The first teeth may be cleaned with water—no toothpaste—and a soft toothbrush, a piece of gauze, or a damp washcloth. Later, a soft toothbrush and no more than a pea-sized amount of fluoride toothpaste are recommended for children over age two. (Toddlers under age two, who are unable to understand the concept of rinsing and spitting out, should use children's toothpaste formulated without fluoride.) Parents can help their young children brush and floss and remind their older children to brush at least twice a day—in the morning and before bed.

Dental visits should begin when a child is three years old or has all his primary teeth. The dentist will check whether or not teeth are coming in properly, clean the teeth, and show the child how to brush and floss.

Immunizations

Immunizations, also referred to as vaccinations, are designed to prevent serious infections and diseases. Many childhood infections are now at their lowest levels in history as a result of routine programs of immunizations and government-funded immunization programs for children in need.

In brief, vaccines work by causing the body to act as though it has already been infected. Vaccines cause the body to create antibodies to fight invading organisms. Once the body mobilizes its defense against the infection, antibodies remain to protect against future infections by the same organism.

When Not to Vaccinate

For most healthy children, the benefits of vaccinations easily outweigh the risks of side effects. Some children, though, have health conditions that may make vaccination inadvisable. If your child has any of these symptoms or conditions, be sure to tell the doctor or nurse before your child is vaccinated.

Inform your doctor if your child:

- Has a serious illness, such as cancer or AIDS (acquired immuno-deficiency syndrome).
- Takes medications for illness.
- Is allergic to eggs (which are used to make some vaccines) or the medications neomycin or streptomycin.
- Has had seizures, or if seizures run in the family.
- Has had a serious allergic reaction (more than pain from the shot or mild fever) from a previous vaccination.
- Has received immune globulin or a blood transfusion recently.

Vaccines contain either a small part of the virus or bacterium or a whole organism that has been killed or weakened. The vaccine is then injected into the body, which reacts by producing antibodies. A person who is vaccinated against a disease gets the benefits of having been exposed to the organism without the risks.

The following list describes vaccines that are known to help prevent infections that were once dangerous and debilitating. (A recommended vaccination schedule is shown in Table 4.1.) Most vaccinations are planned in conjunction with well-baby and well-child visits, with some vaccines given in combination.

TABLE 4.1

Immunization Schedule

Age	DTP	OPV or IPV	MMR	Hib
2 months	✔	✔		
4 months	✔	✔		
6 months	✔	✔*		
12 months				
15 months			✔	
15 to 18 months	✔	✔		
18 months				✔
4 to 6 years	✔	✔		

*In high-risk areas

Source: American Academy of Pediatricians.

DTP Vaccine. The DTP vaccine protects against three conditions: diphtheria, tetanus, and pertussis. All three diseases are serious and can be fatal:

- Diphtheria is caused by *Corynebacterium diphtheriae*. It causes a film to form in the nose, throat, and windpipe and makes breathing difficult. It can affect both the heart and the nerves.
- Tetanus, or "lockjaw," is caused by *Clostridium tetani*. It causes the muscles of the body, including the muscles used for breathing, to go into spasms and stiffen.
- Pertussis, or "whooping cough," is caused by *Bordetella pertussis*. Its common name comes from the fact that infected people cough repeatedly with "whooping" breathing.

One of the recent advances in vaccines is the development of the "acellular" version of the DTP vaccine, called DTaP. The advantage of the acellular vaccine is that it is less likely to cause side effects that may occur from the pertussis part of the vaccine. The acellular vaccine is routinely used today.

Poliovirus Vaccine. Polio, caused by infection with poliovirus, can cause paralysis and death. Before a vaccine was developed in the 1950s, polio was widespread and universally dreaded. There are two types of polio vaccine available today: oral polio vaccine (OPV) and inactivated polio vaccine (IPV). Until recently, most children received OPV. Now, the Centers for Disease Control and Prevention, which monitors the incidence and control of diseases worldwide, offers three different options for vaccinations:

- Two doses of IPV and then two doses of OPV (the first choice)
- Four doses of IPV
- Four doses of OPV

MMR Vaccine. The MMR vaccine protects against three viral infections: measles, mumps, and rubella:

- Measles is characterized by a red rash and fever. It can also cause serious infection that can lead to seizures, brain damage, or even death. The older the child who contracts measles, the more threatening it is.
- Mumps commonly causes swelling of the glands in the cheeks and the lymph nodes under the jaw. Mumps can also cause brain infection (meningitis) and pain and swelling of the testicles in boys and men (infertility is a rare complication).
- Rubella, or German measles, causes a rash and swollen glands. Rubella is very dangerous to pregnant women, because it can infect the fetus. Infected fetuses may die or be born with birth defects.

Unlike polio, which has been nearly eliminated in the United States, measles still occurs. This is mostly due to lack of vaccination or inadequate vaccination. Sometimes the disease is brought into the country by foreign travelers who have not been adequately immunized.

Hib Vaccine. Hib disease is caused by the bacterium *H. influenzae* type b. This infection is the most common cause of the 12,000 cases of bacterial meningitis in young children in the United States each year. It can cause problems such as severe throat infection, a potentially fatal infection called epiglottitis (in which the airway is blocked), pneumonia, and many other serious infections of the blood, skin, bones, and joints.

Available since 1987, the Hib vaccine is one of the newer vaccines offered and is safe to be administered at age 18 months. Approval for earlier administration is expected. A combination vaccine for Hib and DPT may be given, resulting in one less injection. In general, the Hib vaccination causes only mild fever and soreness or redness at the injection site.

Hepatitis B Vaccine. Hepatitis B is a liver disease that is caused by the hepatitis B virus and can lead to liver failure. It can be passed by exposure to body fluids of an infected person and by a mother to her infant at birth. Infants infected at birth have a much higher risk of later developing a serious disease, including cancer, than do people infected later in childhood or as adults. The hepatitis B series of vaccines is usually given in the first year with the first dose offered in the hospital or between 12 and 18 months. (For more about hepatitis B, see Chapter 22.)

Hepatitis B testing is recommended for all pregnant women, and vaccination is recommended for all infants. If a woman tests positive, or if her status is not known, special guidelines for vaccination may be advised (see Chapter 22). The most common side effect of the vaccination is soreness at the injection site, though some children also have a high fever.

Varicella Vaccine. The varicella-zoster virus causes chickenpox, one of the most common childhood illnesses. It is marked by red blotches with clear blisters and is highly contagious. Because it is so common, nearly everyone is infected at some time during childhood. Chickenpox is usually mild in young

wellness tip

If your child is scheduled to receive a vaccination, ask your doctor whether there are any reasons to avoid the particular vaccine. Find out what type of side effects may occur. Most side effects, such as fever or soreness near the site of the injection, tend to be mild, temporary, and can be eased with acetaminophen. Others, such as seizures, are rarer, quite serious, and require a doctor's attention.

children but can be more severe in older children and adults. In severe cases, it can lead to pneumonia or other complications.

The varicella vaccine is the newest vaccine given to children. It is now routinely offered to infants because it is most effective in young children. However, it is still the parent's option, as long-term studies on protection are still in progress. It is about 70 percent effective, and those children who have been immunized and still contract the virus usually have milder cases. Older children and adults who choose to be vaccinated need two shots; infants need only one.

Because the varicella vaccine is new, not as much is known about its potential for rare, serious side effects later in life. Common mild reactions include soreness or redness at the site of the injection and rashes or fever.

Keeping *Your* Child Well

Choosing a doctor for your child and then establishing a positive relationship with that doctor are two of the most important responsibilities for a parent. After selecting a doctor that best fits your child's needs, you can ensure that your child receives routine care, including screening tests and vaccinations, while using doctor visits as opportunities for counseling, information gathering, and consultation about ongoing and future health care needs.

Choosing a Doctor

Children can receive medical care from primary care physicians, family doctors, or pediatricians, doctors who specialize in the care of children. (Chapter 3 provides general information about selecting a doctor.)

Doctors who care for children need special communication skills. A good family doctor or pediatrician understands the nonverbal signals infants and young children use to communicate pain, discomfort, and frustration. She also is able to help children feel as comfortable as possible in the unfamiliar setting of the doctor's office. In addition, a good family doctor or pediatrician is skilled at communicating with children and parents in a friendly, clear, and noncondescending manner.

If you already have a family doctor as your primary care physician, she can provide care for your child as well. There are advantages in having the same doctor care for the whole family. Health problems that affect one member of the family also may affect others. But a pediatrician offers other advantages. You may wish to follow these tips to find the best choice for you and your child:

- Ask for recommendations from family or friends.
- Ask for a recommendation from your internist or obstetrician/gynecologist.

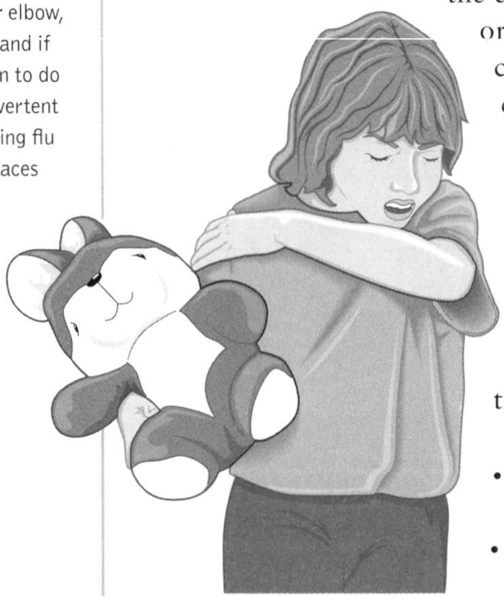

FIGURE 4.3

Preventing the Spread of Colds and Flu

Make it a habit to always cough or sneeze into the inside of your elbow, rather than into your hands, and if you have children, teach them to do the same. This prevents inadvertent spreading of bacteria, including flu germs, to any objects or surfaces you touch with your hands.

search for another doctor. If all goes well, your child's doctor might see her into young adulthood, so the relationship is too important to leave to chance.

What *You* Can **Do**

Good health habits established in childhood can last a lifetime. Providing routine care early in life can prevent many problems and detect others early so that specialized care has the greatest chance for success. Working with your doctor, you can help keep your children happy and healthy—from birth through age ten and beyond:

- Make sure your child has regularly scheduled wellness visits with the doctor.
- Monitor your child's diet, and prepare healthy foods for the whole family.
- Plan physical activities your family can enjoy together, such as taking bicycle rides or swimming.
- Always wear your seat belt when driving. Use the proper safety seat or belt for your child's weight and age.
- Obtain training in CPR and first aid.
- Take your child for recommended immunizations and report any serious side effects. Make sure you receive a record of the immunizations.
- Set a good example of wellness for your children. Children are great observers who learn far more by example than by being told what to do. Remember, when it comes to staying healthy, your actions speak louder than your words.

- Obtain a list, from your health insurance company, of pediatricians who will accept your insurance.
- Interview potential candidates or take your child for one of her well-child visits. Some practices have special visits for expectant parents to describe how the practice operates and to give parents the opportunity to meet particular pediatricians.

Working with Your Doctor

A doctor can only help you keep your children well if you take them to their well-child visits as scheduled. It is most important that you complete your child's schedule of immunizations so that she gets full protection against diseases. If you have to cancel a well-child visit, or if your child is not well at the time of a regularly scheduled well-child visit, reschedule the appointment during the same telephone call you use to cancel, and return to the recommended immunization schedule as soon as possible. It is usually not a problem for any particular immunization to be administered up to a few months after the recommended age.

Take the opportunity during well-child checkups to learn everything you can about helping your child stay well. Your doctor has the experience of caring for many children and will have suggestions for keeping children healthy. She may not volunteer information on her own, because she may be focusing on other aspects of your child's care. Be assertive. Ask questions. If the doctor does not answer your questions in a way that you understand, ask her to restate the information in

another way. If she gives specific instructions about some aspect of care, write down the instructions and repeat them to the doctor so she can make sure you have the correct information.

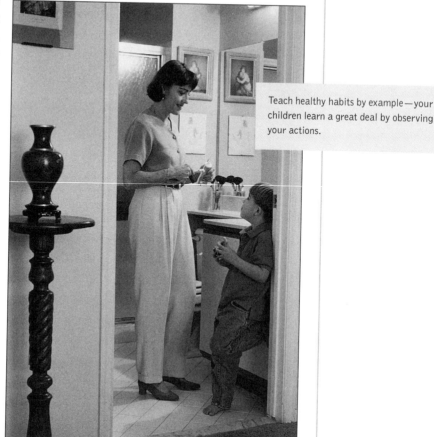

Teach healthy habits by example—your children learn a great deal by observing your actions.

Most doctors embrace their roles as counselors to parents of small children. Unfortunately, though, there are a few who prefer to examine the child and move along to the next patient with a minimum of interaction. If a doctor seems impatient with your questions or makes you feel they are not valid, feel free to express your disappointment either face-to-face or in a letter. If you continue to feel dissatisfied, you should begin the

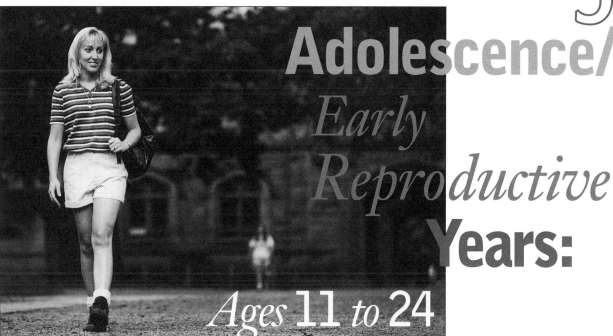

Chapter 5

Adolescence/ *Early Reproductive* Years:

Ages 11 to 24

The early teenage years through young adulthood are filled with change—changes in physical appearance, changes in emotions, changes in the way an adolescent perceives herself and others perceive her. Over these 13 years, a child grows into an adult, reaching and passing a variety of milestones along the way. On this journey, she becomes increasingly responsible for her own health and well-being. Key decisions about lifestyle, such as exercise habits, food choices, and the use or avoidance of alcohol and drugs, help determine whether her life will be characterized by wellness or illness. Periodic physical examinations and counseling from health professionals help the growing, and changing, young woman make appropriate choices.

One of the major changes during this period is the onset of puberty and the surge of hormones it triggers. These are the early reproductive years, the time when young women discover their sexuality and acquire the physical ability to bear children. In addition to possible unwanted pregnancies, choices in sexual behavior may be associated with health risks. Screening for sexually transmitted disease becomes a routine part of a young woman's examination. Counseling educates young women about precautions to take to protect themselves against both disease and unwanted pregnancy. Counseling is especially needed in the early teenage years, when young women may be unaware of sexual health risks.

While parents may still attend doctor's visits with their preteen child, after age 18, most young adults go to the doctor on their own. Therefore, it is important that young women learn how to communicate with physicians and other health professionals about their health concerns.

Regular care with the same doctor since childhood may help the young woman communicate more easily and also helps the doctor more easily recognize

preview

▶ **The Periodic Health Examination**

   Screening

   Counseling

   Immunizations

▶ **What You Can Do**

changes in the patient that may be health-related. Regular checkups also allow the young patient to learn important strategies and gain valuable advice from her doctor about how to keep healthy by:

- Eating nutritiously and avoiding empty calories.
- Engaging in regular physical activity.
- Understanding the physical dangers of substance abuse, including strategies to see how peer pressure may change a person's judgment.
- Learning about sexually transmitted diseases, including precautions to take when becoming sexually active.
- Taking safety precautions to prevent injuries at home and away from home.
- Completing the remaining series of childhood immunizations.

Young women can begin to make their own wise decisions if equipped with the right information. Periodic health examinations and counseling can help them avoid health risk behaviors, and choosing smart health habits will encourage wellness now and in the future. If you are the mother of a daughter, until she is comfortable taking responsibility for her own wellness it is your job to learn all you can and encourage her to learn as well. If you are over the age of 18, you are ready to learn for yourself how to help yourself keep well throughout your life.

This chapter describes what is included in periodic health examinations for females aged 11 to 24 and outlines important concerns during this time. The routine and preventive care described here is designed for young women who are not ill. If a health problem is detected, further care or perhaps referral to another physician may be required.

The **Periodic Health Examination**

During childhood, well-baby and well-child visits to the doctor are considered routine. As children mature into teenagers, both they and their parents may question the need for doctor visits unless they are sick. However, routine well checkups are just as important for adolescents and young adults as they are for infants and toddlers, and perhaps more so. Not only do checkups provide the opportunity for doctors to detect a disease or problem early, they create a time and a place to educate young adult patients about health habits that can become positive lifelong behaviors. The checkups also help adolescents and young adults build a relationship with their physician so that asking difficult questions or discussing sensitive health issues during future visits is not so awkward or intimidating.

Because teenagers may feel uncomfortable going to a doctor whose waiting room is filled with toddlers and young children, now is the time parents usually consider switching from a pediatrician to a primary care physician or family physician. (Some pediatricians accommodate teenagers with special office hours.) This change, along with the parent waiting in the reception area during the checkup, will give the young adult an important and necessary sense of independence and responsibility for her own health care.

While there is no prescribed time period for routine well checkups, most physicians agree that such checkups are most effective when done annually. This spacing allows the doctor to keep up with the many physical changes underway during adolescence. It also allows the doctor to build on discussions of pertinent health issues or update information from the previous visits.

The areas of care that make up a well checkup for adolescents and young adults are shown in the box on this page. They include a physical examination and tests, to screen for illness, health advice and counseling, and immunizations (shots given to prevent infections and disease).

Screening

As with young children, screening detects health risks in adolescents and young adults who have no signs of illness. It is a routine part of any physical examination.

Periodic Health Examination

The following services are performed at each periodic health examination unless a specific age is mentioned.

Screening. The doctor uses these measurements and tests to look for signs of health risks:

- Height and weight
- Blood pressure
- Pap test
- Chlamydia screen
- Rubella serology or vaccination
- Assessment for tobacco use
- Assessment for alcohol or drug use

Counseling. Depending on the patient's age and lifestyle, the doctor will review information relating to potential health risks:

- Fitting in
- Injury prevention
- Substance abuse
- Sexual behavior
- Diet and exercise
- Dental health

Immunizations. The immunizations listed here are recommended for adolescents and young adults:

- Tetanus–diphtheria (Td) booster (11 to 16 years)
- Hepatitis B (11 to 16 years)
- Measles–mumps–rubella (MMR) (11 to 12 years)
- Rubella (12 years plus)
- Varicella (11 to 12 years)

Height and Weight. Measuring height and weight shows an adolescent's growth and development into young adulthood. Adolescents gain about 40 percent of their adult weight and grow about 25 percent of their height during the teenage years. A lack of growth, too little or too much weight gain, or an excess of body fat can be an indication of a disease, or can be a health risk in and of itself.

Weight, in particular, is an important factor in assessing physical health. The U.S. National Health and Nutrition Examination Survey estimates that one-fifth of adolescents between ages 12 and 19 are overweight. These teens are at greater risk for serious diseases, including adult-onset diabetes, hypertension, coronary heart disease, high blood pressure, some forms of cancer, stroke, and high cholesterol, as well as physical problems, such as irregular menstruation, respiratory problems, and flat feet.

While weight gain may be a natural part of puberty (when fat cells in girls tend to develop rapidly), it also may be a result of a poor diet, genetics, or lifestyle choices (such as lack of exercise). In some cases, diet and exercise can help combat obesity (being more than 20 percent overweight). Obesity cannot always be managed, but the earlier in life it is addressed, the greater the likelihood that an obese child will learn the healthy eating habits and food attitudes that may prevent her from growing into an obese adult.

Eating healthy meals and snacks not only helps you maintain an ideal weight but also protects you against certain diseases.

Blood Pressure. Blood pressure is routinely taken during physical examinations to screen for hypertension, or high blood pressure, a leading risk factor for coronary heart disease. Many women with high blood pressure have no symptoms, and screening is the only way it can be diagnosed.

Typically, a doctor or nurse uses a blood pressure cuff to measure a patient's blood pressure. It is important to confirm a high blood pressure reading with additional readings on separate days since transient elevations in blood pressure do not require treatment.

Since hypertension is not common in younger women, an indication that blood pressure is high needs to be followed up with a full examination to determine the cause. Causes might include thyroid disorders, repeated urinary tract infections, kidney disease, use of certain illegal drugs or prescription medications, or pregnancy.

Pap Test. The Papanicolaou Test, or Pap test, screens for cervical cancer. Approximately 16,000 new cases of cervical cancer are diagnosed each year, and about 4,800 women die annually from the disease. All sexually active women with a cervix are at risk for cervical cancer.

The Pap test, also called the Pap smear, can sometimes also detect endometrial, vaginal, and other cancers. It is typically done along with the pelvic examination during a gynecologic visit. Sometimes the results from Pap smears are not clear cut or are difficult to interpret, so a subsequent test is usually ordered. In addition to the Pap smear, other tests for sexually transmitted diseases are sometimes done as part of the pelvic examination. If normal results are received, pelvic examinations are repeated every one to three years. If tests yield abnormal results, pelvic examinations should be performed more frequently.

The First Pelvic Examination

It is recommended that teenage women have their first pelvic examination by age 18, or when they become sexually active, whichever comes first. Although they will most likely be nervous about the procedure, it is not painful. Some teenagers find it uncomfortable, but the discomfort lasts for only a short time.

The examination is done on a medical examination table that has two metal stirrups attached at the end. Prior to the examination, the medical staff asks the patient to undress and put on a dressing robe. For the examination, the young woman lies on her back on the table, with her knees up and apart, and her feet in the stirrups.

The doctor sits on a stool near the patient's feet and illuminates her pelvic area with a bright light. With gloved hands, the doctor inserts a plastic or metal instrument, called a speculum, into the patient's vagina. The speculum is then opened slightly, like a beak. The doctor can now view the inside of the vagina and the cervix, which is the opening to the uterus.

The doctor then uses a spatula, endocervical brush, and/or a cotton swab to swab the cervix and collect a sample of endocervical cells. She also may collect cervical samples, to test for other sexually transmitted diseases, or a vaginal fluid sample, to check for bacteria. These smears and cultures are then sent to the laboratory.

After she removes the speculum, the doctor places one or two gloved fingers into the vagina and her other hand on the abdomen to check the ovaries and uterus for normal shape and size. Finally, the doctor inserts a finger into the rectum to feel the back of the uterus.

Test results are usually received within a few days. The doctor's office notifies the patient of the results; however many women prefer to check with the office as well.

Chlamydia Screen. Chlamydia is the most common bacterial sexually transmitted disease in the United States. Women under age 25 account for the majority of cases of chlamydia, with infection highest from age 15 to 19. It is not uncommon for women to have no symptoms of the disease initially and therefore remain untreated—a dangerous prospect.

Chlamydia causes inflammation of the cervix. If left unchecked, it can infect the uterus and fallopian tubes, a condition called pelvic inflammatory disease (PID). PID often results in swelling and obstruction of the fallopian tubes. The fallopian tubes are very fragile, and once they become infected, the woman may have a high fever and experience extreme pain. She may develop an abscess in her pelvis that requires hospitalization for antibiotic therapy, surgery, or occasionally hysterectomy. Chlamydia is a leading cause of infertility.

Informed Decisions About Medical Tests

When checking a patient's health status, a physician sometimes orders laboratory tests. Before subjecting yourself, or your children, to invasive procedures, it is wise to ask what information the tests will provide, if there is any other way to get the information, and how having that information will affect treatment planning.

By law, health care professionals must provide you with an explanation of the risks and benefits of any test and you must sign a consent form. Patients also have a right to a full explanation of test results. Following are questions you can ask your health professional:

- What is the test designed to show?
- How accurate is it?
- Will the result be definitive?
- What are the possible side effects of the test, and how long will they last?
- What, if any, are the risks of taking the test?
- What are the risks of not taking or delaying the test?
- What is necessary to prepare for the test?
- How much will it cost?

Peer Pressure

Peer pressure, which reaches its greatest intensity during the adolescent and teenage years, can influence teenagers to choose risky behaviors. Many teenagers have heard, "C'mon, have a beer (or a joint). Everyone's doing it." It can be extremely difficult to say no, even when they know they should. If you are a teenager, arm yourself with these strategies to combat negative peer pressure:

- Candidly discuss the negative effects of alcohol and drugs with peers.
- Formulate responses that send a strong "no" message. Role play different situations alone or with friends so that you can practice your responses.
- Use every opportunity to build your self-esteem through community service, good grades, and seeking the approval of people you admire.
- Find a positive peer group, such as one associated with a church, synagogue, or volunteer organization.
- Make friends who also promise to stay alcohol- and drug-free.

Risk factors for chlamydia include having multiple sex partners or new sex partners. Having unprotected intercourse with an infected man is the primary cause of chlamydia. Prevention of sexually transmitted diseases is discussed at length in Chapter 22.

A culture test is the most accurate way to diagnose chlamydia, but it is expensive and requires time for results to be processed. Nonculture tests are available that can detect chlamydia in urethral or cervical specimens. If chlamydia is detected early, antibiotic therapy can be given to eliminate the infection before the fallopian tubes are damaged.

Rubella Vaccination. Although rubella is a mild illness, if a woman gets rubella early in her pregnancy it can cause serious complications, like miscarriage, still birth, and birth defects. The infant may have developmental and growth delays, hearing loss, and heart defects. Due to vaccination efforts, outbreaks of rubella have declined dramatically, but they still occur—often among young adults aged 15 to 29.

Children should have received rubella vaccines early in life. (See Chapter 4 for details.) Unfortunately, the protective antibodies produced by the rubella vaccine may fade over time. Young adults should be screened to determine whether they are susceptible to rubella, or they should just be vaccinated again. This is especially important for young women who are at risk for pregnancy or are planning to become a pregnant.

Drinking, Smoking, Drugs, and Sexual Behavior. In addition to screening for potential disease, doctors also screen for risky behaviors. Adolescence is a typical time for young women to try new things that were previously forbidden them because they were "not old enough." Teenagers often engage in these "adult" behaviors to feel more grown up or to impress their peers.

Doctors ask about alcohol, tobacco, and drug use at each annual examination. They should also ask about sexual behavior and provide information about contraceptive techniques and prevention of sexually transmitted diseases.

Toxicologic tests can provide objective evidence of drug use by measuring concentrations of drugs in blood or urine. Whether these tests are able to detect the drugs depends on the frequency of drug use and the timing of the last use. Marijuana can be detected in urine up to 14 days after use. Cocaine, opiates, amphetamines, and barbiturates are present for a shorter time. The drug tests do not distinguish between abusers and occasional users; they simply report the presence of drugs in the body fluid. False positives may result from other medications being taken and from some substances occurring naturally in foods.

Counseling

Educating young adults is the best way to help them make good health decisions and avoid risky behavior. That is why counseling is such an important part of regular physical examinations. The key is to establish good communication, where there is a give-and-take from both sides. Lectures, where the doctor talks and the patient listens, are less effective.

Fitting In. There is a strong desire among adolescents to be just like everyone else. Adolescents are in the process of building their self-image and their self-esteem. Not only do they emulate their peers, they look to them for approval. They want to fit in. This may continue into young adulthood, and in certain situations into adult life as well.

Counseling can help reassure teenagers that they are making good choices. An adolescent who has adequate self-esteem is better able to resist peer pressure when peer behavior is in conflict with her own definition of appropriate activity. Parents and physicians who listen to the concerns and needs of these young women show them that they have value, further enhancing their self-esteem and good judgment.

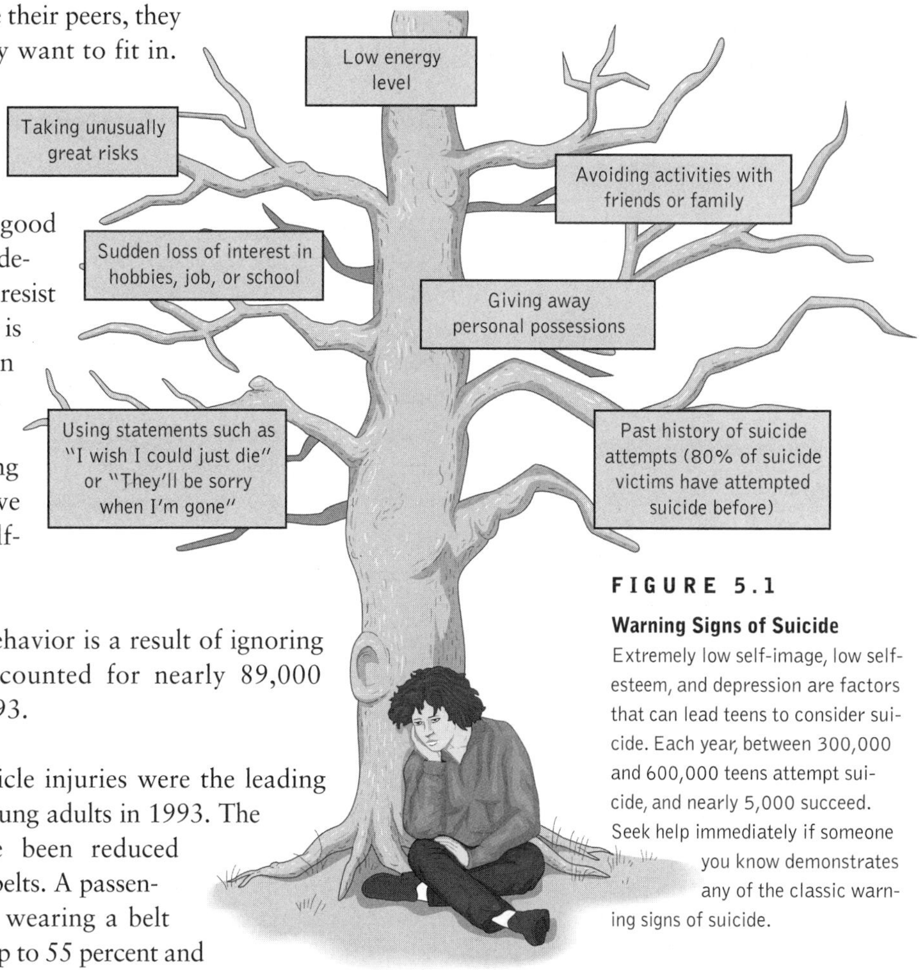

Injury Prevention. Some risky behavior is a result of ignoring safety precautions. Injuries accounted for nearly 89,000 deaths in the United States in 1993.

Lap-Shoulder Belts. Motor vehicle injuries were the leading cause of death in children and young adults in 1993. The number of deaths could have been reduced through the proper use of safety belts. A passenger sitting in the front seat and wearing a belt reduces her chances of injury by up to 55 percent and her chance of death by 40 to 50 percent. Crash victims wearing seat belts at the time of the crash have been shown to have less severe injuries, are less likely to require admission to the hospital, and have lower hospital charges.

Air Bags. While automobile air bags can save lives, they can severely injure or, sometimes kill, passengers. Even though air bags are likely to do more good than harm, take these precautions to lessen the chances of injury or death:

- Move the passenger seat as far back from the dashboard as possible.
- If you are driving, stay as far back from the steering wheel as possible, at least 12 inches.
- If you are under 5 feet 2 inches tall, choose a seat without an air bag. Air bags may hit a short person in the head with enough force to break the neck or fracture the skull.
- Wear your lap-shoulder belt. This will keep you back when an air bag deploys.

Bicycles and Motorcycles. In many states, the law mandates the use of safety helmets when motorcycling or bicycling. Wearing helmets can reduce risk of injury and death. For motorcyclists who wear safety helmets, head injury rates alone are reduced by 40 to 75 percent.

FIGURE 5.1

Warning Signs of Suicide

Extremely low self-image, low self-esteem, and depression are factors that can lead teens to consider suicide. Each year, between 300,000 and 600,000 teens attempt suicide, and nearly 5,000 succeed. Seek help immediately if someone you know demonstrates any of the classic warning signs of suicide.

Labels in figure:
- Low energy level
- Taking unusually great risks
- Avoiding activities with friends or family
- Sudden loss of interest in hobbies, job, or school
- Giving away personal possessions
- Using statements such as "I wish I could just die" or "They'll be sorry when I'm gone"
- Past history of suicide attempts (80% of suicide victims have attempted suicide before)

Underage Drinking

The minimum drinking age in the United States is 21; even so, many U.S. teenagers drink—illegally. Teenagers most at risk include those whose friends already drink, those who are anxious or depressed, and those who do not have strong relationships with their families.

It is never too early or too late to talk to your teen about alcohol use. Here are some tips to prevent and/or curtail underage drinking:

- **Be a good role model. If you drink, chances are your children will want to experiment with it.**
- **Be factual about the effects of alcohol on the body, especially the growing teenage body.**
- **Clearly state your position and rules regarding drinking.**
- **Do not lecture your teenager. Instead respond to her questions about drinking.**
- **Get to know your teen's friends. You will have a better idea about your teen and her lifestyle.**
- **Seek professional help if you suspect your teenager has a drinking problem.**

While motorcycling appears more dangerous than bicycling, bicycling injuries accounted for 550,000 emergency room visits and 1,000 deaths annually before the use of helmets became widespread in the late 1980s. Up to 85 percent of hospitalizations and deaths were a result of head trauma.

Wearing a helmet helps prevent head trauma. Studies suggest that bicycle helmets reduce the risk of head injury by at least 40 percent. In addition, bicyclists can take other safety precautions, such as taking a bicycle training course, avoiding heavy motor vehicle traffic, and staying in a designated bicycle lane, where available.

Smoke Detectors. Fire is a major cause of home injuries. Most injuries and 75 to 90 percent of deaths from fires occur in homes and apartments, rather than in office or commercial buildings.

Installation of smoke detectors is an effective defense against being injured in, or dying from, a fire. Death in a residential fire is two to three times more likely in homes without smoke detectors.

While smoke detectors are effective when they are working properly, smoke detectors fail to operate if they are improperly installed, inadequately tested, or if their source of power (such as batteries) is diminished. That is why it is important to check detectors periodically, and never "borrow" batteries to temporarily operate other pieces of equipment.

Gun Safety. It is not unusual for Americans to keep firearms at home for protection, and the number of homes that contain firearms grows each year. Unfortunately, these firearms are responsible for 12,000 to 13,000 nonfatal injuries per year. In 1993, firearm injuries resulted in 1,740 unintentional deaths. For each case in which a firearm is used successfully for self-protection, there are up to six cases of unintentional death and ten cases of unintentional injury.

According to the U.S. General Accounting Office, nearly one-third of unintentional firearm deaths could be prevented by the use of childproof trigger locks and loading indicators. While it is strongly recommended that firearms not be stored in the home, if a person chooses to have firearms in the home, she should store them unloaded and in a locked compartment.

Substance Abuse. Alcohol, drugs, and tobacco are powerful draws to the teenager and young adult. They seem an easy way to become an instant adult or to gain peer acceptance. Teenagers generally do not think about the health risks they are taking and the future effect drug use may have on their bodies.

Drinking. Though it is illegal to serve alcohol to minors (those under age 21), about half of junior and senior high school students drink—some on a more regular basis than others. Yet adolescents and young adults do not always have a clear understanding of the risks they are taking.

Medical problems caused by alcohol include a variety of serious, and sometimes life-threatening, diseases. Examples include hepatitis (inflammation of the liver), cirrhosis (loss of functional liver cells), pancreatitis (inflammation of the pancreas), neuropathy (a disease of the nervous system), dementia (deterioration of intellectual facilities, such as memory), and heart problems. Intoxication also may lead to unsafe sexual behavior, which puts drinkers at risk for sexually transmitted disease. In addition, pregnant women who drink alcohol put their newborns at risk for birth defects.

Drinking can be extremely dangerous combined with driving a motor vehicle or boat. Drinking and swimming is also a potentially lethal combination.

While use of alcohol by adolescents and young adults has declined over the past decade, it still remains a serious concern. Driving under the influence is more than twice as common with adolescents than with adults. Binge drinking—drinking a lot at one sitting—is especially common among college students.

Recognizing substance abuse is half the problem. Changes in behavior may offer clues that a teenager is indulging in such risky behavior. Warning signs may include new friends, staying out after school, or paying less attention to school work. When a substance abuse problem is recognized or suspected, a variety of strategies can be used, including professional treatment, counseling, and support groups.

Drug Abuse. Abuse of both legal and illegal drugs remains a very serious problem in the United States. An estimated 5.5 million Americans abuse or are dependent upon drugs—and drug use appears to be increasing among teenagers and young adults.

Teenagers typically choose from the following illegal drugs: marijuana, cocaine, heroin, phencyclidine, methaqualone, and hallucinogens. Taking prescription drugs when they are unnecessary is also con-

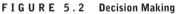

wellness
warning

Alcohol use has been linked to date rape and other sexual assaults. Because alcohol produces mood altering effects, it can reduce inhibitions and increase aggression for both men and women. Alcohol also can make women more vulnerable to assault because it interferes with their judgment about safe environments and decreases their ability to defend themselves if attacked.

FIGURE 5.2   Decision Making
This six-step process demonstrates how to make careful, informed decisions about issues concerning health. Try it the next time a decision has to be made.

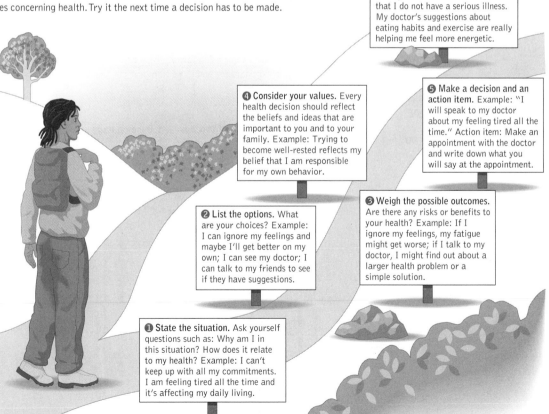

❻ **Evaluate the decision.** How did the decision affect your health? Is your choice working for you or should you make a different choice? Example: I was relieved to learn that I do not have a serious illness. My doctor's suggestions about eating habits and exercise are really helping me feel more energetic.

❹ **Consider your values.** Every health decision should reflect the beliefs and ideas that are important to you and to your family. Example: Trying to become well-rested reflects my belief that I am responsible for my own behavior.

❺ **Make a decision and an action item.** Example: "I will speak to my doctor about my feeling tired all the time." Action item: Make an appointment with the doctor and write down what you will say at the appointment.

❷ **List the options.** What are your choices? Example: I can ignore my feelings and maybe I'll get better on my own; I can see my doctor; I can talk to my friends to see if they have suggestions.

❸ **Weigh the possible outcomes.** Are there any risks or benefits to your health? Example: If I ignore my feelings, my fatigue might get worse; if I talk to my doctor, I might find out about a larger health problem or a simple solution.

❶ **State the situation.** Ask yourself questions such as: Why am I in this situation? How does it relate to my health? Example: I can't keep up with all my commitments. I am feeling tired all the time and it's affecting my daily living.

sidered drug abuse. These drugs include amphetamines, benzodiazepines, barbiturates, and anabolic steroids. In addition, many inhalants, such as amyl and butyl nitrite, gasoline, nitrous oxide, glue, and other solvents, are abused.

While heavy drug users suffer the most medical problems, even occasional drug users can put their futures at risk. Some drugs, like crack cocaine, can cause a heart attack or seizure if smoked even once. Intravenous drug users face the risk of injecting body fluids contaminated with HIV or hepatitis into their bloodstream.

The social consequences of drug abuse are equally devastating. With adolescents, drug use often causes decreased motivation and interferes with school performance. It decreases the likelihood of attending college, increases the likelihood of contracting a sexually transmitted disease, increases the risk of accidental injury, and alienates teens from nonusing peer groups. Young drug users are also more likely to engage in criminal activity related to drug distribution or sale.

Smoking. Smoking accounts for one out of every five deaths in the United States. It is the most preventable cause of premature death. Although smoking has declined in the past three decades, 25 percent of Americans continue to smoke and put themselves at risk for smoking-related diseases and disorders. The majority of smokers started using tobacco as adolescents and young adults. In fact, teenage smokers are so likely to continue smoking that tobacco companies often specifically direct advertising campaigns toward this group.

Tobacco use has been associated with a variety of serious heart- and lung-related diseases. Adolescents who smoke experience increased, and more severe, respiratory symptoms and illnesses, as well as decreased physical fitness.

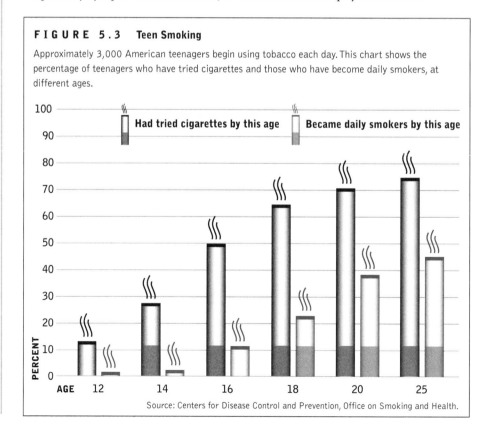

FIGURE 5.3   Teen Smoking

Approximately 3,000 American teenagers begin using tobacco each day. This chart shows the percentage of teenagers who have tried cigarettes and those who have become daily smokers, at different ages.

Had tried cigarettes by this age   Became daily smokers by this age

Source: Centers for Disease Control and Prevention, Office on Smoking and Health.

Longer term effects of smoking include cancer, and not only lung cancer. Smoking has been associated with cancers of the anatomy related to breathing—the trachea, bronchus, larynx, pharynx, oral cavity, and esophagus. In addition, smoking also can cause pancreatic, kidney, bladder, and cervical cancer.

The nicotine found in cigarettes is an extremely addictive drug and difficult to give up. Regular checkups offer the physician a chance to counsel adolescents about the hazards of smoking. Prescribing nicotine products, such as nicotine gum, may help.

Stopping adolescents from smoking before they try their first cigarette is the best route, but may not be realistic. Studies show that approximately 25 percent of 12 to 13 year olds have experimented with cigarettes and 4 percent are regular smokers. Teaching younger children the skills to resist social pressure to try tobacco may be the best alternative.

Risky Sexual Behavior. A young woman's sexual interest begins during her adolescent years. This is the time she first notices the opposite sex (and sometimes the same sex) in a sexual context. It is also the time she begins to experiment, often secretly, with sexual relations. Experimenting with sex can put a young women at risk, not only for pregnancy but for sexually transmitted disease.

Unintended Pregnancy. About 50 percent of young women and 60 percent of young men are sexually active between the ages of 15 and 19—and only one-third of them regularly use birth control. Since most young women have been sexually active for about a year before consulting a doctor about contraception, this is a group that is at high risk for unintended pregnancy.

Because teenagers should not be weighted down with the responsibilities of parenthood, education about contraception—from health care professionals and parents—is important. The education effort should focus on how to practice safer sex. Many parents encourage abstinence, and most schools propose abstinence as the best way to avoid pregnancy and STDs. However, ignoring the possibility that your teen is sexually active places you and your teen at greater risk of having to cope with an unintended pregnancy or disease.

There are many contraceptive options for the sexually active teenager. (See Chapter 17 for a detailed discussion of birth control options.) Teenagers are likely to need guidance in the selection of the right method for them but often do not want to discuss sexual issues with parents for fear of being mistrusted or punished.

Teens and young women may wish to consider the following questions when thinking about birth control options:

- Will I remember to take a pill every day?
- Will I make sure that a condom is used every time?
- Do I feel comfortable inserting a diaphragm?
- Do I prefer a method that I do not have to think about, such as an injection or implant?

Sexually Transmitted Disease. While birth control methods are effective at preventing pregnancy (if used properly), only latex condoms protect against sexually transmitted disease (STD). STDs are infections transmitted through sexual

wellness
warning

Oil-based lubricants can destroy a condom's protective properties. Keep your barrier intact. For lubrication, use water-based gels, foams, and creams instead of oil-based varieties, like baby oil, suntan oil, or Vaseline.

Teen Mothers

The teenage years are challenging enough without having to deal with parenthood. Yet each year nearly a million U.S. teenage girls—or one out of ten young women aged 15 to 19—get pregnant.

In most cases, teenagers do not intend to get pregnant; but, after learning of the pregnancy, about half of them will decide to give birth. In fact, one out of every eight babies born in the United States today has a teenage mother.

Teenage motherhood is not a new phenomenon. However, in the past adoption was much more common, and teens rarely kept their babies unless they were already married. Today, nearly 95 percent of the teenagers who give birth decide to raise the children themselves. These teens are generally single with no real income.

The consequences of teenage motherhood can be devastating. Teen mothers often give up dreams for a career, a happy marriage, or college. Less than one-third of teenage mothers are able to finish high school. Unfortunately, because teenage mothers rarely finish their education, they will earn only about half of the income their peers will earn.

Not only are teenage mothers at a financial and social disadvantage, their babies also may suffer. If a young woman denies she is pregnant, she may not get good prenatal care until late in the pregnancy, placing herself and the infant at risk. Babies born to teenage mothers are more likely to be impoverished, underweight, and chronically ill than children born to women over age 20.

While teenage mothers and their children may feel the negative impact of an unintended pregnancy, so do taxpayers. Tax dollars are used to support the extra services needed by these teens and their children.

There are no upsides in teen pregnancy. However, there are ways to help. Educate preteens and teenagers about how to prevent pregnancy. Help them find appropriate contraception options. Make sure they are comfortable coming to you with their questions. It is never to early to start the dialogue.

For additional information on how to curtail the problem of teen pregnancy, contact the Campaign to Prevent Teen Pregnancies, 2100 M Street NW, Washington, DC 20037.

Source: "The Consequences of Teens and Their Babies." Chicago Tribune, April 30, 1997.

intercourse. One of the most frightening STDs is HIV, the virus that causes AIDS. Other STDs include gonorrhea, syphilis, herpes, and chlamydia. Symptoms of these diseases range from mild irritation to severe pain. Some of these infections can progress to serious illness requiring hospitalization and can even cause life-threatening complications.

Each year in the United States, there are an estimated 12 million new sexually transmitted infections. Adolescents and young adult women are at particular risk for STD. Men and women under age 25 account for two-thirds of all cases of chlamydia and gonorrhea in the United States.

Behavior is the strongest determinant of whether a young woman is at risk for an STD. Having unprotected intercourse or multiple sexual partners puts one at risk. STDs also can be transmitted via intravenous drug use, so taking intravenous drugs or having sexual relations with an intravenous drug user are also risks for STDs.

The most effective way, of course, to protect against STDs is to abstain from sexual relations. But if a young woman has decided to have sexual relations, it is beneficial to maintain a monogamous sexual relationship with a partner who is monogamous with her. Even in a monogamous relationship, however, regular and correct use of latex condoms helps protect against infections that the partner may have acquired by previous sexual contact. It is important to choose latex condoms rather than natural skin varieties. Natural skin condoms do not have the same protective effects and allow transmission of some STD infections, including HIV.

Diet. There is no question that eating a well-balanced diet helps reduce the risk of disease. Poor diet has been linked to major diseases, such as coronary heart disease, some types of cancer, stroke, hypertension, and non–insulin-dependent diabetes mellitus. It is also an issue in other conditions, such as osteoporosis, iron-deficiency anemia, and dental health. (See Chapter 8 for more detailed information on eating for wellness.)

Unfortunately, most adolescents and young adult women do not eat a well-balanced, nutritious diet. This may be due to the temptations of fast foods, poor eating habits formed in childhood, and the prevalence of high-fat prepared foods. It may also be due to the self-imposed restraints of young women who seek extreme leanness for esthetic or athletic reasons.

A teenager not only needs adequate nutrients to maintain her body but also needs the building materials for continued growth. Therefore, an adolescent needs more calories than an adult who is the same height and weight. But even teenagers who are the same age may have different nutritional requirements—because one is experiencing a growth spurt and the other has not yet started puberty. An average young woman in adolescence needs about 2,200 calories daily.

A balanced diet includes carbohydrates (cereals, breads, pastas), protein (meat, fish, eggs), calcium (dairy), fruits and vegetables, some fats, and vitamins and minerals. The proportion of foods from each food group can be altered to accommodate personal tastes and the specific dietary needs at different stages of life.

Fat and Cholesterol. Fats are a problem, not just for adolescents, but for adults as well. Most Americans consume too much fat in their diets, averaging 40 percent or more of their daily caloric input. For a healthy heart, fat calories should amount to less than 30 percent of the total daily calorie count.

Cholesterol is found in many fatty foods derived from animal sources, like red meat, egg yolks, butter, cream, and whole milk. Limiting these foods and substituting foods high in complex carbohydrates helps create a more nutritious diet and healthier lifestyle.

Calcium. Adolescents and young adult women need 1,200 to 1,500 milligrams of calcium per day. Many teens do not meet this standard, and not getting enough calcium puts them at risk for bone density loss later in life.

Encouraging teenagers to add their favorite low-fat dairy products to their diet may help boost their calcium intake. Making these foods a habit can show benefits that last a lifetime.

Eating Disorders. Bombarded by images of ultra-thin models and celebrities, some adolescent girls and young women become obsessed with their weight, equating thinness with happiness and popularity. Most of the time, these are young women whose weight is within normal range, or just slightly above it. Yet some diet incessantly, induce vomiting, and use laxatives until their weight drops to a dangerously low level. Even as their weight drops, their body image stays the same and they continue to see themselves as overweight.

Anorexia nervosa is one type of eating disorder that is increasingly common among young women. Women with anorexia severely restrict their dietary intake to the point of starvation. They often are very secretive about their new eating

wellness **tip**

For women who do not drink or do not like milk, alternative sources of calcium are available. Bulk up on dairy foods other than milk, such as yogurt and low-fat cheeses. Other foods that are high in calcium include calcium-enriched orange juice, broccoli, spinach, sardines, tofu, and salmon. Remember that the benefits of consuming calcium today will last a lifetime.

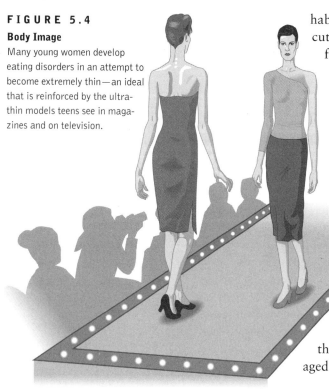

FIGURE 5.4

Body Image

Many young women develop eating disorders in an attempt to become extremely thin—an ideal that is reinforced by the ultra-thin models teens see in magazines and on television.

habits. They may exhibit unusual eating behaviors, such as cutting food in tiny pieces or eating only very low calorie foods. They may decide to call themselves "vegetarian" in order to justify their decreased fat intake (although the true vegetarian diet *is* well-balanced—see Chapter 8). They are obsessed with thinness and/or exercise. They often withdraw from friends and social activities and emphatically deny that there is any problem. They resist any efforts by friends or family to increase their dietary intake or weight.

Bulimia is another common eating disorder. It is characterized by binge eating—eating a lot at one time—followed by induced vomiting, laxative use, or fasting. While the young bulimic's weight remains in the same range over the long term, within days it may rise and fall ten pounds. Symptoms of bulimia include secrecy about eating habits, calluses on the fingers or knuckles that are used to induce vomiting, dehydration, and damaged tooth enamel.

Both anorexia nervosa and bulimia can cause problems with the heart, gastrointestinal system, and endocrine system. They can also delay sexual maturity. It is important to seek professional help to manage eating disorders. These diseases have deep psychological roots that must be addressed, or the problem will never be controlled. Even with professional help, some eating disorder behaviors recur in stressful situations. The most successful treatment plans include psychological counseling and family therapy, nutritional guidance, an appropriate exercise program, and medical checkups.

Exercise. Exercise is an important part of a healthy lifestyle. Regular physical activity and fitness reduce the chances of getting, and dying from, at least six chronic conditions: coronary heart disease, hypertension, obesity, diabetes, osteoporosis, and mental health disorders. Yet 61 percent of women in the United States do not engage in physical activity on a regular basis.

Exercise performed occasionally or seasonally has limited long-term benefits. However, regular physical activity—even moderate activity, such as a walk around the block—can have a tremendous positive effect on health.

For adolescents and young adults, exercise offers additional nonphysical benefits. Engaging in sports teaches teamwork and builds self-esteem. Teenagers also learn how to handle pressure and competition and how to win and lose gracefully.

While vigorous exercise—like running or aerobics—provides more intense cardiovascular benefits, it is often easier to fit moderate exercise into the day. Examples of moderate exercise include any activity that can be easily sustained for 20 minutes. Walking, slow biking, raking leaves, and playing with young children are examples of moderate exercise.

Even in the teenage years, it is important to consult a physician before starting an exercise program. In particular, a doctor will look for any musculoskeletal problems, which may cause injury, and cardiovascular problems, which may limit participation. This complete checkup ensures that the adolescent or young adult is physically fit enough to begin the program.

Dental Health. Many Americans suffer from tooth decay and periodontal disease. This includes cavities, gingivitis (gum inflammation), and periodontis (inflammation of the gum leading to destruction of the bone supporting the teeth). Teenagers and young adults are no exception. In fact, adolescence is the principal time for cavities.

Protect teeth and gums with good daily dental health habits. Brushing with a fluoride toothpaste regularly (three times a day if possible) for a full two minutes at a time will do a great deal toward protecting dental health. Daily flossing in between teeth helps remove bacteria and plaque. Reducing foods with refined sugar and carbohydrates, like cookies, candy, and soda, also protects teeth. A fluoride mouth rinse—if the water supply is not fluoridated—offers increased protection against tooth decay.

Regular visits to a dentist are an important part of maintaining healthy teeth and gums. As with doctor's visits, well checkups to the dentist should be scheduled regularly, usually every six months. At this time, the dentist performs a thorough tooth cleaning, removing plaque and tartar, and fills cavities before they destroy the full tooth. Regular visits also allow the dentist to monitor the health of your teeth and counsel you on steps to take to maintain healthy teeth and gums through the adult years.

Immunizations

While most immunizations are given in the early childhood years, several are administered in early adolescence and the teen years (Table 5.1). Some of these immunizations are a follow-up to earlier injections. Skipping this last set of vaccinations can put your teenager at risk for these diseases. See Chapter 4 for a full explanation of each of these diseases:

- Tetanus–diphtheria (Td) booster (age 11 to 16)
- Hepatitis B (age 11 to 16, if not previously immunized)
- Measles–mumps–rubella (MMR) (age 11 to 12)
- Rubella (age 12 plus)
- Varicella (age 11 to 12)

Consult a health professional for risks and possible side effects that might occur as a result of any vaccination.

Tetanus-Diphtheria (Td) Booster. Because of routine immunization, the incidence of tetanus and diphtheria has dramatically decreased. However, tetanus and diphtheria remain serious infections that can lead to death. The Td booster protects against these diseases.

This is a supplement to the DPT vaccination given in infancy and childhood. The lowercase "d" in the name of the booster signifies a lower dose of the diphtheria

TABLE 5.1

Immunization Schedule

Age	Td	Hep. B	MMR	Rubella	Varicella
11–12		✔	✔		✔
11–16	✔			✔	

vaccine given in childhood. While the DPT also includes a pertussis vaccine, this booster does not.

The Td booster usually is administered between 11 and 12 years of age (although 14 to 16 years is also acceptable). It also may be administered as needed in adulthood, usually about every ten years to maintain its protective effect. If a young adult or adolescent steps on a rusty nail or gets a deep cut, for example, the booster also may be given at that time to prevent tetanus—an often fatal disease where muscles contract and the jaw locks.

Hepatitis B Vaccine. The hepatitis B vaccine protects against severe liver disease. All adolescents not previously immunized against hepatitis B should receive a vaccination. In addition, physicians may recommend booster doses to maintain immunity through adulthood.

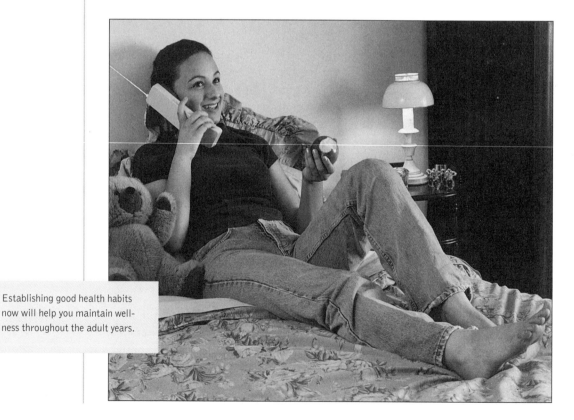

Establishing good health habits now will help you maintain wellness throughout the adult years.

MMR Vaccine. The MMR vaccine protects against three infections: measles, mumps, and rubella. By 11 to 12 years of age, children should have received the second dose of this vaccine.

Rubella Vaccine. Following the MMR immunization, a small percentage of people fail to develop antibodies to protect against rubella. To protect against vaccine failure, many physicians give routine vaccinations through adulthood. A rubella vaccination cannot be given during pregnancy, however, because it may have adverse effects on the fetus. In most cases, a second vaccination is successful, even if the first was not.

Varicella Vaccine. The varicella vaccine protects against the varicella-zoster virus, which causes chickenpox. It is given to children, adolescents, and adults who have not been previously immunized or had the disease. This does not mean they will not contract the disease, but if they do, it will be in a milder form.

It is especially important for young adults to receive this vaccination. In adulthood, the varicella disease is associated with increased risk of serious complications, such as pneumonia and other infections. Adolescents and adults receiving the vaccine receive two doses four to eight weeks apart.

What *You* Can Do

Adolescence and young adulthood is a time of growth and discovery—teenagers should enjoy it. But as they discover who they are and who they want to be, they need to understand why and how many of the decisions they make will affect their future health. They need to establish smart health habits now to maintain wellness in adulthood:

- Schedule regular well checkup doctor and dental visits.
- Get all recommended immunizations. Report any serious side effects.
- Avoid health risk behaviors, such as drinking, smoking, taking drugs, or having unprotected sexual relations.
- Take steps to avoid injury and keep safe.
- Eat a well-balanced diet and avoid becoming overweight. Watch for early signs of eating disorders.
- Look for ways to make moderate exercise a part of daily life.
- Get adequate rest.
- Maintain a balance between school/work and recreation.

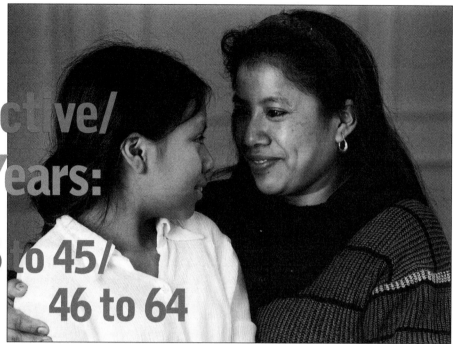

Chapter 6

Later Reproductive/ Mature Years:

Ages 25 to 45/ 46 to 64

If someone gave you the key to perfect health, you would be set to enjoy life to its fullest. Yet the key that opens this door to a lifetime of good health is already in your possession. That key is knowledge. While arming yourself with knowledge cannot promise a lifetime of perfect health, it can dramatically increase the odds of your living an active, satisfying life for a long, long time.

The years between ages 25 and 45, also called the later reproductive years, and between 46 and 64, also called the mature years or leading edge years, are critical ones in terms of planning for wellness. These years will perhaps have the greatest impact on how long, and how well, you live. Health-related decisions you make during the later reproductive years will influence your health literally for the rest of your life. This is the time to build up your body to prepare your muscles and bones for graceful, healthful aging, to take preventive action to avoid chronic disease later in life, and to make taking good care of yourself a high priority among your many responsibilities, such as work and home life. That is why it is especially important to make informed decisions every step of the way.

Just as in early childhood, adolescence, and young adulthood, your body continues to grow and change during this period, although less noticeably so. Ages 25 to 45 are the heart of the reproductive years, and many of you may choose to become pregnant—causing your body to change further to sustain a new life. (See Chapter 18 to find out more about these changes.) Even if you decide not to become pregnant, you may address emotional issues as you plan for family life with or without children. (See Chapter 17 for a detailed discussion of family planning.)

It is especially critical during these years to continue with your regular, periodic well checkups—to ensure health now and in the future. Do not be tempted to skip visits because you feel fine. Regular well checkups allow you to learn important information about staying well and preventing disease and illness. You will gain valuable advice about how to keep healthy by:

- Checking your current health status and screening for any possible complications or areas of concern.
- Discussing limiting use of alcohol, tobacco, and drugs, and receiving counseling on safe sexual practices, all of which may extend your life span.
- Receiving counseling on diet and exercise, including avoiding high-cholesterol, high-fat foods that may present a health risk, and increasing intake of calcium-rich foods or taking calcium supplements to help prevent osteoporosis.
- Encouraging good dental care to enable you to keep your teeth well into your elder years.
- Completing the necessary immunizations to maintain your good health status.
- Receiving reminders on simple lifestyle activities, such as exercising regularly, wearing your seat belt and shoulder harness in the car, and being alerted to new medical conditions.

This chapter describes what you can expect at well examinations during the two life stages, the later reproductive years and the mature years, and outlines important health concerns during this time. The routine and preventive care described here is designed for women who are not ill. If a health problem is detected, further specific care or perhaps referral to a specialist may be required.

The **Periodic** Health Examination

For well examinations, many women use a family practitioner, internist, and/or an obstetrician/gynecologist. The obstetrician/gynecologist can perform a more specialized examination of the female reproductive system, but even a family practitioner or internist is qualified to do basic gynecology, including a Pap smear, though some may prefer to have you see a gynecologist as well. Whatever doctor or doctors you choose, make sure you are comfortable with them and able to ask and have answered any questions without embarrassment.

Periodic health examinations for adult women should be done annually or as recommended. Schedule these well visits, during which full physicals and health assessments are completed, in addition to any sick visits you may have during the year. While you may be tempted to skip an annual checkup—especially if you are feeling well—it is unwise to do so. Maintaining regular contact with your physician will help keep you and her apprised of your usual health condition so even slight changes in your health status can be addressed. It is helpful to schedule your visit in the month of your birthday. That way, you are less likely to forget, and the doctor's office will not be overwhelmed at the start or end of the year.

Screening
Even if you have no signs of illness, you may be at risk for some diseases. Screening can detect potential health risks. As with childhood and adolescent examinations, it is a routine part of any well visit.

Periodic Health Examination

The following services are performed at each periodic health examination unless a specific age is mentioned.

Screening. The doctor uses these measurements and tests to look for signs of health risks:

- Blood pressure
- Height and weight
- Complete lipid profile, including cholesterol, HDL, LDL, and triglycerides (every one to five years, depending on risk)
- Pap test
- Fecal occult blood test (after age 40) and/or sigmoidoscopy (after age 50)
- Clinical breast examination
- Mammogram (ages 40 to 64)
- Assessment for problem drinking, tobacco use, and drug use
- Rubella serology check if vaccination is unknown

Counseling. Depending on your age and lifestyle, the doctor will review information relating to potential health risks:

- Substance abuse (including alcohol, tobacco, and prescription and illicit drugs)
- Diet and exercise
- Injury prevention
- Sexual behavior
- Dental health

Immunizations. The immunizations listed here are recommended for adult women:

- Tetanus–diphtheria (Td) booster (every ten years)
- Rubella (women of childbearing age, if not immune)
- Hepatitis B (by the time they reach adulthood, most people have an immunity to Hepatitis A, so the vaccine for that disease is not usually necessary or recommended for adults)
- Influenza (yearly) if high risk or desired

Blood Pressure. The American Academy of Family Physicians recommends that adults over age 18 be screened for high blood pressure every one to two years. Those at risk—for example, women with a family history of hypertension (high blood pressure) or with hypertension during pregnancy—should be screened more often.

Monitoring blood pressure is important because you probably will not know if you have hypertension; often there are no symptoms. Yet, consistently high blood pressure puts your health at risk, often leading to stroke, heart disease, kidney disease, or, in extreme cases, death. (See Chapter 5 for additional information.)

Moderately high blood pressure can usually be controlled through lifestyle changes, such as optimizing your weight, restricting salt intake, changing your diet, and exercising, and in more serious cases, by using medication. If you are older, and have hypertension and other risk factors which may increase your chances for developing cardiovascular disease (such as smoking, obesity, high cholesterol), your doctor may prescribe medication to lower your blood pressure. To prevent high blood pressure (or treat mild high blood pressure), limit your salt and salty food intake, eat a diet rich in fruits and vegetables and low-fat dairy products, and exercise regularly.

If you do get a reading of high blood pressure during an annual well check-up, ask to have it rechecked on subsequent days. You may not actually have hypertension. Many women suffer from "white coat syndrome," which means they get nervous when they go to the doctor's office—this can increase their blood pressure temporarily. See the Wellness Tip on this page for information about how to get the most accurate blood pressure reading.

Height and Weight. Once you reach the adult years, your height drops one-half inch or more as the effect of gravity compresses the pads between your vertebrae. Height is measured predominantly during this time as a benchmark for weight and osteoporosis. The taller you are, the more you are able to weigh and still remain in a healthy range. Following menopause, if you experience a decrease in height, it may indicate loss of bone mass in the vertebrae as hormone levels drop. Sudden decreases in height, however, signal that the bones are not as healthy as they should be and that osteoporosis screening should be considered.

Weight continues to be an important factor in assessing health. Obesity (meaning a weight that is 20 percent or more above the normal range for your height and body frame) can lead to serious disease and physical problems, particularly when the excess weight is located around the waist. People who are significantly obese—for example, weighing twice as much as they should—are at risk for premature death.

Obesity is a common problem. About one-third, or 58 million Americans, are estimated to be overweight—and this number may be increasing.

Physicians often screen for obesity just by looking at the patient's physical appearance and comparing the patient's weight with the average weight range for her height and body frame. However, more precise tests also are available. For example, doctors can measure skinfold thickness and total body fat.

Detection and intervention can help in many cases. Your physician is likely to recommend diet and exercise as a first-line defense. If that does not work, other interventions, such as counseling or medications to control appetite, may be needed.

Total Blood Cholesterol. Many women already monitor their intake of cholesterol, a fat-related substance found predominantly in foods made from animals or animal products. By monitoring your cholesterol intake, you are decreasing your risk for coronary heart disease.

Cholesterol levels tend to be low in younger women, but increase with age. Therefore, even if you have typically had a low count, it is recommended that you have it monitored periodically as you age. If your family has a history of high cholesterol, or coronary heart disease, it may affect you at a much younger age. The U.S. Preventive Services Task Force recommends routine cholesterol screening for women aged 45 to 65 and for anyone at risk for coronary disease.

wellness **tip**

To get the most accurate blood pressure reading possible, avoid having your blood pressure taken when you are rushed or in pain, or after you have consumed alcohol, tobacco products, or a large meal. When it is time to take your pressure, remain relaxed in a comfortable seated position for several minutes. Do not cross your legs, chew gum, or talk while your blood pressure is being taken. If your pressure still seems abnormal, ask for a retest after relaxing or on a different day.

wellness **tip**

You will need to change your diet at least three days before initiating the fecal occult blood test. Your doctor will give you a list of products to avoid, such as red meat, aspirin, large amounts of vitamin C, and certain fruits and vegetables, which can alter test results. Make sure you follow up with the doctor's office to get your results.

The most common screening test for cholesterol is a blood test, either a finger stick or a blood sample taken from the arm. The test takes just a few minutes in the doctor's office or laboratory, with results often ready the next day. Your test should include not just total cholesterol, but also a breakdown of your lipids, or blood fats, and triglycerides. Ideally you should fast for 12 to 16 hours before the test. If your test results are normal without having fasted, you do not need to repeat the test. If a repeat test is recommended, make sure it is done after fasting for 16 hours.

Your physician's office will help you interpret the test results. Total cholesterol readings above 240 milligrams per deciliter (mg/dL) and LDL above 160 mg/dL are considered high, with readings of 200 to 239 mg/dL and 130 to 160 mg/dL rated as borderline high. If you get a high reading, you may choose to take the test again. Readings can vary due to stress, illness, and even seasonal differences. (See Chapter 20 for further discussion on high cholesterol levels and heart disease.)

Once diagnosed, elevated cholesterol and LDL may be treated with dietary changes, such as avoiding foods high in cholesterol, regular exercise, and/or prescription medication. Reaching and maintaining your optimal weight through diet and exercise also improves your lipid levels.

Pap Test. Women who are either pre- or postmenopausal can be at risk for cervical cancer. As long as you have a cervix, this disease may affect you, though sexual activity increases your risk. The Papanicolaou test, or Pap test, screens for cervical cancer and other related cancers. (See Chapter 5 for a detailed description of Pap testing.)

If cervical cancer is detected and treated early enough, the survival rate is very good—about 90 percent. That is why it is important to be tested as indicated at your well visit. If you have had abnormal Pap smear results in the past, you may need more frequent screening. On the other hand, if you have never had any cervical abnormalities and have had three consecutive yearly Pap smears that are normal, you may need a screening smear less often. But you still need to have the cervix visually inspected annually, or more often if you experience a problem like recurrent vaginal discharge or bleeding after intercourse, between periods, or after menopause.

As part of your Pap test, the physician will do a pelvic examination, examining your internal organs with gloved hands. This examination is conducted to check for uterine or ovarian masses and to see if infection or pain is present.

Screening for Colorectal Cancer. The fecal occult blood test and the sigmoidoscopy are two principle ways of screening for colorectal cancer—the third most common form of cancer in American women. As with many cancers, early detection offers the greatest chance for a cure.

About 55,000 people each year die from colorectal cancer. People at highest risk are those with a close relative with the condition, or with a personal history of colitis, colon polyps, or endometrial, ovarian, or breast cancer.

The fecal occult blood test detects blood in stool samples. This test is a good screening tool because colon cancer is often associated with microscopic bleeding. However, certain foods (those containing substances called peroxidases) and anti-inflammatory medications causing bleeding can produce a positive result that is not caused by cancer.

The fecal occult blood test is a noninvasive procedure that is easy to perform. Stool samples over a time period are smeared onto testing paper that is sent to the laboratory for analysis.

A more invasive test is the sigmoidoscopy, an office procedure where a flexible tube is inserted through the anus, into the colon. The sigmoidoscope allows your doctor to visually inspect the colon for cancerous or precancerous polyps, or growths. While sigmoidoscopes are effective at diagnosing colorectal cancer, they cannot view the entire colon. Therefore, physicians may miss cancerous polyps higher in the colon. These can be checked for by an x-ray test called a barium enema or a full visual examination of the colon, called a colonoscopy.

Mammogram/Clinical Breast Examination. The second most common cancer diagnosed in women is breast cancer. (Lung cancer is the most commonly diagnosed.) There are a number of risk factors, but if you are a female residing in North America or Northern Europe, you are at risk. As your age increases, your risk increases; if you have a family history of breast cancer, you are two to three times more susceptible to the disease. (See Chapter 21 for an in-depth discussion on this topic.)

Breast cancer is treatable and often curable if detected early. That is why screening is so important. In addition to a monthly breast self-examination, it is recommended that you be screened for breast cancer every one to two years with the clinical breast examination and/or the mammogram. If you are over age 50, both procedures are strongly recommended on a yearly basis. Many women in their mid-thirties opt to receive a baseline mammogram for comparison to later mammograms, though its benefit is not clear.

In the clinical breast examination, a physician or medical professional feels the breast tissue and under the arms, checking for lumps—in a similar way to how you should perform a self-examination at home. The difference is that the clinician is specially trained to look for and feel potential growths that may signal cancerous substances. If your doctor finds anything suspicious, she may order a mammogram, regardless of your age or date of last mammogram.

A mammogram is an x-ray of the breast tissue. In order to keep the radiation dose low, your breasts are compressed between glass plates in several different positions to provide different views of the breast. Usually this procedure is performed by a technician in a practice that specializes in breast imaging. The films are read by physicians who specialize in radiology. In some areas, there are highly specialized centers devoted exclusively to breast cancer screening and diagnosis. When your physician refers you to a mammographer, ask whether the center is accredited and whether it uses low-dose equipment. If your doctor does not know, call the facility directly with these questions.

Problem Drinking, Smoking, and Drugs. Drinking, smoking, and drugs are not just problems with adolescents. Many adults engage in these behaviors as well.

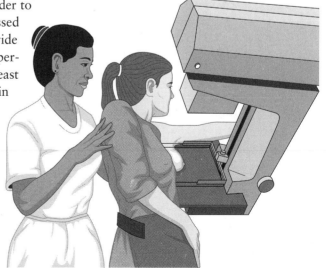

FIGURE 6.1
Mammogram
During a mammogram, the breast is compressed between two glass plates in different positions so x-rays can be taken from several angles.

Just because it is legal for them to drink and smoke does not mean that these are not risky lifestyle habits.

It is difficult, however, to assess these behaviors during a typical physician's visit. Some physicians use screening questionnaires, which are not always effective, or talk at length with their patients, who do not always share the full truth. Real physical changes cannot be detected until your body has been subjected to prolonged, heavy alcohol, tobacco, or drug use.

If you use alcohol, tobacco, or drugs—even socially, not excessively—share that information with your physician. She is under professional oath not to reveal it to anyone without your permission, including your family and employer, and your physician can help determine whether these behaviors are putting your health at risk. Be aware, however, that your medical record may be copied and sent to insurers. However, your records cannot be copied without your express consent.

Rubella. Rubella is not a serious disease but can become so if you contract it when you are pregnant. In that instance, rubella can cause serious complications, like miscarriage, and birth defects, such as hearing loss or heart defects. It is important for every woman of childbearing age to have an immunity against rubella whether she intends to become pregnant or not.(You cannot receive the rubella vaccination while you are pregnant.) Check your immunity status with your physician. If in doubt, ask to be revaccinated with a booster dose.

Counseling

Continuing education about health risks helps you make choices that keep you healthy, now and in the future. That is why counseling is an important part of annual well checkups.

To make sure you are receiving the full benefit of counseling, evaluate the dialogue between you and your doctor. Does your physician spend the time needed to talk things over with you? Do you feel rushed through your examination or does your doctor invite you into her office after the examination for a discussion? Do you feel comfortable asking questions, especially about personal health topics, such as sexual intercourse or an eating disorder? Do you have a give-and-take with your doctor, or does it resemble a lecture with the doctor doing all the talking? Even the most medically-qualified practitioner may not suit your communication style. You will benefit the most by choosing a doctor whose advice you not only trust, but with whom you can easily communicate.

Make sure you provide an opportunity for good dialogue with your physician by scheduling regular well visits, rather than trying to have all your health concerns dealt with at a visit for an acute illness. If you have a number of concerns, schedule one well visit to discuss some of them and have a follow-up visit for the others. That way, both you and your physician can give your concerns the attention they deserve.

Substance Use/Abuse. Many women regularly, and legally, smoke tobacco products, consume alcohol, or take prescription medications. Most women, however, do not realize how easy it is to unconsciously turn occasional use into substance abuse, or risky behavior.

Could You Be Addicted?

If you are like many adults, you have indulged in or at least tried alcohol, tobacco, and/or drugs at some time in your life. But at what invisible point does occasional use turn into dependency and addiction?

More often than not, addiction happens gradually, and you—and your family members—might not even notice. At first, you have a glass of wine or a beer in a social situation, for example. It makes you feel good and helps you relax and make conversation easily, so you try it again at the next social situation. For many people, this is their limit. They have an occasional drink and do not feel the need to drink excessively.

However, sometimes the pleasure or relaxation someone experiences while drinking causes her to indulge more regularly. She may drink after work each day, as well as at social gatherings. Still at this point, she is not addicted. Many people indulge for years at this level, without having a problem controlling their consumption.

The first danger sign is when that woman relies on a drink for emotional support. For example, she had a tough day; she needs a drink. Or her spouse yells at her; she needs a drink. If she is unhappy with the world, she turns to alcohol (or tobacco or drugs) for relief.

At this point, her body begins to change to accommodate the increased intake of the substance. Her body learns to tolerate it. Whereas before, one or two drinks could make her feel better, now it takes three or four.

Further, if she stops her regular drinking habit, she begins to feel sick. This is the point when she has become physically dependent on the alcohol, tobacco, or drug. She continues to drink because she enjoys the sensations it produces, and she wants to avoid the real physical pain or discomfort that would come from stopping or quitting.

The next step is addiction, where the woman's entire life revolves around the drinking, the smoking, or the drug use. Her focus is to obtain it, take it, and get more. All other responsibilities and interests—family, friends, work, even nourishment—fall by the wayside. Unfortunately, some people cannot stop this cycle, which in extreme cases can lead to death.

If you or someone you know is at risk for becoming addicted to alcohol, tobacco, or drugs, take the following precautions:

- **Monitor your consumption.** Keep a log for a month of how often and on what occasions you indulge, how you feel before, during, and after using, and what triggers your use.
- **Try to abstain.** For the next few times, choose to do something else instead of indulging. Remove yourself from the scene. Write down whether you were successful.
- **Consult your health professional.** Dare to be honest about your situation, and take appropriate steps to prevent it from escalating into dependence or addiction.

Tobacco. About 420,000 Americans die each year from smoking. Many more smokers contract a variety of serious heart and lung-related diseases, including cancer. (Lung cancer is the most common form of cancer in women.) If you smoke, you will undoubtedly be counseled by your physician to stop. If you are pregnant, you will be advised to stop immediately, because of the risk to fetal health.

According to the American Lung Association, about 1.5 million adults in the United States quit smoking each year. Although you may not be able to quit on the first try, you are more likely to quit each time you try. (See Chapter 13 for tips on quitting smoking.)

Alcohol. Because adults can consume alcohol legally, with no one to closely monitor their consumption, they may be more at risk for alcohol abuse. This abuse can lead to serious physical conditions, like hepatitis or cirrhosis, as well as emotional problems, such as depression.

The U.S. Department of Health and Human Services recommends no more than two drinks a day for men and one drink a day for nonpregnant women. Your health risks are probably minimal if you drink socially at this level. However, certain health problems are aggravated by even modest use, so if you are at risk for cancer, or liver or heart disease, you should consider alcohol avoidance.

If you drink alcohol on a semi-regular or regular basis, your physician will review with you the quantity and frequency with which you drink, and counsel you accordingly. If you are pregnant, or taking certain prescription medications, she will counsel you not to drink at all. While the level of alcohol that poses a risk during pregnancy has not yet been determined, most clinicians agree alcohol should be eliminated during pregnancy.

If you have an alcohol problem, your physician will recommend a treatment program. Programs vary in their intensity and duration. Some require you to reside at a program site; others require your presence at program meetings. Most involve counseling and advocate lifestyle changes, such as avoiding instances when it is usual for you to have a drink or substituting behaviors for drinking. Some also involve the use of prescription medication. (See Chapter 13 for a discussion of alcohol abuse and treatment.)

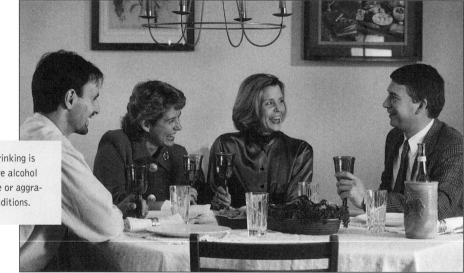

While modest social drinking is generally safe, excessive alcohol consumption can cause or aggravate certain health conditions.

Drugs. About 5 million Americans continue to smoke marijuana once a week or more often, and nearly 1.6 million Americans use intravenous drugs. Illegal drugs include marijuana, cocaine, heroin, phencyclidine, methaqualone, and hallucinogens. In addition, adults who misuse prescription drugs are considered drug abusers. Prescription drugs that are commonly abused include amphetamines, benzodiazepines, barbiturates, and anabolic steroids. Even sniffing glue or paint solvent is considered a drug addiction because it is done to get high.

The "high" of using drugs masks the damage being done to your body. Each time drugs are misused, there is a chance an adverse reaction will occur, such as a brain hemorrhage, heart attack, respiratory problems (if the drug is smoked), or a seizure, to name a few examples. The more often you use drugs, the greater the chance you will experience ill effects, as the drug accumulates in your body.

Drug users place others at risk, as well. If you use illegal drugs, or misuse prescription drugs, you may be tempted to cheat or steal to get money for drugs. If you drive when you use drugs, your reflexes and decision-making skills can become just as hampered as a drunk driver's, and you could cause motor vehicle accidents and injuries. You also may mistreat or neglect family members and friends, as you become obsessed with your drug habit.

Your physician cannot always detect drug abuse in the early stages. Yet this is the ideal time for intervention, as many of the medical problems and adverse effects can be avoided. That is why it is important to be honest with her regarding your drug habits. Remember, she is under professional oath not to share that information with anyone, unless she has your permission to do so. (See Chapter 13 for more information about detecting drug problems and addiction habits early.)

Diet and Exercise. Did you know that an unbalanced or excessive diet is one of the leading causes of illness and death in the United States? Poor diet has been linked to coronary heart disease, cancer, stroke, hypertension, non–insulin-dependent diabetes mellitus, osteoporosis, iron-deficiency anemia, and dental problems, among others. (See Chapter 8 for more detailed discussion of nutrition and wellness.)

It is important to watch your diet throughout your life, as eating habits can have a tremendous impact on how well you feel now and how healthy you will be in the years to come. As you age, you may wish to change your diet to meet certain health requirements. For example, many individuals develop hypertension later in life and may need to limit salt intake, which can raise blood pressure. Other diseases and conditions might require modified intake of water, calories, fat, protein, or calcium, for example. If your doctor does not bring up the subject of your eating habits during your well checkups, ask her if you can talk about any nutritional concerns related to your age group. Feel free to ask questions. Some doctors may not readily bring up the topic of nutritious eating,

wellness **tip**

Constipation is a problem for many women as they become older. If this is a problem for you, consider using diet and exercise, instead of laxatives, to relieve it. Drink plenty of water (six to eight glasses a day), eat a diet rich in fiber, such as fruit and grains, and exercise regularly. You will see a difference shortly. If you continue to have a problem, speak with your physician.

The Benefits of Sports

Joining a sports team, or taking up a sport, is one of the best ways to ensure that exercise becomes a regular part of your lifestyle. Finding a sport that you enjoy could not be easier today. Whether you prefer to exercise alone, or with others, there is a variety of sports activities from which to choose. From basketball to karate to swimming to dance to power walking, there is a sport to fit your lifestyle and fitness level.

Not only are sports fun to do, they provide a wealth of physical and mental health benefits. Here is just a sampling:

Physical Benefits
- Sports help keep you slim and trim, preventing obesity.
- Sports help improve your cardiovascular fitness.
- Sports that incorporate weight-bearing exercises increase your bone mass, reducing the risk of osteoporosis.
- Playing sports reduces stress and tension, which are linked to disease.
- Many women report that exercising decreases their appetite and helps with weight control.

Other Benefits
- Playing sports builds your confidence and self-esteem.
- Sports emphasize teamwork, goal setting, and the pursuit of excellence, skills that apply to other parts of your life.
- Playing sports is a great way to find new friends with a common interest.
- Playing sports and exercising regularly releases the body's endorphins, chemical substances in the body that promote a natural "high."

unless prompted by a patient's questions. Remember, your well checkups are *your* visits; you should feel free to discuss any and all health topics.

Use the well checkup, too, to talk about your exercise habits, or starting an exercise program if you have been inactive. Regular, moderate physical activity reduces the chances of your contracting many serious diseases, such as heart disease, hypertension, diabetes, osteoporosis, and even some mental health disorders, such as depression.

As you age, you may be unable to exercise at the same level and same intensity as when you were younger. That is not a problem. Your practitioner can help you structure an exercise program to maximize your current fitness level and to provide positive health benefits.

Fat and Cholesterol. You are probably quite familiar with the terms fat and cholesterol. In fact, many people look for those words on food labels, even if they do not know exactly what they mean.

Dietary fat is an organic compound found in foods. Cholesterol is not a fat but a substance found in animal products. While both fat and cholesterol are able to be digested by humans, too much of either creates an unhealthy diet. Unfortunately, most Americans consume too much fat, saturated fat, and cholesterol in their diets. Your daily fat intake should be less than 30 percent of all of the calories you consume. Your ideal cholesterol intake varies in terms of your cholesterol blood level, but it too should be kept at a minimum—less than 300 mg a day.

One way to limit fat and cholesterol in your diet is to fill up with complex carbohydrates and dietary fiber instead of fatty foods. Not only does this automatically reduce the fat and cholesterol you consume, it limits the amount of dietary fat absorption and improves your gastrointestinal function as well.

Calcium. Calcium plays an important role in keeping your bones and teeth strong throughout your life. As you age past 30 to 35 years, your bones will become less dense as they lose calcium. This is especially true when you reach menopause. The loss of calcium from bone accompanies the drop in hormone levels at that time. Some bones deteriorate to the point where you might develop osteoporosis, the brittle bone disease that can lead to fractures. Calcium replacement and other therapies to prevent osteoporosis foster bone growth and increase bone density to help reduce the risk of fractures.

How much calcium do you need? The recommended daily dose for women aged 25 to 50 is 1,000 mg of elemental calcium, while for postmenopausal women it is 1,000 to 1,500 mg per day. Pregnant and nursing women are also advised to consume 1,000 to 1,500 mg daily.

Continue taking calcium, especially after menopause. Studies have shown that at least 1,000 mg of calcium each day prevents about one percent of bone loss a year. If you need to take supplements, calcium carbonate, the most common form of calcium, is best taken with food. Calcium citrate and calcium lactate are best taken on an empty stomach.

Physical Activity. In addition to diet, physical activity keeps you healthy, strengthening your heart and bones and improving circulation and overall health. To be effective, however, exercise must be performed regularly. The current recommendation is to exercise moderately every day for at least 20 minutes. Walking, slow biking, gardening, and playing with children are all examples of moderate exercise.

Incorporating regular exercise in your daily routine is the best way to make sure you maintain a physical activity program. However, if you do not have the time to exercise daily, scheduling regular days and hours each week for exercise is the next best option. Your doctor can provide suggestions for a program to meet your individual goals (to keep healthy, lose weight, improve cardiovascular fitness, and so on).

Before you start any program, it is important for you to be checked by your physician for physical fitness. Starting an exercise program without your doctor's OK could put you at risk for injury, and possibly even a life-threatening condition. Use your well checkup to discuss with your doctor your specific plans for exercise, including anticipated time commitment and intensity level. She will alert you to any cautionary measures you should take before beginning your program.

Injury Prevention. Taking simple safety precautions in everyday activities can prevent all sorts of injuries. Injury prevention is an all-too-often overlooked facet of wellness.

Lap-Shoulder Belts. Injuries from motor vehicle crashes are the eighth leading cause of death in the United States. In 1993, 40,115 Americans died in crashes and more than 3 million were injured.

Wearing a lap-shoulder seat belt is a law in many states and should be used by everyone, regardless of your state laws. Studies show that use of lap-shoulder belts greatly reduces injuries and deaths from motor vehicle accidents. In fact, it can cut your risk of serious injury in an accident by 40 to 55 percent.

Not only does the lap-shoulder belt prevent you from crashing into the windshield during a collision, it keeps you and your fellow passengers from being thrown into each other. If you are the driver, it also keeps you behind the wheel so you can steer during an emergency.

FIGURE 6.2
Seat Belt Safety
Wear a lap-shoulder seat belt each and every time you travel in a car. Studies show that use of lap-shoulder belts can cut your risk of serious injury in a car accident by 40 to 55 percent.

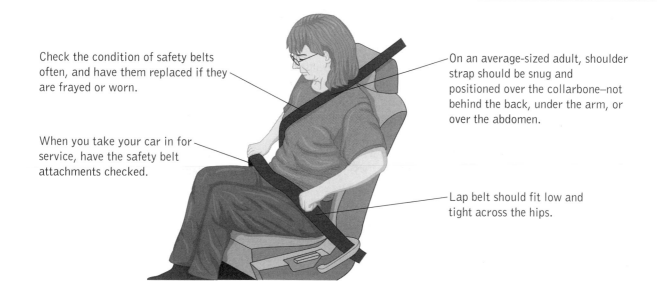

Check the condition of safety belts often, and have them replaced if they are frayed or worn.

When you take your car in for service, have the safety belt attachments checked.

On an average-sized adult, shoulder strap should be snug and positioned over the collarbone—not behind the back, under the arm, or over the abdomen.

Lap belt should fit low and tight across the hips.

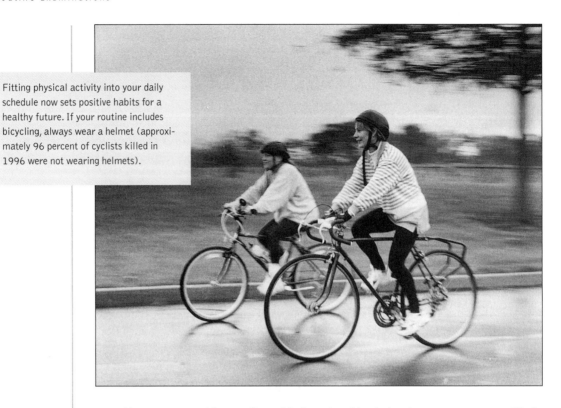

Fitting physical activity into your daily schedule now sets positive habits for a healthy future. If your routine includes bicycling, always wear a helmet (approximately 96 percent of cyclists killed in 1996 were not wearing helmets).

Choose a car with an adjustable lap-shoulder belt, since you are more likely to wear it if it is comfortable. If you are pregnant, wear your belt comfortably below your abdomen, across your upper thighs, for best protection.

Motorcycle and Bicycle Helmets. The death rate from motorcycle accidents is almost 20 times higher than that of car accidents. While no one knows for certain why this is the case, if you ride a motorcycle it makes sense to take safety precautions to reduce the chance of injury or death.

Wearing a motorcycle helmet is one important precaution riders can take. For motorcyclists who wear safety helmets, head injury rates alone are reduced by 40 to 75 percent. Making sure you are drug- and alcohol-free is another important safety measure to take to avoid accidents. Wearing protective clothing and boots will also reduce injuries.

Bicycles, too, require safety measures. While bicycling is a popular children's sport, nearly half of all Americans, including adults, ride bicycles, including the popular mountain bikes with wide-tread wheels. It is not uncommon to see adults cycling to work or riding for pleasure on the weekends. Yet not everyone takes the proper precautions.

Safety helmets alone can reduce the risk of death from bicycle accidents. Between 50 and 85 percent of all bicycle accident fatalities are related to head trauma. Studies suggest that wearing a safety helmet can reduce head injuries by at least 40 percent, and maybe as much as 85 percent.

Many communities require children who ride bicycles and all motorcycle riders to wear safety helmets. In these communities the incidence of injury and death has been shown to be reduced.

Gun Safety. Nearly half of all U.S. homes have some type of gun. One in four homes has a handgun. Yet, according to one survey, 59 percent of parents who said they had a gun in the home admitted to not locking it away from their children. Such carelessness with firearms leads to thousands of unintentional injuries and deaths each year.

It is strongly recommended that guns not be kept in homes, particularly in those where children live or visit. If you must own a gun, store it unloaded and locked up securely, with ammunition stored in a separate location. Childproof trigger locks are available at sporting goods stores, as well as through various health organizations. Parents who own guns must educate their children about the dangers of firearms before bringing a gun into the home. For more information about gun safety and preventing violence, see Chapter 14.

Smoke Detectors. Smoke detectors are an essential safety precaution in the home. Death in a residential fire is two to three times more likely in homes without smoke detectors. Older adults are especially at risk in house fires. In fact, fires and burns are the leading cause of accidental death in older adults, who may have impaired vision, hearing, and mobility. Make sure to check the smoke detectors in your home monthly to make sure they are working (on the first of each month, so you remember), and change the battery each year.

Carbon Monoxide Detectors. While many people have smoke detectors installed in their homes, few have carbon monoxide detectors. These devices detect carbon monoxide, a colorless, odorless gas that is extremely poisonous. Carbon monoxide may be released via a gas stove or fireplace, whether in your home or in an adjacent structure. Using carbon monoxide detectors can save you from preventable carbon monoxide poisoning.

Sexual Behavior. The years between age 25 and 64 are sexually active ones for most. Sexual contact may put you at risk for sexually transmitted disease (STD), and your doctor can counsel you on safe sexual practices.

STD Prevention. Sexually transmitted diseases (STDs) are infections transmitted through sexual intercourse. Examples include human immunodeficiency virus (HIV), the virus that causes AIDS, and gonorrhea, syphilis, herpes, viral warts, and chlamydia.

Symptoms of these diseases range from mild irritation to severe pain. In other cases, you will notice no symptoms at all until the disease progresses to a more serious stage. (That is why annual screening for STDs during your well visit is so important.) Some of these infections can progress to serious illnesses requiring hospitalization and can even cause life-threatening complications. Be aware that STDs are more easily transmitted from a man to a woman than vice versa and may have more serious consequences for women than for men.

Each year in the United States there are an estimated 12 million new cases of sexually transmitted infections—and of these, 40,000 to 80,000 are new transmissions of HIV. Yet, high-risk behaviors—such as engaging in sexual relations with more than one partner and without the regular use of a latex condom—continue among women and their partners.

wellness **tip**

Are you over 40? Do not think you are no longer at risk for an unintended pregnancy. Remember, as long as you are menstruating, even irregularly, you can become pregnant. Until you have reached menopause (one year of having no periods), take appropriate precautions if you do not want to get pregnant.

You can be sexually active and still take precautions to prevent the spread of STDs. These precautions include abstaining from actual sexual intercourse or limiting sexual relations to one partner who is also monogamous with you.

Using a latex condom each time you have intercourse further protects you from STDs. (Other birth control methods do not.) Only *latex* condoms have this protective effect. Natural skin condoms allow viruses, like HIV, to penetrate.

Make sure, however, not to use a latex condom with an oil-based lubricant, like Vaseline. This destroys the condom's protective effect. Instead, choose a water-based lubricant. Your physician can recommend several choices.

Unintended Pregnancy. The risk of unintended pregnancy is by no means limited to the teenage years. About two-thirds of American women are at risk for unintended pregnancy. These are women who are engaging in sexual relations but who do not want children at this time in their lives, or possibly not at all.

Unintended pregnancy can be avoided, of course, through regular use of contraception, such as oral contraceptives, like the pill; barrier contraceptives, like the condom or diaphragm; and other options, including intrauterine devices (IUDs), implants, injections, abstinence, or sterilization. (See Chapter 17 for a detailed explanation of contraceptive options.) Choose a birth control method with which you are comfortable and that fits your lifestyle.

Brushing and Flossing Your Teeth

As long as your natural teeth are in your mouth, you will need to brush and floss them daily to prevent tooth decay. If plaque is not removed each day, it hardens on your teeth as tartar. Not only does tartar lead to tooth decay, its presence can cause gum disease, infection, and tooth loss.

But if you are like many Americans, you are not brushing or flossing well enough, or long enough. Here are some tips:

- Choose a soft bristle brush and fluoride toothpaste.
- Gently brush teeth on all sides, using circular and short back-and-forth strokes.
- Take special care to brush along the gum line. Ask your dentist or hygienist to show you how to hold the brush.
- Lightly brush your tongue to remove food residue and plaque that may have accumulated there.
- Brush for a full two minutes. (Consider using a kitchen timer to ensure you have brushed for the full length.)
- Floss each time you brush, or at least at bedtime. Floss between each tooth, on the top and bottom of your mouth.
- To make flossing easier, use a floss holder, or experiment with the new, easy-gliding flosses available.
- If brushing or flossing results in persistent bleeding, pain, or irritation, consult your dentist.

Whatever contraceptive method you choose, make sure you know how to use it correctly. Many times, unintended pregnancies result when a birth control product is used incorrectly. Ask your physician or clinician if you are at all unsure about a birth control method or product.

Dental Health. Most women in the United States suffer from some form of tooth decay and/or periodontal (gum and bone) disease. The average adult has between 10 and 17 teeth that are either missing, decayed, or filled. About half of all adults have inflammation of the gums, called gingivitis, and 80 percent have periodontis, an inflammation of the gums leading to destruction of teeth-supporting bones. Older adults have an even greater prevalence of periodontal disease.

Daily dental hygiene habits can help prevent oral disease. This includes brushing your teeth regularly with a fluoride toothpaste, for a full two minutes three or more times a day if possible. Flossing between teeth daily removes the bacteria and plaque that can irritate gums. Regular use of a fluoride product, such as a rinse, also is helpful in providing a protective effect for your teeth. (This is especially important if your water supply is not fluoridated.)

Your food choices also can play a role in the health of your teeth and gums. Products with refined sugar and carbohydrates, such as crackers, cookies, candy, and soda, tend to stick to the teeth. Reducing the frequency with which you consume these types of foods can increase the health of your mouth.

No matter how well you clean your teeth, you will benefit from regular dental checkups and a professional cleaning every six months. Regular visits allow the dentist or dental hygienist to remove tartar that you could not remove; review dental hygiene, such as proper flossing technique; and monitor your overall dental health and pinpoint possible concerns for the future.

Immunizations

Your basic immunizations will have been completed by the time you reach adulthood. This does not mean that you are done with immunizations, however. Often, you will need booster immunizations to make sure your defenses against disease are strong. The following immunizations are commonly given to adults. See Chapter 4 for a full explanation of each of these diseases:

- Tetanus–diphtheria (Td) booster
- Rubella booster
- Hepatitis A and hepatitis B
- Influenza

Interestingly enough, most adults have not been immunized by their physicians according to the most current guidelines. This may be because many adults are at relatively low risk for contracting some diseases or because of the cost of administering the vaccines. Yet, routine vaccination throughout adult life is an important part of preventive health care. Check with your physician to make sure you are up-to-date on all immunizations.

Tetanus–Diphtheria (Td) Booster. Tetanus and diphtheria remain serious infections that can lead to death. The Td booster protects against these diseases.

wellness **warning**

Do your gums bleed easily? You may have gingivitis, an inflammation of the gums that can lead to periodontal disease. Brushing your gums and flossing between your teeth regularly can help. Talk to your dentist about other actions you can take.

Myths About Vaccinations

Some people choose to forego vaccinations because of certain misconceptions. Below are six popular myths about vaccinations and how medical practitioners respond to these myths.

Myth:
Many diseases are not common today, not because of vaccinations but because of better sanitation and hygiene.
Better sanitation and hygiene certainly have contributed to prevent the spread of disease. However, if you examine historical evidence, incidence in disease dropped most dramatically when the various vaccines were introduced. If vaccines were eliminated, incidence of disease would likely rise, despite good sanitation. For example, when Great Britain, Sweden, and Japan cut back on the pertussis (whooping cough) vaccine, there was an epidemic of more than 100,000 cases.

Myth:
Diseases for which we have vaccines have been practically eliminated from the United States. Therefore people do not really need to be vaccinated.
It is true that the incidence of many of these diseases in the United States is very low. However, many of these diseases still are quite common in other parts of the world, and U.S. travelers can easily bring them back into the country. If no one were vaccinated against them, the country would likely face an epidemic.

Myth:
Vaccinating someone for multiple diseases at the same time increases the risks of side effects.
Studies show that combination vaccinations are safe and effective and pose no increased risks of side effects. In fact, people expose themselves to many more foreign antigens and bacteria each day, simply from eating food.

Myth:
There are dangerous batches of some vaccines that cause adverse reactions and deaths.
Vaccine batches, or lots, are tracked for serious, adverse side effects. If a vaccine batch were to be found defective, the Food and Drug Administration would immediately recall it. That has not occurred in this century. Many adverse effects may be coincidental and not related to the vaccine at all. Others may be a matter of allergic reaction, which cannot be predicted.

Myth:
Vaccines cause serious side effects, including sickness and death.
Vaccines are very safe. If they do cause side effects, these are minor and temporary, such as a low fever or discomfort at the injection site. Serious side effects are extremely rare. As for death caused by vaccination, it is so uncommon that it always makes the news. However, it is caused by severe reactions that may have occurred with exposure to the illness as well. Only one death is believed to be possibly associated with a vaccine between 1990 and 1992. The Institute of Medicine reports the risk of death from vaccination as "extraordinarily low."

Myth:
Most people contract diseases even though they have been vaccinated.
Vaccines are not 100 percent effective for everybody. For example, many are effective for 85 to 95 percent of the recipients. That means that some people who are vaccinated could contract the disease. Because most people in the United States have been vaccinated, if an epidemic strikes, some of those people will be at risk. Of course, if no one were vaccinated, everyone would be at risk for the disease.

The Td booster usually is administered every ten years to maintain its protective effect. If you have not received your Td booster within this time frame, you are at risk for contracting the disease if you receive a puncture wound or any type of injury where the tetanus bacteria can enter your system. This is serious, as death occurs in 19 to 24 percent of all tetanus cases, and chances of death increase with age.

The Td booster however, is highly effective in preventing tetanus and diphtheria. There are few side effects, although many people experience temporary inflammation where the vaccine was administered.

Rubella Booster. Rubella is a relatively mild disease, but not so if you are pregnant, as the illness can cause severe fetal abnormalities and fetal death. If you had a rubella vaccination during childhood, it is a good idea to receive a booster during adulthood to ensure that you are not susceptible to the disease. You can also check your immunity to rubella through a simple blood test, to determine if a booster shot is necessary. Both precautions must be taken, however, *before* you become pregnant. Pregnant women who may be susceptible to the disease can receive a vaccine injection during the first few days after they deliver the baby.

Hepatitis A and Hepatitis B Vaccines. Hepatitis A and hepatitis B are both serious viral inflammations of the liver. Hepatitis A is spread through infected food or water; hepatitis B is spread through bodily fluid contact, such as in sexual relations, or with poorly sterilized needles or dental instruments. Hepatitis A is generally milder than hepatitis B. Both can cause liver damage and, with more serious complications, can even lead to death.

Vaccines now are available for both Hepatitis A and hepatitis B. Vaccinations are recommended if you are at high risk for contracting either disease. For hepatitis A, this may include frequent travelers, people living in areas where the disease is present, or those who work in a hospital or laboratory where exposure to the infection could occur. For hepatitis B, high risk groups include intravenous drug users, sexually active adults with multiple partners, blood recipients, and health care workers with frequent exposure to blood products.

Influenza Vaccine. While influenza, commonly known as the flu, can incapacitate you for several days, it also can cause death. Each time there is a flu epidemic, 20,000 or more deaths are reported. Influenza crosses all age barriers, affecting adults as frequently as children. The elderly, and those with chronic conditions, such as severe asthma, cystic fibrosis, and diabetes, are especially at risk.

Getting an influenza vaccination can prevent the illness or, at a minimum, reduce its severity in healthy adults regardless of age. This in turn reduces hospi-

wellness
warning

The influenza virus is expelled into the air each time an infected person sneezes, coughs, or even talks. It can be inhaled by anyone who walks close by or spread by hand contamination. To prevent your risk of contracting the disease, stay at a distance from any infected person. If you are caring for someone with the flu, it is recommended that you wear a surgical mask in the presence of the person who is ill and avoid direct hand contact. Frequent hand washing is advised to prevent viral spread.

A Healthy Example

The healthy choices that you make can extend to your family as well. Encouraging others, such as your spouse, partner, siblings, parents, or children, to join you in healthy habits and activities is a natural extension of your own program. Plus, making changes for the better is easier and more fun when you do it with others.

Remember, however, that each age group has special health needs. (Consult other chapters in Part II for specifics on each age group.) Your children's needs will be different from yours, as will your parents' needs. Get to know the health needs of all members of your family so you can encourage them toward a positive, healthy lifestyle.

talization rates and deaths. Because the strain of influenza changes each year, the influenza vaccine is reformulated each year. The recommended time to receive a flu vaccination is in the fall, at a time when you are healthy, and before the official start of flu season.

Most people experience no adverse reactions from the influenza vaccine. Some may experience mild, local side effects or feel achy for a few hours. Though uncommon, there is the possibility of an allergic reaction.

What *You* Can Do

Good health is no accident. It is up to you to choose each element of your own healthy lifestyle, tailoring those choices to meet your own health and wellness needs. Smart choices during your later reproductive years will create a strong foundation to help you enjoy your mature years and reduce your risk of chronic disease. You will feel better and look better and have more energy. Do what you can during this critical time to stay well and healthy:

- Schedule regular well checkup doctor and dental visits.
- Protect yourself from infection by getting recommended immunizations, throughout your adult years.
- Avoid smoking, excessive drinking, and taking drugs.
- Take precautions to avoid injury and stay safe.
- Eat a well-balanced diet and make exercise a part of your daily life.
- Make healthy choices that are right for you.
- Set a good example to help others follow a healthy lifestyle.

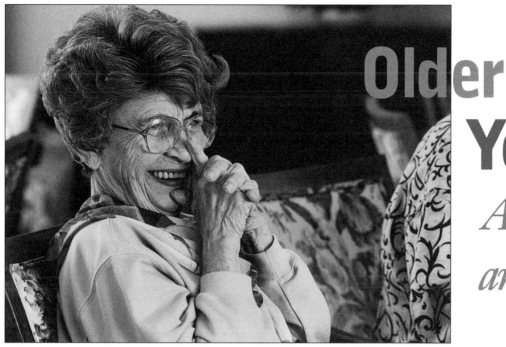

Older Years:
Ages 65 *and* Over

Decades ago, few people focused on the special health needs of the elderly, mainly because it was uncommon for anyone to live that long. At the turn of the twentieth century, the average life expectancy for women was only 48 years, barely what we consider now as middle age.

Today, however, thanks to medical and scientific advances, the average life expectancy has increased to 75.7 years. In fact, the most rapidly growing age group in the United States are men and women aged 85 and older, who represent about 3 million people. Of that group, about 35,000 are 100 years old or older.

What do these statistics mean for you? Essentially it means you are likely to live far into your elder years. Whether you spend these years feeling well and enjoying a rewarding healthy lifestyle, or suffering from physical ailments and chronic disorders, is largely up to you. If you choose now to adopt a lifestyle focused on wellness, take care of yourself, and follow recommended preventive services, you have a good chance of staying energetic and healthy into your elder years. If, on the other hand, you avoid exercise, eat poorly, smoke cigarettes, and neglect medical checkups and screening tests, then you may find the elder years marked by a decrease in energy and chronic or debilitating health problems.

It is never too late to begin a healthy lifestyle. While poor choices made early in life might have negative consequences regardless of changes made later, improving your eating habits and engaging in physical exercise will better the quality of your life at whatever age you choose to begin.

Regardless of your health regimen, the process of aging naturally brings with it potential health problems. For example, after decades of use, your vision and hearing inevitably weaken. The persistent wear and tear on your body and decreasing hormone levels can cause your bones to weaken. Since your immune system is not as vigorous as it once was, incidents that you easily weathered when you were younger take a heavier toll now. It may take longer to recover from a bout of influenza or a simple skin infection, for example. One of the single most important practices to adopt as you reach the elder years is to educate yourself about your body's changing needs so you can provide better care for yourself.

The best way to learn what to expect as you age is to plan regular wellness checkups with a helpful physician. Such checkups allow you to learn important strategies and gain valuable advice about how to keep healthy by:

- Keeping a close watch on your physical condition, screening for potential areas of concern, and treating acute and chronic medical conditions as they arise.
- Encouraging you to follow a healthy diet, adding supplements as needed for your age and medical condition.
- Monitoring your exercise program to make sure your activities are safe and beneficial.
- Encouraging good dental care to enable you to keep your teeth well into your elder years.
- Offering advice on injury prevention, including how to safeguard against falls and injuries which may be more devastating as you age.
- Providing counseling on the impact of alcohol, tobacco, and drugs (both legal and illegal) on your health.
- Monitoring your mental status, including evaluating signs of memory loss, inappropriate behavior, Alzheimer's disease, or dementia.
- Evaluating your emotional health, including coping skills, dependency issues, depression, and anxiety.
- Providing counseling and treatment for infectious diseases, such as influenza, pneumonia, and STDs, which remain a risk if you remain sexually active.
- Completing the available immunizations to prevent avoidable diseases and maintain your health status.

This chapter describes what you can expect during wellness checkups beginning at age 65, and it outlines what you can do to maintain optimal health. The routine and preventive care described here is designed for women who are not ill. If a health problem is detected, further care or perhaps referral to another physician may be required.

The **Periodic** Health Examination

It is not unusual for older people to depend on more than one health care provider. Usually one doctor is in charge, acting as a generalist, while the others specialize in different areas related to particular health needs.

While you may visit specialists on a regular basis to monitor aspects of your health or address specific conditions, these appointments do not take the place of a complete, periodic health examination. The specialist focuses on only one area of your body, while your primary care physician considers all the factors affecting your health.

Your Aging IQ: How Much Do You Really Know About Getting Older?

You are getting older, so that automatically qualifies you as an expert on aging, right? Take this quiz and find out how much you really know.

1. Are urinary accidents normal for older adults?
No, urinary accidents (incontinence) are a symptom of a weakness of bladder control, infection, or disease or are a side effect of medications. Medical treatments and over-the-counter medications are available to stop this problem. Urinary leakage does not need to be accepted as a consequence of aging, nor need it interfere with your freedom to be active.

2. Will you take more medications now that you are older?
Yes, you probably will take more medications now than you did when you were younger. Check with your pharmacist or doctor to make sure none of the medications interact with each other to produce undesirable results.

3. Will you gain weight as you age?
Yes, weight gain is likely unless you make the proper caloric adjustments to prevent unwanted weight gain. Because of decreasing physical activity and changes that slow your metabolism, you will need fewer calories as you age. It is a good idea to look for ways to consume fewer calories, reduce fat intake, and remain physically active.

4. Will you begin to lose interest in sex as you age?
No, many people enjoy healthy, satisfying sexual relations well into their elder years. Like many other activities, continued sexual activity is the key to continued interest. Make time and plan to enjoy sexual relations, just as you would other special activities.

5. Should you avoid extremes of heat and cold, which can be dangerous as you get older?
Yes, your body is less able to adapt to heat and cold as you age.

6. Will you sleep less as you age?
No, but your sleep may become more fragmented. For example, you may sleep less during the night but take naps during the day. (See Chapter 10, on sleep disorders, to determine whether you are sleeping normally.)

7. Are you less likely to get heart disease than men of your age?
No, by age 65, women have an equal chance of contracting heart disease—about one in three—as men. Not smoking, following a healthy low-fat diet, and remaining physically active can help reduce this risk.

8. Can you reduce your risk of osteoporosis through diet and exercise?
Yes, eating foods rich in calcium, taking supplements, and exercising regularly (using weight-bearing techniques) help keep your bones strong and reduce the risk of osteoporosis. Medications or estrogen replacement therapy further reduce your risk. Ask your doctor about screening for osteoporosis to see if you would benefit from these additional therapies. (Chapter 25 discusses osteoporosis at length.)

9. If you live long enough, will you become confused and forgetful?
No, confusion and forgetfulness are related to specific conditions, such as strokes, Alzheimer's disease, minor head injuries, poor nutrition, drug reactions, and depression, among others.

The periodic health examination usually is performed by a primary care practitioner who might be an internist (who specializes in internal medicine), a family practitioner, or, for some women, a specially trained obstetrician/gynecologist. Internists and family practitioners have a broad knowledge of medicine and are best suited to provide an overall analysis. However, a periodic health examination may also be performed by a gerontologist, a doctor who specializes in geriatrics (the medical problems of older people).

Whichever kind of doctor you choose for primary care, make sure she is someone with whom you can easily communicate. If your doctor asks about your medical history, gathers records from other physicians, listens patiently to your questions, and answers each one to your satisfaction, then you have found someone you can work with for many years. If, on the other hand, your doctor is not interested in test results of other physicians, fails to ask about your medical history, condescends to you, or seems to think your questions and concerns are trivial or unimportant, you are wise to seek another.

As you age, you will find that the physicians you choose will be younger, often significantly younger, than you are. While you may feel more comfortable with a doctor closer to your own age, remember that you trade the experience of older doctors for the newest screening methods and treatments that younger doctors have been taught. Medical schools today include topics such as preventative medicine, early screening, and geriatrics in the curriculum. Regardless of your doctor's age, it is important that you trust her expertise and feel comfortable in her presence.

Screening

Screening is a traditional part of any general physical examination. In screening, the doctor examines you for potential health risks. Specifically, she checks blood pressure, vision, hearing, and other areas that may be a particular concern for your age range. Following are descriptions of each area traditionally screened during older age.

Blood Pressure. An estimated 43 million Americans suffer from high blood pressure, also known as hypertension. It puts them at risk for coronary heart disease and other serious conditions, including stroke. However, there are often no symptoms associated with hypertension, and researchers suspect that many Americans have undiagnosed high blood pressure.

A medical professional should take your blood pressure using a blood pressure cuff during each doctor's visit. During the annual physical examination, she may take it more than once to obtain an average reading. Make sure she checks both arms and that blood pressure is taken in both a sitting and standing position. Dramatic drops are common in the elderly upon standing. Also ask to have the blood pressure checked by palpation as well as by stethoscope to make sure older and rigid blood vessels do not show artificial elevations of pressure.

The blood pressure results taken are not always accurate. Mechanical errors may influence the outcome. Your body position (if your legs are crossed), anxiety level, and what you ate for lunch can affect a reading. Remember that you can request a reading later in the examination or on a subsequent day if you believe it to be incorrect.

If you are diagnosed with hypertension, it can be treated. One way to control mild hypertension is by eating a diet that is rich in fruits, vegetables, and low-fat dairy products, and low in sodium and saturated fats. Even in cases of more significant high blood pressure, a healthy lifestyle that includes establishing a regular moderate exercise regimen can lower blood pressure. Be sure to ask your doctor about the latest research on diet and exercise and request help in choosing a diet that might make medication unnecessary.

Periodic Health Examination

The following services are performed at each periodic health examination unless a specific age is mentioned. Many physicians will complete portions of this examination at each of several follow-up visits during the year, while others will complete all of them during one visit.

Screening. The doctor uses these measurements and tests to look for signs of health concerns or problems:

- Blood pressure
- Height and weight
- Fecal occult blood test and/or sigmoidoscopy
- Mammogram/clinical breast examination
- Pap test
- Vision screening
- Hearing assessment
- Complete physical examination
- Screening blood tests for blood sugar and kidney function; complete lipid profile
- Electrocardiogram (EKG)

Counseling. Depending on your age and lifestyle, the doctor will review information relating to potential health risks:

- Substance use
- Diet and exercise
- Injury prevention
- Dental health
- Sexual behavior

Immunizations. The immunizations listed here are recommended for older adult women:

- Pneumococcal (once)
- Influenza (yearly)
- Tetanus–diphtheria (Td) booster (every ten years)

Mental Health. Screening for Alzheimer's disease and stress-related conditions.

More serious cases of high blood pressure put you at risk for stroke and heart failure and may need to be treated with medication along with the lifestyle recommendations. Your doctor will help you decide what kind of medication and how much is appropriate for you.

If you have other risk factors—high cholesterol, obesity, or a smoking habit—your doctor may prescribe treatments or drugs to help solve these problems and lower your blood pressure. Remember that if your physician puts you

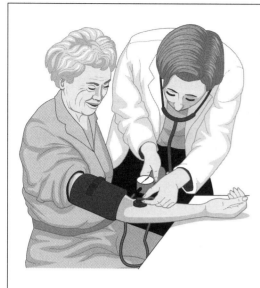

- Do not smoke or drink caffeine within 30 minutes before the measurement.

- You should be relaxed, having rested for at least five minutes before the reading.

- Your legs should not be crossed, and your bladder should be empty.

- Do not speak or chew gum during the measurement.

- Make sure you are seated with your bare arm supported and at heart level.

- Make sure to have two or more readings taken at two-minute intervals. The results of the readings should then be averaged. If the first two readings differ by more than five mm Hg, additional readings should be obtained.

- Your doctor may check your blood pressure in other positions, such as standing, especially if you are on blood pressure medication.

FIGURE 7.1
Blood Pressure Reading
Follow these tips to ensure an accurate blood pressure reading. If you think your reading is incorrect, ask to have it checked at a subsequent visit.

on medication for hypertension, it may be temporary—from a few months to a few years—or the treatment may be long term. Be sure to discuss any medication with your physician so that you can better understand how long you may have to take the medication and what will need to happen in order for you to be able to go off the medication. After taking the medication for a while, be sure to review the dosage and side effects with the doctor so that any adjustments and changes can be made. If you have lost weight, stopped smoking, and/or increased your exercise, you may be able to reduce or stop the medication.

Height and Weight. It is not unusual to gain a few pounds as you get older because your metabolism slows and you may reduce your activity level. To maintain an ideal weight, you will need to watch your eating habits more carefully than ever. If your weight measurements indicate you are not within normal range, but are in fact overweight, you will need to take steps to reduce your weight in order to reduce the amount of wear and tear on your bones, joints, and body functions. Obesity can lead to serious disease and physical problems, including arteriosclerosis and hypertension.

Your physician can advise you about steps you can take to reduce your weight. There are sometimes side effects with major lifestyle changes. Low calorie diets, for example, may cause dizziness, fatigue, or hair loss. Drugs may cause chest pain, palpitations, shortness of breath, headaches, or insomnia. Be sure to ask your doctor about a safe regimen for your particular circumstances. Prescription drugs and surgery, which sometimes help women lose weight, are rarely recommended for elderly patients.

Your height is also likely to change as you age. Most people experience a loss of one-half to one inch as gravity compresses the pads between the vertebrae. Following menopause, bone begins to deteriorate, which can make you shorter as bones compress or your spine becomes curved. Ask your doctor to assess whether your weight and height are within normal range. A significant loss of height is a sign of osteoporosis (see Chapter 25).

Screening for Colorectal Cancer. Each year, about 55,000 people die from colorectal cancer, the third most common form of cancer in American women. People over 50 years of age are especially at risk for this disease. As with many cancers, early detection offers the greatest chance for a cure.

The fecal occult blood test and the rectal examination are two principal ways of screening for colorectal cancer. (See Chapter 21 for more information on these tests.) The fecal occult blood test detects blood in stool samples, which can signal the presence of colorectal cancer. The rectal examination and sigmoidoscope allow your doctor to visually inspect the anus, rectum, and colon for cancerous or precancerous growths, by using a gloved finger and a flexible tube inserted through the anus into the colon.

These tests are important because there may be no detectable symptoms of colorectal cancer. While there are no clear-cut guidelines on how often these tests should be performed, fecal occult blood tests can be done annually, and a rectal examination can be scheduled every three to five years. If the specialist finds abnormalities indicating disease, she will order an x-ray of the colon and a colonoscopy for a complete evaluation of the colon.

People generally are willing to undergo the rectal examination and fecal occult blood test, a noninvasive procedure involving smearing stool samples onto testing paper. They often shy away from the sigmoidoscopy, because it can be uncomfortable and embarrassing, with modest expense. However, improvements in technology, such as flexible fiber optic sigmoidoscopes, have made the procedure less invasive and more acceptable. Fear of discomfort and embarrassment, though understandable, can be dangerous and deadly. Remember, colorectal cancer can be treated if caught early.

Mammogram/Clinical Breast Examination. Breast cancer, the most common cancer diagnosed in women, is usually detected by the mammogram, which is a special x-ray of the breast tissue, or during the clinical breast examination, when a doctor's palpates the breast tissue with her fingers and hands. (See Chapter 21 for more detailed information on preventing and screening for breast cancer.)

During the clinical breast examination, a physician or medical professional looks at and feels the breast tissue, checking for lumps, abnormal texture, enlarged lymph nodes, and skin changes. The examination is similar to the monthly self-examination you do at home. When you go for a mammogram, a trained technician operates equipment to compress your breasts in different positions between glass plates, and x-rays are taken of each position. A trained mammography radiologist reviews the x-rays and reports to your doctor. Additional x-rays may be required if signs of potential cancer appear on the routine mammogram.

It has been proven that women between ages 50 and 70 benefit greatly from routine screening for breast cancer because of the increased likelihood of breast cancer and because there is a greater chance for a cure if the cancer is detected before it has spread to other parts of the body. The benefits of routine screening in women over the age of 65 have not been studied extensively, but it is believed that this age group of women, too, can benefit from breast cancer screening, since the incidence of breast cancer increases with age. If you are in your older years, therefore, you should be routinely screened for breast cancer every one to two years with both the clinical breast examination and the mammogram. If you are at a higher risk for breast cancer because you have a family history of the disease or are on prolonged hormone replacement, for example, more frequent screening is recommended.

Pap Test. About 16,000 women each year are diagnosed with cervical cancer; 4,800 die from the disease. Yet, if it is detected early, the survival rate is about 90 percent.

The Papanicolaou test, or Pap test, screens for cervical cancer. (See Chapter 5 for a detailed description of Pap testing.) As long as you are sexually active, you are advised to have the Pap test once a year. If you have had a hysterectomy where your cervix also was removed, you are not at risk for cervical cancer, and you do not need this screening test.

If you are elderly, are no longer sexually active, and your annual Pap smears have consistently been normal, you are at very low risk for cervical cancer and probably do not need this screening test. However, if you are in your older years and have not been regularly tested for cervical cancer, you may have undiagnosed cancer. Some women have never had a Pap test, and others have had an average of only one per decade. If this is the case, make sure you are tested promptly, and thereafter schedule annual examinations. After three normal tests, if you are no longer sexually active, you are considered at a low risk for cervical cancer and can talk to your doctor about the need for further Pap tests.

Vision Screening. As you age, it is likely that your vision will begin to worsen. While this is naturally frustrating, it also may be quite dangerous. For example, decreased vision increases your risk of falling or of getting into a car accident. You may misread important instructions, such as on medicine bottles, or you may stop reading altogether.

After decades of almost constant work, your eyes begin to lose elasticity and they become more susceptible to disease. For example, most older people suffer from presbyopia, which occurs when the eye lens loses elasticity, making it to difficult to focus clearly when looking at things close at hand. Presbyopia also makes it difficult for some people to see at night and when lighting is dim. Reading glasses and bifocals solve most problems with this very common disorder.

A more serious eye problem faced by many older people, cataracts cloud the eye lens or surrounding membrane and obstruct the passage of light. Cataract sufferers lose clarity in their vision. Age-related macular degeneration causes the loss of central vision (the ability to see straight ahead), and glaucoma, where increased pressure within the eye results in damage to the optic nerve, are both relatively common among the elderly. (For more information on these eye conditions, see Chapter 24.)

Loss of visual acuity can often, but not always, be treated either with a prescription for glasses or contact lenses, or through medication and/or surgery. Unlike traditional surgery, which requires a hospital stay, many eye surgeries can now be performed on an outpatient basis.

In the case of glaucoma, or retinal detachment, early detection helps prevent further, irreversible vision loss. With other eye conditions, such as cataracts, treatment is best begun when they interfere with daily life for the patient. There is currently no real advantage to early detection of cataracts.

The Miracle of Lasers

If you need to have eye surgery, chances are it will be done with a laser—an intense beam of light that can cut like a scalpel. Unlike a scalpel, a laser can cut a single cell without damaging surrounding cells, allowing the surgeon to do precise work.

The term laser is actually an acronym for "light amplification by stimulated emission of radiation." The laser device itself uses electricity, mirrors, and a crystal or a gas to generate a single narrow beam of light of a single type, as compared to sunlight, which has a variety of light wavelengths. Lasers are regulated by the Food and Drug Administration and must meet strict safety standards for surgery.

In eye surgery, the pupil acts as the window through which the laser light can enter and reach cells that are deep within the eye. Because the surgeon does not have to cut the eye, laser surgery poses fewer risks and less chance of infection than traditional surgery. It also allows the patient to have surgery in a clinic, an ambulatory center, or a physician's office.

Laser surgery most often is used to correct cataracts, glaucoma, and retinal tears, but it has the potential to treat the majority of eye disorders. Experts predict lasers eventually will be used to correct nearsightedness, farsightedness, astigmatism, and the degeneration of vision after age 65.

wellness **tip**

Are you squinting to see clearly? Do you sometimes have trouble focusing your eyes? Do little flecks or spots invade your vision? These can indicate deteriorating vision or more serious disease. Schedule an eye examination as soon as possible. Don't neglect the wellness of your eyes.

Unfortunately, many women do not like to admit that they are suffering from vision loss. Studies have shown that a quarter of the older population is wearing incorrect eyeglass prescriptions and that uncorrected vision is common among nursing home residents. That is why it is important to schedule regular checkups with an optometrist to check your prescription and/or with an ophthalmologist, a physician who specializes in diseases of the eye. There is no formal recommended time frame for screening, although many ophthalmologists suggest visits every two years.

Hearing Assessment. As you age, your hearing also may deteriorate. In your older years, a partial hearing loss is common, although approximately 25 percent of women retain full, normal hearing in at least one ear their whole lives. Most hearing loss begins early in a woman's life, when she is exposed to recurrent loud noises or inner ear infections. Such minor loss may not be noticeable because the rest of the ear is in good working order. But as women age, and as other parts of the hearing system deteriorate, they notice more hearing loss.

If your hearing is gradually diminishing, you may not notice the loss. A periodic hearing test is a good way to evaluate your hearing ability. A formal test is not usually performed annually. Instead, many doctors prefer to question patients about their hearing. Some physicians use a technique where they whisper a question, out of the line of vision, to determine the patient's hearing ability. Patients who show a potential for hearing loss are tested, either in the physician's office or at a hearing testing center. Patients with hearing loss are then counseled about their options, including the techniques available to better understand others, prevent further loss, treat reversible problems, or investigate the wide range of hearing aids available to amplify sound.

wellness **tip**

If you suspect you may have a hearing problem, do not wait for your next general checkup. Contact your physician or a hearing examination center to set up a hearing test. Early analysis of the cause may lead to treatment that will improve hearing or prevent further loss.

Even with the advent of more and more sophisticated hearing aids, few work as well as the natural ear. Protection against hearing loss is of paramount importance. Women of all ages are encouraged to avoid exposure to loud noises, to treat ear infections promptly, and to limit the use of such devices as headphones, which are generally much louder than most people realize.

Physical Examination. A general but thorough physical examination is a part of every periodic checkup. The doctor will carefully assess your entire body, including skin, eyes, ears, nose, throat, chest, heart, lungs, and nervous system.

Screening Blood Tests. Routine blood tests help your doctor screen for medical problems that sometimes occur without symptoms. Blood tests can reveal a number of problems, such as anemia, blood disorders, diabetes, kidney disfuction, or risk for heart disease.

EKG. An electrocardiogram (EKG or ECG) shows the electrical impulses from your heart. This test can alert your doctor to heart muscle damage or problems in your heart's electrical system. (See Chapter 20 for more information on screening for heart problems.)

Counseling

One of the greatest benefits of routine, periodic checkups is the opportunity to speak with your physician and glean her medical expertise on everything from how to structure your daily exercise routine to what you can eat for maximum energy. During this "counseling" session your physician evaluates your overall lifestyle, takes into consideration any special stresses or unusual circumstances that may be occurring in your life, and makes appropriate suggestions to ensure your wellness. Whether or not you intend to follow the doctor's advice exactly, listen carefully to her comments, do your own reading, and make your choice based on sound knowledge and your own best judgment. As you gain knowledge and perspective, you can empower yourself to take control of your life and health to meet ever-changing needs as you age.

Substance Use. While few people in their older years are illicit drug users, many are frequent consumers of tobacco and alcohol. If you are like many in this age range, you grew up smoking cigarettes and drinking socially before the harmful health effects of tobacco and alcohol were known.

Used in moderation, these substances may not present a health risk. However, older people who have been using these products for many years, and those who use them to excess, may compromise their health and quality of life. (Turn to Chapter 13 for self-assessment tests to see if you may be at risk for a substance abuse problem.)

Tobacco. One out of every five deaths in the United States is caused by the consequences of smoking. Each of these deaths might have been prevented had the smoker taken steps to quit. While it is not easy to quit, experts agree that the health benefits are tremendous—even if you have had a long history of smoking. After ten years of not smoking, your risk of getting lung cancer is 30 to 50 percent lower than it would be if you continued to smoke. Studies have shown that your risk of dying prematurely also is substantially reduced, even if you quit after age 70.

If you smoke, please talk to your physician about quitting. She can offer medicinal support, such as prescription nicotine gums or patches to reduce the effect of tobacco withdrawal on your body, or non-nicotine medication to help your body deal better with withdrawal side effects. She may also be able to recommend smoking cessation programs, which offer emotional support for people who are trying to quit smoking. You may not be able to quit on the first try, but every time you attempt it, you learn how better to control the urge to smoke so that on the second, third, or fourth try, you are more likely to be successful.

Alcohol. Even if you drink infrequently or at a moderate level you still may be at risk, not for alcoholism, but for alcohol-related accidents, which can be just as dangerous. Alcohol impairs your ability to make decisions and slows your physical reaction time. That means if you are drinking in conjunction with any activity that requires coordination, good reflexes, careful attention, and sound judgment you could be putting yourself and others at risk for injury.

Most older women who drive depend on their cars for a sense of independence, and they want to continue to drive for as long as possible. It is difficult sometimes for women to come to terms with the fact that reflexes, coordination, and reaction time are affected by aging, but it is important to realize that driving requires more concentration as we get older. Though drinking and driving are to be avoided at any age, older people must be particularly aware that consuming alcohol before driving can cause accidents that may lead to injury and death.

The responsible and safe choice is to avoid alcohol in situations where driving or other physically and mentally demanding activities are planned. Allowing two hours to recover from a drink is wise. Remember that women generally have a greater susceptibility to alcohol because their livers take longer to break it down.

wellness
warning

Combining alcohol with prescription drugs often has unexpected results. Driving after even one drink can be particularly dangerous if you also take medication.

Medication's Changing Effects as You Age

Take a five to ten milligram dose of Valium at age 35, and you will feel relaxed or have relief of muscle spasm. Take the same dose at age 75, and you will become sleepy and groggy, and you may lose muscle control to the extent that you cannot stand up. As you age, your muscle tissue diminishes, your liver slows down, and your kidneys do not work as efficiently as they once did. As a result, medicines stay in your system longer. A dosage that was just right for you as a young person, then, may be too strong for you in your elder years.

Drug manufacturers are beginning to research how medicines work differently in people of different ages. The Food and Drug Administration, which approves all drugs on the U.S. market, is working on regulations for drug manufacturers that will include a special section on geriatric reactions for each drug approved.

Make a point of discussing this issue with your doctor and with every specialist you see. Whenever a doctor prescribes a new drug for you, make sure you understand when and how to take it and how to store it properly. Be sure each doctor knows of any other medications you are taking, and ask each to check to be sure there are no risks involved in mixing them. Then, alert your doctor if you experience incontinence, indigestion, confusion, sleeplessness, or other changes. Do not assume that a symptom is not related to the drug you are taking. The doctor might be able to recommend a different medication.

wellness **tip**

Consuming adequate protein is especially important for elderly women, even those on a diet. The Recommended Dietary Allowance (RDA) of protein for women is 50 grams. For example, if a woman eats a small serving of chicken breast (30 grams of protein), an eight-ounce glass of skim milk (8 grams), and 1 cup of low-fat yogurt (12 grams) in the same day, she will meet the RDA.

Diet and Exercise. As you age, a nutritious diet and a regular exercise program become critically important. Both have an impact on your continued health throughout your older years. If you follow a healthy regimen of diet and exercise, you actually can improve your health and guard against many ailments, including coronary heart disease, cancer, stroke, hypertension, and diabetes.

Take your age and medical condition into account when making food choices and devising a moderate exercise program. For example, if you have high blood pressure you will need a diet low in sodium and fat and with plenty of low-fat dairy products, fruits, and vegetables. Your physician may counsel you on nutrition or refer you to a nutritionist, a registered dietitian, or a nurse who has studied nutrition.

As you age, you may be unable to exercise at the same level of intensity and duration as when you were younger. Structure an exercise program that meets your current fitness level and that includes activities you enjoy. Make sure your doctor knows your usual activity level, your exercise program, whether you have made any changes in the last year, and whether you have any symptoms—such as shortness of breath, increased fatigue, or chest, arm, or throat discomfort—with activity. They may signal the onset of heart disease and require further tests.

Fat and Cholesterol. A nutritious diet limits the intake of fat and cholesterol. Fat, an organic compound found in foods, and cholesterol, a substance found in animal products, have been linked to such serious illnesses as heart disease and certain types of cancers.

If you are like most Americans, you already consume too much fat and cholesterol. Try this experiment to find out. Monitor your fat intake and your total calories for one day on your regular diet by reading food labels and writing down the information you find there. Your daily intake of dietary fat should be less than 30 percent of total calories consumed. If it is not, you need to change

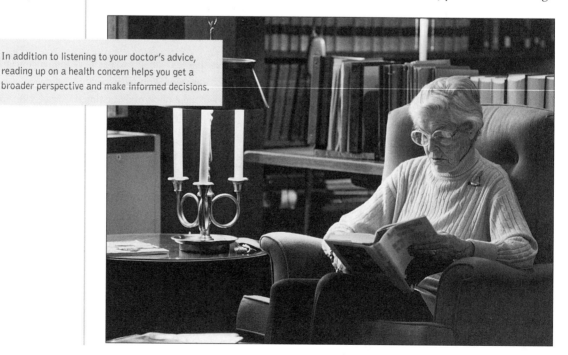

In addition to listening to your doctor's advice, reading up on a health concern helps you get a broader perspective and make informed decisions.

your eating habits. Similarly, you can monitor your daily saturated fat and cholesterol intake. It is important to get your lipids tested, including LDL (harmful) and HDL (good) cholesterol and triglycerides, to determine whether you need to limit your intake even more. (See Chapter 8 for more information on limiting fat and cholesterol in your diet.)

One way to limit fat and cholesterol in your diet is to follow the American Heart Association recommendation of five to six servings of fruits and vegetables a day in order to fill up with foods high in complex carbohydrates and dietary fiber and to cut back on fatty, processed, and packaged foods. Eating whole grain foods and cereals, combined with fruits and vegetables, not only automatically reduces the fat and cholesterol you consume, it improves your gastrointestinal function too, which is a concern to many people in their older years.

Calcium. It is no secret why some women maintain strong bones and teeth throughout their lifetimes. It is almost certain that they consume a sufficient amount of dietary calcium to offset their body's calcium loss. As you age and your bones become less dense, calcium's protective effect becomes especially important. Consuming adequate calcium strengthens your bones and can help reduce fractures and other complications from osteoporosis—brittle bone disease—as well as tooth loss.

Physical Activity. Americans are, on the whole, notoriously sedentary, and they become even more so as they age. Yet physical activity is a necessary part of wellness throughout life. It aids in retaining agility and helps ensure the strength and stamina necessary for independent living. (See Chapter 9 for more detailed information on this topic.)

If you already exercise, ask your physician to evaluate your program to make sure it is meeting your needs. Remember that exercise does not have to be strenuous to be effective, but it does need to be done on a regular basis. Any moderate activity carried out for 30 minutes a day is a good choice. The Surgeon General advises that the 30 minutes of activity can be completed throughout the day, though continuous activity is more beneficial. Many older women enjoy walking, which they can do at their own pace, at convenient times, and either alone or with others.

If you do not already exercise, speak with your physician about starting an exercise program. Always get a checkup to make sure you are physically able to exercise. Initiating a program without such a checkup could put you at risk for injury and possibly even a life-threatening condition. Share with your doctor your specific plans for exercise, including the anticipated time commitment and intensity level. She will alert you to any cautionary measures you should take before beginning your program.

Make exercise an enjoyable part of your daily routine. Choose a time of day when your energy level is typically high. This is the most effective way to make sure you exercise regularly and have the energy to do so. The safest time to take a daily walk is in the early morning when the air is cleaner and there is less traffic. Walking in the morning also allows you to get your body moving early and helps you be more productive throughout the day. If, however, you receive treatment for a heart condition, it is better for you to wait and exercise later in the day.

Calcium Supplements: A Good Idea at Any Age

Whether or not you have regularly consumed calcium in the past (through food or dietary supplements), it is never too late to start. Studies have shown that, even after menopause, 1,000 to 1,200 milligrams (mg) of elemental calcium each day prevents about one percent of bone loss a year. In fact, you should be consuming 1,000 to 1,500 mg of elemental calcium per day. If you are not getting enough in your diet, make sure you take a calcium supplement. These are available without a prescription. Your physician or pharmacist can recommend a calcium formulation.

Depending on your other medical conditions and medications, you may get your elemental calcium from calcium carbonate, calcium lactate, or calcium citrate. (See Chapter 8 for a list of calcium-rich foods and for specifics on choosing a calcium supplement.)

wellness **tip**

Avoid muscle strain and low back pain by maintaining proper posture. If you stand and walk properly, you will be amazed at the difference in your energy level.

FIGURE 7.2
Preventing Falls

Falls are the leading cause of injury and unintentional death among older people in the United States. Take these precautions to reduce the risk of falls in your home.

Injury Prevention. As you age, you also become more susceptible to injuries. Impaired vision or hearing, decreased bone density, diminished muscle strength, and other factors associated with aging can increase your risk of injury. There are many precautions, however, that you can take to prevent such injuries from occurring. During your regular well checkups, your doctor can counsel you on steps you can take both in and out of your home to ensure your safety.

Lap-Shoulder Belts. Deaths from motor vehicle accidents are highest among young adults and the elderly. While drivers older than 65 cause fewer accidents, those who are involved in accidents have a greater likelihood of experiencing serious injury.

Many older people began driving before seat belts were required equipment in American automobiles, and they have never developed the habit of buckling up. However, using a lap-shoulder belt reduces the risk of injury and death from motor vehicle accidents by 40 to 55 percent. Not only does it prevent you from crashing into the windshield during a collision, it keeps you and your fellow passengers from being thrown into each other. If you are in the driver's seat, using a lap-shoulder belt keeps you firmly behind the wheel so you can steer during an emergency. Make wearing a safety belt a habit whenever you step into a motor vehicle. In most states, it is the law.

Motorcycle and Bicycle Helmets. Many adults continue to enjoy such activities as bicycling and motorcycling throughout their older years. If you participate in these activities, remember to take the necessary safety precautions. In most states

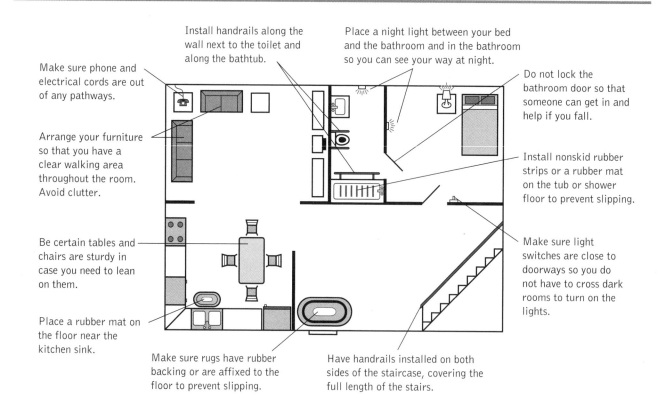

Install handrails along the wall next to the toilet and along the bathtub.

Place a night light between your bed and the bathroom and in the bathroom so you can see your way at night.

Make sure phone and electrical cords are out of any pathways.

Do not lock the bathroom door so that someone can get in and help if you fall.

Arrange your furniture so that you have a clear walking area throughout the room. Avoid clutter.

Install nonskid rubber strips or a rubber mat on the tub or shower floor to prevent slipping.

Be certain tables and chairs are sturdy in case you need to lean on them.

Make sure light switches are close to doorways so you do not have to cross dark rooms to turn on the lights.

Place a rubber mat on the floor near the kitchen sink.

Make sure rugs have rubber backing or are affixed to the floor to prevent slipping.

Have handrails installed on both sides of the staircase, covering the full length of the stairs.

it is illegal to ride a motorcycle without a helmet, but it is equally important to wear a helmet while bicycling. For bicycle riders, studies suggest that wearing a safety helmet can reduce head injuries by at least 40 percent, and maybe as much as 85 percent. If you ride, invest in a comfortable, well-fitting helmet to ensure that you will wear it. It may save your life.

Preventing Falls. Falls are the leading cause of nonfatal injuries and unintentional deaths among older people in the United States. Hip fractures from falls result in 250,000 hospital admissions each year. Falls are especially dangerous if you are elderly, as they often result in broken bones or other serious complications that can change the quality of your life. For example, half of serious falls among the elderly result in admission to a nursing home for continual care. After recovering from a hip injury, only half of elderly patients regain full function.

Often, falls are caused by physical changes in your body that cause you to be less agile, such as instability in your posture, gait, or balance, diminished strength in your muscles, poor vision, or cognitive impairment from medications you are taking. Falls may also result from inadequate lighting and incorrect footwear. Areas where falls often occur include stairs, irregular pavements, slippery surfaces, and loose rugs.

Gun Safety. No one is immune to firearm injuries. Each year, firearms are responsible for 12,000 to 13,000 nonfatal injuries and many fatal ones. (See Chapter 5 for additional statistics on firearm injuries and deaths.)

Safety precautions can reduce this risk. While it is recommended that you do not keep firearms in the home at all, if you choose to do so, keep the guns unloaded and stored in a locked compartment. Store ammunition separately. Use trigger locks and loading indicators and learn safe firearm practices. If you have grandchildren who visit you, it is your responsibility to be sure firearms are not where they can reach them.

Smoke Detectors and Carbon Monoxide Detectors. Smoke detectors and carbon monoxide detectors are two essential safety items for the home. If you have not already had them installed, make them a high priority for reducing your risk of injury. Smoke detectors signal the presence of smoke and the possibility of fire. Carbon monoxide detectors signal the presence of a colorless, odorless gas that is extremely poisonous.

Smoke detectors are important because older adults are especially at risk from fire. Burns and smoke inhalation are a primary cause of accidental death in older adults. If a fire begins in your home, your reduced ability to see and hear, along with decreased mobility, may make it difficult to act quickly enough to escape.

Carbon monoxide detectors, too, are essential for all adults. If carbon monoxide is released in your home—via a gas stove or fireplace for example—you may not know it, yet you could die as a result.

Both smoke detectors and carbon monoxide detectors work by emitting a loud shriek when smoke or carbon monoxide is detected. If your hearing is impaired and you believe you may not hear the warning, consult your local hardware store manager. Some new models are available that also use bright lights as an alert.

Preventing Falls in the Home

You can take precautions in your home to eliminate falls:

- Remove or secure loose rugs, cover slippery areas, and improve the lighting in your home, especially in hallways and stairwells.
- Choose comfortable footwear that provides stable footing, and wear it whenever you walk around the house, even at night. You may also consider an external hip protector, which can reduce the chances of hip fractures if you do fall.
- Discuss other ways to reduce risk of falls with your physician. She can check your ability to walk safely and recommend aids. Accepting the necessity for a cane or a walker to prevent falls will go far in reducing the risk of injury.

Hot Water Heater. How hot is the water in your water heater? If it is too hot, it could put you at risk for scalding. Scalding burns account for 42 percent of hospitalizations for burn injuries in people over age 65. Scalding burns are caused by tap water or by food and drinks that are too hot.

Turning the temperature down on your hot water heater is an easy way to prevent these types of burns. Set your water heater at or below 120 to 130°F. Even at this lower temperature, you will find your water is heated adequately. You will also save money by lowering the cost of heating water.

CPR Training. CPR, or cardiopulmonary resuscitation, is a technique designed to revive a person who stops breathing. You can be trained in CPR at your local chapter of the American Heart Association, your local hospital, and at many nonprofit groups or community programs.

CPR is an especially important skill to have if you live with another person, or if you interact regularly with others, especially those who are elderly. It is not uncommon for people over age 65 to choke and stop breathing when eating. Choking is responsible for 2,500 deaths in this age group annually. CPR training includes lessons in the Heimlich maneuver, a technique that uses compression under the rib cage to eject the foreign object or food particle from a person's windpipe. Knowing CPR and the Heimlich maneuver may help you save a loved one's life. You can also encourage those who live with you to learn these techniques in the event that you need help.

Dental Health. There is no reason why you cannot keep your original set of teeth well into old age. You just need to take the time to care for them. The regimen for healthy teeth is no different when you are older than it was when you were younger. Flossing and brushing daily and visiting your dentist regularly for cleanings and checkups continue to be the rule.

Yet, if you are like most older adults, you probably already suffer from some form of tooth decay and/or periodontal (gum and bone) disease. In fact, 95 percent of elderly people have periodontitis, or inflammation of the gums leading to destruction of teeth-supporting bones. More than one-third have periodontal disease where at least one tooth has begun to be detached.

While you cannot reattach a tooth that has become detached, you can protect the remaining teeth and gums through daily health habits. This includes brushing your teeth regularly with a fluoride toothpaste for a full two minutes, three or more times a day if possible. It is also recommended that you floss between teeth daily to remove the bacteria and plaque that can irritate gums. Special brushing devices may be used to aid in gum and tooth health. Regular use of a fluoride product, such as a rinse, is also helpful in providing a protective effect for your teeth. (This is especially important if your water supply is not fluoridated.)

Changing your diet also can have an effect on your dental health. Reduce your consumption of products with refined sugar and carbohydrates, such as crackers, cookies, and candy, which tend to stick to teeth. Substitute raw fruits and vegetables, which provide a natural cleansing effect each time you eat them. The nutritional steps you take to prevent bone loss associated with osteoporosis will also help protect you from periodontal disease.

Visit the dentist regularly so she can evaluate your teeth and gums. She may recommend a specialist to treat periodontal disease, or provide a regimen of antiplaque and antigingivitis agents to help keep your teeth strong and healthy.

Sexual Behavior. Women rarely experience any loss of sexual capacity as they age. In some cases, an ailment, such as arthritis, may impact your ability to function sexually because it is difficult to move, but pain relief medication and other treatments can help you feel more comfortable and at ease.

If you remain sexually active after menopause, you are no longer at risk for an unintended pregnancy, but you are still at risk for sexually transmitted diseases (STDs). STDs are infections transmitted through sexual intercourse. Examples include human immunodeficiency virus (HIV, the virus that causes AIDS), gonorrhea, syphilis, herpes, chlamydia, and genital warts. Symptoms range from mild irritation and discharge to severe pain with intercourse, urination, and even during usual, daily activities. In some cases, you will notice no symptoms at all until the disease progresses to a more serious stage. That is why regular screening for STDs continues to be important as long as you remain sexually active. (See Chapter 22 for more information on STDs.)

You can avoid STDs with some simple precautions. Avoid high-risk behaviors that may lead to the transmission of STDs. These include engaging in sexual relations with more than one partner or with partners whose sexual or drug use history is not known. Be as certain as possible that your partner is monogamous with you and insist that he use a latex condom if there are any doubts. (Natural animal skin condoms do not offer the same protection.) Otherwise, you can choose to abstain from sexual relations altogether to avoid STDs.

Immunizations

Periodic immunizations can go far toward preventing common illnesses among older adults. Immunizations may be given seasonally, as at the start of cold and flu season, or on an as-needed basis. Many older women have not received a full set of immunizations. If you have not been immunized recently, check with your physician. Specifically, the following immunizations are commonly administered throughout your elder years:

Pneumococcal Vaccine. The pneumococcal bacteria causes the lung infection commonly known as pneumococcal pneumonia. It also sometimes causes meningitis, an inflammation of the brain and/or spinal cord. Pneumococcal disease is common among older adults and is responsible for a number of deaths. You are at risk for pneumococcal disease if you are 65 or older. If you also have chronic cardiac or pulmonary disease, diabetes, reduced immunity, or sickle cell disease, or if you lack a functioning spleen, you are at even greater risk.

The pneumococcal vaccine has been shown to be effective in building up resistance to this disease among the elderly, unless they are immunocompromised. For example, the vaccine will not work in a woman who is undergoing chemotherapy or who has chronic renal failure or an immunoglobulin deficiency.

The length of the vaccine's protective effect is not known, but it may be five to ten years or greater. Discuss with your doctor whether this immunization is right for you.

wellness **tip**

Starting over? Remember that a sexual relationship with a new person can put you at risk for a sexually transmitted disease (STD). Before engaging in heavy petting or intercourse, share sexual histories and discuss STDs. For each encounter with a new partner, use a latex condom unless you have proof your partner is not infected.

What to Expect from the Flu Vaccine

Getting an influenza vaccination can prevent this potentially debilitating illness or reduce its severity if you contract it despite the vaccine. Physicians recommend annual immunizations, in fall or early winter, for all women aged 65 and older.

You probably will experience no significant adverse reactions from an influenza vaccination. Most people report soreness or achiness at the site of the injection, but it can be relieved with aspirin or acetaminophen taken prior to receiving the vaccination. Occasionally, there are mild, systemic side effects, such as mild body aches, for the 24 hours after the vaccination, which can usually be relieved by over-the-counter pain medication. Reduced dosages of the vaccine are also available for those susceptible to side effects.

Influenza Vaccine. Influenza, though a common illness, is not to be taken lightly. It can lead to more severe illness, hospitalization, or death. Each time there is an influenza, or flu, epidemic, 20,000 or more deaths are reported in the United States. Flu is not, as commonly thought, simply a severe form of a cold. It is caused by a different virus and affects the entire body. This illness is especially dangerous for older people. Young people who get the flu generally become incapacitated but recover within a few days. Among older people, the flu takes a greater toll on the body and requires a longer recovery time. You are more at risk for the flu if you have a chronic condition, such as severe asthma, heart disease, or diabetes.

Tetanus–Diphtheria (Td) Booster. Tetanus, also called "lockjaw," is a disease that causes your voluntary muscles to contract spasmodically. Diphtheria is a disease that causes a severe sore throat with a false membrane that forms in your throat, as well as inflammation of your heart and nervous system. Both are serious infections, which can lead to death, and they can occur at any age. Chance of death, however, increases with age.

The Td booster protects against both of these diseases. There are few, if any, side effects, although many people experience inflammation and/or soreness where the vaccine is administered. Td boosters retain their protective effect for approximately ten years. If you have not received a Td booster within this time frame, you are at risk for contracting the diseases if you receive a puncture wound or any type of injury where the tetanus or diphtheria bacteria can enter your system.

Mental Health

Many events common to old age can create stress or strain on your mental health. Your doctor will work with you to help you assess the need for care if you lose function due to illness or mental anxiety.

Alzheimer's Disease. In recent years, Alzheimer's disease has been recognized as a common cause of loss of mental function in older adults. While rare in people under age 50, Alzheimer's strikes ten percent of those over age 65 and almost half of those over age 85. Because the symptoms are sometimes attributed to "normal aging," researchers suspect that many cases of Alzheimer's go undiagnosed.

Alzheimer's is a condition caused by damage to the nerve cells in the brain. In a healthy adult, the brain sends orderly messages across neurons. For example, if you touch a pin and it hurts, the brain transmits that signal to your finger. In Alzheimer's patients, the messages cannot get through because the neurons become tangled and twisted. As they stop being used, they start to decay. The decaying neurons become stuck in an abnormal protein produced by the body, forming "plaques" in the brain. As more neurons are destroyed, the Alzheimer's sufferer's condition worsens.

The early signs of Alzheimer's include memory loss, especially forgetting about recent occurrences. For example, sufferers forget the names of people they just met, places they have recently been, or even what they have just said. Changes in personality often follow. Irritability and depression are common. Eventually, Alzheimer's sufferers lose intellectual capacity—the ability to think and speak—and physical function, such as the ability to control their bladders and bowels. There is no test available to confirm a diagnosis of Alzheimer's disease. However, most clinicians are able to diagnose the disorder from a patient's behavior. Treatment with medications to slow memory loss is available, but results are variable.

What causes Alzheimer's remains a mystery. Medical experts theorize that it may be a gene, an illness, or a natural, degenerative effect of aging. Research continues in the hopes of finding ways to treat and prevent Alzheimer's.

Small Strokes. Atherosclerotic plaque and emboli, or blood clots, can reduce the flow of blood to areas of the brain, causing the loss of small areas of brain cells, or small strokes. Individually, these strokes rarely cause symptoms or problems, but when several occur, the brain's ability to compensate for loss of function is overwhelmed. Changes in mood, memory, and behavior (called dementia) may be identical to Alzheimer's disease. Testing with CAT or MRI scans will show evidence of small strokes, however.

Recent research has shown that small strokes accelerate the damage and memory loss caused by Alzheimer's. Postmenopausal hormone replacement has been seen by some to reduce the development of both Alzheimer's and small strokes. Thus far, this is the most promising therapy for women. However, further research is needed before we have definitive proof of its efficacy.

Depression and Stress-Related Disorders. The death of a spouse, the loss of friends and loved ones, and your own illness or disability are high on the list of stressful events you may experience as you grow older. While stress is a natural response to situations such as these, stress that is frequent, chronic, or prolonged can impact your health. It can cause depression, sleeplessness, a change in eating habits, lack of energy, and decreased interest in sexual relations. Emotional stress can also cause or aggravate such physical ailments as migraine headaches, high

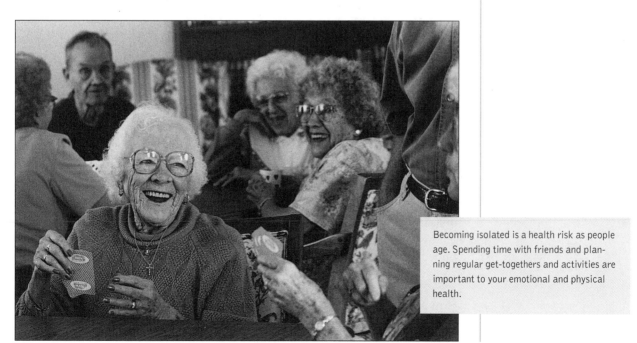

Becoming isolated is a health risk as people age. Spending time with friends and planning regular get-togethers and activities are important to your emotional and physical health.

How to Reduce Stress in Your Life

Try these techniques to reduce the stress in your life.

1. Exercise more frequently. Release the stress through physical activity, such as walking, running, swimming, or working around the house or in the garden.

2. Share your feelings of stress with someone else. Talk about your situation with a family member or close friend. Sharing the stress relieves some of the tension.

3. Take time to laugh and cry. Make sure you have time to play and have fun. Laugh a little, and it will help. Similarly, allowing yourself a good cry also releases tension and can even help prevent headaches.

4. Take good care of yourself. Make sure you eat well and get enough sleep. This will make you better equipped to deal with stressful situations.

5. Prioritize your responsibilities. You may find your list of responsibilities over-whelming. Prioritize the most important tasks, and work on those first. Then, you can tackle the remaining tasks.

6. Do not depend on alcohol or over-the-counter drugs to deal with stress. Alcohol and drugs only provide temporary relief from stress and in the long run can become habit-forming. Take drugs sparingly and only if your doctor recommends them.

7. Learn how to relax. Schedule time just to relax. Do not make any demands on yourself during this time. Choose a pleasurable activity that will help you forget your worries. Focus just on the activity, and enjoy yourself.

8. Seek professional help. If stress still seems overwhelming, seek professional help. Your physician can recommend a counselor who can help you cope and work through your situation.

blood pressure, bowel problems, backaches, ulcers, or even heart disease. It is important to make your physician aware of stress factors in your life as they develop. She can recommend the most effective ways to relieve stress.

What *You* Can Do

Make smart choices based on what you have learned about healthy living in your elder years. Enjoy this period of your life, when responsibilities to children and work may have lessened and you have more time to pursue your own interests. You want to maintain the highest possible quality of life for as long as possible. It is not as difficult as you may think. Review what you can do to stay healthy and avoid health risks. If you follow this prescription for healthy living, you will increase the chance that your elder years will be the best they can be.

- See your doctor for your regular preventive checkups. Don't wait until you need treatment for illness or for chronic illnesses.
- Schedule all recommended screenings and immunizations.

- If you smoke, stop. If you drink alcohol, limit your consumption.
- Maintain a nutritious diet and a regular exercise program to keep you strong and healthy.
- Take precautions to avoid injury, in and away from your home.
- Protect yourself from sexually transmitted diseases.
- Practice good dental hygiene, and visit the dentist regularly.
- Watch for signs of stress that can impact your good mental health. Limit your exposure to stressful situations, including friends and family members that make you feel angry or tense.
- Order your affairs so that you do not have to worry about the disposition of your property or money after you are gone. Worrying about these issues can be a major source of stress for women who have previously depended on spouses.
- When you have problems of any kind, acknowledge them, and don't hesitate to seek the help you need.
- Maintain healthy relationships with others who share common interests with you.
- Set a healthy example for others with your lifestyle.

PART III

A Healthy Lifestyle

A healthy lifestyle. You've read about it in magazines. You've heard about it on TV and the radio. It's almost a cliché. Yet behind every cliché is an important grain of truth. A healthy lifestyle can change your health now and for the future. Unfortunately, too many women today shun a healthy lifestyle because they are overwhelmed by one of two ideas: either that they are going to have to suffer for it, that they are going to be deprived of good food, good fun, and so on, or that it is too complicated, just "more things to do" in an already busy life.

The truth is that once you examine the key elements of a healthy lifestyle as outlined in Part III, you will see that shaping your current lifestyle into a healthier one does not need to leave you feeling shortchanged. For example, when it comes to nutrition and healthful food choices, the key is moderation. If you love butter, you don't have to give it up entirely. When it comes to exercise, again, moderation is the name of the game. With the exception of smoking, excessive alcohol consumption, drugs, and unsafe sex, there is very little you have to eradicate from your life completely—and much you

can do to improve the good habits you probably already have in place.

Armed with all the knowledge, facts, and amazing results that medical research has uncovered, there is no reason not to take responsibility for your own future and feel proud that you are doing it. One of the primary benefits of leading a healthy lifestyle is in the mental health department. You will get a tremendous boost of self-esteem and a dramatic sense of control and independence when you make choices such as eating better, quitting smoking, becoming more physically active, creating good sleep habits, avoiding harmful substances, safeguarding your home and family against injury, communicating more effectively with loved ones and coworkers, taking steps to prevent violence against yourself and others, and making and reaching goals related to sexuality, family planning, pregnancy, and menopause.

Part III synthesizes all the information, guidelines, tips, and advice you need to make your own decisions about shaping a healthier lifestyle—starting right now.

Eating *for* Wellness

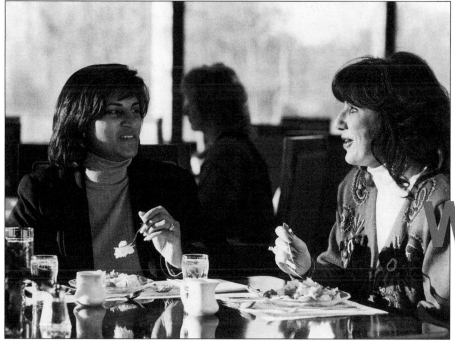

It seems that almost every day some new study or new finding about the relationship of food and health hits the newsstands. One day we read or hear about a food item that is good for us or one that is not, only to learn weeks later that the rules have changed. Salt, once blamed for increasing the risk of high blood pressure, stroke, and heart disease, has now been cleared of most charges except in salt-sensitive individuals. The fat in avocados, once believed to be as dangerous to your health as the fat in beef, is now categorized among the fats that are good for you. Small wonder that many women have problems choosing the right foods and eating a balanced diet.

One step toward achieving nutritional health is to learn how food works in the body and how to find an appropriate balance in the foods you choose. Another is to make intelligent use of the mass of information available to you—and sift out that information that most directly pertains to you and your age group and lifestyle. Americans have more nutrition information at their fingertips than ever before—witness the nutrition labels on packaged foods and the nutritional analyses in many cookbooks. This chapter helps you make sense of all that information and helps you understand the relationship between diet and health so that you can make informed decisions about the food you eat every day.

Here are three general, easy-to-remember guidelines that will help you establish healthful eating habits:

- Use moderation as your guide in eating and drinking.
- Vary the types of food you choose and the preparation methods you use.
- Balance your diet: too much of even a good thing could be too much.

Washing Produce

It is important to wash fruits and vegetables to remove dirt, bacteria, and residual pesticides. Wash with water, not with soap or detergent. Water is just as effective as soap at removing particles, and it does not leave the residue that soap can leave. While some liquid cleansers are being marketed specifically for washing produce, they have not proved more effective than water at cleaning fruits and vegetables.

Moderation, variety, and balance. This chapter explains how these three rules related to healthful eating can help you achieve and maintain your ideal weight.

The **Elements** of **Good** Nutrition

Nutrition—the science of food—looks at how the body is supplied with what it needs for life, health, and growth. Food does far more for your body than satisfy hunger. It supplies fuel for energy, protects against disease, and plays an essential role in overall health and vitality.

Unlike the koala bear, which can survive on a diet comprised solely of eucalyptus, humans need a variety of foods. Different types of food provide different types of nutrients, which in turn play different roles in the body. The nutrients are converted into energy and body "building blocks" (chemicals that can be used by cells) through a process known as metabolism, which occurs as food moves through the digestive tract.

Too little or too much food—or too little or too much of a particular nutrient—can have a negative effect on health: malnutrition and overabundance of calories or nutrients are contributing factors in many of the leading causes of death and disability. These negative outcomes can easily be prevented. Knowledge is the key: understanding the basics of nutrition puts you in control of getting the proper moderation, balance, and variety in your diet. These choices will improve your health and the quality of your life.

The basics of a good diet include adequate amounts of carbohydrates, proteins, and fats to help meet your daily energy requirements. In addition, other elements, such as vitamins and minerals, fiber, and water, are essential for good health.

Carbohydrates

Carbohydrates are your main source of energy so foods containing carbohydrates should be a major part of your diet. Foods that are high in carbohydrates include grains, vegetables, fruits, dry beans, and peas. To maintain energy, you need carbohydrates throughout the day.

There are two kinds of carbohydrates. Simple carbohydrates are sugars, such as the fructose and glucose found in fruits and vegetables, the lactose found in milk, and the sucrose found in sugar cane and beets, which is made into refined sugar. Complex carbohydrates are starches and dietary fiber found in rice, potatoes, bread, vegetables, beans, and grains.

Carbohydrates provide the body with energy through a process called oxidation. When carbohydrates are oxidized (burned up), they are converted into a simple sugar called glucose. Simple carbohydrates—sugars—can enter the bloodstream quickly and can provide a quick burst of energy. Complex carbohydrates—starches—on the other hand, take longer to convert, so you gain energy from starches over a longer period of time.

In addition to providing energy, carbohydrates play an important metabolic role. If your body's supply of glucose is low, the body must tap into its supply of fat and protein for alternative sources of energy. Dietary carbohydrates must be present for this fat-burning process to take place.

It is generally recommended that you get 55 to 60 percent of your total daily calories from carbohydrates, with an emphasis on complex carbohydrates. No more than 15 percent of your daily calories should come from simple carbohydrates.

Many women believe that they must cut down on carbohydrates if they want to lose weight. In fact, potatoes, pasta, and many other carbohydrate-rich foods are not high in calories. Because they are bulky and slow digestion, they actually reduce hunger and total caloric intake. The way they are prepared makes them fattening. Here are some suggestions for preparing foods high in carbohydrates without adding the fats that raise the calorie levels:

- Try pancakes without butter. Top them with low-fat yogurt and fresh fruit or reduced fat margarine products.
- Substitute mushrooms or peppers for meatballs with pasta.
- Replace whole-milk ricotta in lasagna with low-fat cottage cheese.
- Trade potato chips for a bowl of freshly popped popcorn, without salt and butter. For flavor, try a dash of cayenne pepper.
- Make macaroni salad, but hold the mayonnaise. Add low-fat yogurt instead.

Most supermarkets and health food stores carry a wonderful selection of grains that provide complex carbohydrates. Try different varieties of white and brown rice, jasmine, arborio, and basmati rice, kasha, polenta (a cornmeal food), couscous, amaranth, and grits. And don't forget the beans; dried beans are a rich source of fiber, vitamins, minerals, and protein as well as complex carbohydrates.

Proteins

Proteins are essential for building and repairing body tissues. The body uses proteins in skin, hair, nails, teeth, muscle, and many other components. Proteins are constantly being broken down in the body and need to be replaced.

Proteins are made up of chemicals called amino acids. Some amino acids can be produced in your own body, while others—known as essential amino acids—must by obtained from your diet. Essential amino acids are found in fish, meat, poultry, eggs, milk, and cheese. These foods are said to have complete proteins.

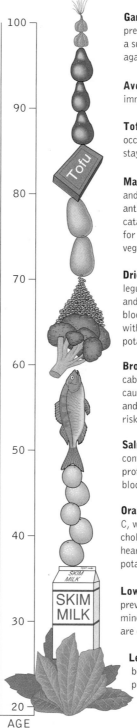

Garlic. Studies show garlic may help prevent some types of cancer, and contains a substance that may provide protection against heart disease.

Avocados. Vitamin B₆ helps boost your immune system.

Tofu. Soy products contain naturally-occurring estrogen that helps your bones stay strong and are rich in protein.

Mangoes. This tasty fruit is rich in niacin and beta-carotene, a substance that has anticancer properties and may help prevent cataracts and lung infection. This also goes for other yellow, orange, and red fruits and vegetables.

Dried Beans and Peas. Rich in fiber, legumes may lower your risk for colorectal and breast cancers and may lower your blood cholesterol. Legumes are also packed with B vitamins, calcium, iron, zinc, and potassium.

Broccoli. Along with other members of the cabbage family (kale, brussels sprouts, and cauliflower), broccoli contains antioxidants and other substances which may reduce the risk of certain cancers.

Salmon. The fat in this fish is good! It contains omega-3 fatty acids, which may protect against heart attacks and high blood pressure.

Oranges. Oranges are packed with vitamin C, which helps raise HDL, the "good cholesterol," and thus may help prevent heart disease. Oranges also contain potassium and beta-carotene.

Low-fat dairy products. The calcium helps prevent osteoporosis. Other vitamins and minerals, such as vitamin D and riboflavin, are essential for good health.

Leafy greens. Rich in folate, fiber, iron, beta-carotene, and calcium, these powerhouse vegetables are classic disease prevention foods, including cancer and heart disease.

FIGURE 8.1 **Foods for a Long Life**

Each of these foods contributes to longevity in a different way. Memorize these top ten heavy hitters—nutrient-dense foods that are recommended for a longer, healthier life.

Vegetarian Diets

Vegetarianism, once considered an "alternative" dietary lifestyle, has gained a great deal of popularity and is now considered mainstream. But vegetarianism is more than just a trend. Recent studies have shown that vegetarian diets can have significant health benefits. Vegetarians generally have lower blood pressure and cholesterol levels than most meat-eating Americans. As a result, they are less likely to develop heart disease or diabetes. Vegetarian diets are also beneficial to the digestive system, lowering the risk for both serious digestive problems (such as colon cancer) and minor ones (such as constipation and diverticulitis).

People choose to become vegetarians for a variety of reasons, ranging from wanting to improve their health to upholding religious or ethical beliefs. And while the term vegetarian is used to describe the diets of all these groups, there are actually many different types of vegetarians. Following are the general categories of vegetarianism:

- **Vegans** do not eat any foods of animal origin, including milk and eggs; they eat only foods from plant sources.
- **Lactovegetarians** avoid meat and eggs but consume dairy products as a source of protein.
- **Ovovegetarians** avoid meat and dairy products but consume eggs as a source of protein.
- **Lacto-ovovegetarians** include eggs and dairy products in their diets, but they do not eat meat.
- **Semivegetarians** usually maintain a diet of fruit, vegetables, grains, and dairy products, but they occasionally eat poultry, fish, and sometimes meat.

If you or someone in your family is, or is planning to become, a vegetarian, it is important to plan meals carefully. Vegetarians, and vegans in particular, must be sure to consume foods that contain the nutrients they would otherwise get from meat or dairy products. Following are the primary nutrients that strict vegetarian diets usually lack:

- **Calcium.** It is essential that women get adequate amounts of calcium to protect against osteoporosis. While calcium is found primarily in dairy products, it is also found in plants such as broccoli, kale, and collard greens. Eat foods rich in vitamin C to improve your body's absorption of calcium. You can also obtain calcium from calcium-fortified foods or from calcium supplements.
- **Iron and Zinc.** Iron and zinc are more readily absorbed when they are obtained from meat. Vegetarians need to obtain sufficient quantities of these minerals from plant foods. Iron is found in legumes, the skin of potatoes, fortified grain products, and dried fruit. Zinc is found in such foods as wheat germ, peas, and lentils.
- **Vitamin B$_{12}$.** Lack of vitamin B$_{12}$ can cause anemia and problems with the central nervous system. Vitamin B$_{12}$ is found only in animal products, so strict vegetarians must take supplements or eat fortified foods to get the proper amount.
- **Vitamin D.** Vitamin D helps the body absorb calcium and prevent bone mineral loss. Fortunately, your body can produce the necessary amount of vitamin D through occasional exposure to the sun. Supplements are also available and are frequently found with calcium.
- **Protein.** Unlike the protein found in fish and meats, the protein in legumes and grain products is incomplete, meaning it lacks one or more of the essential amino acids. By combining a number of protein-rich products, you can get the amount of protein your body requires.

Balance and variety are the keys to a healthy vegetarian diet. By eating a wide range of nutrient-rich foods, such as legumes (beans), vegetables, fruits, and whole-grain breads and cereals, you can easily obtain all the nutrients necessary to eat for wellness.

~~~~~~~~~~~~~~~~

Other foods, including dry beans and peas, nuts, seeds, vegetables, and grains, contain some but not all of the essential amino acids. They are said to provide incomplete proteins. You can get all of the essential amino acids, however, by combining certain incomplete proteins. For example, a peanut butter sandwich, which combines grain and peanuts, provides all the essential amino acids. You could also combine beans with rice, or dry beans with grains or nuts. Incomplete proteins do not need to be combined in the same dish, or even at the same meal. You just need to eat them during the same day. Knowing the correct combinations is particularly important to vegetarians who tend to avoid some or all of the foods that contain complete proteins.

Your body cannot store protein, so you need to eat adequate amounts of protein every day. How much protein do you need? The Recommended Dietary Allowance (RDA) for protein is based on a person's age and weight. A healthy adult needs 0.8 grams for each 2.2 pounds of body weight. This translates into about 44 grams for a 120-pound person and 55 grams for a 150-pound person. (Note that 55 grams of protein is roughly the amount found in two 2- to 3-ounce servings of lean cooked chicken or fish.) Most Americans eat far more protein than they need.

Fats

Fats can be stored by the body and can be used as a source of reserve energy. Fats also play a vital role in transporting and storing other nutrients, in insulating the body and protecting internal organs from injury, in maintaining healthy skin and hair, and in regulating body temperature.

Fats are found in many types of food. Foods that are especially high in fats include butter, cream, milk, cheese, some meats, nuts, fried foods, and many processed foods. Some fats, such as the fat in bacon or the cream cheese on a bagel, are easy to see. Other fats are less obvious. Did you know that avocados contain fat?

On news programs, in magazines, or on food labels you may have seen dietary fats classified as either saturated or unsaturated. Saturated fats are found in meat, whole milk, butter, coconut oil, and palm oil, and are generally solid at room temperature. Hydrogenation converts a liquid saturated fat to solid at room temperature. Unsaturated fats, found mainly in vegetable oils, nuts, and seeds, remain liquid at room temperature.

Americans are generally advised to restrict their intake of saturated fats to a maximum of ten percent of total calories. This is because saturated fats are associated

wellness **tip**

It is important to remove the skin from chicken before serving, since chicken skin is 85 percent fat and there is a high concentration of fat between the skin and the meat. It is not necessary to remove the skin before cooking, however, as studies have shown that fat from the skin does not migrate to the meat during cooking.

Heart-Healthy Eating Tips

1. Use the new Nutrition Facts label as a tool. The labels provide information about calories, fat, and sodium.
2. Keep in mind that the advice to keep calories from fat to less than 30 percent does not apply to individual foods but to your entire diet over a period of a week.
3. The body needs polyunsaturated fats and fat-soluble vitamins; include fats, such as liquid oils and margarine, in a heart-healthy diet.
4. Watch serving portion sizes, particularly of protein. Three ounces of cooked meat is about the size of a deck of cards.
5. To reduce your intake of cholesterol-laden egg yolks, mix one egg yolk with two to three egg whites.
6. Try fat-free versions of your favorite foods. Use cooking spray to reduce fat when sautéing and to oil baking pans.
7. Make vegetables, grains, beans, peas, and fruit—which are naturally low-fat—the center of the meal; use meat as a side dish.
8. When eating out, don't be afraid to make special requests (for example, ask that dressings be served on the side).
9. Look for words that signal that a food is high in fat: buttered, fried, creamy, with gravy, au gratin, scalloped.
10. Make the transition to a new heart-healthy diet slowly by adding or replacing one or two items at a time.

Source: Adapted from "Guide to Heart Healthy Eating," available from the American Medical Women's Association, 801 N. Fairfax Street, Suite 400, Alexandria, VA 22314.

**15 Easy Ways to Cut
Fat Consumption**

1. **Read labels when you shop,
   avoid foods high in fat.**
2. **Choose cooking oils that
   are low in saturated fat.**
3. **When buying meat,
   choose lean grades.**
4. **Use skim or low-fat milk
   instead of whole milk or
   cream; use low-fat and
   part-skim milk cheeses.**
5. **Use fish or poultry in
   place of meat in main
   dishes.**
6. **Replace high-fat ingredients with low-fat ones.**
7. **Broil, bake, or roast meat
   instead of frying.**
8. **Use cooking spray instead
   of butter, margarine, or oil
   to coat pans.**
9. **Trim fat from meats and
   remove skin from poultry.**
10. **Use a low-fat spread, like
    jelly, on toast or bagels.**
11. **Avoid cream-based recipes.**
12. **Eat fruits, vegetables, or
    popcorn for snacks.**
13. **Avoid high-fat breads, like
    croissants and sweet rolls.**
14. **When dining out, request
    vegetarian dishes.**
15. **Choose green salad with
    low-fat dressing as an
    appetizer.**

with high levels of cholesterol and an increased risk of cardiovascular disease, as well as certain cancers. (Cholesterol is discussed in more depth later in this chapter.)

Unsaturated fats can be divided into two types: polyunsaturated fats, such as corn, safflower, sesame, and sunflower oils, and monounsaturated fats, such as olive, peanut, and canola oil. The distinction between the two types is significant: polyunsaturated oils tend to lower the amount of LDL ("bad") cholesterol in the bloodstream but also reduce levels of HDL ("good") cholesterol. Monounsaturated fats reduce LDL levels without producing a corresponding reduction in HDLs. Thus, olive, peanut, and canola oil are the preferred oils in a healthy diet.

How much fat do you need in your diet? Nutritionists generally recommend that healthy individuals get no more than 30 percent of their total calories from fat, and that they try to get most of those calories from unsaturated fats. Consuming enough fat is not a problem in this country; most Americans eat more fat than they need and more than is good for them. Excess fat in the diet contributes to obesity and to high cholesterol levels, which in turn contribute to a variety of serious health problems. However, some healthy oils found in margarine products, mayonnaise, and nuts have healthy fat soluble nutrients and antioxidants, which have been shown to reduce heart disease.

Vitamins and Minerals

Vitamins and minerals are often referred to as micronutrients because they are needed in very small quantities. Nonetheless, they are essential for good health. A well-balanced diet rich in fruits and vegetables generally provides all the vitamins and minerals you need, though pregnant or lactating women may be advised to take supplements.

Vitamins help certain chemical reactions take place in the body and facilitate other processes, such as bone formation and the immune response. Minimum amounts of vitamins needed to prevent certain diseases have been established by the U.S. Food and Nutrition Board. These RDAs are sufficient to create substantial stores in the body. Supplements that exceed RDA levels do not have any value for the average American. However, daily supplements that modestly exceed RDA doses are not harmful either. High doses of certain vitamins (such as vitamin A) can actually be toxic, while a lack of any one vitamin (such as vitamin C) can produce a specific deficiency disease. Descriptions of the sources of vitamins and minerals, their functions, RDAs, and associated deficiency disorders appear in the boxes on pages 151 and 152.

Minerals are substances that form part of many tissues, help regulate fluid levels, maintain a healthy nervous system, and keep various body processes operating smoothly. The body constantly absorbs, uses, and excretes minerals, so they need to be replaced regularly.

Minerals occur naturally in the earth. They pass from soil to plant to animals. A varied and balanced diet that includes plant foods and plant-eating animals normally provides sufficient quantities of all of the necessary minerals except, perhaps, calcium. Women are often advised to take calcium supplements to build up their bone stores as a safeguard against osteoporosis later in life. Some women choose to supplement their diet with other minerals as well.

Once a mineral is absorbed in the body, the blood carries it to the cells for use, where it competes with other minerals for absorption. Be aware that too

Vitamins

Vitamin A. Helps promote healthy hair, teeth, and nails. Vitamin A also contributes to eye function. Night blindness, dry eyes, dry skin, and reduced growth in children are signs of a deficiency. Overdosing with vitamin A can lead to painful joints, rashes, diarrhea, hair loss, dry skin, and fatigue. Beta-carotene, a precursor to vitamin A, is water soluble and does not accumulate in dangerous levels. It is found along with vitamin A in low-fat dairy products, green and deep yellow vegetables, yellow or orange fruits, and organ meats. RDA: 4,000 IU.

Thiamine (vitamin B_1). Contributes to nerve function and digestion and enhances appetite. In extreme cases of deficiency, it can cause beriberi, muscle wasting, and heart failure. It is available in pork, grains, cereals, and seafood. RDA: 1.5 mg.

Riboflavin (vitamin B_2). Needed to metabolize foods and maintain mucous membranes. Important for the formation of red blood cells. Deficiencies manifest as visual problems and difficulty in swallowing or eating. It is available in meat, fish, chicken, leafy greens, beans, and nuts. RDA: 1.2 to 1.3 mg. No toxic effects have been reported in higher doses.

Niacin (vitamin B_3). Required for enzymes to convert food into energy. Enhances nerve function, appetite, and digestion, and lowers cholesterol. Detoxifies body of effects of drugs. Deficiencies manifest as skin problems, diarrhea, and mouth sores. It is available in poultry, seafood, nuts, potatoes, cereals, and fortified whole grain breads. RDA: 13 to 15 mg. More than 100 mg can cause flushing, itching, diarrhea, and ulcers (in amounts greater than 100 to 300 mg). Higher doses are sometimes used to lower cholesterol but in susceptible individuals can cause liver abnormalities. Niacin should be used for this purpose only under a doctor's supervision.

Pantothenic acid (vitamin B_5). Essential for converting food to forms accessible by the body. No known deficiencies; it is manufactured in the intestines. RDA: 10 mg.

Pyridoxine (vitamin B_6). Essential for protein metabolism and absorption and red blood cell formation. Deficiencies manifest as anemia, depression, confusion, inflammation of mucous membranes of the mouth, and convulsion in infants. It is often used to alleviate premenstrual symptoms and, when taken with B_{12} and folate, may reduce the risk of heart disease by decreasing homocysteine levels. It is available from meats, fish, poultry, grains, cereals, bananas, prunes, and watermelon. RDA: 1.4 to 1.6 mg. Irreversible nerve damage has been reported at doses in the 150-200 mg. range.

Vitamin B_{12}. Important for building genetic material (nucleic acid), blood cells, and nerves. Deficiencies cause pernicious anemia (a chronic, sometimes fatal, form of anemia) and progressive nerve damage, not all of which is reversible. Some people cannot absorb B_{12} from dietary sources and need to receive it in injectable form. Available in meats, poultry, and eggs. RDA: 2.0 mcg. No toxic effects have been reported in higher doses. It is used with B_6 and folate to reduce the risk of heart disease.

Vitamin C. Promotes healthy cell walls and gums. Helps the body resist infection. Can help overcome stress and improve disease resistance. Acts as an antioxidant, which may reduce the risk of heart disease and cancer. Deficiencies manifest as dry skin, slow healing, and in extreme cases, scurvy. Available in citrus fruits and juices, strawberries, watermelon, cabbage, broccoli, peppers, and plantains. RDA: 60 mg. Excess vitamin C is promptly excreted in the urine and it can be used to make the urine acidic to fight infection. More than 1,000 to 2,000 mg can impair immunity and cause kidney stones.

Vitamin D. Helps maintain healthy bones and strong teeth by affecting calcium metabolism. Deficiency manifests in children as rickets. Vitamin D is available in egg yolks, fish oils, fortified milk, and butter but is also made in the skin from occasional exposure to the sun. RDA: 200 to 400 IU. Overdosing can cause diarrhea, drowsiness, nausea, vomiting, and loss of appetite. In susceptible persons, more than 1,200 IU can lead to kidney stones or calcification of soft tissue.

Vitamin E. Helps form red blood cells, muscles, and tissues and acts as an antioxidant. It improves circulation, promotes normal clotting, repairs tissue, and is helpful in treating fibrocystic breasts and alleviating premenstrual syndrome. It also reduces the risk of coronary heart disease. Zinc is required to maintain the proper levels of vitamin E in the blood. It is available in poultry and seafood, nuts, wheat germ, eggs, and vegetable oils. Tocopherols, chemical compounds that have the same effect on the body as vitamin E, can be found in oil, nuts, wheat germ, and antioxidant supplements. Few women have diets with sufficient caloric intake to provide adequate levels of vitamin E. However, diets rich in natural sources of vitamin E (margarine products, nuts, and oils) protect against heart disease. RDA: 12 IU. Doses over 800 IU can cause excessive blood thinning and bleeding tendencies.

Vitamin K. Required for blood clotting, contributes to bone formation, and helps prevent osteoporosis. It is found in alfalfa, broccoli, dark green leafy vegetables, and soybeans. RDA: 55 to 65 mcg. It reverses the effect of the blood thinning drug coumadin (warfarin) so large amounts should not be consumed by individuals on that medication.

Minerals

Calcium. Helps build strong bones and teeth. Important for nerve and muscle function. Deficiencies manifest as rickets in children and osteoporosis in adults. Available in milk and milk products, canned salmon with bones, oysters, broccoli, and tofu. It is more effective when taken in smaller doses throughout the day and with small amounts of fat. It works less effectively when taken all at once. Nonmenstruating female athletes and women going through menopause require greater amounts owing to decreased estrogen effect, which causes greater bone loss. RDA: 800 to 1,200 mg; 1,200 to 1,500 mg in postmenopausal, pregnant, or lactating women.

Chromium. Required to metabolize glucose and important in the synthesis of cholesterol, fats, and protein. Chromium (also known as glucose tolerance factor) maintains stable blood sugar levels in people with diabetes and hypoglycemia. Found in raw sugar, water, meat, cheese, whole grains, and fortified cereals. Two out of three Americans are chromium deficient, owing to a depletion of chromium from soil and the water supply and diets high in refined sugars and flours. Cutting down on refined sugars and augmenting chromium levels with supplements may prevent susceptible adults from developing adult-onset diabetes. RDA: 800 to 1,200 mg.

Folic acid (folate). Folic acid is required for the formation of red blood cells and is necessary for DNA synthesis. It may be helpful in treating such diverse conditions as anxiety, depression, and cervical dysplasia. It helps regulate embryonic function and is essential for fetal nerve cell development. Neural tube defects (NTDs) in newborns have been linked to folic acid deficiencies. Mild folic acid deficiencies can lead to spontaneous abortion, low birth weight, and growth retardation. It is available in barley, beans, dates, chicken, whole grains, pork, root vegetables, spinach, wheat germ, salmon, tuna, milk, and oranges. Recently, scientists confirmed that folic acid can protect us from heart disease by reducing the production of homocysteine, a blood vessel irritant. Standard replacement dose for deficiencies is 400 to 1,000 mcg. Use of oral contraceptives and certain antiseizure medication may increase the need for folic acid. RDA: 400 to 800 mcg.

Iodine. Important for thyroid function. Deficiency manifests as goiter (enlarged thyroid gland) and underactive thyroid function with weakness and lethargy. Available in iodized salt, seafood, or vegetables from iodine-rich soil or the sea (kelp, seaweed). RDA: 150 mcg.

Iron. Important for manufacture of hemoglobin. Essential to red blood cell function and oxygen transport. Deficiencies manifest as fatigue, shortness of breath, and iron-deficiency anemia. Available in red meats, shellfish, legumes, fortified breads and cereals and from cooking with cast iron pans. Found in supplements with sulfates and gluconates and is best absorbed with foods containing vitamin C. RDA: 18 mg.

Magnesium. Promotes bone growth. Activates enzymes to release energy. Deficiencies manifest as cramps, muscle weakness, and heart rhythm disturbances most commonly seen in alcoholics, people on diuretics, and kidney patients. Magnesium deficiencies in pregnancy are associated with high blood pressure and toxemia. Available in leafy vegetables, beans, nuts, oysters, and scallops. Often used as a supplement in the treatment of premenstrual syndrome. RDA: 400 mg.

Phosphorous. Converts food to energy to form healthy bones and teeth, and helps maintain proper kidney function. Deficiencies are rare. Balance should be maintained among magnesium, calcium, and phosphorous. Insufficient or excess amounts of one of these will affect the body adversely. Excess amounts of phosphorous can interfere with calcium uptake. Available in dairy products, egg yolks, meat, poultry, and fish. RDA: 1 g.

Potassium. Important for a healthy nervous system and a regular heart rhythm. Essential for hormone secretion, normal cell and muscle function. With sodium, potassium is found in the body's water supply. Regulates the transfer of nutrients to cells and cellular impulses. Available in dairy, fish, fruit, legumes, meat, vegetables, and whole grains, especially apricots, bananas, blackstrap molasses, nuts, potatoes, oranges, raisins, tomatoes, winter squash, wheat bran, and yams. Potassium levels can be depleted by diabetes, kidney disorder, diarrhea, use of diuretics, and laxatives. Stress can cause an imbalance in the potassium-sodium ratio. RDA: 1,600 to 2,000 mg minimum.

Sodium. Important for normal cell and nerve function and fluid balance. Deficiencies cause seizures and weakness. Found as a supplement in most processed foods and in vegetables from the sea (kelp, seaweed). Most Americans get too much sodium. Excess sodium can cause high blood pressure in sensitive individuals, swelling, or fluid retention. RDA: 2400 mg or less.

Zinc. Important for bone growth, digestion of protein, metabolism of energy through action on thyroid hormone conversion and insulin. Also important for sense of taste, wound healing, maintaining levels of vitamin A in the blood, and overcoming anorexia. Found in eggs, poultry, wheat germ, milk, beans, liver, oysters, and crabmeat. RDA: 15 mg.

Units of Weight
g = gram (a U.S. nickel weighs 5 grams)
mg = milligram (1,000 mg = 1 g)
mcg = microgram (1,000 mcg = 1 mg)
IU = International Unit (arbitrary value, not based on weight)

much of one mineral can deplete another. For example, excessive amounts of calcium inhibit magnesium absorption. If you do feel that you need to add minerals (or vitamins) to your diet, consider a multiple vitamin/mineral supplement. This way, you will be assured that you are receiving the RDA for the necessary vitamins and minerals, without taking toxic (too much) or inadequate (too little) amounts. Multiple-dose vitamin/mineral supplements that allow you to take more than one dose per day help maximize absorption and are usually recommended to be taken with meals.

Fiber

Fiber is not strictly a nutrient, since it cannot be absorbed by the body, but it plays an essential role in the digestive process. Sources of fiber include fruits and vegetables (especially the peels and seeds), oat and wheat bran, dried beans and peas, barley, and whole grains.

There are soluble and insoluble fibers. Soluble fibers bind with water to form gels, which soften stool and relieve constipation. Soluble fibers have also been shown to lower blood cholesterol levels and slow the entry of glucose into the bloodstream, reducing the risk of diabetes.

Insoluble fibers increase stool bulk, helping it pass through the digestive tract more efficiently. Insoluble fibers may also help alleviate certain digestive disorders (see list below) and are believed to help prevent colon cancer.

A high-fiber diet can protect against or help ease the following conditions:

- **Chronic constipation** by increasing the bulk of stool, softening stool, and by stimulating contractions of the bowel.
- **Diverticulosis** (a condition in which tiny sacs called diverticula form in the wall of the colon) by reducing the muscle contraction pressure of the intestines needed to push stool through the bowel. This reduces the chance of developing diverticulitis, a condition in which the diverticula become infected or inflamed.
- **Irritable bowel syndrome** (irregular contractions of the bowel muscles, resulting in diarrhea, constipation, bloating, pain, or other abdominal disorders) by increasing the bulk of stool and reducing muscle contraction pressure needed to move stool through the bowel.
- **Colon cancer.** Further research is needed, but it is widely believed that a high-fiber diet helps protect against colon cancer by speeding the movement of toxins through the bowel to reduce contact with tissue, or through other means.
- **Heart disease.** Some of the soluble fibers, such as pectin (in many fruits) and oat and wheat bran, have been shown to lower cholesterol absorption from dietary sources. High cholesterol can lead to cardiovascular disease.
- **Diabetes.** In some studies, patients with diabetes who ate moderate amounts of oatmeal as part of a high-carbohydrate, high-fiber diet required less insulin than patients on regular diets. By slowing absorption of food, fiber reduces the insulin the body needs to produce at any one time and stabilizes blood sugar after eating.
- **Weight control.** Many dietary aids are actually various types of fiber. They work by adding bulk to the diet and providing a feeling of fullness. High-fiber foods also reduce caloric intake by moving foods through the digestive tract more quickly and by blocking the action of digestive enzymes, which cause breakdown and absorption of food calories.

Canned or fresh?

Which is better: canned or fresh fruits and vegetables? While some nutrients are lost during the canning process, new technologies allow canned fruits and vegetables to retain most of their vitamins and minerals. On the other hand, most "fresh" fruits and vegetables that you find at the supermarket are actually picked before they are ripe, shipped thousands of miles, and stored for long periods of time—all of which lead to significant nutrient losses. Choose fruits and vegetables that are locally grown when you can—or grow your own.

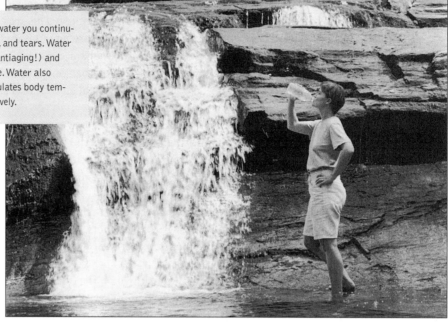

Eight glasses of water a day replaces the water you continually lose through your breath, urine, sweat, and tears. Water hydrates your skin from within (good for antiaging!) and prevents dehydration, which causes fatigue. Water also transports nutrients, lubricates joints, regulates body temperature, and helps eliminate waste effectively.

Water

Nearly 70 percent of your body weight consists of water. Water makes up approximately 75 percent of muscle tissue and about 25 percent of body fat. Even bones are 20 percent water. Water is involved in nearly every body process, including digestion, circulation, and excretion. It is essential for maintaining a normal body temperature. Although you could survive for weeks without food, you could not survive without water for more than a few days.

Your body loses water continually through breathing, sweating, and elimination, so you need to constantly replenish the water in your body. The best way to do this is to drink plenty of water—nutritionists generally recommend six to eight glasses a day for good health. You need more than that when the weather is hot or when you exercise or do physically demanding work. Water has other advantages too: it is free, contains no calories, helps you feel full, and speeds the digestive process. Excessive water intake can lower your blood sodium level and cause weakness and seizures. If there is excessive loss of sodium in sweat, salt tablets are sometimes taken, along with water replenishment.

Developing *a*
Balanced Diet

It is one thing to know the basics of nutrition but quite another to put that knowledge to use. How do you make sure you are getting all the essential nutrients in the right amounts? How do you achieve the proper moderation, variety, and balance? Where do you begin? Various guidelines, ranging from simple to quite complex, have been developed to help you.

Using the Food Guide Pyramid

One recommendation is that you use the Food Guide Pyramid. A simple method designed to help people choose and create balanced meals, the Food Guide Pyramid was developed by the U.S. Department of Agriculture (USDA). It recommends specific numbers of daily servings from each of these five main food groups:

- Bread, cereal, rice, and pasta
- Fruits
- Vegetables
- Meat, poultry, fish, dry beans, eggs, and nuts
- Milk, yogurt, and cheese

A sixth group, consisting of fats, oils, and sweets, is to be used sparingly.

The Food Guide Pyramid demonstrates graphically how many daily servings you should choose from each food group. The base of the pyramid represents the largest amount of food needed; the top of the pyramid represents the smallest amount needed. Notice that the foods at the base of the pyramid are those that are high in complex carbohydrates, low in fat, and often high in fiber. You need between 6 and 11 servings of the foods in this group every day. As you move up the pyramid, the number of recommended servings gets smaller. At least 5 servings of fruits and vegetables are recommended daily to reduce the risk of cancer and heart disease and provide vitamins and nutrients to the diet. At the top of the pyramid are fats, oils, and sweets, for which there are no recommended servings,

FIGURE 8.2
Food Guide Pyramid
The Food Guide Pyramid helps you create a balanced diet by giving the suggested number of daily servings from each food group.

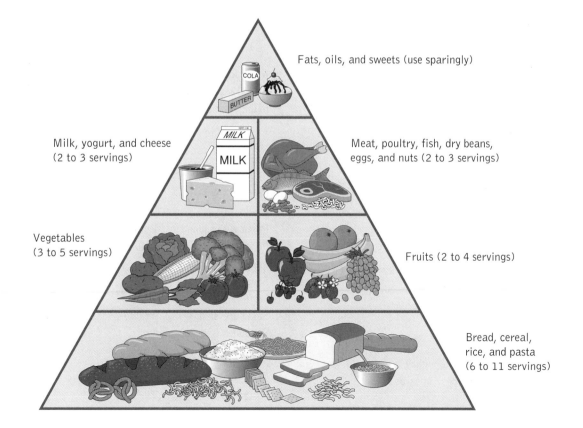

Fats, oils, and sweets (use sparingly)

Milk, yogurt, and cheese
(2 to 3 servings)

Meat, poultry, fish, dry beans, eggs, and nuts (2 to 3 servings)

Vegetables
(3 to 5 servings)

Fruits (2 to 4 servings)

Bread, cereal, rice, and pasta
(6 to 11 servings)

in part because you will get as much as you need of these foods from the foods in the other pyramid boxes.

One key to using the Food Guide Pyramid successfully is understanding serving sizes. The serving sizes are *small*. In the bread, cereal, rice, and pasta group, for example, a single slice of bread represents one serving. Five or six small crackers represent one serving. A half-cup of cooked cereal is one serving. When you realize how small the servings are, you begin to see that eating 6 to 11 servings in one day would not amount to a great deal of food. The box "What Constitutes a Serving?" gives examples of servings for each of the five recommended food groups.

Another key to using the Food Guide Pyramid successfully is to focus on variety. Make sure that your five servings of fruits and vegetables consist of *different* fruits and vegetables: maybe banana on your breakfast cereal or yogurt; lettuce and bean sprouts on your sandwich at lunch; and then carrots and broccoli for dinner. By focusing on variety you make sure that you get all the nutrients you need.

The Food Guide Pyramid, when used intelligently, represents a simple way of bringing moderation, variety, and balance to your diet.

What Constitutes a Serving?

There are a number of misconceptions about what "one serving" really is. While most people believe that a serving is enough food to satisfy their appetite, serving sizes—as defined by the Food Guide Pyramid—are relatively small portions. Following are sample serving sizes from each food group.

Bread, Cereal, Rice, and Pasta

1 slice of bread
1 medium muffin
$^1/_2$ of a bagel or English muffin
$^1/_2$ cup of cooked cereal, rice, or pasta
1 cup of cold cereal

Fruits

1 whole medium fruit (apple, banana, orange, etc.)
$^1/_4$ cup of dried fruit
$^1/_2$ cup of canned or chopped fruit
$^3/_4$ cup of fruit juice

Vegetables

1 cup of raw leafy vegetables
$^1/_2$ cup of cooked vegetables
$^1/_2$ cup raw chopped vegetables
$^3/_4$ cup of vegetable juice

Meat, Poultry, Fish, Dry Beans, Eggs, and Nuts

3 oz. of cooked lean meat, poultry, or fish
(about the size of a deck of cards)

1 egg
$^1/_2$ cup of cooked legumes
$^1/_2$ cup of nuts or seeds
4 tbsp. peanut butter

Milk, Yogurt, and Cheese

1 cup of milk or yogurt
2 slices ($1^1/_2$ oz.) of cheese
$^1/_2$ cup of cottage cheese
$1^1/_2$ cups of ice milk or frozen yogurt

Now look at some of these serving sizes compared to what a typical restaurant serves, and you will see why Americans tend to underestimate what they eat by as much as 50 percent!

	Official USDA Serving	Typical Restaurant
Bagel	2 oz.	4–5 oz.
Chips	2 oz.	3 oz.+
French fries	3 oz.	6–8 oz.
Ice cream	$^1/_2$ cup	1 cup+
Pasta with sauce	1 cup	3 cups
Popcorn	2 cups	8–12 cups
Meat	3 oz.	6–16 oz.
Soda	8 oz.	16 oz.+
Muffin	2 oz.	4–6 oz.
Salad dressing	2 tablespoons	4 tablespoons
Sandwich	4 oz.	9–12 oz.
Pizza slice	5 oz.	9 oz.+

Source: Berkeley Wellness Letter, University of California, September 1997.

Using the Dietary Guidelines

General dietary guidelines were published by the U.S. Department of Agriculture and the U.S. Department of Health and Human Services in the mid-1990s. The guidelines are intended to help Americans choose foods that will meet their nutrient requirements, promote health, support active lives, and reduce the risk of developing a chronic disease. The guidelines make the following suggestions:

1. Eat a variety of foods.
2. Balance the food you eat with physical activity.
3. Maintain or improve your weight.
4. Choose a diet with plenty of grain products, vegetables, and fruits.
5. Choose a diet low in fat, saturated fat, and cholesterol.
6. Choose a diet moderate in sugars.
7. Choose a diet moderate in salt and sodium.
8. If you drink alcoholic beverages, do so in moderation.

Notice how the guidelines emphasize moderation, variety, and balance—the three basic rules outlined at the beginning of this chapter. Notice too, the emphasis is on foods high in carbohydrates and low in fats—which mirrors the Food Guide Pyramid. And notice the attention to weight control and physical activity—important components of any sensible health plan or wellness program.

Using Nutrition Labels

New labeling regulations for packaged foods were introduced in the mid-1990s. Almost all processed foods and some raw foods must carry a Nutrition Facts label that lists the major nutrients, both in grams and milligrams, and also as a percentage of the recommended daily value (see Figure 8.3). The daily values, listed in the columns in the lower half of the label, are the recommended amounts of nutrients for a person who needs 2,000 calories a day. Some labels also list the daily values for a person who needs 2,500 calories a day. (Individual caloric needs are discussed later in this chapter.)

Listed on the labels are the amounts per serving of calories, fat, cholesterol, sodium, carbohydrate, and protein. Percentages for vitamins A and C, for calcium, and for iron are also provided. The amount of fat in the food is broken down to show how much of that fat is saturated fat—an aid for those who are carefully controlling their intake of fat.

Using nutrition labels enables you to make sure you get the daily nutrients you need and dissuades you from choosing certain foods when you see just how many calories, how much fat, or how much sodium, they contain. And be sure to check the serving size at the top of the label before you look at the percentages. You will be surprised at how many servings some containers hold.

Other types of food labels are also subject to regulation. The language that labels can use has been strictly defined, though the unwary consumer could still be fooled. The American Heart Association offers the following definitions:

- **Calorie-free** actually means fewer than 5 calories per serving.
- **Light** means $1/3$ fewer calories or no more than $1/2$ the fat of the higher-calorie, higher-fat brand, or no more than $1/2$ the sodium of the higher-sodium brand.

Hidden Sugars

Sugar in processed foods is hidden under many names:

- caramel
- corn sweetener
- corn syrup
- dextrin
- dextrose
- fructose
- fruit juice
- glucose
- honey
- invert syrup/sugar
- lactose
- lycasin*
- malt
- maltodextrin
- maltose
- mannitol*
- sorbitol*
- sorghum syrup
- sucrose
- xylitol*

* Sugar alcohol, derived from monosaccharides. Sugar alcohols have the same number of calories as sugar.

FIGURE 8.3

Nutrition Labels

Take time at the supermarket to read food labels to make healthful food choices and control your intake of fat, sugar, and sodium.

- **Fat-free** means less than 0.5 gram of fat per serving.
- **Low fat** means 3 grams (or less) per serving.
- **Sodium-free** or **no sodium** indicates that there are less than 5 milligrams of sodium per serving, and no sodium chloride.
- **Very low sodium** means that there are 35 milligrams of sodium or less per serving.
- **Low sodium** means that there are 140 milligrams of sodium or less per serving.
- **Reduced sodium** or **less sodium** indicates that there is at least 25 percent less sodium per serving than the higher-sodium brand of that product.
- **High fiber** indicates that there are 5 grams or more of fiber per serving.
- **Good source of fiber** indicates that there are 2.5 to 4.9 grams of fiber per serving.

Nutrition Facts

Serving Size 1/2 Cup (49g/1.8 oz.)
Servings per Container About 10

Amount Per Serving	Cereal	Cereal with 1/2 Cup Vitamins A & D Skim Milk
Calories	190	230
Fat Calories	25	25

	% Daily Value **	
Total Fat 3.0g*	5 %	5 %
Saturated Fat 0.5g	3 %	3 %
Cholesterol 0mg	0 %	0 %
Sodium 120mg	5 %	8 %
Potassium 120mg	4 %	10 %
Total Carbohydrate 39g	13 %	15 %
Dietary Fiber 3g	12 %	12 %
Soluble Fiber 1g		
Sugars 12g		
Other Carbohydrate 24g		
Protein 4g		

Vitamin A	15 %	20 %
Vitamin C	4 %	6 %
Calcium	2 %	15 %
Iron	10 %	10 %
Vitamin D	10 %	25 %
Thiamin	25 %	30 %
Riboflavin	25 %	35 %
Niacin	25 %	25 %
Vitamin B6	25 %	25 %
Folate	25 %	25 %
Vitamin B12	25 %	35 %
Phosphorus	10 %	20 %
Magnesium	10 %	15 %
Zinc	25 %	30 %
Copper	4 %	6 %

*Amount in cereal. One half cup of skim milk contributes an additional 65mg sodium, 6g total carbohydrate (6g sugars), and 4g protein.
**Percent Daily Values are based on a 2,000 calorie diet. Your daily values may be higher or lower depending on your calorie needs:

		Calories	2,000	2,500
Total Fat	Less than		65g	80g
Sat. Fat	Less than		20g	25g
Cholesterol	Less than		300mg	300mg
Sodium	Less than		2,400mg	2,400mg
Potassium			3,500mg	3,500mg
Total Carbohydrate			300g	375g
Dietary Fiber			25g	30g

Calories per gram: Fat 9 • Carbohydrate 4 • Protein 4

Servings. The label shows both the size of one serving (in customary and metric measurements) and the number of servings contained in the package. Many packaged foods contain more than one serving.

Calories. This section gives the total amount of calories in one serving and the number of calories that come from fat in that serving.

Nutrients. The amount of each nutrient a serving contains is given in grams or milligrams.

Percent Daily Value. This section also shows the amount of each nutrient as a percentage of the daily value. The percent daily value is a recommendation of health experts based on a 2,000 calorie daily diet.

Daily Values. These are the recommended amounts of each nutrient for a 2,000 and 2,500 calorie daily diet. The percent daily values are derived from these recommendations. Daily values are given as either a maximum or minimum amount.

Conversion Guide. This section provides information about the number of calories in 1 gram of fat, carbohydrate, and protein.

What About Cholesterol?

Cholesterol is fat that the body must use to maintain proper nerve function and healthy cells. It is also essential for the formation and regulation of hormones, such as estrogen. In the liver, your body actually manufactures all the cholesterol it needs for this job.

Cholesterol in the diet is derived mainly from animal sources, such as red meat. When you consume more cholesterol than your body can use, the extra cholesterol attaches itself to proteins and lipids (fats) in your bloodstream, where it becomes a lipoprotein. There are two major kinds of lipoproteins: high-density lipoproteins (HDL, the "good" cholesterol) and low-density lipoproteins (LDL, the "bad" or harmful cholesterol). LDL actually circulates cholesterol through the bloodstream, where it is oxidized and enters cells attached to the walls of your arteries—called plaque. A buildup of cholesterol deposits in plaque leads to hardening of the arteries and a condition called atherosclerosis. HDL actually removes LDL cholesterol from your bloodstream and from plaque, by transporting it to your liver, where it can be eliminated from your body.

Blood Lipid Levels. It is important to have your blood lipid levels (the levels of cholesterol and other fats in the blood) measured by a doctor to determine if you are at risk for atherosclerosis, which can lead to coronary artery disease or heart attack. Do not get your cholesterol tested with a quick finger-stick test at the mall—these tests may be less accurate or misleading if the breakdown of LDL and HDL is not given. For best results, get tested in your doctor's office and fast for 12 to 16 hours before the test with nothing to eat or drink except water. If you have a family history of early atherosclerosis or high cholesterol, have your blood lipid levels tested soon.

Triglycerides are another common type of fat derived from vegetable and animal sources. They are stored in the body as a fat and at high levels increase a woman's risk of diabetes, pancreatitis, and atherosclerosis. High blood levels of triglycerides are a risk factor for heart disease, especially in women. They often accompany other known risk factors for heart disease, such as diabetes, obesity, hypertension, and low HDL. In fact, women with diabetes who have high triglyceride levels are especially susceptible to cardiovascular disease. It is believed that high triglycerides make LDL cholesterol more likely to enter plaque and lead to atherosclerosis.

Lowering Cholesterol Levels. Fortunately, cholesterol can be lowered in most situations through diet. A diet low in saturated fats and cholesterol can reduce your cholesterol levels and lower your risk of heart attack by two to three percent for every one percent drop in total serum cholesterol. The American Heart Association has established dietary guidelines in the form of Step I and Step II Diets (see box on next page). You may also try the following:

- Eat fewer foods that are high in saturated fats, such as fatty meats, whole milk, and saturated oils (coconut, palm, and palm kernel oils).
- Eat more fruits, vegetables, and whole grains.
- Choose foods low in cholesterol.
- Eat foods high in fiber.

wellness
warning

Although a food label may claim "No Cholesterol," this food may still not be a good choice for you if you already have high cholesterol. Avoid palm and coconut oils—although they do not contain cholesterol, they are still saturated fats and can promote atherosclerosis. Even fat-free products should be looked at carefully, as these may be high in calories.

A Fish Story

You may have heard that eating fish will lower your cholesterol. This is true in part. Fish oils, particularly the omega-3 fatty acids found in tuna, cod, mackerel, herring, sardines, anchovies, and salmon, can lower your triglyceride levels, but they may also increase your total cholesterol levels. Eating large quantities of fish can also interfere with the normal clotting process of blood. A study of Eskimo populations found a lower incidence of heart attacks, but an increased incidence of strokes, owing to the Eskimos' high consumption of fish.

The current recommendation is to eat fish high in omega-3 fatty acids twice a week. In fact, a recent study published in the *New England Journal of Medicine* found that people who ate at least 8 ounces of fish a week had a 40 percent lower risk of fatal heart attack than those who ate no fish. According to the American Heart Association, fish oil supplements should only be taken under medical supervision.

Dietary Recommendations of the American Heart Association for Lowering Cholesterol

Step I Diet

This is the first level diet to reduce cholesterol levels and reduce your risk of heart disease.

- Your total intake of fat should not exceed 30 percent of your total daily calories. Of this, at most 8 to 10 percent may come from saturated fat.
- Eat less than 300 milligrams of cholesterol per day.
- Eat only enough calories per day that you need to reach or maintain a healthy weight.
- If you have questions, see your doctor, a registered dietician, or a nutritionist.
- If the Step I diet does not sufficiently lower your cholesterol within three months, your doctor may recommend the Step II Diet.

Step II Diet

This is a more restricted diet, used to reduce cholesterol when the Step I Diet is not successful.

- Your total dietary intake of fat should be 30 percent or less.
- Less than 7 percent of your day's total calories should come from saturated fat.
- Eat less than 200 milligrams of cholesterol per day.

- Avoid alcohol, especially if your doctor has told you that you have high triglyceride levels.
- Avoid table sugar, soft drinks, and corn syrup. (Real maple syrup is a healthier choice.)

In addition to diet, there are several things you can do to improve your cholesterol and, thereby, decrease your risk for heart disease:

- If your physician has prescribed a cholesterol-lowering agent for you, take your medication daily.
- Stop smoking. If you stop smoking, you can raise your good cholesterol (HDL). HDL helps protect against atherosclerosis.
- Exercise regularly. Exercising, such as a brisk walk for 20 to 30 minutes a day, can decrease the levels of fats in your blood and increase your HDL.
- If you are postmenopausal, speak with your doctor about postmenopausal hormone replacement, which restores the healthier lipid levels premenopausal woman have and dramatically reduces the development of coronary heart and other blood vessel disease.

Medications. Only about one-third of your blood cholesterol comes from diet. Your body makes the rest. Some people have high LDL cholesterol and triglycerides even if they follow a low-fat diet, exercise, and maintain ideal weight. Medications to lower LDL and triglycerides and raise HDL reduce the risk of coronary heart disease and prevent recurrent heart attacks and cardiac death in women. If you have a high LDL and/or triglyceride level, and a low average HDL, speak to your doctor regarding medication options.

What About Snacks?

At least 60 percent of Americans eat between meals. There is nothing wrong with snacking, provided you choose the right kinds of foods to snack on. Unfortunately, many people choose processed foods, such as potato chips and cupcakes, that are high in calories and low in nutrients.

A better approach is to choose snacks that will help you meet your daily quota of servings from the five food groups. A little preplanning will enable you to have these snacks around and available so you do not substitute the unhealthy processed foods. Here are some suggestions for healthy snacks:

- A banana, orange, apple, or any other fresh fruit
- Prepeeled carrots, available in grocery stores in small bags
- Dried fruit (watch the calories!)
- Rice cakes
- Low-fat yogurt
- Whole-grain bread with peanut butter
- Raw vegetables and yogurt dip
- Celery sticks with low-fat cream cheese
- Dry-roasted unsalted nuts
- Popcorn (without butter or salt)

wellness **tip**

Popcorn is a particularly good choice for a snack. It is filling, nutritious, full of fiber, and low in calories if you pop your own with an air popper and hold off on the butter. To add taste, experiment with herbs and seasonings, such as cayenne pepper.

Is Your Snack Food Tricking You?

When you grab a bran muffin instead of a candy bar, you might think you are making a smart snack choice. Watch out for the hidden ingredients in these "healthy" snacks:

- Store-bought muffin or quick bread (such as banana bread)—if it feels heavy and has a shiny surface, it probably has as much fat and calories as a cupcake, a downside that far outweighs the benefit of any ingredients such as bran, banana, or carrots.

- Granola bar—most granola bars today are chock full of candy bar ingredients, such as chocolate chips or marshmallow bits, saturated oils, and sugar; look for more "pure" granola bars at your local health food store and read the label carefully.

Remember that low-fat or fat-free foods may be high in calories. Read the label and pay attention to the serving size.

What About Fast Foods?

You are in a hurry and you have less than 20 minutes to grab something to eat. What better than a fast food place? Until fairly recently, fast food meant high-calorie, high-fat, high-sugar food. Fast food places were not for the nutrient-conscious and weight-conscious.

Now that is changing. Consumer demand for healthier fast foods has led to salad bars, broiled instead of fried foods, low-fat desserts, low-sugar preserves, pizza topped with vegetables, and many other items that a nutrition-conscious person can eat with confidence. And many fast food chains provide nutritional information about their menu offerings. Of course, those old standbys—burgers and fries, milkshakes, and deep fried chicken—are still available. But now you can check the nutritional information before you make your choice. Do you really want all those empty calories?

Making Chinese Take-Out Healthier

Following are some tips for making your Chinese take-out experience healthier:

- Drain the sauce from stir-fried dishes, since that is where much of the fat is located.
- Leave the last inch of sauce-saturated food in the container.
- Order steamed dishes and request that food be prepared in a low-fat manner.
- Since portions tend to be large, eat primarily the vegetables and the rice.
- If you are with a group, order fewer dishes (including at least one of steamed vegetables) and share them.
- If you are alone, order one steamed vegetable dish and one meat or fish dish. Then combine part of each with rice, and save the remainder for another one or two meals.

Nutrition *and* Weight Control

With all the low-fat, no-fat foods available, and all the nutrition labeling, and the ever-present focus on controlling calories, you would expect Americans to be in better shape than ever before. Diet books still top the bestseller list. Millions of dollars are spent on diet aids and weight loss equipment. Yet in fact, more than 55 percent of American women are overweight, and obesity (generally defined as more than 20 percent above recommended weight) is a serious and growing problem. Obesity among children is of particular concern: approximately 80 percent of children who are obese at ages 10 to 13 will be obese as adults. We are paying the price for our more sedentary lifestyle and for the availability of so much food—especially rich, fatty food.

Why the concern about becoming overweight? Apart from the negative effect it has on self-esteem and social life, being overweight or obese is associated with a number of serious diseases. High blood pressure, cardiovascular disease, and diabetes are more prevalent in people who are overweight. The risk of developing certain cancers is also higher in overweight people. For all these reasons, achieving and maintaining your ideal weight is highly recommended.

Determining Your Ideal Weight

It is no accident that ideal weight tables are published by life insurance companies. These tables help insurers assess a person's likelihood of dying early. The insurers know that people who are overweight generally have shorter life spans than those who maintain their ideal weight.

Weight is not really the issue, though. Weight is easy to measure, so it tends to be the focus of attention, but what is more important is body composition—and specifically the proportion of body fat to other tissues. It is that extra fat that puts a strain on the heart, reduces energy levels, and contributes to the diseases listed above.

Of course, the body needs some fat. Fat cushions and protects internal organs and helps the body metabolize nutrients. And women need more fat than men (about 12 percent of total body weight compared with 3 percent for men). In fact, more than 25 percent of the average American woman's body weight consists of fat.

There are various ways to measure the amount of body fat. The skinfold measurement technique uses calipers to measure the amount of fat under the skin at specific body sites. You do not really need fancy measurements, though. A full length mirror tells you what you need to know.

Weight centered around the waist and abdomen is a particular risk, especially for heart disease. If your waist-to-hip ratio is greater than or equal to 0.8 for a woman (and greater than or equal to 1.0 for a man) you are at increased risk for heart disease. For example, a woman whose hips are 36 inches should have a waist of 28.8 inches or less. (A man with 34-inch hips should also have a waist of 34 inches or less.) Losing this localized weight through diet and exercise will reduce your risk, more so if you can get that ratio below 0.8.

TABLE 8.1

Metropolitan Life Height and Weight Table for Women

Height in Feet/Inches	Small Frame (pounds)	Medium Frame (pounds)	Large Frame (pounds)
4' 10"	102–111	109–121	118–131
4' 11"	103–113	111–123	120–134
5' 0"	104–115	113–126	122–137
5' 1"	106–118	115–129	125–140
5' 2"	108–121	118–132	128–143
5' 3"	111–124	121–135	131–147
5' 4"	114–127	124–138	134–151
5' 5"	117–130	127–141	137–155
5' 6"	120–133	130–144	140–159
5' 7"	123–136	133–147	143–163
5' 8"	126–139	136–150	146–167
5' 9"	129–142	139–153	149–170
5' 10"	132–145	142–156	152–173
5' 11"	135–148	145–159	155–176
6' 0"	138–151	148–162	158–179

Weights at ages 25 to 59 based on lowest mortality. Weight in pounds according to frame (in indoor clothing weighing 3 lbs. for women; shoes with 1" heels). Reprinted courtesy of Metropolitan Life Insurance Company, *Statistical Bulletin.*

wellness **tip**

Many people believe that starchy foods are more fattening than high-protein foods. In fact, both simple and complex carbohydrates contain the same number of calories (4 per gram) as protein. It is the butter and sauce that add fat and calories.

How Many Calories Do You Need?

If you are already at your ideal weight and want to maintain that weight, you need to consume as many calories each day as you use. Your body uses a certain number of calories to maintain the healthy function of such processes as circulation, respiration, and metabolism. So even when you are resting, your body is using calories. A physically active individual has a higher metabolic rate, so she burns more calories even at rest. Your caloric needs are also determined by your age. Growing children, for example, need more calories than adults. Pregnant and lactating women, and people recovering from injury or surgery, need more calories than other individuals. Caloric needs also vary with climate. People who live in colder climates need more calories to maintain a normal body temperature than people in warmer climates.

Your daily activities also determine how much you need to eat to maintain your current weight and supply the energy you need. A woman who rides the elevator to the tenth floor and then sits behind a desk all day needs fewer calories than a stay-at-home mother of three who lugs loads of laundry to and from the basement, walks the dog twice a day, and works out three times a week. (The box on page 165 explains how you can figure out your daily caloric requirement to maintain your current weight.)

If you want to lose weight, you need to take in fewer calories than you use. For most women, a combination of eating less and exercising more is the healthiest and most successful combination. The number of calories you will burn during a given exercise is determined by your current weight and activity level and the duration and intensity of the exercise. For example, a moderately active woman weighing 120 pounds and walking at 5 miles per hour on level ground would burn 77 calories for each 10 minutes she walks. Walking uphill, walking faster, or carrying weights will increase the number of calories used.

Designing Your Weight-Control Program

If you determine that you need to lose weight, you need to develop a program that will work for you. More diets are started then stopped because the plan was not well thought out. It is recommended that you start with small changes and focus on losing no more than one or two pounds per week. Remember that losing weight slowly and keeping it off is a long-term process and is healthy; rapid weight loss and yo-yo dieting are actually harmful. You need to be willing to make permanent changes in your diet and lifestyle.

Begin with Small Steps. Here are some suggestions of small, easy changes that you can take one step at a time:

- **Reduce your intake of fat.** Switch from butter to low-fat margarine products, from ice cream to ice milk or nonfat frozen yogurt, from cakes and cookies to fresh fruit. Try meat-free meals, then meat-free days. Dribble a few drops of salad dressing on your salad and toss well, rather than pouring it on.
- **Increase your intake of fiber to help you feel full.** Try raw vegetables or a low-fat granola bar instead of a chocolate bar or potato chips.
- **Drink plenty of water.** Avoid high-calorie sodas and fruit juice and empty-calorie alcohol.
- **Eat three regular or six smaller meals per day at the same time each day.** Avoid skipping a meal—doing so may cause you to become hungry and overeat later in the day. Frequent small feedings enable you to satiate your hunger with less food.
- **Eat small portions of a variety of foods each day.** Use the Food Guide Pyramid to guide you. Use smaller plates and do not leave serving dishes on the table. Do not feel you have to eat everything on your plate.
- **Choose low-calorie snacks.** If you do become hungry between meals, reach for raw vegetables or fresh fruit.
- **Do not crash diet.** Losing weight rapidly puts a strain on your heart, makes your skin sag, and saps your strength. Slow, permanent weight loss is the goal, even if it is only a few pounds.
- **Exercise.** Aim for a minimum of 20 to 30 minutes of moderate exercise each day. (See Chapter 9 for an in-depth discussion of exercise.)
- **Enlist the help of your friends and family in your diet.** Avoid people who try to sabotage your efforts by offering high-calorie food. If you must eat a high-calorie food, make it part of your diet, limit the size, and make it a special occasion. One piece of chocolate savored can save a diet, while a whole candy bar gobbled up can wreck it.

Determining Your Daily Caloric Requirement

To maintain a normal basal metabolic rate, women require between 10 and 20 calories a day for each pound of body weight, depending on age and level of activity. For example, a 30-year-old woman who weighs 140 pounds and is sedentary needs 1,400 calories a day (140 x 10 = 1,400). If she is physically active and wishes to *maintain* her weight, she needs to consume enough extra calories each day in addition to her baseline requirement, to offset the calories burned during exercise. If she chooses to expend 360 calories a day walking before work, she will need to consume 1,760 calories a day (1,400 + 360 = 1,760) to maintain her weight. If she wishes to exercise to lose weight, she would not consume the extra calories.

The older you get, the fewer calories you need. For each decade after age 30, subtract two percent from the calories you required at age 30. A 40-year-old woman who weighs 140 pounds and is sedentary would subtract two percent of the 1,400 calories (or 28 calories), arriving at 1,372. If she exercises and wishes to maintain her weight, she will add calories to offset the calories expended during exercise.

Avoid Fad Diets. They usually promise more than they can do and more than most people can accomplish. About 90 percent of people who lose weight following "wonder" regimens regain the weight, sometimes even more than they had originally lost. If you are tempted to try a specific weight-control program, ask the following questions before you sign up:

- What are the health risks associated with this diet?
- What data can you show me that prove that your program actually works?
- What percentage of your customers kept off the weight that they lost after they completed the diet program?
- What are the costs for membership, weekly fees, food, supplements, maintenance, and counseling? What is the payment schedule? Will my health insurance cover any of these costs? Do I get a refund if I drop out or fail to lose the expected weight?
- Do you have a maintenance program? Is it included in the fee or does it cost extra?
- What kind of professional supervision is provided? What are the credentials of these professionals?

Any weight-loss program that sounds too good to be true probably is. Even zero-calorie fat replacers have turned out not to be the magic bullet so many had hoped. Olestra, for example, a synthetic chemical made up of sugar and vegetable oil that is not absorbed by the body, was recently approved by the Food and Drug Administration (FDA). Some objectors called the replacement fat dangerous, citing that excess use can lead to bloating and diarrhea, as well as loss of fat soluble vitamins. Although the FDA states that the substance is safe, foods containing the product must bear a label warning of possible gastrointestinal problems, such as diarrhea and bloating.

Increase Your Activity Level. Exercise is an essential partner to good nutrition in any weight-loss program. In addition to burning calories, regular exercise can decrease the levels of fats in your blood, increase your ability to burn calories, lower your normal heart rate, lower your blood pressure, relieve tension, help you sleep better, and increase muscle mass, which also burns more calories.

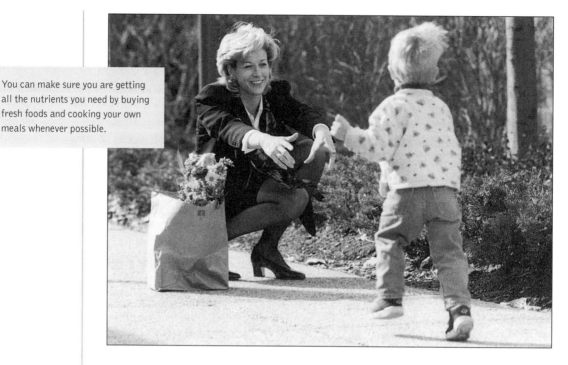

You can make sure you are getting all the nutrients you need by buying fresh foods and cooking your own meals whenever possible.

However, it is essential to check with your physician before you begin any exercise program, especially if you are middle-aged or older and have not been physically active. When you have been given the green light, follow these simple rules from the American Heart Association:

- Establish an exercise schedule. Choose a specific time of day, such as before breakfast, for your exercise. Set aside a number of days per week for your chosen activity.
- Exercise with a friend for moral support and to avoid skipping a day.
- Vary your routines to prevent boredom or overuse of certain muscles.
- Allow your body to become conditioned. Take it slowly at first.
- Do not stop suddenly after you exercise, but allow your body to adjust to the decreased rate of activity. Increase your exercise no more than ten percent a session to avoid serious injuries.
- Try an exercise, such as brisk walking, hiking, jogging, swimming, or bicycling, that will increase blood flow to your working muscles to ensure cardiovascular fitness.
- Include low-intensity activities in your routine, such as slow walking, gardening, or dancing.

Reward yourself with a new pair of sneakers or jogging shoes or a warm-up suit. Above all, make exercise a regular and permanent part of your life. (See Chapter 9 for more information on exercise.)

Do You Need to Gain Weight?

If your body weight is below average for a woman of your height and frame size, your doctor may recommend that you gain weight. Some women are underweight because they have a high, or "fast," metabolism; others are underweight because they do not get enough calories due to illness or poverty. Following are eating and exercising tips to help you gain weight slowly and safely:

- Eat consistently. Be sure to eat at least three full, well-balanced meals and two nutritious, high-calorie snacks a day.
- Eat larger portions. A slight increase in portion size at each meal adds a significant number of calories.
- Eat healthy foods that are high in calories. Cranberry juice has 50 percent more calories than orange juice; granola and nut cereals have two times the calories as other cereals.
- Periodically substitute high-calorie liquids, such as fruit juice or milk, for water, which has no calories. Be sure to still drink eight 8-ounce glasses of water each day.
- Start doing resistance exercises, such as weight lifting and push-ups, to build muscle mass and increase your appetite. Increase calorie intake, though, or you could lose weight.

Before making any extreme alterations to your diet and exercise regimen, consult your doctor.

Source: Adapted from Clark, Nancy, MS, RD. "How to Gain Weight Healthfully." Health Net. http://www.health-net.com/gain.htm. (June 17, 1997).

Meeting *Special* Dietary Needs

Most women require a special diet at some point in their lives. Athletes, for example, need diets that increase their strength and endurance as well as energy stores. Postmenopausal women require a calcium-rich, low-fat diet that offers protection against osteoporosis and heart disease. Women with serious illnesses require diets that provide them with sufficient energy and help strengthen their immune systems.

Female Athletes

Exercise does not increase your requirement for vitamins or protein. The American diet is already high in protein, and vitamins do not play a role in improving performance. Athletes may, however, have to maintain higher than average stores of fats to avoid losing weight. If you are an athlete, you will require the same distribution of dietary calories as any healthy adult, that is, more carbohydrates than fats or protein. Complex carbohydrates should make up 55 to 65 percent of your diet, fat should make up 25 to 30 percent, and protein 12 to 15 percent. Carbohydrate loading (consuming large quantities of carbohydrates) should be practiced only before endurance events, such as long-distance running. High-carbohydrate meals should be taken two or three days before competition, following a low-carbohydrate, high-protein, high-fat diet. Limit your practice of carbohydrate loading to three or four times a year or only when absolutely essential. Pregame meals may also be high in carbohydrates to provide ready fuel for competition.

Proper hydration—adequate fluid intake—is essential for the athlete. If your exercise regimen will be unusually intense and if you have to work out or play a game or match in hot, humid conditions, electrolyte replacement fluids are a good idea. Beverages that are ten percent sugar will improve endurance, provide carbohydrates for muscles, and prevent depletion of glycogen stores. Beverages

**Do You Need
a Supplement?**

**You may be a candidate for
vitamin or mineral supplements if you are:**

• **Dieting.**
• **Skipping meals.**
• **Eating irregularly.**
• **Pregnant.**
• **Nursing.**
• **A vegan (strict vegetarian,
  eating no meat, fish, or
  dairy products).**
• **Avoiding dairy products.**
• **A smoker or heavy drinker.**
• **Elderly.**
• **Chronically ill.**
• **Exercising vigorously to
  lose weight (without con-
  suming enough nutrient-
  dense foods to balance the
  effort).**

with more than ten percent sugar may cause cramping and diarrhea. Perspiration causes sodium and potassium loss. Replace these nutrients by eating lightly salted and potassium-rich foods and beverages. Salt tablets are not a good idea except in extreme situations. They can cause nausea and stomach upset.

Postmenopausal and Elderly Women

Women may lose two to three percent of their bone mass per year in the first years after menopause, rather than the usual one-half to one percent of annual bone loss as they age. While postmenopausal hormone replacement is one option to address this, a calcium-rich diet is usually recommended as well, to prevent further bone loss. Soybeans may also prevent the bone loss that increases a woman's risk of developing osteoporosis. Researchers recently found that by eating two ounces of soy protein a day (which contains 92 milligrams of phytoestrogens—naturally-occurring estrogen), postmenopausal women were able to increase their bone density by 2.2 percent over a 6-month period. Consuming soy protein was also associated with an eight percent drop in LDL ("bad" cholesterol) and may decrease the risk of heart disease in older women. (See Chapter 19 for a complete discussion of menopause and further dietary recommendations.)

Many elderly women are overweight, which increases their risk of degenerative diseases, such as diabetes and heart disease. A woman who is mildly overweight may not be at increased risk for degenerative disease; however, an older woman who is 20 percent above her desirable weight should lower her weight. An underweight elderly woman should gain weight to improve her overall health. Other conditions of the elderly, such as depression, mental disorders, confusion, memory loss, and fatigue, can often be improved with proper nutrition and supplementation.

The most common dietary danger zones in elderly women include:

• Insufficient protein intake.
• Insufficient water intake. The same amount of water (six to eight 8-ounce glasses per day) is recommended for all women.
• Insufficient vitamin and mineral intake. The body's ability to manufacture some vitamins, such as vitamin D, slows down with age. Dietary sources of vitamin D are especially important for elderly women. Older women usually spend less time in the sun (one way the body gets vitamin D). Unless older women drink four glasses or more of fortified nonfat milk daily, they will need vitamin D and calcium supplements.
• Vitamins C and E are important to keep the eyes healthy and prevent cataracts. Elderly women should take 400 IU of vitamin E and 500 mg of vitamin C daily. In one study, senior citizens on vitamin E supplements showed improvements in depression, mental alertness, and motivation.
• Elderly women also have a decreased ability to absorb B vitamins. Foods such as beans, liver, and some other meats are rich in B vitamins and may be helpful. Supplementation may also be necessary.

Women with Compromised Immune Function

Women with suppressed immune function, such as those with HIV or cancer, are likely to have a decreased ability to absorb vitamins and minerals, resulting in weight loss. As these diseases progress, malnutrition further weakens the body's defense systems. A low-fat diet supplemented with B vitamins, vitamin A, selenium, and zinc may help strengthen the immune function. Above all, it is important for these women to maintain a desirable body weight. Alcohol and tobacco products should be avoided.

Overcoming
Negative *Body* Images

Many American women are obsessed with their weight. Some blame the media's hyped images of ultrathin models or bad eating habits learned in childhood. Regardless of the cause or causes, approximately 25 percent of women who are concerned about their weight suffer from anorexia or bulimia. These disorders are characterized by an unrealistic fear of becoming fat and a refusal to gain weight and maintain a normal body weight. Women with anorexia try to attain the "perfect" body through excessive dieting and exercise. Many women who suffer from anorexia believe they are overweight, but in reality they are seriously underweight. Bulimia is characterized by excessive and compulsive eating, followed by purging in the form of vomiting and abuse of laxatives and diuretics to lose weight. Many women suffering from anorexia or bulimia cease to menstruate.

Eating disorders occur more often in women (less than ten percent of cases are in men). These disorders were once thought to be chiefly associated with adolescent girls and young adult women, but they are now being observed in older women as well. Although the exact cause of eating disorders is unknown, it may be associated with genetic or psychological factors that occur at puberty, as well as unrealistic goals and expectations. Eating disorders can be carried to such an extreme as to result in death. Early identification of an eating disorder can help bring about recovery, but controlling these disorders is usually a lifelong process.

Light therapy studies have shown a beneficial effect on women with bulimia. The women were exposed to bright light for 30 minutes a day over a period of two weeks. Subjects whose symptoms usually worsen during the winter months (a condition called seasonal affective disorder) showed the greatest improvement in overcoming bulimia.

There is also evidence that eating disorders may be associated with zinc deficiency. Zinc deficiency can result from poor diet, excess fiber consumption, stress, vomiting, and diarrhea, or the demands placed on the body for zinc during the teenage years. In a study of 62 patients, zinc deficiencies were documented in 54 percent of anorexics and 40 percent of bulimics. In another study, zinc sulfate supplementation (45 to 90 micrograms per day) was associated with significant weight gain in 20 patients with anorexia, 13 of whom returned to normal menstruation within 1 to 17 months.

Women are more prone to stress-related zinc deficiencies than men, possibly because men can store high concentrations of zinc in their prostate glands and can draw upon them during times of stress. Women, on the other hand, do not have prostates and must draw zinc from other tissue, such as muscle tissue and bone. Anorexics can wind up using their own tissue to gain nutrients missing from their diet. When the heart muscle, which is one percent zinc, is tapped for further stores of zinc, heart function can be seriously compromised, contributing to arrhythmias and eventually heart failure. Once the heart muscle has been damaged, any weight a recovering woman regains will stress her heart muscle further. Professional treatment, possible hospitalization, and expert consultation should be sought by women who have muscle weakness, irregular heartbeats, cramping, and poor mental function.

What *You* Can Do

Just as there is no question that smoking leads to lung cancer, there is no dispute that making simple improvements in your diet, based on the three rules of moderation, variety, and balance, is one of the most important factors in improving your wellness. Understanding the ways your body uses different foods allows you to make smart, informed food choices that help you enjoy a healthy life. Following are some general guidelines for using nutrition to your advantage:

- Eat a balanced diet. Choose from among the five food groups. Limit fats, sweets, and oils.
- Eat high-quality foods. Cook your own meals whenever possible, using fresh foods and produce. Avoid canned and processed foods.
- Avoid smoking.
- Drink in moderation. Do not drink at all if you are pregnant or nursing or sensitive or easily addicted to alcohol.
- Try to meet your vitamin needs through food. Take vitamin supplements only when necessary or as recommended by your physician. Many women need zinc, calcium, and iron supplements if their diets are not adequate.
- Drink six to eight 8-ounce glasses of water daily.
- Reduce your caloric intake and exercise to lose weight. Avoid fad diets.
- Know what you are eating; read food labels.

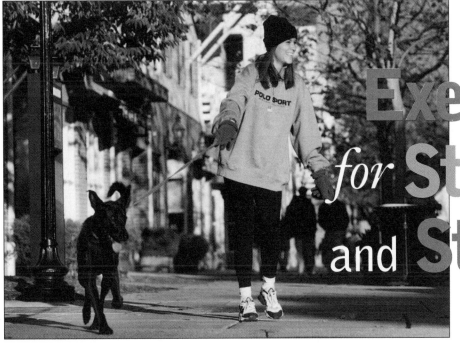
Exercising *for* Strength *and* Stamina

Experts agree—exercise is an important part of a healthy lifestyle. Regular exercise lowers the risk of certain chronic diseases, improves mental health and general well-being, promotes weight control, and helps build muscle strength and flexibility. Despite the known benefits of exercise, however, millions of adults in the United States remain inactive.

In fact, more than 60 percent of American adults do not participate in regular physical activity, and 25 percent of all adults are not active at all, according to a 1996 report issued by the office of the Surgeon General. The report, titled Physical Activity and Health, was researched by the Centers for Disease Control and Prevention along with other federal agencies, as well as the American College of Sports Medicine and the American Heart Association. All participants in the study agreed that physical activity does not have to be vigorous to provide health benefits. A key finding of the report is that people of all ages can improve the quality of their lives simply by starting a lifelong practice of moderate physical activity. As little as 30 minutes a day of moderate exercise—even if activities are spread throughout the day—can offer health benefits. The more activity, the more benefits, but the greatest benefit is gained with the first 30 minutes of exercise. Women who are already physically active will benefit more by increasing the intensity, frequency, or duration of their exercise.

Doctors previously recommended that women and men participate in exercise that elevates the heart rate at least three times weekly for 20 or more continuous minutes each time. This is still a healthy recommendation, but for many people, work and family commitments do not allow for such a structured goal. For busy people, formal exercise programs with gyms and equipment present a hurdle to health that is often too high to overcome. Therefore, the current recommendation is to start with 30 minutes of moderate exercise that can be accomplished throughout the day.

Moderate exercise includes a surprisingly wide range of common activities. Here are a few examples:

- Climbing stairs (instead of taking the elevator)
- Walking short distances (instead of driving)
- Housework
- Gardening
- Lawn care, such as raking leaves
- Carrying packages or a small child
- Playing actively with children
- Painting your bedroom
- Peddling a stationary bicycle
- Dancing, either for recreation or in a class setting

The Physical Activity and Health report concludes that the cardiorespiratory benefit from physical activity over several short sessions appears the same as when the same total amount and intensity of activity occurs in one longer session. For example, three 10-minute stair-climbing sessions at work should offer all the same benefits as 30 minutes on the Stairmaster in the gym.

This new recommendation encourages women (and men) to make physical activity an integral part of their everyday lives, without the necessity for special equipment, the expense of joining a gym, or the hassle of signing up for classes. When you do choose special physical activities, look for those that promote cardiovascular conditioning, muscle strength, and weight control.

Health Benefits
of Exercise

Cardiovascular disease is the leading cause of death among women as well as men in the United States. Regular physical activity greatly reduces the risk of cardiovascular disease for both women and men. Physical activity also reduces the risk of developing diabetes, hypertension, obesity, osteoporosis, and colon cancer. It improves mental health and mental clarity, reduces the negative effects of stress, and can help improve sleeping habits. It builds strong muscles, bones, and joints and improves overall endurance and energy.

Lack of physical activity, on the other hand, has been linked to a higher death rate at earlier ages. It has been estimated that 250,000 deaths per year in the United States might be avoided if more people engage in regular physical activity.

According to the Institute for Aerobics Research, people who are fit live longer and the quality of their lives is better. In fact, strength training and other forms of regular, moderate activity in older adults often help make it possible for them to live independently, which enhances the lives of older Americans and their families. Physical training is becoming an important economic as well as personal issue as the "baby boomer" generation ages.

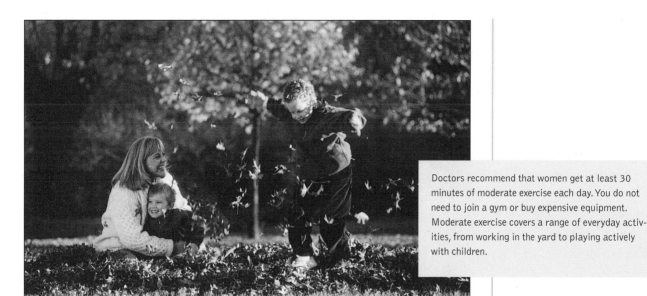

Doctors recommend that women get at least 30 minutes of moderate exercise each day. You do not need to join a gym or buy expensive equipment. Moderate exercise covers a range of everyday activities, from working in the yard to playing actively with children.

Cardiovascular Health

Lack of exercise produces the same risk for heart disease in women as do high cholesterol, hypertension (high blood pressure), and cigarette smoking. Conversely, regular physical activity benefits a woman as much as does quitting cigarette smoking does.

How does physical activity improve your cardiovascular health? Exercise enhances the body's ability to take in oxygen and transport it to vital tissues. This process helps prevent coronary artery disease, which can lead to angina (chest pain) and heart attacks. Angina and heart attacks are usually caused by a condition called atherosclerosis. Cholesterol deposits called plaque gradually thicken the walls of blood vessels. The openings narrow, restricting blood flow to the heart, which causes discomfort known as angina. If the cholesterol deposit, or plaque, suddenly ruptures and forms a clot that blocks the blood flow completely, a heart attack occurs. Atherosclerosis can also lead to stroke when the same process causes a blockage in the supply of blood to the brain.

The risk of heart disease is inversely related to one's activity level. That is, risk decreases as activity increases. In a study of Harvard University alumni, moderate activity reduced the risk by 29 percent, and high levels of activity reduced the risk by 46 percent. The risk for low activity alumni was 2.4 times that of active alumni who engaged in vigorous sports. Regardless of whether exercise is job-related, recreational, or sports-related, to be beneficial it must become a regular habit. When exercise stops, the risk of heart disease increases once more.

Several factors that are linked to a higher risk for heart disease are listed below. In every case, exercise has been shown to decrease the risk.

Blood Lipids. Fats in the blood are called lipids. They include cholesterol (lipoprotein) and triglycerides, both of which are related to the risk of heart disease. There are two major forms of cholesterol: low-density lipoprotein (LDL) is the "bad" form that promotes the thickening of the lining of blood vessels that

**Are You at Risk
for Heart Disease?**

If any of these factors apply
to you, an exercise program
combined with lifestyle
changes can help protect
against heart disease:

- Overweight
- Elevated blood lipids
  (cholesterol and
  triglycerides)
- High blood pressure
- Physical inactivity
  (sedentary lifestyle)
- Insulin resistance or
  elevated blood sugar
  (diabetes)
- Smoking
- Diet high in saturated fat
  and salt
- Family history of early
  heart disease (before age
  40 in male relative or age
  50 in female relative)
- African-American ethnic
  background

occurs with atherosclerosis; high-density lipoprotein (HDL) is a "good" form of cholesterol that helps remove LDL. Exercise increases HDL cholesterol and decreases LDL cholesterol and triglycerides, thus lowering the risk of heart disease. Activity, weight loss, and a low-fat diet help lower LDL levels. High LDL cholesterol can be inherited. For those with a family history of high LDL cholesterol levels or heart disease, regular physical activity is even more important.

Hypertension. Regular physical activity reduces the risk of developing hypertension, or high blood pressure. Exercise also helps lower blood pressure in people with hypertension. Why is hypertension dangerous? High blood pressure puts stress on the heart and blood vessels, which can lead to damage to the heart, brain, and organs, such as the kidney. Exercise helps the blood vessels open and the heart and entire body work more efficiently and thus reduces blood pressure. Weight loss, another benefit of exercise, can also help lower blood pressure. In many cases, exercise can help lower blood pressure in patients with hypertension to the point that the need for medication is lessened or eliminated.

Blood Clotting and Poor Circulation. A blood clot can be dangerous if it lodges in a narrowed blood vessel. A clot can prevent blood and oxygen from reaching the heart, brain, or other vital organs. Regular exercise increases the body's ability to break down blood clots and keep blood flowing efficiently throughout the body. It also increases the flow of blood to muscles used during exercise and promotes better circulation, even when you are not exercising.

Glucose Intolerance and Insulin. Glucose is a sugar that is the body's main source of fuel. Insulin is a hormone that helps move glucose into the cells, where it can be used for energy. When the body doesn't make enough insulin or when insulin is not used properly, the level of glucose in the body becomes too high. This condition, called hyperglycemia, is the basic abnormality in diabetes. The diabetic condition is not simply an abnormality of glucose metabolism, however. A patient with this condition also has lipid metabolic problems that increase her risk of atherosclerotic heart disease, obesity, and hypertension. Regular exercise reduces glucose intolerance and insulin resistance, reducing the amount of insulin needed to keep blood glucose levels normal.

Overweight

Obesity (being 20 percent over optimum weight) is at an all-time high in the United States. Being overweight, in fact, has become a major health issue. A recent study conducted by Louis Harris and Associates, and commissioned by the American Medical Women's Association found that, based on height, weight, and body frame type, over 55 percent of American women are overweight. Fewer than 49 percent claim to exercise for at least 30 minutes twice a week or more often.

Several life-threatening diseases are linked with obesity, including diabetes, heart disease, and some forms of cancer. Regular exercise results in a leaner, trimmer, healthier body. Sustained exercise burns calories from fat stores, promoting weight loss and a reduced risk for such diseases. As exercise burns excess fat and builds muscle, it can alter the body's metabolism so it uses fat more effectively.

This process increases the body's ability to burn calories and fat, even when the body is at rest or not exercising.

Muscle, however, weighs more than fat. In fact it is twice the weight of fat per unit volume. Therefore, when a woman begins to exercise and build muscle, she may lose fat without losing weight. She will notice a difference in her body shape, however. It will become leaner, especially in the abdominal area, which further reduces cardiac risk.

Women who are dieting—that is, they are consuming fewer calories than are being used by the body—should combine their efforts with an exercise program to burn fat, build muscle, and increase cardiovascular fitness. Weight loss from dieting alone can weaken muscles, resulting in fatigue and less stamina for physical activity. Too rapid a weight loss can rob the body of muscle mass and actually harm your health. Aim for gradual weight loss of one pound a week. This gradual weight loss is less harmful to the body and more likely to be permanent. Repeatedly losing and then gaining weight, the so-called "yo-yo" weight cycle, is more harmful than never losing weight.

Diabetes

As stated earlier, the hormone insulin allows the body to convert glucose in food into energy. If the body does not produce enough insulin, or if the body is not using it correctly, glucose levels rise and become potentially dangerous. This condition is called diabetes. There are two different forms of diabetes: Type 1 diabetes occurs when the pancreas is unable to make insulin and requires insulin to be taken daily. Type 2 diabetes occurs through a process called insulin resistance—when the body is unable to lower blood sugar with available insulin.

Type 2 diabetes is often referred to as non–insulin-dependent diabetes mellitus, or NIDDM. Though oral medications are frequently needed by NIDDM patients, it can often be controlled by diet, exercise, and weight management. Regular exercise lowers the risk of developing NIDDM. It makes cells less insulin resistant and insulin more efficient in promoting movement of glucose to the muscles cells where it can be used. Exercise can also be helpful in the control of insulin-dependent diabetes, often eliminating the need for other treatments.

In people who are obese and develop diabetes, the fat cells themselves may contribute to the insulin resistance. Diet and exercise can help these people attain normal body weight—and normal blood sugar levels. In some cases, insulin and other medications may no longer be needed.

Cancer

Regular physical activity may lower the risk of colon cancer. Exercise improves the digestive system, resulting in more efficient processing of food and faster transport

wellness **warning**

A round body shape with a high concentration of abdominal fat (a "pot belly") and a waist measurement to hip measurement of greater than 0.8:1 in women (1:1 in men) increases the risk of cardiovascular disease. Reducing the waist-to-hip ratio actually lowers cardiac risk even more than weight loss alone.

Calories

What we usually refer to as a calorie is really a kilocalorie. It is the amount of heat required to raise the temperature of one kilogram (one liter) of water by 1°C. It is necessary to reduce your calorie intake or expend about 3,500 calories to lose one pound of fat. Depending on the intensity of exercise, it takes an hour to use 300 to 600 calories. Jogging one mile burns about 100 calories. Following are examples of calories burned per minute by other activities for an average woman (132 to 154 pounds):

Activity	Calories burned per minute
Cleaning windows	3.7
Walking	4.0
Gardening	5.6
Cycling (9.4 mph)	7.0
Tennis	7.1
Shoveling snow	7.5
Climbing stairs	8.4
Swimming (slow)	11.5

through the colon. Exercise does not, however, appear to have a positive effect on rectal cancer. Some studies have shown a weak link between exercise and a lower risk of breast and prostate cancer, but these areas require further research. Postmenopausal breast cancer statistically appears to occur less frequently in lean women, but the reason is not clear.

Muscle and Bone Strength

Exercise not only keeps your heart fit, it keeps your musculoskeletal system fit, too, increasing your strength and stamina. When you repeatedly contract a muscle against resistance (such as weights or water in a swimming pool), the muscle develops more tissue and is capable of greater force or strength. Directing an exercise to a specific part of the body builds muscle there. Increased muscle strength can help support other parts of the body and its activities. For instance, stronger abdominal muscles help support the back and prevent pain and injury. If you exercise regularly, and then stop, muscle tone will begin to lessen within two weeks. If physical activity is still not resumed, the beneficial effects disappear within two to eight months.

Bone is continually being broken down and remade. During childhood, bone growth is faster than bone loss, so bone mass increases (which is important for body growth). Good bone density depends on adequate calcium in the diet and exercise in childhood. After skeletal growth is complete, bone continues to be broken down and remade, but at a slower rate. The rate of bone rebuilding is related to the amount of "pull" by the muscles, so stronger, more active muscles result in stronger, denser bone. On the other hand, when bone breaks down more rapidly than it rebuilds, density decreases with age.

Decreased bone density results in osteoporosis, a condition that leads to disabling bone fractures and affects older women seven to eight times more frequently than older men. (Osteoporosis is discussed later in this chapter.) Weight-bearing exercises, in which the weight of the body comes to bear on bones and muscles, helps maintain bone density and prevent bone loss.

Ligaments connect bones to bones within joints, and tendons connect muscles to bones. Warming and stretching muscles before, during, and after exercise helps keep muscles, ligaments, and tendons more flexible. Flexibility helps prevent injury, such as torn ligaments, tendon rupture, or muscle strain.

Flexibility is especially important for older people and those with arthritis because it keeps joints mobile and helps people stay active. Regular physical activity and stretching can also improve balance, coordination, and agility in elderly women, which in turn can help prevent falls, fractures, and injury and prolong independent living.

Mental Health

Physical activity can relieve anxiety, depression, and the negative effects of stress. Even in women who are not experiencing serious mental conditions, exercise can lift the spirits, clear the head, improve concentration, and help them maintain a positive mood and outlook. Mastering a specific physical activity generally improves self-image, which in turn improves confidence. The benefits of physical activity are felt by women who begin to exercise at moderate levels, and they increase at greater levels.

Anxiety. Anxiety is an unpleasant emotional state in which a woman feels fear for no apparent reason and experiences physical symptoms, such as rapid heart beat and sweating. Anxiety is a normal reaction to stressful or threatening circumstances, and can actually improve performance in some cases. When anxiety is out of control, however, or when it occurs repeatedly in response to things that most people do not find frightening, it becomes a mental disorder (see Chapter 12). Improved fitness can help reduce anxiety and is effective when combined with mental health therapy.

Depression. Depression is a sense of sadness, low self-esteem, pessimism, hopelessness, and despair. Although mild depression may go away on its own, evaluation and treatment with medication are often needed if symptoms persist. Studies have shown that physical activity reduces or relieves depression in all age groups and at all fitness levels. Regular exercise may also help prevent depression, although researchers are less clear on the cause and effect relationship. It is thought that exercise may prevent depression in healthy individuals, and it may relieve some symptoms in those with mild to moderate disorders.

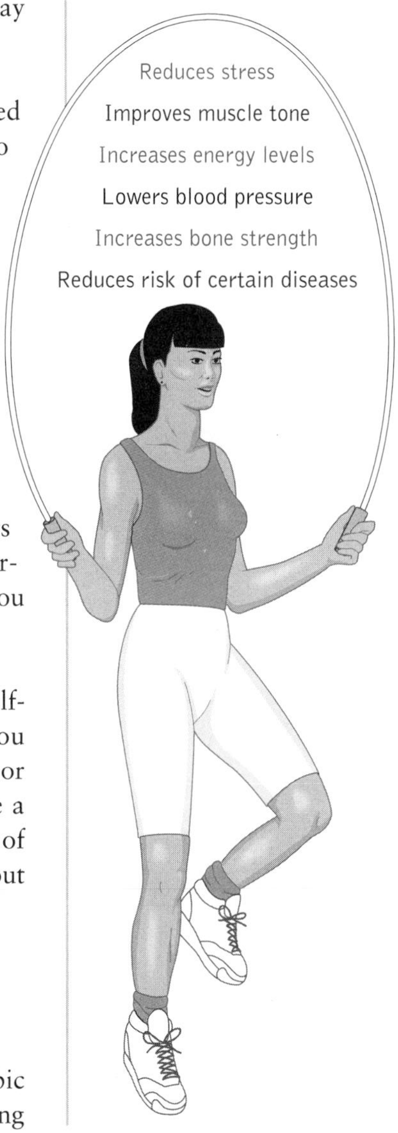

Stress. Your body has an immediate response to a perceived threat; it is called the fight-or-flight response. It triggers changes in the body that cause senses to sharpen, the blood supply to large muscles to increase, and blood pressure and heart rate levels to rise. The fight-or-flight response is considered a positive form of stress, dating back to the time when early humans had to either kill or run from dangerous animals and other physical threats.

While these physiological reactions help prepare the body for a crisis, they can negatively affect your physical and mental health if that response occurs repeatedly. Over time, stress can break down the immune system, increase susceptibility to disease, and disturb attention, concentration, and sleep patterns. It can also cause migraine headaches, chronic fatigue, gastrointestinal disturbances, and many other health problems.

Exercise is an excellent stress management tool for most people. It lowers blood pressure, eases tension in muscles, and helps reduce blood clotting. During exercise, the body also releases endorphins, natural chemicals that make you feel good and help alleviate the emotional symptoms of stress.

Self-Efficacy. One measure of sound mental health and high self-esteem is self-efficacy, the ability to produce or achieve a desired effect or goal. When you work up to 50 sit-ups from 25, add an extra half mile to your morning walk, or increase your dumbbell weights from three to five pounds, you experience a boost in self-efficacy and a heightened sense of mastery. These positive feelings of competence may extend to other areas of your life. In short, feeling good about yourself physically helps you feel good about yourself in general.

Types *of* Exercise

When it comes to exercise, there is literally something for everyone. Aerobic exercise builds cardiovascular strength. Endurance training (including walking

FIGURE 9.1
Health Benefits of Exercise
Regular physical activity has a positive impact on many aspects of your physical, mental, and emotional health.

Reduces stress
Improves muscle tone
Increases energy levels
Lowers blood pressure
Increases bone strength
Reduces risk of certain diseases

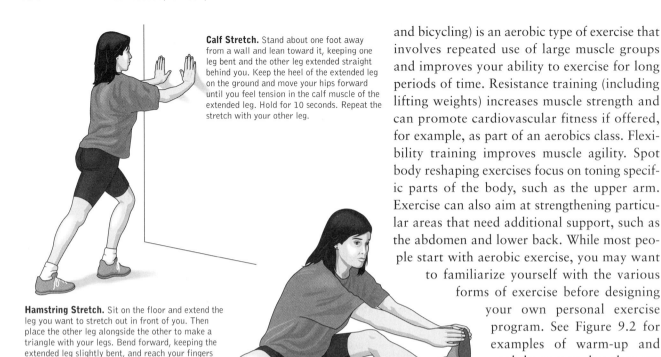

Calf Stretch. Stand about one foot away from a wall and lean toward it, keeping one leg bent and the other leg extended straight behind you. Keep the heel of the extended leg on the ground and move your hips forward until you feel tension in the calf muscle of the extended leg. Hold for 10 seconds. Repeat the stretch with your other leg.

Hamstring Stretch. Sit on the floor and extend the leg you want to stretch out in front of you. Then place the other leg alongside the other to make a triangle with your legs. Bend forward, keeping the extended leg slightly bent, and reach your fingers toward your toes until you feel slight tension. Hold the position for 20 seconds. Repeat the stretch with your other leg.

Arm stretches. For the first stretch, reach your arm under your chin and across your other shoulder. Gently push the arm back with your free hand until you feel a slight tension. Hold for 15 seconds. Repeat the stretch with your other arm. For the second stretch, raise one arm and bend it behind your head to touch your other shoulder. Use your free hand to gently pull the elbow downward. Keep your hand away from the elbow joint. Hold for 15 seconds. Repeat the stretch with your other arm.

FIGURE 9.2
Remember to Stretch

To lower your risk of injury during any type of physical activity, be sure to stretch your muscles before and after you exercise. Here are a few simple warm-up and cool-down stretches you can do.

and bicycling) is an aerobic type of exercise that involves repeated use of large muscle groups and improves your ability to exercise for long periods of time. Resistance training (including lifting weights) increases muscle strength and can promote cardiovascular fitness if offered, for example, as part of an aerobics class. Flexibility training improves muscle agility. Spot body reshaping exercises focus on toning specific parts of the body, such as the upper arm. Exercise can also aim at strengthening particular areas that need additional support, such as the abdomen and lower back. While most people start with aerobic exercise, you may want to familiarize yourself with the various forms of exercise before designing your own personal exercise program. See Figure 9.2 for examples of warm-up and cool-down stretches that can help prevent injury during any type of exercise.

Aerobic Exercise

Repeated exercise removes oxygen from the body. In response, the body increases blood flow and increases the ability of the cells to store oxygen. The higher the level of exercise, the greater the response. The ability to store oxygen at the cellular level is called aerobic capacity.

The term aerobic literally means "in the presence of oxygen." During aerobic exercise, energy is produced when energy stores, such as fat and carbohydrates, are oxidized. As exercise continues, the use of oxygen increases until the amount of oxygen available in the blood is depleted. The exercise is then called anaerobic, or "without oxygen." Lactic acid builds up in the blood and muscles when energy is used faster than it can be produced aerobically. Lactic acid and high levels of carbon dioxide produced in response to intense exercise can result in fatigue, difficulty breathing, and muscle discomfort or cramps.

Aerobic exercise produces positive effects; anaerobic exercise is detrimental to your health. To avoid turning aerobic exercise into anaerobic exercise, make sure you work out at a level at which you can breathe comfortably and take time to stretch and rest muscles to rid them of lactic acid buildup.

Aerobic capacity can be assessed most simply by measuring the heart rate during exercise. As the body develops a greater need for oxygen, the heart beats faster. With increased training and aerobic ability, the heart becomes more efficient, pumping more blood with each beat. Therefore, the heart rate of a fit per-

Target Heart Rate

The target heart rate is the level that gives you the best workout. It is about 60 to 80 percent of your maximum heart rate, the fastest your heart can be expected to beat. The maximum heart rate is determined by subtracting your age in years from 220 (220 - age in years = maximum heart rate). Following are some general guidelines for finding the target heart rate for nonpregnant women:

Age (years)	Average maximum heart rate (220 - age in years)	Target heart rate for exercise (60–80% of maximum heart rate)
20	200 beats per minute	120–160 beats per minute
30	190	114–152
40	180	108–144
50	170	102–136
60	160	96–128
70	150	90–120

Source: The National Institutes of Health, National Heart, Lung, and Blood Institute.

son rises more slowly than that of an unfit person. Also, a fit heart returns to resting levels more quickly than an unfit one. The exercise level that provides the best workout for aerobic fitness is called the target heart rate. This heart rate allows most people to exercise optimally as they progress from being novices at exercise to veterans. People who have cardiac conditions or who are taking heart medications need to check with their doctor before using the target heart rate and exercise programs.

Endurance Training

Endurance is the ability to perform well over a period of time. You can improve your cardiovascular endurance through repeated aerobic exercise, which enhances the function and capacity of the heart and lungs. It also improves the ability of muscles to use oxygen and produce energy aerobically.

Endurance training involves alternately contracting and relaxing the muscles and using large muscle groups to put stress on muscle fibers. As tiny tears in the muscles repair themselves, muscles strengthen. A continuous supply of energy to fuel this activity is provided to muscles by the conversion of fat and carbohydrates to energy. Trained muscles go through changes that enable them to better use oxygen from the blood and energy stores. This increased efficiency results in greater endurance. Endurance activities include walking, running, swimming, cycling, and cross-country skiing.

Resistance Training

Resistance exercises are designed to build muscle strength by contracting groups of muscles against some type of resistance (like stretching a rubber strip or tube). Strength is the maximum force that can be exerted in a single voluntary muscle contraction. It can be measured and developed in various ways through resistance training. The type of training depends on the purpose and area to be targeted. Because lifting, moving objects, and moving oneself are important parts of

The Gender Gap

Women are different from men when it comes to endurance and strength. Understanding these differences can help you structure an exercise program that is best for you.

Aerobic fitness and strength are about the same for boys and girls until after puberty. At puberty, levels of the hormone testosterone rise in males, resulting in the growth of long bones and an increase in muscle mass and size. As they move through adolescence, many girls become far less active than boys, therefore reducing further their comparative aerobic ability.

Women have twice the body fat men have (some of which is necessary for reproductive function and health), so they have less lean body weight to support strength and aerobic

fitness. Also, on average, women have smaller bodies than men, and muscle strength is related to size.

Interestingly, pregnancy enhances women's endurance levels to the extent that after pregnancy, women are close to men in terms of endurance. The effect of this change is seen best in distance runners, who have dramatically improved endurance after their first pregnancy.

It is important to realize that differences between men and women are relative and that comparing your strength and endurance to a man's is not productive. Gaining more strength relative to your current level is all that really matters.

daily function, a loss of physical strength interferes with independent living. Resistance training targets specific muscles in order to increase strength but does not necessarily have the aerobic benefits associated with endurance training. Swimming is an excellent form of exercise that provides resistance for many muscle groups at once, and provides an aerobic workout without putting too much stress on bones and joints.

Isotonic Strength. Isotonic, or dynamic, strength is the maximum weight a muscle can support at one time. The most common form of isotonic exercise is weight lifting. Isotonic strength is measured as the hardest part of the lift, at the very beginning, when resistance is high. Weight lifting machines or free weights can be used to target specific muscles. Weights do not have to be heavy to be effective for women. One- to five-pound free weights are adequate for most active women. Multiple repetitions of isotonic exercise at lower weights build strength and muscle tone, while increasing the weight increases muscle size and strength with fewer repetitions. Many women prefer the look of more toned, less bulky muscles obtained with lower weight exercises. It is wise to work out under the supervision of a professional if you wish to use heavier weights. Start at low levels and increase the weights slowly. As with all exercise, isotonic exercises demand good posture and breathing technique.

Isometric Strength. Isometric or static strength is the exertion of maximal force or muscle contraction against an immovable object. Isometric exercises are often used in physical rehabilitation or along with weight lifting. These exercises, which were popular in the 1960s, are now believed to have limited use and benefit. The most popular isometric exercises for women today are Kegel exercises—used to strengthen the muscles in the lower pelvis to prevent incontinence after childbirth or with age.

Flexibility Training

Flexibility helps improve performance in endurance and resistance training while improving range of motion and, usually, posture. It is recommended that warming up and stretching the muscles be done before and after exercise. Before exercise, stretching prepares the muscles for activity and helps prevent injury. After exercise, a cool-down period of stretching helps prevent flexibility-limiting muscle soreness and tension that can occur when an exercise session ends abruptly.

Several forms of exercise are geared specifically toward improving flexibility, and they offer other benefits to the mind and body as well. Yoga, which incorporates concentration and meditation techniques, is the most popular and accessible of these practices and can lead to impressive gains in flexibility. Classes are offered at most gyms and at many community centers and YWCAs, as well as in private yoga centers. Videotapes and books are also available that describe postures and the philosophy of yoga. Many participants find yoga not only healthful for the body, but helpful in reducing stress, as well.

Pilates is a stretching and strength-building technique that focuses on the important muscles that create good posture and body alignment. Developed by German fitness expert Joseph Pilates in the 1920s, the method was originally used by dancers but is gaining mainstream popularity. The original method required equipment called the Universal Reformer, but many gyms and dance studios today offer a modified Pilates class that can be done on floor mats.

Musculoskeletal Exercises

Almost any type of physical activity will improve the health of your musculoskeletal system. However, there are specific musculoskeletal exercises that are designed to strengthen the knees, lower back, and other areas of the body where muscles and bones work together. These exercises can be performed at home, in a more formal setting, such as a gym or community education class, or under the supervision of a physical therapist or trainer.

FIGURE 9.3

Abdominal Strengthening

This exercise is based on the Pilates method, a movement technique that focuses on building sleek muscles and supporting good posture.

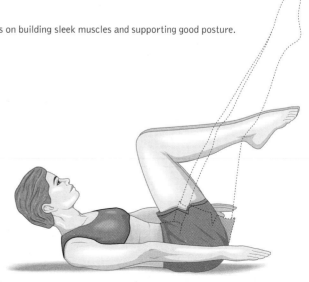

STEP 1 Lay on your back with head lifted and knees bent into the chest. Raise your arms slightly off the floor, palms down. Contract your abdominal muscles and press the small of your back into the floor. Point your toes.

STEP 2 Straighten your legs toward the ceiling, then lower slightly, making sure lower back stays pressed against the floor. Raise your arms 1–2 inches off the floor. Breathe in through your nose, counting to five, then out through your mouth, counting to five, while gently pumping straightened arms up and down with each count. Do 10 reps.

Levels of
Exercise

How hard should I exercise? How long should each exercise session last? How often should I exercise? Women commonly raise these questions as they begin to design their own fitness program. Since every woman is different, it is important for every woman to work at her own level. Understanding the concepts of intensity, duration, and frequency will help you make these important decisions about your program.

Intensity

Intensity refers to how physically demanding, or how hard, an exercise or physical activity is. The intensity of exercise needed to improve physical conditioning varies with the individual based on her age, general health, body weight, level of fitness, and other factors. When you rely on low-intensity exercises, you will require more time to increase your aerobic capacity than when you engage in high-intensity exercise. However, please note that although high-intensity activity provides greater conditioning in shorter time, it poses a higher risk of joint or musculoskeletal injury or damage than low- and moderate-intensity exercise, especially if you are beginning an exercise program after a period of inactivity.

Exercise is often categorized as high-, low-, or no-impact, depending on how much weight is brought to bear on supporting limbs. High-impact exercise involves jumping or jumping-like movements in which both feet leave the floor at

Intensity of Exercise

Moderate-level physical activity expends approximately 200 calories per day in a 30-minute session. To achieve the same benefit with light-level activity, you need to perform the activity more often or for longer periods or both. Following are examples of activities based on the calories expended per minute.

	INTENSITY	
Low (about 300 calories/hour)	**Moderate** (400 calories/hour)	**High** (500-600 calories/hour)
Walking	Walking briskly	Walking briskly uphill or carrying weights
Cycling, stationary	Cycling for pleasure or transportation	Cycling fast or uphill
Swimming, slow treading	Swimming, moderate	Swimming, fast
Golf, power cart	Golf, carrying clubs	
Boating	Canoeing, leisurely	Canoeing, rapidly
Carpet sweeping	General cleaning	Moving furniture

once. Running is high-impact. Low-impact exercises involve movements in which only one leg or foot leaves the ground at any time. These exercises are better tolerated by most women and pose less risk of injury or damage.

Most aerobics programs offer high- and low-impact classes. If you take a low-impact class, you can still get a high-intensity cardiovascular workout if the choreography causes your heart rate to elevate, for example, by using strong, "pumping"-type arm movements.

Swimming is a no-impact form of exercise. It is preferred by people with joint problems or arthritis and those who cannot tolerate the weight-bearing forms of exercise. Non-weight-bearing forms of exercise, such as swimming and some forms of yoga, do not reduce osteoporosis risk and should be supplemented with weight bearing exercises, if possible.

Duration

Duration refers to how long you exercise. For example, running up three flights of stairs is exercise of short duration. Taking a 60-minute aerobics class is exercise of long duration.

The number of calories expended is a function of duration and intensity of exercise, along with other factors. For example, activities that expend 200 calories daily in a total of 30 minutes (1,400 calories per week) have been shown to provide additional health and fitness benefits. Longer duration training improves fat metabolism and weight control and lowers blood lipids. In the study of Harvard University alumni mentioned earlier, health and fitness levels were highest among those participants whose activities expended 2,000 calories per week.

Frequency

Frequency refers to how often exercise or physical activity takes place. Previously, experts recommended 20 or more minutes of endurance exercise that elevated the heart to its target rate three or more times per week. Although this frequency produces valuable health benefits, it is now generally accepted that the same benefits can be achieved by participating in moderate-intensity physical activities outside of formal exercise programs for a total of 30 minutes daily, even if the activity is broken into smaller segments.

Preventing *Injuries*

As everyone knows, exercise poses some risk of injury along with the benefits to health. Minor injuries can be avoided by taking common sense precautions, such as double-knotting shoelaces to avoid tripping and wearing a bicycle helmet. Major injuries are rare for someone who is engaged in a moderate exercise program, and they can usually be prevented altogether when she is aware of potential danger.

Musculoskeletal Injuries

The most common injuries associated with physical activity are musculoskeletal injuries, that is, injuries to the skin, bones, muscles, tendons, and ligaments. These include bruises, blisters, sprains, and strains. Such injuries can occur with

Exercise and the Risk of Heart Attack

Although the risk of heart attack and sudden death increase slightly with physical exertion—even for women who are physically active—the benefits of exercise far outweigh the risks. Your exercise program can be structured to fit any level of fitness. If there is any sign of increased risk of a heart condition—family history, previous heart attack or angina, or warning symptoms with exertion—consult your doctor for help designing an appropriate and safe exercise program.

excessive amounts of activity or with suddenly beginning too high a level of activity for which the body is not conditioned.

Following a rigorous weight-bearing exercise routine for many years can result in damage to the joints unless you remember to pace yourself and take steps to avoid overworking your musculoskeletal system. For example, some runners and aerobic instructors who do not heed this kind of advice find that they fall victim to arthritis and chronic pain as they grow older. Again, the goal in exercise is to feel better, to maintain healthy systems, and to enjoy a high quality of life. You are wise not to "compete" with people doing similar exercise, a tempting practice that often leads to injury. Offer yourself a reasonable challenge whenever you exercise, but remember that moderation is the healthiest approach to keeping fit for life.

Overexertion

Injury can result from overdoing an exercise. It is best to start gradually and avoid high-impact exercise initially. Always drink plenty of fluids to avoid dehydration. Be aware of bodily responses. It is important to watch for signs of overexertion. Pain should not be a part of a fitness program. Fatigue, pain, or rapid heart rate may mean that you are overdoing and should decrease the intensity of exercise before overexertion occurs. Any activity that is practiced to the extreme can result in injury.

An important part of exercise is to continuously monitor the feedback your body is giving you, both while exercising and throughout the day. Watch for the following signs of overexertion:

- Inability to finish the exercise
- Inability to talk during the exercise
- Faintness or nausea during or after the exercise
- Persistent or increasing fatigue
- Sleeplessness
- Persistent aches and pains in the joints

Heart Attacks and Sudden Death

The occurrence of heart attacks and sudden death are rare during exercise. These incidents are more likely, however, in sedentary people with advanced or unrecognized heart disease who engage in strenuous activity to which they are unaccustomed. Sedentary people, with or without known heart disease, who wish to increase their physical activity need to build up their level of activity gradually.

Special *Concerns* for Women

A woman's body, her metabolism, her endurance, and her strength differ fundamentally from a man's. Therefore women must approach physical training differently. Most women do not require large, bulging muscles, for example, to feel physically fit. They are more interested in achieving their ideal weight, moving freely, remaining disease-free, and looking and feeling healthy.

Safety Guidelines

The following guidelines, developed by The American College of Obstetricians and Gynecologists, are designed to help women develop a safe and healthy exercise program.

Aerobic Exercise

- Limit exercise routines that involve repeated foot impacts to 30 minutes of duration and work at a level that does not raise the heart rate to more than 75 percent of the maximal. There should be a day of rest between such sessions.
- Select a resilient floor or surface for exercise that involves repeated foot impacts. If such a surface is not available, modify the exercise routines to ensure that the feet remain close to the floor throughout the program.
- Precede all aerobic exercise with a gentle warm-up routine that uses the full range of motion of the joints. This increases the elasticity of the muscles and will help prevent injury.
- Stretch the muscles that are used repeatedly during aerobic exercise after each session.
- To reduce the severity of impact shock on the lower extremities, avoid jumping on the same foot more than four times in a row.
- Avoid extremes of joint motion and extension (such as deep knee bends and hyperextension of the knee).
- Keep your feet moving throughout the session to prevent cramping in the muscles of the foot.
- Avoid rotating the trunk while on your feet with your hips or lower spine flexed. Rotational activity in this position puts a high level of stress on the disks in the back.
- Follow every period of intense physical activity with a cool-down period that involves at least ten minutes of lighter activity. Do not stop exercising abruptly. It is best to avoid hot showers and baths immediately after intense physical activity, because it may cause weakness or fainting.
- Learn to assess your physical status and progress while you are engaged in vigorous aerobic exercise. Measure your heart rate during peak levels of exercise to ensure that the intensity of activity is within the desired range. If you measure the recovery heart rate after exercise, you can document your progress in improving cardiovascular fitness. Failure to progress as measured by this method may indicate the need for more intense activity during the aerobic phase or may signal the presence of other problems.

Strengthening Exercises

- Always skip a day between sessions when lifting weights or doing other strengthening exercises.
- Stretch and warm up your muscles gently before doing any resistance training, and again after each session.
- When lifting weights, working with elastic bands, or using any other type of strengthening equipment, exercise in a slow and controlled manner. Ballistic (rapid or jerky) movements increase the risk of injury.
- The most efficient way to improve strength is to repeat a movement (such as lifting a weight) ten or fewer times per set. Allow brief rest periods between sets, and limit yourself to three sets for each different exercise.
- When the strength of one muscle or muscle group is disproportionate to that of the opposing muscle or group, work for a while exclusively on the weaker muscle to restore balance around the joint.
- Never hold your breath during strength-training exercises. Always exhale during the exertion phase of each repetition.

Stretching Exercises

- You can perform stretching exercises as often as you wish; one session a day is recommended for maximum flexibility.
- Warm up the entire body before muscles are stretched.
- Avoid rapid, jerky movements, and do not hold your breath while stretching.
- Stretch muscles only to the point where you feel tension. If you experience pain, the stretch has gone too far.
- Hold each stretch at a gently challenging point until you feel the muscles relax. In this way you achieve the maximum benefit from the stretch.

Source: Women and Exercise. Washington, DC: ACOG; 1992. The American College of Obstetricians and Gynecologists Technical Bulletin 173.

Before embarking on an exercise program, it is wise to take some time to assess the special exercise needs relating to breast care, bone mass, hormonal changes, pregnancy, and age. Taking appropriate precautions and making modifications to individual exercise programs can help women participate in physical activity at appropriate levels throughout their lives.

Breast Care

A woman's breasts are made up mostly of fatty tissue. They are not easily injured during sports and do not require any special protection beyond basic support and comfort. A woman's pectoral muscles are not usually very strong, so they do not provide good support for the breasts during exercise. The breast ligaments provide only modest support.

All this does not mean that exercise will cause breasts to sag—that is a factor of breast size, weight, age, and lack of support. It does mean that a bra that provides good support—without wires or seams—will make exercise more comfortable and avoid stretching ligaments and tissues. A sports bra should be made of a light and breathable fabric, and it should be well-fitted to prevent bouncing. Sports centers and specialized shops can provide advice and fittings.

Friction during exercise, such as jogging or high-impact aerobics, can cause chafing and irritation of the nipples. A tight-fitting bra will help prevent this problem. Special pads to prevent chafing and applying lanolin to the nipples to keep them soft may prevent or relieve any discomfort.

Menstrual Cycle

In women, too much exercise can cause hormonal changes resulting in changes in menstruation. Some woman who exercise to excess even stop having menstrual cycles altogether, a condition called amenorrhea.

Exercise-induced amenorrhea is brought on by a complex set of changes that affects the hormones that regulate the function of the ovaries. These changes interrupt production of the hormone estrogen, which is produced in the ovaries. The fertility of a woman with amenorrhea may be affected, but will probably return to normal when ovarian function returns. Long periods of low estrogen production can interfere with the building of strong bones or can result in loss of bone density similar to that which occurs in postmenopausal women.

The good news is that exercise-induced amenorrhea occurs only with extreme amounts of exercise, usually during professional or Olympic training of runners, gymnasts, and figure skaters. Running 20 to 30 miles a week can cause menstrual irregularities, and periods usually stop in women who run more than 40 miles per week. A woman in training who misses or has irregular periods should see a doctor and consider reducing her exercise schedule or taking an estrogen supplement to protect her bones.

On the other hand, moderate exercise can offer benefits to women during menstruation. Many women who experience cramps during their periods have reported that exercise often alleviates the pain and discomfort.

Pregnancy

Pregnant women are encouraged to be active and to exercise. An active lifestyle can ease some of the discomforts of pregnancy. It also helps build stamina, muscle tone, and coordination.

Changes That Affect Exercise. There are some key changes that take place in the body during pregnancy, which a woman is advised to take into consideration when planning an exercise program.

Safety Guidelines for Exercise During Pregnancy

- Exercise regularly, rather than intermittently.
- Avoid the supine (flat on the back) position after the first trimester.
- Modify the intensity of exercise based on how you feel. Avoid becoming overtired or overheated.
- Avoid activities that pose a risk of loss of balance or abdominal trauma.
- Make sure you eat an adequate diet to support the extra 300 calories per day required by pregnancy.
- Drink lots of fluids and avoid exercising in hot weather.
- You can resume a more active exercise program slowly four to six weeks after delivery, with the guidance of your health care provider.

Weight Gain. Doctors advise women to plan to gain between 20 and 35 pounds during pregnancy. As she steadily gains, the pregnant woman needs to exercise at a slower pace than she might earlier have done. It is considered unwise for a woman to exercise with the goal of losing weight while she is pregnant. However, exercise may help a pregnant woman use calories more efficiently and help her avoid excessive weight gain. Because of increased weight and cardiovascular changes, however, care must be taken to monitor the heart rate to ensure there is not too much stress placed on the heart by exercising too strenuously.

Balance. As her abdomen grows, a pregnant woman's center of gravity changes. Her posture and the curvature of her spine also may change. For these reasons, activities, such as bicycling, that rely on balance and sudden stops are not recommended.

Core Body Temperature. Even a moderately high core body temperature during pregnancy can harm the fetus. Doctors usually advise women to avoid the use of hot tubs, saunas, and steam rooms during pregnancy. However, the core body temperature can also reach 101°F or higher during strenuous exercise in a hot environment. Although there is usually no reason for women who have engaged in strenuous activity before pregnancy to discontinue the exercise, it is recommended that they work out in a cool environment and check their body temperature at the end of each exercise session. Warning signs of overheating include a higher than usual heart rate and more sweating than usual, as the body tries to get rid of excess heat. Checking one's temperature with an oral thermometer at the end of an exercise session is recommended to help women make sure that they are staying in a safe range.

Hormonal Changes. The tremendous hormonal changes during pregnancy help prepare a woman to give birth. One effect of hormones on the body is the relaxing or loosening of ligaments that hold the pelvic bones in place, which enable the pelvis to widen when the baby is born. Other tendons and ligaments also are affected by this process, however, most notably those in the ankles. Just when a woman needs more support to accommodate weight gain, the ankles are, in fact, at a higher risk for sprains during pregnancy. Care is advised when putting strain on any ligaments and tendons during exercise.

Suitable Exercises for Pregnant Women

Very few exercises are inappropriate for pregnant women. A woman who was active before she became pregnant can continue to be active during her pregnancy. Swimming is a good choice because it is not weight-bearing and usually can be performed throughout pregnancy with little risk of injury. Downhill skiing, on the other hand, poses a significant risk of accidental injury, and the low oxygen levels associated with high altitudes may be harmful to those not acclimated. Water skiing, surfing, parachuting, jumping, and deep sea diving are also not recommended. Otherwise, almost any exercise program that does not cause you to become overheated or unduly exhausted can be continued.

Enjoying Exercise

Since you want to make exercise a part of each day for the rest of your life, make sure your fitness program includes exercises or activities that you enjoy. Look for exercises or activities you are confident you can comfortably do, or learn to do.

If you like to be outdoors, join a walking group, hike on the weekends, or learn how to cross-country ski. If you find it hard to get motivated at home alone with an exercise video, invite a friend over. Better yet, look into a community or adult education organization for beginner or intermediate level aerobics instruction, and enroll with your friends.

Keep the intensity low or moderate; you are more likely to continue your program if it is not overly demanding. Setting realistic goals, monitoring your progress, and providing self-reinforcement rewards (a new leotard or a night out at the movies) all contribute to keeping your motivation and enjoyment high.

Risk Factors and Exercise. There are some women who should not exercise during pregnancy. If any complication occurs in the course of your pregnancy, ask the doctor specifically about the advisability of resuming exercise. In general, women with the following conditions are wise to avoid exercise:

- Vaginal bleeding at any stage of pregnancy
- Preterm labor (in the current or a previous pregnancy)
- Pregnancy-induced increases in blood pressure
- Medical problems that restrict exercise when not pregnant

Osteoporosis

Osteoporosis is a painful, disabling condition in which decreased bone density (brittle bones) can lead to bone fractures. All women have a higher risk for osteoporosis than men, and certain women are most at risk. Prevention of osteoporosis begins in childhood, when adequate calcium intake and physical activity build good bone density.

During the period from puberty to menopause, women with normally functioning ovaries are somewhat protected from osteoporosis if they had normal bone development during childhood. As women age, calcium intake, weight-bearing impact exercise, such as walking with weights or jogging, and estrogen therapy all play important roles in general health maintenance and osteoporosis prevention. However, calcium loss from bones can still occur, especially during menopause. Non-weight-bearing forms of activity, such as swimming and bicycling, are excellent forms of cardiovascular exercise, but they do not prevent osteoporosis or bone loss.

What About the Kids? Fitting Exercise into Your Day

Women with young or school-age children may find it almost impossible to make time to exercise. Consider these solutions to see if one or more might work for you:

- Wake up 30 minutes before the rest of the family does. Turn on an exercise video without the sound, and work out while the sun rises. (Be sure to warm up on cold mornings.) Other quiet early morning activities include yoga and Tai Chi.
- If you have a partner at home to watch the kids, consider taking a brisk walk. If you make a daily plan to meet a walking partner, you are much less likely to roll over and go back to sleep or have other excuses, knowing she is out there waiting.
- If your kids are older, try to find activities you can do together, such as bicycling, skating, or tennis.
- Swap childcare with a neighbor who has children about the same age of yours. (Many parents today handle babysitting needs this way.) You exercise Tuesday and Thursday mornings or evenings; she exercises Wednesday and Friday. If you're married, swap childcare with your husband in the same manner.
- Find a gym or aerobics program that offers free childcare.
- Remember that exercise does not have to be structured to "count." A brisk walk with the baby in a stroller, playing with the kids on the front lawn, or running around a playground for 20 minutes are all viable forms of exercise.

Walking Your Way to Health

Walking is free. It can be done any time, any day, with no special equipment other than a pair of comfortable walking shoes. Walking can be a healthy form of exercise for nearly everyone. It is low-impact and poses very little risk of injury. Small wonder that walking is by far the most popular form of exercise among American women. Research shows that a brisk walk can keep a woman's heart in shape. A study of over 84,000 female nurses between the ages of 40 and 65 found that brisk walking (roughly four miles per hour) for three hours a week lowered their risk of developing heart disease by 40 percent. Even leisurely walking has more benefit than no walking. Here are some tips for walking your way to health:

- Start slowly with a 15-minute stroll if you have not been exercising regularly.
- Measure how far and how fast you walk so you can gauge progress.
- Keep the activity interesting; walk with a friend, vary the route, explore neighborhoods other than your own.
- Swing your arms to get a full body workout.
- Maintain good posture to help strengthen back muscles.
- If the weather is bad, move indoors to a shopping mall, indoor track, or treadmill.

Designing Your
Personal Exercise Program

Today, there are many options for developing a personal fitness program. Your program can incorporate moderate daily activity if you are just starting out, and this can be supplemented by more structured and/or longer-duration activities. You can exercise at home, in a gym, or with friends. In most cases, physical activity does not require any special equipment or training. Although you can invest in "high-tech" equipment, it is not essential to a healthy and enjoyable exercise program.

Overcoming Obstacles

There are barriers to exercise that interfere with starting or maintaining an exercise program. Among the most difficult barriers for women are lack of time (due to work or family commitments) and lack of appropriate childcare. (See the box on page 188 titled "What About the Kids? Fitting Exercise into Your Day" for some suggestions if you have children.) Other barriers include lack of equipment, lack of walking trails and other recreational facilities, bad weather, and an unsafe environment.

A daily exercise regimen is ideally something to look forward to. If you are constantly facing such obstacles to enjoyment, you will be less likely to continue. Sometimes you have to be creative. If walking is your exercise of choice, but you have no safe place to walk or the weather is bad, consider going to the mall. A great many large malls open their doors before shopping hours begin just for the benefit of walkers who use the main floor and mezzanines as a track. The main thing is to arrange a daily program that involves the fewest possible impediments, so that it can quickly and easily become a routine.

Most people who do not exercise claim they are too tired at the end of the day or say they cannot find time for it. One way to overcome such obstacles is to schedule an exercise program at a more convenient time of day, such as early in the morning before showering. People who exercise in the early morning find that it helps wake them up, clears their minds, and gives them a chance to plan their day before beginning other activities. Early morning exercisers often find that they have more time during the day and feel good about themselves, because while others are just starting their day, they already have an important thing done.

Getting Started

Most healthy adults do not need to receive a medical checkup before beginning an exercise program. Generally, though, women who are just beginning an exercise program are advised to start slowly. Women over age 40 who plan a vigorous program, and those who have either a chronic disease or risk factors for a chronic disease (such as heart disease or diabetes), should consult a physician to help them develop a suitable exercise program. An exercise test may be recommended if a woman appears to have a risk of heart disease that could complicate her exercise program. Women who are pregnant should follow the special guidelines that appear earlier in this chapter.

Getting Equipped

It is important to select the proper footwear based on the activity to be performed. Shoes are available for walking, running, dancing, aerobics, tennis, basketball, or a combination of sports (cross-training). While it is not necessary to invest in top-of-the-line footwear, for strenuous or high-impact activities, higher-quality footwear is recommended. Proper fit is important. The staff at a sporting goods or shoe store should be able to provide advice. The sole of the shoe should be thick and strong, but flexible, and designed for the surface on which it will be used. Check for adequate arch support, and always wear socks to prevent blisters.

No special clothing is required for exercise; however, it is best to wear clothing that is designed for comfort and ease of movement. Avoid clothing that rubs or binds. For outdoor activity, wear light clothing in warm weather. In cold weather, several thin layers are preferable to a single thick layer. Polypropylene is a synthetic material that wicks (draws) moisture away from the skin. It is a good choice for underwear as well as for socks. Avoid rubberized sweat suits because

Exercise Guidelines

Following are some general guidelines for common-sense exercise from the American Heart Association:

- Exercise only when you're feeling well. Wait until symptoms and signs of a cold or the flu have been absent for two days or more before resuming activity.
- Do not exercise vigorously soon after eating. Wait about two hours after eating to ensure that blood flow can be directed from digesting food to supplying working muscles.
- Adjust exercise to the weather. If the air temperature is over 70°F, slow the pace, be alert to signs of heat stress, and drink adequate fluids to prevent dehydration. If you

experience a headache, dizziness, faintness, nausea, cramps, clammy skin, or heart palpitations, you may be suffering from heat stress. Stop exercising immediately, find a cool place to rest, and take fluids until you feel better.
- Slow down for hills. When ascending hills, decrease speed to avoid overexertion.
- Wear proper clothing and shoes. Clothing should be loose-fitting, comfortable, and able to "breathe." Shoes should be appropriate for the exercise. (See the section on this page titled "Getting Equipped.")
- Be alert to your body's feedback. Stop exercising at the first sign of overexertion (discomfort in the upper body, faintness, shortness of breath, discomfort in the bones and joints).

The Cost of Fitness

As with any major purchase, it is important to consider service, warranty, and ease of operation. But it is not necessary to spend a fortune for fitness. The best choices for you may be the most basic ones.

- **Jump rope:** A length of number 10 sash cord can be purchased at a local hardware store for under $10. The ends of the rope should reach your armpits when you loop the rope beneath your feet. A rope is highly portable, and skipping can be done anywhere for a workout that builds aerobic capacity and coordination.

- **Exercise videos:** Many programs are offered for about $20.

- **Free weights:** A set of weights ranging from feather weight to over 40 pounds can be purchased for about $40. Individual pairs of dumbbells from one to five pounds cost about $10 a pair, while heavier weights cost more. A set of 300-pound free weights with adjustable dumbbells and a basic bench runs around $300. A better investment may be a higher-quality bench that is adjustable and comes with leg-extension and leg-curl attachments. It is recommended that most women start with rubber- or plastic-coated dumbbells ranging in weight from three to eight pounds.

- **Bicycle:** For about $200 you can buy a stand for a regular bicycle and turn it into a stationary bicycle. Otherwise, you can get a nonmotorized stationary bicycle for under $500. It should be comfortable and easy to adjust. Digital displays and computer graphics add to the price but not to the quality of the workout.

- **Stair machines:** Lower priced (under $500) stair machines are hydraulically powered and may worsen knee problems. A sturdy unit that operates smoothly may cost around $1,000.

- **Treadmill:** Lower level machines under $500 do not come close to offering the smoothness or durability of higher-priced machines, which cost about $1,000.

- **Multi-station weight machines:** A multi-station weight machine should be easy to use and comfortable. A high-quality unit costs at least $1,000, so it is best to try out six to eight repetitions per exercise before you decide on one.

Other types of equipment include cross-country ski devices, which provide a full-body workout, arm and leg combination machines, and rowing machines. These machines are complex and expensive but can provide a good workout if they are used regularly.

they interfere with the body's natural way of removing heat. Cottons and synthetic materials that are "breathable" are best.

Choice of Activity

Choosing the best activity for you depends on your specific health needs, the availability of equipment, and which activities you enjoy. For example, if you want to strengthen your back, look for a gym with a professional who can tailor your workout with exercise equipment that focuses on the appropriate muscles. If you want to improve overall cardiovascular fitness, look for aerobic and endurance training exercises, activities, or classes. If you enjoy team sports but do not want to work out in an overly competitive environment, look for a local volleyball or softball league that meets informally once or twice a week.

By varying the type of activities you choose over the course of a week, you can develop a well-rounded program for optimum health.

Aerobic Endurance. Good choices for promoting aerobic endurance include swimming, running or jogging, bicycling, walking, skiing, and aerobic dance. Team sports also may be effective if they involve prolonged activity. Swimming provides conditioning of upper and lower extremities as well as aerobic condi-

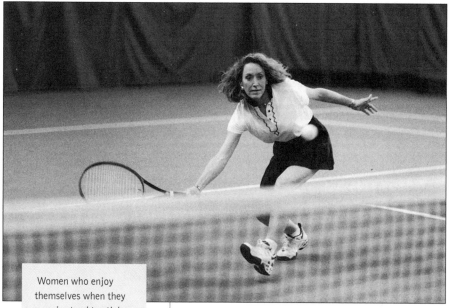

Women who enjoy themselves when they exercise tend to stick with it longer than those who find it boring or difficult. Vary your physical activities so you don't get bored, or exercise with a friend to make the time more pleasurable and social.

tioning with minimal impact. The water buoyancy makes swimming a good choice for women with orthopedic problems, pregnant women, and some older women. Bicycling, if performed at an active pace, conditions the abdomen, lower back, and parts of the upper body as well as the legs. Jogging and brisk walking are the most common forms of aerobic activity. They can be performed almost anywhere, in any weather, and at your own pace.

Strength and Toning. Exercises directed to strengthening muscles include free weights, isotonic exercises, elastic resistance (using large rubber bands or tubes), body-weight resistance (push-ups), or weight-training machines. Weight training can also be used for toning or increasing muscle mass and shape. These programs are best done under the direction of a trainer or in a class setting.

Home Exercise Equipment. Home exercise equipment is becoming increasingly popular as a means of helping busy people design an exercise program to be carried out in the comfort and convenience of their home (no babysitter or weather problems). The equipment is generally easy to use. Complex equipment may help you through all phases of an exercise program—aerobic, strengthening, and stretching. Many people, however, find it difficult to get motivated to exercise on their own. For some, listening to music or watching television helps. When purchasing home exercise equipment, it is best to look for the basics, with only those features essential for the intended use. Try using a friend's equipment a few times to see if it works for you. Such testing will help you buy equipment that you enjoy using.

Individual and Team Sports. Many women think of exercise only in terms of exercise classes or working out at a gym. As you design your own personal fitness program, consider individual and team sports, too. For many women, the term sports is an immediate turn-off. They think, "Oh, sports are for men. Sports are competitive, and I want to have fun while I exercise." However, informal community-based women's team sports offer a fun, social way to incorporate fitness into your life. With a little investigating you can almost always find a team that is appropriate for your level. Joining a team guarantees that you will get out of the house and exercise. Consider the following sports options—they may help you rethink your approach to sports as a means of helping you become fit:

- Check the local paper for news of running clubs.
- Check the "Y" or a local pool for adult swimming teams.

- Consider joining a tennis or racquetball club where matches are planned.
- Look for community league volleyball, softball, or soccer teams.

What *You* Can Do

Talk to any woman who was once inactive and is now committed to an exercise program, and she will tell you that the change was hard at first. However, she will almost certainly add that after a few weeks of regular exercise, she reached a "point of no return." That is, she found that the pleasure she received from carrying out her daily routine was much greater than the inconvenience, sore muscles, or feelings of awkwardness that accompanied the start of her program. You, too, can reach that point. Where once you couldn't imagine 30 minutes of aerobic activity a day, in a few weeks you can be saying, "I can't do without it!"

- **Think of exercise as cumulative during the day.** When you choose a parking space at a distance from your destination; when you choose the stairs over the elevator; when you choose to walk to the corner store instead of driving—remember that every five minute period of exertion leads you toward your goal of 30 minutes a day.
- **Challenge yourself.** Taking it too easy will not yield results, and you may feel you are wasting your time.
- **Know your limits.** Overdoing the challenge will leave you tired, sore, and frustrated. Start slowly and build to greater challenges over time.
- **Find an exercise partner.** Knowing someone is waiting for you to join her will get you out the door.
- **Plan a realistic time for exercise.** Can you get up 30 minutes before your family to go for a walk or work with an exercise video? Can you exercise at night while watching your favorite programs on television? Can you walk during your lunch hour at work? Make sure the time you choose is a time that will be consistently available to you.
- **Take precautions.** Find a safe environment to exercise in, and choose activities, clothing, and equipment that will protect you from injury and make exercise a pleasant experience. If you are overweight or have reason to worry about high blood pressure or heart problems, check with your doctor before beginning your program.
- **Enjoy yourself.** Any challenging program will have moments of frustration and even discomfort. But at the end of your sessions, if you feel more discomfort than pleasure, or if you find you do not look forward to exercise after the first few weeks, then try out new activities until you find the ones that you truly enjoy.

Sleeping Peacefully

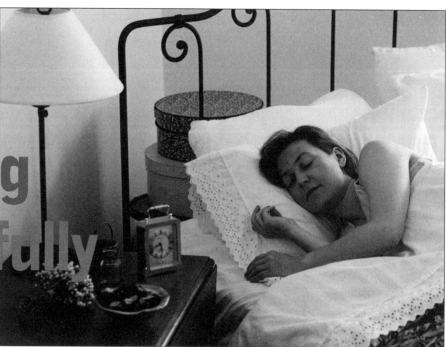

Scientists used to think of sleep as a simple loss of consciousness. A century ago, sleep was thought to be caused by either reduced or increased blood flow to the brain. In ancient Greece, the philosopher Plato suggested that sleep was caused by stomach vapors clogging the pores of the brain.

The time you spend asleep is as important to your wellness as the elements of a healthy lifestyle, such as good nutrition and regular exercise. Sleep provides a period of rest necessary for restoration of the body and the mind. A good night's rest is critical to mental alertness and overall energy, as well as to the proper functioning of the cardiovascular and endocrine systems. Sleep also helps maintain the body's natural immune system, which helps combat disease. When a woman gets run down from lack of sleep, she is more susceptible to disease and infection. Getting enough rest is a matter of determining how much sleep your body needs to function well and then learning good sleep habits.

The old adage says a person spends nearly a third of her life asleep. In today's busy world, however, many people feel like they do not sleep as well—or as long—as they would like. In fact, as a nation, we are sleeping nearly an hour and a half less each night than we did a century ago. Remarkably, most people forego sleep on purpose, in order to "make more time." Researchers point out that sleep deprivation—not getting enough sleep—afflicts a majority of Americans, over and above the 35 million with insomnia (difficulty falling asleep) or other sleep disorders.

Why We *Sleep*

Scientists know a great deal about sleep but still know very little about why we sleep. Experts agree that we need sleep in the same way that we need air, water, and food. Broadly speaking, sleep is considered an active state in which the body and mind "repair" themselves. If we get inadequate sleep over a long enough period of time, our bodies and minds stop functioning properly.

Behavioral psychologists, neurophysiologists, and other sleep researchers have studied how the central nervous system regulates sleep and waking. Psychiatrists have studied whether dreaming is a physical need. While theories and research results abound, there is no generally accepted explanation of the function of sleep.

Definitions of Sleep

Just what is sleep? In simple terms, sleep is a state of suspended consciousness, in which the body can respond to external stimulation but much less readily and much less efficiently than when awake. Physically, the muscles are relaxed; mentally, the brain is electrically active—in a pattern distinct from the awake mode—but seldom conscious of external or internal stimuli.

Circadian Rhythms

Circadian rhythms, sometimes referred to as your "body clock," are daily cycles that regulate changes in body temperature, cardiovascular rates, and endocrine (hormonal) activity. These rhythms originate in an area of the brain called the suprachiasmatic nucleus (SCN), a small cluster of nerve cells located near the hypothalamus.

Circadian rhythms do not follow a 24-hour cycle, like our solar day; they are actually closer to a 25-hour cycle. The reasons for this discrepancy are unclear. However, humans have essentially trained themselves to operate on a 24-hour schedule, based on their perception of light and dark and on other lifestyle factors. Infants, for example, must "settle in" to the day/night cycle, a welcomed milestone for new parents. For adults, lifestyle factors, such as setting your alarm clock and when you eat dinner, also help you keep in tune with a 24-hour schedule, but light is the most important regulator. Most people find it difficult to sleep in bright light, perhaps because it suppresses the body's release of melatonin, a natural substance in the body that helps you sleep.

There are high and low points in the daily circadian cycle—periods of increased or decreased activity, concentration, and work capacity. For example, most people find it very hard to stay awake and function well in the middle of the night (a low point from roughly 2 to 6 A.M.). Traffic and industrial accidents occur more often during this period. There is also a period of decreased alertness after lunch, between 1 and 4 P.M. This "post-lunch slump" is actually caused by a dip in circadian rhythms, not the digestive process. Many countries, such as Spain and Italy, continue to have afternoon nap times (siestas) during which businesses are closed, perhaps reflecting a more realistic adaptation to normal circadian rhythms. On the other hand, most people experience a high point in the morning and early evening. Most adults find it hard to stay asleep during this period, particularly between 9 and 11 A.M. and between 7 and 9 P.M.

Dreams

Everyone dreams—in fact, studies have shown that you need to dream—but not everyone remembers dreams. Here are some interesting facts about dreams:

- People who wake directly from REM sleep are most likely to remember their dreams.
- To help remember dreams in the morning, some people keep pen and paper by the bed so they can jot down key events as soon as they awaken.
- Dream interpretation is the subject of an entire library of books.
- Some people are able to learn how to have lucid dreams, in which they consciously steer where the dream goes.
- People who are blind from birth have dreams that consist of sound and tactile sensation rather than images. In REM sleep, people who are blind do not have the eye movements characteristic of the phase.

How Sleep Works

Researchers have identified several stages people go through during sleep. These include a transition period from waking to sleeping, four stages of non-REM (rapid eye movement) sleep, and REM sleep. Over a typical night's sleep, you will go through the cycle several times, with each cycle lasting about 90 to 100 minutes.

Restful Wakefulness

The first stage of sleep, which typically lasts about five minutes, is called "restful wakefulness." During this stage, your muscles begin to relax and your brain waves slow as concentration, memory, and other cognitive processes become less efficient. Although you can be easily aroused from this stage of sleep, your decreased attention and memory make it difficult to carry on a conversation. Sometimes during this stage, you may feel your body jerk slightly, almost as if you are falling.

Non-REM Sleep

Non-REM sleep, the second stage, consists of four substages. You progress forward through the four substages of non-REM sleep and then go in reverse through substages 3, 2, and 1 before entering REM sleep. Researchers measure non-REM sleep with an electroencephalograph (EEG), a machine that monitors brain waves. Brain waves behave differently during each stage of non-REM sleep.

Substage 1. During substage 1 sleep, you gradually become drowsy and begin to drift off to sleep. Your muscles relax, your breathing and pulse rates decrease, and your brain waves slow. Since the EEG measures these brain waves as theta waves, substage 1 sleep is also known as theta sleep. This substage usually lasts 2 to 5 minutes.

Substage 2. During substage 2, your brain waves slow even further as you fall into deeper sleep. Bursts of electrical activity, called spindles, are visible on the EEG during this time. This substage usually lasts 15 to 30 minutes.

Substages 3 and 4. During substages 3 and 4, the periods of deepest sleep, the heart rate and breathing slow further, and body temperature and movements decrease slightly. Researchers believe that the body "repairs" itself during this period, because more infection-fighting antibodies are produced. Brain waves also slow significantly during substages 3 and 4. Scientists sometimes refer to this period as delta sleep, because the brain's electrical activity during this period is recorded in delta waves. These substages normally last a total of 30 to 40 minutes during your first sleep cycle, but become shorter as REM sleep increases.

REM Sleep

REM sleep, or active sleep, is named for the rapid side to side eye movements that characterize it. During REM sleep, blood and oxygen flow to the brain increases. The activity of the central nervous system is similar to when you are awake. Your pulse rate increases, your breathing becomes irregular, and your muscles twitch, although a biochemical switch prevents you from consciously moving your muscles. Most significantly, the electrical activity in your brain increases, as you dream most often and most intensely during REM sleep. This stage lasts 11 to 25 minutes and occurs at the end of a full sleep cycle. REM sleep increases in frequency as you progress through a night's sleep.

As you grow older, your REM patterns change. Infants, for example, can move quickly into periods of prolonged REM sleep. With age, however, your duration of REM sleep may diminish significantly. Elderly women may lose REM sleep entirely.

Waking

At the end of a sleep cycle, your body temperature starts to rise and your respiration and pulse rates start to stabilize. Researchers know more about how we sleep than about how we awaken, but they do know that typically it takes some time to overcome the inertia associated with sleep. When you wake up abruptly, such as when your alarm clock goes off, it is often at the end of a period of REM sleep, when dreams may be recalled with great clarity.

How Much
Sleep You **Need**

Many people perceive the ability to get by on less sleep as an admirable quality. People who do not need a lot of sleep are considered efficient, organized, or competitive. Many people fight their body's need for sleep, citing other demands on their time, whether at work or at home. Sleep, however, is a biological requirement, like good food and water, and everyone needs a certain amount of sleep to be well rested and function at their best. The amount varies from person to person, so needing more or less sleep is an individual characteristic.

Many women are chronically sleep deprived. Adolescent girls are at particular risk, since excessive social demands and homework may shorten the amount of sleep they get at a time when they need substantial sleep.

Since World War II, we have become a 24-hour society. Some 15 to 20 percent of all people in the workforce operate on schedules that differ from the traditional 9 to 5 day, many of them on shifts that interfere with natural sleeping schedules. Studies of sleep patterns in environments regulated only by natural light, without clocks, show that our natural daily sleep requirement approaches 10 hours.

With such high value placed on time in our 24-hour society, many women sacrifice sleep in order to fit more into their already busy schedules. In fact, women today sleep an average of 1 1/2 hours less each night than they did a century ago.

General Recommendations

On average, a person needs close to 8 hours of sleep a night to feel well rested and alert throughout the day. The requirement varies with the individual, from 6 to 9 hours usually, although some people require as much as 10 hours of sleep.

wellness warning

Depriving your body of the amount of sleep it needs can be dangerous. You cannot train yourself to get by on less sleep or trick yourself into needing less sleep.

Effects of Sleep Deprivation

Some estimates suggest that one-third to one-half of all Americans have experienced occasional periods of sleep deprivation. Almost everyone has experienced some form of insomnia at some point in their lives. Short-term sleep deprivation is not especially harmful. But chronic, regular lack of sufficient sleep can have significant mental and physical effects, because sleep loss is a cumulative process.

Sleep deprivation affects your mood first, making you irritable. It becomes difficult to concentrate and stay alert. Your short-term memory is impaired, as is your general performance: your reaction time, your ability to think clearly. Your ability to make decisions is also affected. Substantial sleep deprivation over a long period can lead to hallucinations. Sleep-deprived people may not be aware of how lack of sleep is affecting them, contributing to small mistakes or mishaps, such as placing a mug of hot coffee too close to the edge of the counter, or major disasters, such as car accidents. For example, the investigation of the Challenger shuttle explosion found that NASA managers involved in making the decision to launch had been sleeping less than the bare minimum of 5 hours a night for several days. Sleep deprivation has been linked to the accidents at the Three Mile Island and Chernobyl nuclear power plants and the Bhopal chemical plant, as well as the Exxon Valdez oil spill.

Sleep is a critical physical need. Sleep deprivation can seriously impair your wellness and ability to function. The best way to prevent or overcome sleep deprivation is to make sure you get enough good sleep on a regular basis.

Physical Factors That Affect Sleep

How well you sleep is affected by a variety of physical factors—age, diet, exercise, stages of the reproductive cycle, including pregnancy or menopause, and medical conditions.

Age. The amount of time we need to sleep changes as we age. Infants and small children sleep longer than adolescents, and adolescents sleep longer and awaken later than most adults. As we age, the timing in our circadian rhythms shifts, so that we fall asleep earlier and wake up earlier.

Diet. When you eat, what you eat, and how much you eat can affect how well you sleep. Eating heavy meals prior to bedtime may disrupt your sleep. Also, eating foods, such as chocolate or other caffeinated items, that contain mild stimulants may keep you from falling asleep. Some women find that certain foods, particularly those that contribute to heartburn or reflux (stomach acid rising into your esophagus), hinder their ability to fall asleep easily. Being overweight can cause sleep disruptions, such as loud snoring and sleep apnea (difficulty breathing during sleep).

Exercise. Regular exercise improves the quality of sleep and can help you fall asleep faster. But because body temperature drops in the early stages of sleep, and exercise raises your core body temperature, it is important not to exercise too close to bedtime. Ideally, you should not exercise within three hours of going to sleep.

Menstrual Cycles, Pregnancy, and Menopause. Hormone levels fluctuate during the reproductive cycle, affecting the quality of sleep. In the first part of the menstrual cycle, progesterone levels are lower and women typically sleep less deeply. Ovulation brings higher levels of progesterone, causing more sleepiness. Progesterone levels drop again with the onset of bleeding, and many women have some difficulty falling asleep at this time. Women who are pregnant often have difficulty falling asleep as they adjust to the changes in their body, and their growing abdomen and softening pelvic bones may make it difficult to find a comfortable sleeping position. Also, they may feel the need for more sleep to compensate for the extra energy their bodies are expending. During perimenopause (the stage just prior to menopause), classic symptoms, such as hot flashes and night sweats, often occur with the onset of REM sleep, making the quality of sleep less restful.

Mood Disorders. Mood disorders, such as depression, can have a great impact on sleep. Women with depression often complain of having difficulty falling asleep or remaining asleep. (Anxiety can also cause difficulty in falling asleep.) Depression is also characterized by general fatigue and difficulty concentrating, symptoms that may worsen with irregular sleep patterns. More serious depression can cause frequent awakenings or early morning awakenings (3 or 4 AM).

On the other hand, certain disorders have been known to cause fatigue or extreme sleepiness. Seasonal changes in mood, atypical depression, and manic depressive illness have been known to cause hypersomnia, or excessive sleep. Chronic fatigue syndrome, a debilitating disorder that affects women in particular—many of whom also suffer from depression—can cause a constant state of tiredness that lasts months to years. With this syndrome, exerting even small amounts of energy can cause exhaustion. Researchers suspect a connection between depression, chronic fatigue syndrome, and the immune system.

Seasonal Affective Disorder. Seasonal changes have been known to affect the amount of time a person sleeps. During the winter, people with seasonal affective disorder (SAD) sleep longer and are more lethargic when awake. In spring and summer months, people with SAD tend to sleep less and have significantly higher energy levels during the day. SAD tends to affect women more than men. The severity and frequency of SAD cases vary with geographic location. SAD is more prevalent in higher latitudes, due to the decreased amount of daylight in such locations. People with SAD-associated sleep disorders have responded to therapy with bright light, especially early in the morning.

Infections and Illness. Sleep can be disrupted by a variety of medical conditions, as well as by the medications used to treat them. Urinary tract infections, for example, can cause frequent awakenings during the night, reducing the overall quality of sleep and leaving you groggy and still tired in the morning.

Lifestyle Factors That Interfere with Sleep

Lifestyle also affects the quality of sleep. A variety of factors, including shift work, jet lag, smoking, and alcohol consumption, can interfere with sleep.

wellness **tip**

Many people find that a light snack of milk and toast helps them fall asleep, because carbohydrates and milk increase the levels of tryptophan, serotonin, and melatonin—compounds that have been associated with improved sleep onset.

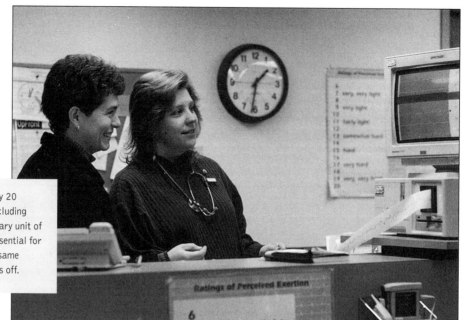

It is estimated that approximately 20 percent of the U.S. workforce, including these nurses in the cardiopulmonary unit of a hospital, works at night. It is essential for shift workers to sleep during the same hours each day, even on their days off.

Shift Work. People who work on shifts, especially on night shifts—which conflict with natural circadian rhythms—must fight sleep deprivation constantly. It is recommended that night shift workers maintain their sleep patterns on their days off as well, in order to keep their body clocks synchronized. People who work on rotating shifts, such as police officers and hospital doctors and nurses, may find it impossible to settle into a steady pattern and are at increased risk for many chronic illnesses. To stay alert on the job, shift workers must make sure to treat their daytime sleeping period as a requirement.

Jet Lag. What travelers know as "jet lag" is actually the effect of the body's circadian rhythms being out of synchronization with the local night and day times. The effects of sleep deprivation still occur during the circadian low period, so travelers who cross several time zones may find themselves groggier during the day and wide awake at night. For several days before their trip, travelers who want to avoid jet lag can try to gradually adjust their mealtimes and bedtimes to match the time zone they are traveling to. Once they arrive, exposure to daylight will help "reset" their circadian rhythms. Those who arrive in the morning will adjust most quickly if they wait until the local nighttime to sleep. Because the 25-hour circadian clock makes it easier to stay up late than to go to sleep earlier, it is easier to adjust to local time after flying west than after flying east.

Caffeine. Because caffeine is a mild stimulant, it can affect how easily you fall asleep and remain asleep. Not only coffee and tea, but many soft drinks, chocolate, and some over-the-counter pain relievers contain caffeine. In addition, caffeine used in conjunction with other medications may affect the onset of sleep. If you have any type of sleep problems, it is recommended that you avoid drinking caffeine close to bedtime. Sensitive women may need to avoid caffeine for 8 to 12 hours before bedtime.

Smoking. Like caffeine, nicotine is also a stimulant and affects how well you sleep. Smoking also restricts air flow to the lungs, which can cause problems similar to those of sleep apnea (inadequate oxygen and frequent incomplete awakenings) and thus less restful sleep. Nicotine withdrawal during sleep can also cause you to awaken partially. Researchers have found that heavy smokers do not sleep as deeply during the non-REM delta sleep stage.

Alcohol Consumption. Because alcohol is a sedative, it may initially cause sleepiness. Eventually, however, it leads to arousal and awakening, as your blood alcohol level decreases, your metabolic activity increases, and you experience mild withdrawal symptoms. Since alcohol blocks REM sleep, frequent awakenings can occur. The result is shallower and less restful sleep. Heavy drinkers may experience a dramatic increase in dreams or arousal. During the period of withdrawal, heavy drinkers may also experience insomnia and disturbing nocturnal hallucinations.

How to Improve
the *Quality* of Your Sleep

Good sleep habits are not difficult to develop, but they must be practiced regularly in order to be effective. If changes in your lifestyle—such as avoiding naps and caffeine—do not improve the quality of your sleep, behavioral modifications and medications may be necessary.

Sleep Habits

People who sleep peacefully maintain regular lifestyle habits that help them get enough sleep in a comfortable environment. Following are some tips for good sleep:

- Establish a routine of getting up at the same time every day and going to bed at the same time every day.
- Allow yourself at least one hour before bedtime to unwind. Consider this a transitional period each evening before engaging in a relaxing before-bed ritual, such as a warm bath or a period of meditation.
- Keep your bedroom dark, quiet, and at a comfortable temperature (60 to 65°F).
- Lie down intending to go to sleep only when drowsy. There is no reason for going to bed if you are not sleepy; it will only make you worry about your inability to sleep.
- Make sure you have a comfortable, supportive mattress.
- Sleep only as much as you need; oversleeping can make you feel less well-rested.
- Avoid napping.
- Get regular exercise, which eases muscle tension, but avoid exercising less than three hours before bedtime.
- Avoid large meals close to bedtime.
- Make sure you are getting appropriate amounts of B-vitamins, calcium, and minerals in your diet.

Mattresses

Most Americans sleep on traditional innerspring mattresses, but there are alternatives. Besides waterbeds and futons, there are high-density contour foam mattresses and air mattresses. Whatever kind of mattress you choose, test it out in the store by taking your shoes off and lying down on it. Flip your mattress at home occasionally—both top to bottom (e.g. putting the end at the head of the bed down at the foot of the bed) and upside down—to prolong its life.

The Better Sleep Council suggests that you need a new mattress if you answer yes to these questions:

- **Do you wake up sore or stiff, or with back pain?**
- **Does the surface of your mattress look uneven?**
- **Are there sagging spots where you lie, or around the edges of the mattress?**
- **Are some spots more comfortable than others?**
- **When you roll around do you hear creaks or crunches?**
- **If you sleep with a partner do you both roll toward the middle of the bed?**
- **Have you used the bed nightly for 8 to 10 years?**

- Avoid caffeine, alcohol, and smoking four to six hours before bedtime.
- Try not to worry about personal problems or time commitments right before sleeping. In the late afternoon or early evening, make a list of things to do, ideas to think about tomorrow, or feelings you are trying to work out.
- Use your bedroom only for sleep and sex, avoiding any stressful activities (such as work or study). Do not watch television in the bedroom.
- If sleep evades you for more than 20 minutes, get up and do something boring to encourage drowsiness. Tossing and turning encourages insomniac behavior.
- Do something relaxing to signal your body that the day is over.
- Spend only as much time in bed as you actually need to sleep.

Relaxation Techniques

Try to leave your frustrations and anxieties outside the bedroom. Deep breathing, yoga, or massage can encourage a calm state of mind. If it is difficult to relax enough to get a good night's sleep, you may want to try some form of relaxation technique before going to bed. Training is available in a variety of methods, all designed to relieve tension and encourage sleep.

Behavioral Modification Techniques

Establishing good sleep habits may require changing some of your behaviors, such as avoiding working or studying in bed. But people who still have trouble sleeping may need to try more specific types of behavioral modification. Some therapists, for example, suggest limiting sleep in order to ensure sleepiness at bedtime. For people who have trouble sleeping at appropriate hours, whether as a result of jet lag or not, delaying bedtime by a few hours each day may help synchronize their internal body clocks with local time.

Medical Intervention

Sleeping medications can help you sleep, but they can have unwanted side effects, including addiction. Studies suggest that although sleeping pills may help you fall asleep, they do not help you sleep better.

Prescription Drugs. For serious sleeping problems, your physician may prescribe certain medications. People who have trouble sleeping as a result of other condi-

FIGURE 10.1
Relax Before Bedtime
This relaxation technique, called the Bellows, can relax you before bedtime and help you sleep more soundly.

STEP 1 Lie on your back on the floor or a firm mat. Begin breathing deeply, slowly, and regularly.

STEP 2 As you exhale, pull your right knee gently toward your chest. Breathe gently and deeply several times. With each exhalation, allow your legs, shoulders, back, and face to relax.

STEP 3 As you inhale, straighten your right leg. Exhale and pull your left knee toward your chest. Repeat as with your right leg.

STEP 4 Pull both knees toward your chest. Repeat as with your right leg.

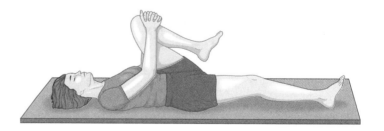

Repeat the entire cycle at least three times and as many as eight times. Move very slowly and rhythmically, and keep your eyes closed.

tions (mood disorders, infections, and other medical conditions) may benefit from the temporary use of such medications.

Nonprescription drugs. Over-the-counter sleeping medications are widely available, but many contain antihistamines, such as those in allergy and cold medicine, which have a mild sedative effect. Some may cause lingering fatigue after you wake up. Some can make you agitated, rather than sleepy. Supplements of melatonin, the hormone that encourages drowsiness, have become popular as a natural sleeping aid, but the effects of taking melatonin have not yet been studied thoroughly. Researchers caution against overusing it because it is not regulated and the long-term effects are not yet known. Melatonin does make you drowsy, but it may not help you sleep through the night. GABA (gamma aminobutyric acid), a neurotransmitter that acts as a sedative, is another over-the-counter preparation, typically available in health food stores, that seems to promote sleep but is not yet well-studied. An occasional standard aspirin or acetaminophen may be your best bet for nonprescription help in sleeping. It does not make you drowsy, but it can help you sleep longer and wake up less often if mild pain or discomfort distracts you.

Sleep *Disorders*

Everyone has trouble sleeping at some point. It can be a temporary disruption of sleep or a sleeping disorder. If your sleeping problem persists and interferes with daily function, seek professional help.

Warning Signs
Women who regularly get a good night's sleep wake up feeling rested and refreshed. If you have problems falling asleep, sleeping through the night, or waking up, even an appropriate amount of sleep will leave you feeling tired. Sleep problems and disorders are categorized as related to falling asleep (such as insomnia) or related to awakening (such as sleepwalking). Some are transient, short-term changes in sleep patterns; some are more serious and are best treated by a physician.

Common Problems Related to Falling Asleep
Dyssomnias, or trouble falling asleep, cover a broad range of difficulties—from simple circadian rhythm disorders, in which a person's internal clock differs from the external time, to mysterious conditions like narcolepsy, in which a person can fall asleep instantaneously at any time.

Circadian Rhythm Disorders. Circadian rhythm disorders occur when the external cues that cause sleepiness are changed—usually to later in the evening—resulting in a delay in falling asleep and waking. For example, many adolescents experience sleep delays because of their busy schedules and the peer-induced trend to stay awake longer. This results in a progressively later bedtime and a prolonged period of sleepiness early in the morning. Their sleep schedules also gradually drift out of sync because, as stated earlier, our biological clocks run on a 25-hour cycle and the world runs on a 24-hour clock. People with circadian

I'm So Sleepy: Diagnosing Hypersomnia

Hypersomnia—excessive sleepiness—is measured by a change in a person's normal sleep patterns. For example, if you usually needed eight hours of sleep each night, and now are consistently tired despite getting your usual eight hours, you could have hypersomnia. Besides experiencing excessive daytime sleepiness, people with hypersomnia are also fatigued and have difficulty concentrating.

Hypersomnia can be caused by circadian rhythm disorder, seasonal mood disorder, sleep deprivation, or other sleep problems. In addition, infectious diseases that affect areas of the mid-brain can cause "sleeping sickness."

If you suspect that you have hypersomnia, keeping a sleep calendar may help you discover the cause of your sleepiness. Each day, record your bedtime, the hours you spend sleeping, and the time you wake up. Also record the times you consume caffeinated or alcoholic beverages and how close to bedtime you exercise. Be sure to record any naps you take, since frequent napping has been known to cause hypersomnia. On the other hand, a 10- to 15-minute nap might help get rid of sleepiness. Discuss your sleep habits and any prospective changes with your physician or sleep specialist.

In extreme cases of hypersomnia, your physician may recommend a polysomnography, or sleep EEG. This procedure requires an overnight stay in a sleep laboratory, where doctors measure your brain waves, eye movements, respiratory patterns, and muscle activity. Sleep apneas, periodic leg movements, and disturbance in normal sleep patterns can be diagnosed with this procedure.

Source: Adapted from "Hypersomnia Information." The Sleep Well. http://wwwleland.stanford.edu/~dement/hypersomnia.html. (October 16, 1997).

rhythm disorder need to transition back to a normal day/night cycle by going to bed slightly later each night and awakening slightly later each morning. This slowly readjusts the timing of the individual's sleep clock.

Narcolepsy. A chronic, often inherited genetic disorder affecting the part of the brain that regulates sleep and wakefulness, narcolepsy affects a very small percentage of the population. The condition typically presents itself in adolescence, although it can occur at any time throughout life. Narcoleptics fall asleep suddenly and without warning at all times of day in any circumstances. These "sleep attacks" can be as brief as 30 seconds or longer than one-half hour. They are often accompanied by a loss of muscle control, especially when the person is excited or laughing. Symptoms of narcolepsy include:

- Excessive sleepiness.
- Temporary decrease or loss of muscle control, especially when getting excited.
- Vivid dreamlike images when drifting off to sleep or waking up.
- Waking up unable to move or talk for a brief time.

Insomnia. Occasional difficulty falling sleeping or staying asleep is perhaps the most common sleep-related problem. Insomnia is often caused by a disruption in your regular sleeping schedule, by stress, or by consumption of too much alcohol or caffeine. There are three basic types of insomnia:

- **Transient insomnia** lasts for just a few nights.
- **Short-term insomnia** lasts two to three weeks, and can be caused by life changes, such as job changes, a new baby, divorce, grief, or simply by worries about health or finances or a big meeting at work, that keep you from relaxing at bedtime.

- **Chronic or long-term insomnia** lasts three weeks or longer, even for months or years, and can be caused by shift work; high noise levels; chronic substance abuse, including drugs and alcohol; mood disorders, including depression; or certain medical conditions, such as heart disease, arthritis, diabetes, asthma, chronic sinusitis, epilepsy, and ulcers.

Good sleep habits can help you overcome short-term bouts of insomnia. See the standard suggestions described earlier in the chapter. If you have any of the following daytime symptoms, you may need professional help to treat your insomnia:

- You feel sleepy and find it hard to stay awake.
- You have trouble performing your work or daily tasks.
- You have trouble concentrating.
- You feel disoriented, anxious, or irritable.
- You have trouble remembering things.
- You have an accident or near-accident caused by drowsiness.

Common Problems Related to Waking

Parasomnias cover a range of disorders related to trouble waking up fully. They include sleep inertia, sleepwalking and talking, night terrors, leg cramps, apneas, and snoring. Some are triggered during the shift from non-REM to REM sleep. Instead of making that transition smoothly to activate the eyes to create a dream, the feet or mouth or some other body part is activated. It is recommended that people suffering from parasomnias avoid any activity that makes the first hour of sleep deeper (such as use of sedatives) and try not to exercise near bedtime.

Sleep Inertia and Sleep Paralysis. Little research has been done on the physiology of waking, but it is known that the body wakes up in stages, just as falling asleep occurs in stages. Sleep inertia, or sensation of sluggishness, can last 10 or 15 minutes after you begin to awake, impairing your body's reaction time. Sleep paralysis is a more severe state, in which the biochemical switch that prevents you from consciously moving your muscles during REM sleep continues to act as you awaken. Waking dreams in this state can cause feelings of frantic inability to move; the sensation that someone is in the room is not uncommon. Because the eyes and tongue are not affected by the REM sleep biochemical switch, blinking and moving your tongue may overcome the sensation of paralysis. If the condition occurs regularly, medication may be necessary.

Sleepwalking, Sleeptalking, and Sleep Eating. People who walk, talk, or get up and eat in their sleep are responding to commands their sleeping brains send to their muscles, commands which healthy sleepers cannot respond to. Researchers believe that although people in such states appear to be asleep, their brains must be processing at least some visual information, to enable them to negotiate stairs, open refrigerator doors, or even drive a car without crashing.

Sleep Terrors and Nightmares. Sleep terrors and nightmares are two different experiences, both related to "bad dreams." Sleep terrors most often occur in chil-

wellness
warning

If a sleepwalker exits the house or has frequent episodes in which injuries occur, it is imperative that she seek professional help from a sleep disorder center. There have been fatalities associated with some sleepwalking incidents.

dren and usually disappear during adolescence. During sleep terrors, which occur during delta wave sleep, the person's eyes are typically open. Sufferers scream or hyperventilate, and their heart rates increase dramatically. They are in an obvious state of panic and disorientation but cannot identify what brought it on; often they have forgotten the entire event in the morning. Sleep terrors may be caused by stress. Stress management techniques and establishing a regular sleep pattern can alleviate the condition.

During nightmares, a person's eyes may be closed. People who have nightmares wake up with a feeling of relief; they realize they were dreaming and they usually remember the nightmare. Several types of medications can cause strange dreams or even nightmares: some antihypertensive medications, beta adrenergic blockers, L-DOPA (used for treating symptoms of Parkinson's disease), and some antidepressants.

Disorders Affecting the Limbs. Abrupt, involuntary movements of the legs while sleeping, medically referred to as nocturnal myoclonus—can occur at varying intensities. Periodic limb movements during sleep, common among people aged 65 and over, occur every 30 seconds or so and may continue for hours. These movements cause frequent brief awakenings that hinder the quality of sleep. In its severest form, restless leg syndrome, crawling, tingling, or prickling sensations in the legs force the sleeper to move or rub the legs for relief, even to get up and walk around.

REM Sleep Behavior Disorder. If the biochemical switch that prevents conscious muscle movement during the REM phase malfunctions, sleepers may find themselves physically acting out events that occur in their dreams. People deprived of REM sleep act out some of their dreams when they are awake.

Sleep Apneas. Apneas are disturbances in breathing while asleep that typically make people stop breathing momentarily, often hundreds of times a night. Apneas, one of the most common disorders, are caused by a restriction in the breathing passages. They can lead to chronic cardiovascular disease and high blood pressure because they reduce the amount of oxygen in the blood.

There are two commonly diagnosed types of apnea: obstructive and central. Obstructive sleep apnea, the most common type, occurs when tissue in the throat blocks the air passage, often when the person is snoring. It can be due to being overweight, excessive alcohol consumption, or physical characteristics. Central sleep apnea occurs when the body has a decreased sensitivity to rising carbon dioxide levels, delaying the brain's signal to take a breath.

Apneas have several common symptoms:

- Loud snoring
- Waking up unrefreshed
- Difficulty staying awake during the day
- Waking up with headaches
- Waking up during the night choking
- Waking up sweating

Apneas occur most often in middle-aged men who are overweight, but anyone who starts snoring louder or more often than usual or who wakes up often struggling to breathe should get help from a physician, since apnea can be potentially fatal.

Snoring. Snoring is caused by air passing over soft tissue in your throat, causing a vibration. Some estimates suggest that nearly one out of every seven women snores regularly. Snoring can be a sign of more serious sleep problems, such as apneas. People who are overweight or drink alcohol close to bedtime tend to snore more, as do people who sleep on their backs, because that position allows the tongue to slide back into the air passage. Dental devices, such as jaw positioners or tongue retainers, can help keep the airway clear. Sewing tennis balls into the back of a pajama top can discourage you from sleeping on your back.

Teeth Grinding. Some people clench their teeth together while they sleep, usually early in the sleep cycle, sometimes grinding them loudly enough to wake their partners. They also may wake up with jaw pain or earache. This disorder, which occurs in about 15 percent of the population, is sometimes caused by an irregularity in the way the upper and lower jaws meet when the mouth is closed but more often occurs when the sleeper is anxious, tense, or angry. Alcohol consumption can aggravate the condition. Occasional mild tooth grinding is not harmful, but frequent, even violent episodes can damage the teeth. Relaxation and stress management techniques may resolve the problem. More severe cases may require the use of a dental guard.

Sleep Clinics

Occasional sleepless nights during stressful periods are no cause for alarm. For problems that recur or that continue for more than a few weeks, you may want to ask your physician to refer you to a specialist at a sleep disorders clinic.

Sleep specialists use an electroencephalograph to measure brain activity, body temperature, breathing rates, and muscle movements during sleep. They may also monitor eye movements, evaluate airway obstructions, and measure the amount of oxygen in the blood.

What *You* Can Do

Sleep is an important aspect of physical and mental health. It helps the immune system fight off disease, allows you to feel rested and renewed, and keeps the mind sharp. Factors that disrupt sleep also disrupt other aspects of a woman's wellness. Women need to pay attention to developing positive sleep habits just as they would other aspects of their health.

- Be aware of how much sleep you need to function well.
- Establish a sleeping schedule that ensures you get enough sleep and stick to it.
- Practice good sleeping habits.
- Get help if you cannot sleep.

Fostering *Good* Relationships

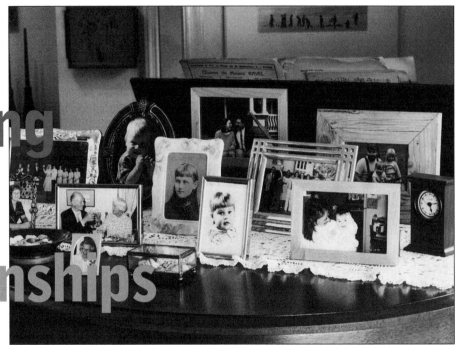

An interesting aspect of wellness is the ability to learn and use the skills that help individuals establish and maintain successful relationships. Why are relationships part of wellness? Learning how to establish and maintain positive relationships helps promote both mental and physical health. Without an emotional support system, people are actually at greater risk for illness and death. Studies have shown that socially isolated people have higher rates of tuberculosis, accidents, and psychiatric disorders. Survival rates for heart patients are significantly lower when they live alone or do not have a close personal tie to a companion, friend, or spouse. Other studies show that the stress people experience when key relationships in their lives are strained can manifest itself in neck and back pain, headaches, irritable bowel syndrome, and other disorders.

Communication lies at the heart of good relationships. There are many styles of communication, and no one style is effective for everyone. Individual styles of communication are rooted in the family relationships one experiences in childhood. Early interpersonal skills, such as learning to share, show affection, make friends, and ask for help, are developed through the interactions a child has with her complex network of parents, siblings, and other people (such as caregivers and relatives) who are significantly involved in her life. When the communication skills modeled for a child are appropriate, the child learns how to form healthy relationships.

Girls and boys, regardless of their family background, exhibit marked differences in how they relate to others. In general, traditional society has conditioned females to be nurturing and to focus on feelings; males are expected to be action-oriented. Little boys are encouraged to be more independent and little girls to be more compliant. People talk to boys and girls differently and accept different ways of talking from them. Even parents with firm intentions to avoid raising their children according to gender stereotypes may subconsciously encourage differences in behavior and communication. In studying how parents talk to young children, psycholinguist Jean Berko Gleason found that fathers give more commands to their children than mothers do, and they give more commands to sons than to daughters.

In her popular book *You Just Don't Understand: Men and Women in Conversation*, linguistics professor Deborah Tannen says, "Girls and boys grow up in different worlds of words." Girls tend to play in pairs or small groups in which they use language to promote connection and intimacy. "Let's try this" or "Let's go over there" are common phrases among girls playing together. Boys, in contrast, play in large groups that are structured hierarchically. They use words to jockey for status, issue challenges, boast, and argue about who gets to play with what (or with whom) and who is best at what. Boys are more likely to use language to give orders, such as "Gimme the ball" or "Get out of the way." Boys are more threatened by anything that challenges their independence, while girls are more threatened by a rupture in their relationships. Also, boys are taught to be "tough" and suppress their feelings. In games, if a boy gets hurt he is expected to get out of the way and stop crying so the game can go on. With girls, the game stops while everyone gathers around to help the one who is crying.

Researchers have noted gender differences in communication styles in children as young as age three. This research parallels other studies that show boys' and girls' gender identity (how they have been conditioned socially to act as a boy or girl) is essentially in place by age three.

Regardless of one's experiences, however, it is possible at virtually any time in one's life to develop the skills needed for successful relationships. In fact, improving interpersonal skills is a lifelong process. Each stage of life brings its

Fostering Good Self-Esteem

When parents love and accept their children for who they are, they go far toward helping their children develop good self-esteem. People with healthy self-esteem feel good about themselves, relate well to different kinds of people, and believe they are competent to cope with life's challenges.

Even when disciplining children for inappropriate behavior, parents can let children know they are loved. In order to develop positive self-esteem, children need to recognize that mistakes are learning experiences and do not make them "bad."

Even as an adult, if you feel you have low self-esteem you can work to improve your feelings of self-worth by following these recommendations:

- Think about the kind of person you want to be. Act consistently with that image. Looking for positive role models can help.
- Minimize negative thoughts about yourself. Shift your attention to something else.
- Focus on your successes. Congratulate yourself for the things you have handled well during the day rather than dwelling on mistakes.
- Use affirmations. Come up with short statements about your positive qualities and repeat them to yourself—especially in moments of doubt or stress.

own challenges, in both personal and professional contexts, for building relationships, such as acquiring childhood playmates, dating, marriage, establishing adult friendships, parenting, maintaining family bonds with siblings and aging parents, and interacting with bosses, coworkers, and clients. This chapter identifies the skills that foster good relationships, the danger signs that indicate that a relationship is taking a turn for the worse, and strategies needed to keep a relationship successful or rebuild a relationship that is faltering or failing.

The Power of
Good Interpersonal Skills

Often you meet or hear about a particular person who has good interpersonal skills—meaning she can interact with all types of people, generating admiration for herself and leaving others feeling good about themselves. You probably also have met someone who you would describe as having poor interpersonal skills. She "rubs people the wrong way," leaves people cold in conversation, or holds her opinions above all others. Positive interpersonal skills are the building blocks for good relationships. They are not inborn; they are learned.

The first step in learning good interpersonal skills is to turn outward—acknowledging that you stand on common ground with the people you meet and trying to understand their viewpoints. When you communicate with others using this open approach, you will most certainly improve your relationship-building skills.

Recognizing the Need to Be Appreciated

William James, the American educator, once said that "the deepest principle in human nature is the craving to be appreciated." This fundamental truth lies at the heart of all good relationships. People want to be valued, to feel they are important, and to be respected. That is why people are usually far more motivated by praise than by criticism. Receiving sincere, honest appreciation reinforces a person's self-esteem and makes her more responsive and open to a relationship.

Recognizing the Need to Be in Control

Another basic need is to feel a sense of control. That does not mean being in charge of everything all the time, but simply a desire for the independence and self-reliance to manage important aspects of one's life. Threats to feelings of independence and control can generate conflict and damage one's self-esteem. Part of the give-and-take inherent to most human relationships occurs because a person's need to resist being controlled by others paradoxically coexists with—and often conflicts with—the need for involvement and caring.

Heightening Self-Awareness

Recognizing that these needs—the need to be appreciated and the need to feel in control—are common to all human beings is an important basis for good interpersonal skills. For the next few weeks, as you interact with those around you, be aware of how your actions and words affect others' needs for appreciation and control. Strive to heighten your awareness of yourself; it can allow you to evaluate and learn from your experiences.

Understanding the Other Person's Point of View

When we see someone is having a problem, a natural impulse is to rush in and offer advice before taking the time to really understand the difficulty from that person's perspective. Or, when we argue or disagree with someone, our first tendency is to try to get them to hear us, to "win them over" to our side. However, Dale Carnegie, a pioneer in teaching successful personal skills, says the key to success in life is the ability to understand the other person's view and see things from that person's angle as well as your own. If you are in a disagreement, or are wanting to help someone with a problem, try to grasp their point of view first before expressing your own. Stephen Covey, author of *The Seven Habits of Highly Effective People*, says that the single most important guideline he has learned in the field of interpersonal relationships is "seek first to understand, then to be understood."

Resisting the Desire to Change Others

Another habit that stands in the way of successful interactions is wanting to change others' behavior or attitudes. No one can make another person change. You can, however, change the way you react to someone, and that in turn often triggers a change in their behavior or attitude. Recognizing one's own ability to change and taking responsibility for personal choices and actions, instead of focusing so much on trying to change others, are basic qualities of people with good interpersonal skills.

These principles are the foundation of good interpersonal skills. To really make relationships work you must have an understanding of the essentials of good communication and the ability to put them into practice.

Positive *Communication*

An irony of modern life is that with the development of technologies for global communication—computers, satellites, television, radio, telephones, the Internet—communication on a personal level still remains very difficult. Ineffective communication can create problems in all facets of life: loneliness, family problems, stress, job dissatisfaction, even illness. Although we often think of "talking" as communication, in actuality communication encompasses far more than the spoken word. Communication experts estimate that only 10 percent of communication is represented verbally, that is, by what people actually say. Another 30 percent is represented by tone of voice and 60 percent by body language, including eye contact, posture, and gestures. These aspects of communication are sometimes referred to as the Three V's: verbal (words), visual (body language), and vocal (tone of voice).

Another element of communication is conversational style—a combination of pacing, volume, sentence structure, intonation, word choice, and other factors that form each person's unique way of communicating. As linguist Deborah Tannen explains in *That's Not What I Meant,* many times what is perceived as rudeness, stubbornness, inconsiderateness, or refusal to cooperate really represents differences in conversational style. If your words and your body language are sending conflicting messages, people will respond more strongly to your nonverbal messages than to your verbal ones. This unconscious characteristic of conversation is often used to create rapport, guard against confrontation, or avoid hurting others.

Each person's conversational style is determined by many factors, including family environment, the region where she grew up, and gender. As stated earlier in the chapter, men and women essentially grow up in different cultures and thus communicate differently. This idea was popularized in the book *Men Are from Mars, Women Are from Venus* by relationship expert John Gray. Because women are deeply driven by a need to form connections, they seek to share feelings and develop rapport through conversation. For women, the essence of friendship is talk. But men use talk as a way to preserve independence and maintain status in a hierarchical order. That is why their talk often focuses on providing information and solutions. To a man, giving information to another sends a message of superiority. Many men are reluctant to ask for help or directions, for example, because it would conflict with their perception of themselves as self-sufficient. Women generally do not mind asking for directions, because in their view, seeking and receiving help establishes positive bonds between people. Women avoid using talk to demonstrate superiority, because it conflicts with their need for connection.

Good communication involves learning two key skills: listening and expressing. Once learned, these skills can be applied to all kinds of relationships.

Listening Skills

A study of people in various occupations found that 70 percent of their waking moments was spent in communication, and 45 percent of that time was spent listening. Only 30 percent was spent talking; the rest was taken up with reading and writing. But few people are truly good listeners. Experts estimate that 75 percent of spoken communication is ignored, misunderstood, or soon forgotten.

What is good listening? Good listening is more than merely hearing what is said. It is trying to understand what the speaker is saying and the feelings behind it—without judging, evaluating, making assumptions, or concentrating on how to respond. Covey calls this listening with the intent to understand, "empathic

FIGURE 11.1
Attentive Listening
Listening is equally important to talking. Practice these attentive listening skills.

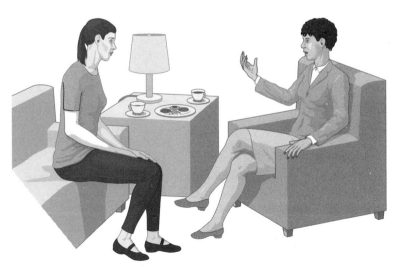

Assume a posture of relaxed alertness, indicating that you feel comfortable with the other person and that you are interested in what she is saying.

Incline your body toward the speaker, rather than leaning back in the chair, to display your attentiveness.

Face the other person squarely and keep your eyes on the same level.

Do not cross your arms or legs, as these positions can communicate defensiveness or inflexibility.

Position yourself an appropriate distance from the other person. Three feet is usually a comfortable distance.

Maintain eye contact. Avoid focusing on distractions, such as talk in another part of the room or a ringing telephone.

Keep physical barriers from coming between you and the speaker. At work, this means moving from behind your desk or offering your visitor a seat alongside you.

listening." "Empathic listening," he says, "gets inside the other person's frame of reference. You look out through it, you see the world the way they see the world, you understand their paradigm, you understand how they feel." Empathic listening is characterized by patience and openness. This approach to listening not only increases your chances of getting accurate information, it also offers the other person the affirmation that you are paying attention to them.

Attending. In his book *People Skills,* communications specialist Robert Bolton divides listening skills into three categories: attending skills, following skills, and reflecting skills. "Attending" refers to nonverbal communication that shows the other person has your full attention. Here are a few specific suggestions to show that you are listening:

- Be alert, yet relaxed, a posture that suggests you feel at home with the other person but also that you sense the importance of what you are hearing and are intent on understanding.
- Incline your body toward the speaker, which communicates more attention than does leaning back or sprawling in the chair.
- Face the other person squarely with your eyes on the same level.
- Keep an open body position, with arms and legs uncrossed. Tightly crossed limbs can communicate inflexibility or defensiveness.
- Position yourself an appropriate distance from the other person; either being too far away or too close can increase anxiety levels. The "right" distance varies, of course, from culture to culture; in American society, about three feet is considered a comfortable distance.
- Use appropriate body motion. Good listeners move their bodies in response to the speaker; ineffective listeners move in response to unrelated stimuli—they may jingle coins, drum their fingers, twirl a pencil, or shift their weight often.
- Maintain eye contact, which expresses interest and a desire to listen. Many people have trouble doing this; think about how uncomfortable you feel when talking to someone who keeps glancing around the room. For effective eye contact, focus softly on the speaker and occasionally shift your gaze to another part of the body, such as a gesturing hand, and then back to the face and eyes.
- Avoid environmental distractions, which may mean turning off the television or asking that telephone calls be held.
- Keep physical barriers from coming between you and the speaker. In offices, the desk is a common barrier. When possible, move from behind the desk and use two chairs for the conversation, or, if the room is small, pull the visitor's chair up alongside the desk.

Following. Following involves skills that encourage the speaker without getting in her way. Unfortunately, the average listener tends to interrupt often to interject points or ask questions. For the best results, listeners should use these techniques:

- **Door openers.** These are nonthreatening invitations to talk, such as "You seem like you have had a bad day. Want to talk about it?" or "Is there anything that's bothering you? If you'd like to talk, I'm here to listen." If you offer a door opener and are not taken up on it, it is best to let it go. Avoid roadblocks that shut down communication. Roadblocks include judgmental statements such as "What happened? You look like you just lost your best friend" as well as advice and comments intended to be reassuring like "Cheer up" or "I'm sure it can't be anything that bad."

- **Brief indicators that you are staying with the speaker.** Short comments, such as "mm-hmm," "really?" or "go on," do not imply that you agree or disagree with what the speaker has said, simply that you are hearing the speaker and want to keep listening.
- **Open-ended questions.** Questions that cannot be answered with a simple yes or no are best because they allow the speaker to explore her thoughts. "What was it about the job that intrigued you?" is an example of an open-ended question. "Did you like the way they described the job?" is an example of a closed question. However, if the listener asks too many questions, she dictates the direction the conversation takes rather than allowing the speaker to lead.
- **Attentive silence.** This is a positive type of brief silence that gives the speaker time to think about what she is going to say and lets her proceed at her own pace. Bolton notes that, in his communication workshops, most people are uncomfortable with silence at first. Those on the listening end may feel so ill at ease "that they have a strong inner compulsion to shatter the quiet with questions, advice, or any other sound that will end their discomfort by ending the silence." In a short time, however, most people can become more comfortable with silence. During pauses, a good listener will observe the other person's body language for clues to the message being delivered and think about what the speaker has said and is feeling.

Reflecting. The empathic listening described by Covey is a "reflecting skill." Bolton explains that when the listener reflects, she restates the feeling and/or content of what the speaker has communicated in order to show that she understands and accepts the information or message. Reflective responses are nonjudgmental and concise, and they attempt to mirror or summarize what the other person is thinking and experiencing. When the listener reflects, the speaker is given the chance to assess whether the listener has interpreted the message appropriately. If she has not, the speaker can rephrase or explain further. It is not necessary to use reflective listening for every occasion, but it is especially helpful to use when you are listening to someone who has a problem or is looking for solutions. Reflective listening can be broken down into four types—although a reflective response often fits into more than one category.

- **Paraphrasing** is making a succinct response that restates the core content of the speaker's message or expressed thought, in the listener's own words. For example:

    SUE: I don't know whether I should quit my job. I enjoy it and we can use the money. But I feel guilty about leaving my baby in day care and I feel cheated for missing out on so much time with her.

    CHERYL: You like your work but you're torn between your job and your wish to spend more time with the baby.

- **Reflecting feelings** means using concise statements to mirror to the speaker the emotions she is communicating. This skill calls for the listener to be attuned to body language, tone of voice, and "feeling" words. In the following exchange, Mary picks up on Keiko's unhappiness but misses the frustration. Based on Mary's reflective response, Keiko further clarifies her feelings:

  KEIKO: I'm so miserable, Craig and I just broke up. I had hoped he'd be "the one" and now I'm alone again. I don't know if I'll ever find the right person.

  MARY: You're unhappy about losing Craig and being alone.

  KEIKO: Well, sure I'm unhappy, but more than that, I feel so frustrated about the whole dating scene.

- **Reflecting meanings** involves joining feelings and facts in one succinct response. Bolton suggests using this structure: "You feel . . . because . . ."

  PILAR: My husband yelled at me last night for backing into a parking meter. He was standing there waving his arms—I assumed he'd tell me when to stop, but he didn't. Now he's furious at me.

  SARAH: You feel hurt because he's blaming you, even though hitting the meter wasn't altogether your fault.

- **Summative reflections** restate the main themes and feelings the speaker expressed over a longer stretch of conversation. These statements may tie together several recent comments or recap key issues and feelings. Because they highlight things the speaker has emphasized throughout the conversation, summative reflections give the speaker an integrated snapshot of what has been communicated. Phrases that can lead effectively into summative reflections include "As I've been listening, your main concern seems to be . . . " or "I'm hearing a central theme that you keep coming back to, which is . . . ."

Expressing Skills

Everything you say is subject to interpretation. You can, however, increase the likelihood that what you say and what the listener understands will be close by utilizing good expressing skills. Expressing yourself with clarity and precision means that you know what you want to communicate and that your words and nonverbal cues convey the same meaning. There are four kinds of information conveyed when you express yourself:

1. **Observations.** You report the facts about things you have seen, heard, read, or experienced, without stating opinions or making inferences. "The President's state of the union address focused on gun control, crime, and public education."
2. **Thoughts.** You offer opinions, generate theories, and come to conclusions. "I think that you have a lot of options you haven't considered yet."
3. **Feelings.** You express the emotions you are experiencing. "I feel hurt and angry."
4. **Wants and needs.** In a sense, expressing wants and needs is making both an announcement and a request. Communicating your wants and needs is

wellness **tip**

Reflective listening is an excellent skill to have in your communications storehouse, but be careful not to overdo it. Reflective listening takes effort. It is best employed when the other person's needs or problems signal an invitation for intense listening.

critical in intimate relationships. "I need you to call when you're going to be more than 20 minutes late, so I don't worry unnecessarily."

Expressing Yourself Clearly

When you choose to express a thought, feeling, or idea, you can use different communication strategies. If you keep the following guidelines in mind, you will have a better chance of minimizing confusion and communicating effectively:

- **Know your intent.** Before you speak, ask yourself, "What is my real purpose for saying what I am about to say? What result am I aiming for?" This may require preparation or even rehearsal, especially with a sensitive issue.
- **State your intent up front.** This is especially important in emotionally charged situations. For example, if you are angry with a friend, instead of launching into how upset you are, you could say "I feel upset about something and would like to clear the air so we can enjoy our day together."
- **Be clear and straightforward instead of indirect.** This can be difficult for women, since they tend to link directness with being demanding. A man is likely to be more comfortable asking straight out, "Would you please run to the store?" whereas a woman might say, "I really need some things from the store, but I am so tired," hoping that the listener will empathize and offer to go. The risk of being indirect is that you may be misunderstood or the request underlying your statement may not be picked up, resulting in either or both parties feeling annoyed.
- **Be tactful and respectful.** You can be honest and direct without hurting someone's feelings. Avoid sarcasm and acknowledge the other person's feelings, even if you do not agree with him or her.
- **Monitor your tone of voice.** This is particularly important for women, who tend to use sharp or high-pitched tones unknowingly, especially in stressful situations. If you hear yourself sounding "out of sync" with your intent, explain. For example, say "I know I sound angry, but that is because this issue means so much to me."
- **Use "I" statements.** In structuring statements this way, you express your viewpoint without trying to criticize others. (See the following section for more information about "I" statements.)

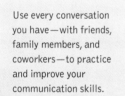

Use every conversation you have—with friends, family members, and coworkers—to practice and improve your communication skills.

Using "I" Statements

"I" statements are an effective way to express yourself without judging others or putting them on the defensive. "I" statements provide disclosures to others about your feelings, likes and dislikes, beliefs, needs, reactions, attitudes, and intentions. They can be as simple as "I like the way our meeting went today," "I feel tired," or "I enjoy swimming."

The most effective "I" statements focus on feelings rather than thoughts or opinions. Saying "It's mean of you to say that" is far less productive than "I feel hurt by what you said."

Many experts advocate three-part "I" statements, especially in situations where you are trying to get the listener to change a specific behavior. These statements consist of a disclosure of feeling, a behavior description, and a tangible physical or psychological effect. The structure goes like this: I feel [emotion] when you [behavior] because [effect]. Some examples are:

- I feel annoyed when you take money out of my wallet without telling me because then I'm caught without enough cash when I need it.
- I feel frustrated when you pick me up late because it shortens our evening.

To try to bring about a specific behavior, you can follow the three-part "I" statement by a request:

- I feel frustrated when you walk away when we disagree, because then we can't solve the problem. Would you please stay?

Equally effective are statements like these:

- I'm upset that you didn't pay me back on time because I needed that money to pay my rent.
- I'm angry that I wasn't consulted about the new hours because they affect my employees.

A Woman's
Key Relationships

The most basic step we can take to get along with others is to give them the benefit of the doubt whenever possible. Even if you end up hurt or angry, assume that your reaction was not necessarily what was intended. Once the person communicating with you learns how you feel, and realizes it was not what she intended, the speaker has the opportunity to clarify what she meant.

Women especially need to focus on their reactions during interactions with the people in their key relationships—family, friends, and coworkers. Rather than accept emotional reactions, such as guilt or intimidation, as inevitable and unavoidable, it is more effective to step back and observe what is going on. Explore your reaction and think of solutions for avoiding a similar reaction in the future. This type of reflection gives you emotional distance. If your boss constantly makes you feel belittled, it is your responsibility to examine why your boss is making you feel that way and to do something about it. Depending on the situation, solutions could range from letting your boss's words roll off your back to asking for a brief meeting to discuss how you feel. Remarkably, there is a very good chance your boss has no idea you are feeling the way you are.

"Win-win" is another effective philosophy for women to practice in interpersonal relationships. Win-win is based on the belief that human interactions should be cooperative rather than competitive—it means constantly seeking mutual benefit. Everyone benefits, and one person's success does not have to be achieved at the expense or exclusion of others. With the win-win frame of mind, you evaluate potential actions to determine if they are acceptable and satisfying for all parties involved. Using the win-win approach might mean, for example, carefully planning your words and the order of what you will discuss in order to prevent a negative or hurtful response from the listener; or it might involve planning questions to ask the listener to make sure that she too feels involved and heard. According to Covey, having a win-win mindset requires a high level of maturity—a balance between the courage to take the action necessary to reach a goal and the consideration to think of others' welfare. A win-win attitude makes its easier to get others to cooperate, because they see there is something in it for them.

A less constructive mindset is "win-lose," which is considered by communication experts to be an authoritarian style. Covey notes that many people have been "scripted" in the win-lose mentality since birth. For example, those raised with conditional love—not loved for who they are, but for what they do—tend to be threatened by the successes of others and to see life as a win-lose situation. Thinking win-win and giving others the benefit of the doubt are simple approaches that can enhance the success in all key relationships in a woman's life.

Family Relationships

Relationships with family members are often the most emotionally rewarding as well as the most difficult in a woman's life. In childhood, family interactions are a practice ground for future relationships. In our adult lives, it may be difficult (but certainly not impossible) to alter these learned roles and behaviors.

Parents. The first exposure a child has to building and maintaining relationships is with her mother and father. When these two relationships are grounded in trust, positive communication skills and relationship skills can be nurtured as the child grows.

Mother-Daughter Relationships. Children look to their mothers to meet their needs for survival and to provide approval, comfort, and reassurance. They identify with her and learn from her example. A child is attuned to what makes her mother happy, because when things go well for her they are likely to be more pleasant for the child as well.

Many women maintain healthy, loving, supportive relationships with their mothers. When some daughters grow up, the relationship with their mother evolves into a peerlike friendship. Some mother-daughter relationships are mutually protective and nurturing. Others are characterized by dysfunction and

Teaching Children About Feelings

Parents have many opportunities to promote children's emotional stability and give them the foundation they need to grow into emotionally healthy adults:

- **Give unconditional love.** Let your child know that your love is constant and steady. Your love should not depend on the way your child looks or behaves, nor should your love be used as a reward or held back as a threat. The more secure a child feels about your love, the better she will feel about herself as she grows up. Express your love through words, touch, affection, and attention.

- **Communicate well.** Communication is one of the most important skills you teach your child, so try to be understanding, patient, honest, and open. Express your feelings, ask questions, and consider what you are about to say before the words leave your mouth. Frequent criticism and phrases like "Don't bother me" or "That's a stupid thing to say" can make a child feel hurt, unwanted, or worthless.

- **Encourage happiness.** You cannot teach a baby to be happy, but you can create an environment in which natural joyfulness can emerge. Encourage your child to explore the world with curiosity and to express natural exuberance. Show your child what you love about the world. Focus on the positive.

- **Respect children's feelings.** Let them know that all feelings are healthy and important.

- **Talk about feelings.** Children experience many emotions for which they do not have the language skills to name. You can help children recognize and label them while learning that it is good to talk about them. Say things like "I wonder if you're angry" or "You look like you're happy."

- **Share your own feelings.** This helps broaden children's understanding and language skills.

- **Use closeness and reflecting responses** to affirm your child's feelings. Be willing to touch or hold your child as she shares joyful or difficult feelings, and reflect her feelings through such responses as "It sounds like you're frustrated," or "I know you're angry right now, and I'm going to stay with you."

- **Respect nonverbal communication.** Do not demand that children explain their feelings in words before they are ready. If a child is crying and you ask why, she may not answer because she is expressing herself through her tears.

- **Differentiate between feelings and behavior.** You can stop a behavior like hitting, kicking, or throwing things while still respecting the feelings behind it.

- **Separate your feelings from your children's.** Sometimes listening to children's emotions sparks intense feelings in parents. Try to keep the two separate so you can continue to give productive attention to your child.

- **Enjoy and nurture your child's individuality.** Discover individual needs and strengths, moods and fears, and sense of humor and playfulness. Recognize that your child is unique and appreciate those special qualities.

- **Be a good example.** Children show their love for you and learn how to conduct themselves by imitating you. Model acceptable ways to express feelings. Your examples become permanent images that will guide their behavior and attitudes throughout life.

- **Help develop coping strategies.** Your child needs to learn constructive ways to handle anger, conflict, and frustration. Help your child sort out her feelings and encourage your child to come to you with problems. Model good skills for coping with change and give your child emotional support to adapt to new challenges.

- **Be realistic.** Even the best parents get exhausted or cranky. When it is hard to listen or support your children's feelings, you can take breaks without making them feel their feelings are wrong. "I guess you still need to cry. I am going to give my ears a rest and come back in a few minutes to make sure you're OK" is an example of how to do this.

pain. Most clashes between mothers and daughters stem from trying to maintain a high level of intimacy while at the same time allowing separateness. The strong identification daughters have with their mothers has the potential for strong conflict. Following are several suggestions for improving a strained mother-daughter relationship:

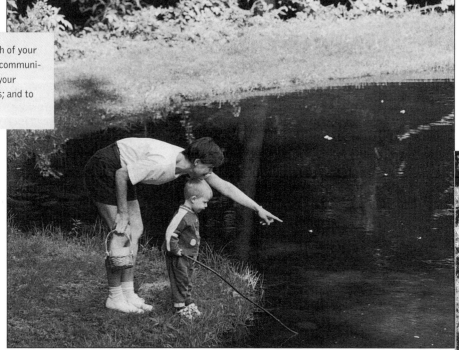

Be sure to spend individual time with each of your children. You can take this time to foster communication, love, and self-esteem; to listen to your child's feelings and ideas, and share yours; and to discover your child's individuality.

- **Remember that you cannot change your mother;** you can only change yourself. When you try new strategies for interacting with your mother, her responses are likely to change accordingly. For example, if you always lash out defensively when she criticizes you, try silence. Refuse to give her a willing opponent.
- **Set limits.** These can involve time, space boundaries, advice, even gift-giving. Find tactful, diplomatic ways to enforce limits, such as ending a telephone conversation firmly but pleasantly after 15 minutes rather than letting your mother tie you up for an hour. If she asks how your love life is and you do not want to discuss it, say "Fine" and take the initiative to change the subject. With time, she will learn to deal with you on your own terms.
- **Do not argue with your mother.** If she harps on an issue, such as how she wishes you would not ride a motorcycle, let her know you understand her concerns. You could say, "Yes, you've mentioned that before. It seems to make you anxious. I appreciate your concern for my well-being."
- **Focus on the positive.** Tune in to what is most noble and nurturing in your mother's communications and do not dwell on the more negative parts.
- **Look for the love.** Try to identify the positive emotional intent behind your mother's behavior by putting yourself in her shoes. For example, when you give someone you care about advice, it is probably because you want them to be safe or successful. You do not intend to give the message "you are incompetent." It is the same with your mother.
- **Stop blaming your mother.** Let go of your anger about her mistakes—no mother is perfect, endlessly nurturing, or all-knowing. Accept responsibility for the person you have become.

The healthiest adult mother-daughter relationships are based on mutual respect and are characterized by the ability of both mother and daughter to move easily between states of dependence, independence, and interdependence.

Father-Daughter Relationships. Fathers often feel a special protectiveness toward daughters. Some classic patterns in father-daughter relationships include the father who treats his daughter like an adored princess, the father who solves his daughter's problems, and the father who sees his daughter as a lifelong pupil. There are also patriarchs who bring in the paycheck and settle disputes but are otherwise detached or uninvolved, and "invisible" fathers who are physically present but emotionally disconnected.

Today, a style of involved, nurturing fatherhood is emerging. Men are taking a more hands-on role in caring for their children, are more open about expressing their feelings, and are more conscious of how they can help daughters foster independence and high self-esteem. Fathers who take their daughters seriously help a daughter feel she is a person of consequence. Often this is accomplished through participation in activities like extracurricular programs, weekend classes, parent days at school, girls' sports leagues, and so on.

In adulthood, even very close, loving father-daughter relationships tend to focus on activities, information exchange, and problem-solving. Stock market tips or how to find a good mechanic are generally the domain of the father. Typically, the mother remains the parent with whom daughters probe feelings and talk about relationships.

Siblings. Siblings can be considered our first partners in life. Through our relationships with siblings, we learn about intimacy, conflict, and cooperation. From their brothers, girls find out about the opposite sex and get lessons about what it is to be male. With their sisters, girls tend to have close, emotionally intense relationships. Researchers have found that in middle adulthood and old age the closest, most long-standing sibling relationships are between sisters. Traditionally, sisters are seen as the ones who keep a family together throughout life.

There are many unanswered questions about sibling relationships, how siblings influence each other, the impact of gender and birth order, and how parental attitudes affect siblings. Although siblings are raised in the same family, each child's experiences may be dramatically different. Essentially, each child is born into a different marital environment, because the environment is influenced by each new addition to the family. It is human nature that all siblings squabble and jockey for their parents' approval. Sibling rivalry has a powerful effect on the development of one's identity. A woman's personal identity evolves to a large extent from a simultaneous desire to be like brothers and sisters as well as to be different from them. Through adolescence and early adulthood, siblings can be role models, sounding boards, and support systems; unfortunately, they can also become such a source of hurt or humiliation that the relationship temporarily or permanently ends.

When adult siblings are friends, they can serve as wonderful allies, helping to sort out conflicts. They know family dynamics, family history, and the hot buttons of other family members. They have unique insights and perspectives on the family. As aunts and uncles, siblings can fill a special place in the lives of their nieces and nephews and serve as positive adult role models in the extended family.

Even adults who have become distanced from their siblings may find themselves trying to renew the bonds in midlife, a time when people have developed a strong sense of self and are reaffirming the value of family. The illness or death of a parent can put new stresses on sibling relationships—bringing them closer together or creating distance when there is long-standing hurt or anger. By the time adults reach old age, most will say they feel closer to siblings than to any other relatives except their own children. Though sibling rivalry may remain strong in early and middle adult years, by the later adult years most feelings of envy and resentment have faded and emotional support gains greater importance.

Spouses, Lovers, Lifelong Partners

"I have always been struck by the difficulty of predicting how any individual will behave in a love relationship," says psychologist Michael Broder in his book *The Art of Staying Together*. He sees many people who are inept when it comes to intimacy but are "brilliantly in charge of their lives in every other area."

In healthy love relationships, each partner makes a commitment to care about the other, as well as about oneself and the relationship. Both partners work at developing good communication skills and maintaining goodwill. Each partner must value and respect the other for who he or she is—not who the partner thinks the other should be. In solid marriages and love relationships the fundamental needs for approval and appreciation are met for both partners.

Relationships require "maintenance." Little matters left unattended can require larger energies that disrupt communications and reduce pleasure in the relationship. Watch for these signs that your relationship needs attention:

- You do not look forward to spending time with your spouse and find your time together less interesting than almost any other activity.
- You are either passive or irritable around your spouse. You bicker constantly.
- You do not confide your inner feelings to each other.
- The activities you do together are monotonous and routine, even if there are a lot of them.
- You do not deal with difficult issues (like money).
- There is a powerful inner fear that the marriage will come apart if something provocative is brought up.
- You complain about your spouse to other people, but you have stopped talking to your spouse. You are no longer interested in trying to make things better.

Friendships

When psychotherapist Lillian Rubin interviewed 300 men and women ages 25 to 55 to study the nature of friendship, she heard a recurring theme: "Friends accept me for who I am." Even those study participants who said they love their families deeply noted that it is much easier to be themselves around friends. They repeatedly talked about how friends allow them to test out various parts of themselves and find strengths that had not been tapped into before. In her book *Just Friends*, Rubin quotes a 32-year-old anthropologist:

I didn't really know I was smart until I became friends with Myra, who's a brilliant woman. I'd say something to her and she'd look impressed, like, "Wow, that's clever," and I used to be surprised. It was my friendship with her that enabled me to go back to graduate school, get my Ph.D., and become a college professor.

Rubin reports that women choose female friends who seem to bring out their best qualities, while accepting their flaws. Generally, women's friendships with each other are characterized by shared intimacies, self-revelation, nurture, and emotional support.

Women with close male friends note that those relationships are different from the ones they have with women. And, many women maintain strong friendships with men other than their husbands. Conversations with these male friends tend to focus more on ideas and problem solving, with little sharing of feelings or exchange of personal information.

Female friendships are tremendously compelling. Women friends confide in each other with an ease that often astounds men. Women friends provide a sympathetic ear and an outlet for feelings—a kind of safety valve—that friendship with a male may not provide. "Many women insist that, rather than being a strain on the marriage, their friendships are an important source of support for it," Rubin says. "Woman after woman told of the ways in which friends fill the gaps the marriage relationship leaves, allowing the wife to appreciate those things the husband can give her rather than to focus on those he can't." Throughout life, women have more friendships than men do, and they continue to make new friends, while most men lose old friends without replacing them. In an essay on friendship, Pulitzer Prize-winning author Anna Quindlen wrote:

Female friendships can be rich and rewarding.

In our constantly shifting lives, our female friends may be the greatest constant and the touchstone not only of who we are but who we once were, the people who, taken together, know us whole, from girlfriend to wife and mother and even to widow. Children grow and go; even beloved men sometimes seem to be beaming their perceptions and responses from a different planet. But our female friends are forever.

The concept of "best friends" is particularly strong among women. Best friends are drawn together in much the same way as lovers—an attraction almost impossible to put into words. Something clicks. Although best friendships may come and go rapidly in childhood or adolescence, they are fairly stable in adult-

Getting Along with Your Boss

- **Stop trying to change your boss. Work on understanding your own behavior to have a better relationship.**

- **Make sure you are fully aware of what your boss is trying to accomplish. Do not assume you know her goals. If you are not sure, ask.**

- **If you are having difficulty prioritizing your work, ask for your boss's help. This actually may help her realize how many tasks she is asking you to accomplish simultaneously.**

- **Focus on solutions, not problems. If there is a problem with which you need your boss's assistance, be prepared to suggest ways of solving it.**

- **Study your boss's personality, style, and preferences. Know the best way and time to present information to your boss to get approval for something you want.**

- **If your boss does not accept a suggestion, try to look at the decision from your boss's point of view. If you do not readily under-stand her reasoning, ask her to explain her rationale.**

hood. The intensity of the emotional relationship can lead to rivalries, like those between siblings. Best friends have tremendous power to help and to hurt. Rubin notes that the most bitter complaints she heard in her research had to do with intimate friendships that failed. Women try to make sense of the experience, but often find no clear-cut reasons. Some causes of strain include changes in one or both friends, poor adjusting after one or both of the friends marry, lack of time, competition, and unresolved conflicts.

For best friendships to survive, friends have to learn to meet today's needs rather than those of the past and to tolerate the changes that inevitably occur. They also must withstand the periods of distance in today's busy lives, when work demands and family obligations may cause friendships to be put on the back burner for a time.

Sometimes, you may feel it is better for you emotionally to end a friendship. For example, some friendships become out of balance. One friend does all the giving while the other does all the taking. Perhaps there is not enough common ground to sustain the relationship. Or the friend has become so negative and crit-ical you feel dragged down. The friend may have a perception of you that makes you feel constrained—perhaps you have changed, and the friend is not ready to accept the change. If you are unsure about the wisdom of maintaining a friend-ship that is requiring much effort and energy, do a "cost-benefit" analysis to determine whether the price of continuing it outweighs the payoff of ending it. Ask yourself:

- Am I obsessing about the situation to a point where it is destructive?
- Are the emotional frustrations worth it?
- Are there key reasons why I need to preserve the relationship?
- Is there a realistic way to solve the problems we have?
- Do I feel like cutting my losses and moving on?

If you decide to end the relationship, give yourself permission to let go.

Workplace Relationships

An estimated 80 percent of people who have difficulty in their jobs do so because they relate poorly to others. Good interpersonal skills are at the core of success in the workplace. Teamwork is essential in the business environment. On a good team, the results surpass the sum total of each individual's talents and efforts.

The Workplace Tie to Your Emotional Past. The emotional dynamics between people at work often resemble those of a family. This may not be apparent in workplaces where conflict is low, but when stress escalates, we often revert to the coping strategies we learned as children. Falling back on defensive, unhealthy behavior patterns can be costly, both emotionally and financially. You become more susceptible to anxiety, hurt, and anger; you feel powerless, you are less pro-ductive, and it is harder to feel accepted and fulfilled. Ultimately, if these patterns continue, your health and self-esteem can suffer.

Some red flags that suggest you have lapsed into unproductive strategies in the workplace include: feeling like you are fighting the same battles over and over, blaming others, or having the sense of being stuck in a rut. If you detect such signals, try to step back and become an objective observer of the situation. What seems to be going on? Do you recognize familiar patterns? Are you playing out roles you filled at home, such as being the scapegoat or the martyr? Become aware of your thoughts, feelings, and behaviors without judging yourself too harshly. Ask yourself if a person you are having trouble with reminds you of someone in your family. Sometimes, women who have unresolved emotional issues with a parent will have a hard time coping with a boss of the same gender. And sometimes, women may try too hard to please their female bosses or depend too heavily on the response they receive in return.

The new awareness you get from assessing your behavior patterns and automatic responses in the workplace can help you identify times when you need to alter your communication style or use conflict resolution skills (discussed later in the chapter). It is important to recognize that all parties involved share in the responsibility for what happens at work; not any one person is entirely at fault. As you interact with others at work, ask yourself, "What do I want the other person to understand about me right now?" Then act and communicate in a way that achieves the understanding or impression you are seeking.

Women Working with Women. Women, because of their deeply ingrained drive to bond with other women and fill a nurturing role, sometimes find the workplace to be an interpersonal obstacle course. Women may be critical or mistrustful of women who focus on productivity, finance, or other bottom-line issues without reaching out to share emotionally with their female coworkers.

Jealousy is another hot spot for women in the workplace. One survey found 25 percent of women participants agreed that jealousy is a problem for women who work with women, as is a tendency to take things personally. Some women feel threatened when other women appear exceedingly competent or have achieved a higher level of career success. Another problem for women is that they tend to back away from the prospect of competing with other people. When they do compete, women often try to maintain a supportive, cooperative environment, which, although laudable, can be emotionally draining and create obstacles to basic corporate objectives, such as sales goals and budget negotiations with vendors.

Some strategies that women who work with other women can use to foster productive workplace relationships are as follows:

- Be aware of the tendency to personalize workplace interactions. To avoid overpersonalizing, keep a distance between what you produce and who you are. Not reaching your sales target, or getting feedback that suggests improvement is needed in the department you run, has nothing to do with whether you are a good person or how people feel about you. Try to look at your own business behavior objectively.
- Balance politeness and directness. Although women tend to be uncomfortable with directness, it must be used when we supervise or instruct others. Practice being direct. In speaking and in writing, use short, concise sentences when making requests. Do not apologize for rational, logical, business-oriented requests. Do not cajole and do not act coy.
- Accept the fact that not everyone will like you. This is a big one. Not everyone

will become a fast friend, but they can still respect you and work well with you. Women have diverse styles and approaches, all of which have their own validity.

- If you dislike someone you work with, step back, study her style, and try to separate irritating behaviors from skills and abilities. Does she remind you of some significant person in your past with whom you have had problems? What does she do well, even if you do not like the way she does it? Focus on her strengths. Think about what is at stake if you do not get along with her, and how you can both benefit if you do get along.

- If you feel irritated or offended, pause first to reflect on the feeling rather than responding. This is referred to as "taking a walk" with the feeling. As you calm down, think about the appropriate behavior for your response. Emotionally charged confrontation is bad communication.

- If you want to acknowledge discomfort with a fellow worker, do not ask why she does not like you, which puts her on the defensive. Emphasize behavior rather than feelings by saying, "I've noticed that when I [behavior], that seems to make you uncomfortable." This may open the door to constructive feedback.

- Precede requests to female staff members with personal conversation, however brief. According to Pat Heim, author of *Smashing the Glass Ceiling,* women employees resent being given direct requests by women supervisors or bosses without the expected bonding and sharing opportunity.

Repairing
Relationships

Relationships are hard work, and they do not always go smoothly. When conflicts and misunderstandings arise, feelings get hurt. There is no simple formula for handling every situation. The communication skills and suggestions described earlier in this chapter are a good place to start, however. Here are more techniques to draw upon in difficult situations.

Conflict Management

Women, more often than men, tend to cringe at the thought of conflict or confrontation. Many women grow up being taught that conflict, like anger, is to be

Crying at Work

Women are more likely than men to cry in emotionally charged situations. The source of tears is usually unrecognized anger or frustration and comes from feeling out of control. Women are usually appalled at the thought of crying at work. If you feel tears coming on, you can say, "Excuse me, I need to get a drink of water," and then bring the water back with you. It is almost impossible to drink water and cry at the same time. Or you can say, "This conversation is really upsetting me. I need some time—could we meet again later?" Then go to a private place where you can decide what the tears are about and how to deal with the situation constructively.

avoided and denied. As women mature, they assume the role of peacemaker and soother of feelings; the people who make sure that everyone is happy. Situations involving conflict cause fear, anguish, and stress. Many women equate conflict with the feeling that they do not know what will happen, that they might lose or forfeit control, and that the relationship will worsen if there is conflict.

Conflict, like change, is unavoidable in life. Conflict arises when we have different needs, goals, values, approaches, or interests. In its mildest form, conflict can be disruptive; at its worst, conflict can be destructive. But conflict also has a positive side. It allows us to learn, change, and grow. It stimulates creativity, compromise, negotiation, understanding, and problem solving.

Certain skills and attitudes can prevent needless conflict. Nonproductive behaviors like threatening, judging, and insulting others should be avoided. Using good communication skills is essential in resolving conflict. Shouting at someone may release your tension, but it is likely to increase the other person's. Being aware of behaviors that have caused conflict in the past, and being sensitive to telltale signs of impending conflict, can help you diffuse confrontations and practice productive ways of dealing with angry or hurt feelings. Constantly repressing such feelings can lead to psychological problems and psychosomatic illness. Some women have been taught to do everything they can to avoid confrontion. They may withdraw emotionally or patch things up without working through the underlying issues. Giving in, or capitulating, is fine sometimes, but women who do this repeatedly go through life without getting their needs met. They often become angry and resentful; they are at increased risk for depression, substance abuse, or stress-related physical illness.

It is also unhealthy to dominate others when conflicts arise. Forcing solutions onto others breeds resentment. In fact, a major contributor to conflict is the drive to "be right." To manage conflict in a positive way, you must let go of your need to have your principles and convictions win out, and instead look at how to reach a common ground with the other person.

Not every conflict needs to be resolved—some just are not that important in the grand scheme of things. A good yardstick is the level of commitment involved. Ask yourself, "Is this a conflict I need to tackle or can I let it go?" Think about whether the conflict will still feel important, still make you angry, in 24 hours. If the answer is yes, you need to deal with it.

When conflict arises and you think it needs to be resolved, the best approach is to act, not react. You have the power to choose your response to what you experience in life. Following are some key strategies for handling and resolving conflict:

- **Treat the other person with respect.** To do this you must recognize that other people have a right to their own beliefs and values. The heat of conflict, unfortunately, tends to promote angry, disrespectful outbursts and biting comments. Body language and facial expressions can easily convey all kinds of unspoken criticisms. It takes willpower to maintain equilibrium and mutual respect.
- **Use effective listening.** This is probably the most important conflict resolution skill of all. Practice the reflective, empathic listening skills described earlier in the chapter.
- **Briefly state your views, needs, and feelings.** Say what you mean clearly. Use "I" statements to communicate your feelings.

• **Avoid using accusatory terms.** Phrases such as "you always" or "you never" put the other person on the defensive. Rephrase your thoughts to focus on a specific incident as an example.

Using these strategies allows both parties to appreciate each other's viewpoint. Clearing the air may diffuse the problem. Or it may motivate one or both of you to change, thus bringing peace without further discussion. Also useful are collaborative problem-solving techniques (see sidebar).

Managing Anger

Anger is usually a secondary feeling that covers up deeper emotions, like fear, rejection, hurt, or embarrassment. Some women would rather express anger than let others see their vulnerability. Others are taught that anger is bad and that if they feel angry, they certainly should not express it. Women tend to communicate anger indirectly through sarcasm, put-downs, sabotaging people's efforts, blame, ridicule, criticism, or making complaints to a third party. Women who do not express their anger may feel anxious, depressed, or restless, or develop physical problems, such as headaches. Taking the following steps can help you begin to deal with anger constructively:

• Recognize and accept your anger, and allow yourself to feel it.
• Learn to express anger in ways that do not damage valuable relationships (use "I" messages).
• Get in touch with the underlying feelings your anger may represent.

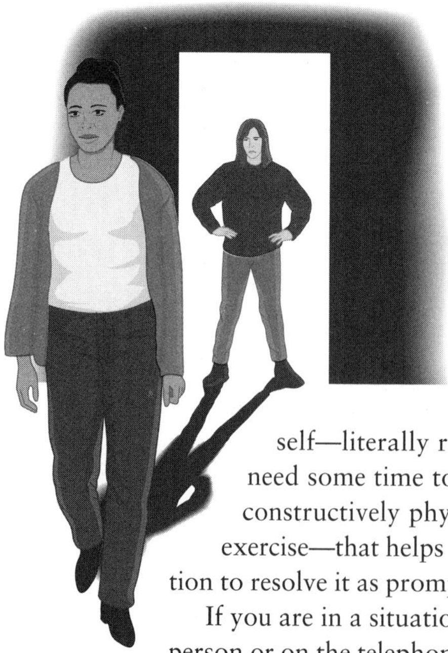

Have you ever wondered why, when you are angry, you sometimes act impulsively or blurt something out without considering the negative consequences of your actions or words? Interestingly, the brain's architecture is such that sensory signals reach the center of emotions, the amygdala, before they finish traveling through the neocortex, or "thinking" part of the brain. Based on the input to the amygdala, a woman may leap into action before the neocortex has had a chance to digest the information and initiate a calmer plan of action.

It is important to acknowledge anger, but responding in the heat of anger is not usually a good idea. Some experts recommend a version of "time out" to give your rational thinking process a chance to function. If, for example, you feel an argument coming on with your husband or child, stop yourself—literally remove yourself from the situation. You might say, "I need some time to think about this. Can we talk later?" Do something constructively physical—clean your desk, wash the car, take a walk, go exercise—that helps the angry tension dissipate. Always return to the situation to resolve it as promptly as you can, however.

If you are in a situation where another person is angry and yelling at you, in person or on the telephone, let her continue until she runs out of steam. Hurling

FIGURE 11.2

Managing Anger

The first step to resolving a heated conflict is removing yourself from the situation until your anger is under control. Try one of these suggestions to help dispel your anger:

• Exercise

• Listen to quiet music

• Take a long bath or shower

• Talk about it with a friend

• Sit quietly for half an hour

• Take a walk

Collaborative Problem Solving

Collaborative problem solving means getting both or all parties involved in identifying and carrying out a solution to conflict. Here are the key steps:

- **Define the problem in terms of needs, not solutions.** For example, if your children are fighting over who gets to use the computer, each one will probably say "I need to use the computer." But if one child says "I need to do my homework," and the other says "I need to send an E-mail message to my girlfriend," solutions start to surface. Sometimes you need to encourage the people involved to pinpoint their needs.

- **Brainstorm possible solutions once each person's needs are stated.** Remember that no idea is a bad idea. Never criticize anyone's idea during a brainstorming session. Sometimes the most far-fetched idea turns into the best solution. Record all ideas and expand on them. Do not limit yourselves by thinking there is only one right solution.
- **Clarify options and select the best solution or combination of solutions.** Rather than eliminating solutions one by one, see which choices coincide, and identify the ones that seem best. Then settle on the solution jointly, so it meets everyone's needs as much as possible.
- **Put the plan into effect—plan who will do what, the methods to be used, and the deadlines.** Follow up later and assess how well the solution is working out.

accusations in response or defending yourself will only fuel her anger. When she calms down, say, "I'm willing to have a discussion with you, but only when it's a respectful conversation for both of us." (This should not be said condescendingly or it will just upset the person more.) Then set up a time to get together and talk. Following are more constructive tactics for dealing with another person's anger:

- **Protect yourself through visualization.** Imagine the anger coming toward you like a beam of negative energy, then striking the ground and dissipating. Or run your hands across the top of your head, imagining you are clearing away the negative energy. Think up a visualization technique that works for you.
- **Cut the person down to size in your mind.** Imagine she is getting smaller and smaller and her voice is growing fainter.
- **Focus on what you are learning from the situation.** Ask yourself, "What can I take away to help me deal with future situations like this? How can I make sure I do not get stuck in a situation like this again?"
- **Realize that the other person is responsible for her own anger.** You are only responsible for managing your reaction to the anger. Do not buy into her anger. Remain calm. This can be extremely difficult, but it is very effective.

Criticism as a Force for Change

Some women tend to think of criticism as pointing out flaws in others. Other women associate criticism with insults and pain, hearing about something they did wrong or receiving harsh judgments. But the ability to give and receive criticism in an appropriate manner is a key attribute of successful people.

"Most people respond to criticism as if someone is throwing a knife at them," says psychologist Hendrie Weisinger, author of *The Critical Edge*. "They duck and dodge, trying to avoid it. Or they take it to heart and let it hurt them." And sometimes they respond by throwing a "knife" of their own—trying to hurt back. In order to avoid such hurtful retaliation, the first step is to change your definition of criticism. Think of it as evaluative information that is communicated in a way that lets you use it to your advantage. Of course, not all criticism is delivered in a constructive manner, but even when it is not, you can regard it as information that may help you grow.

Avoid viewing criticism as an issue of being right or wrong or as a put-down. Keep your emotions in check by breathing deeply and slowly. The more emotional you become, the more your body tenses and prepares to attack or withdraw in the "fight or flight" response. This tension becomes part of your nonverbal communication and may be interpreted as anger. Listen carefully to what is being said rather than concentrating on defending yourself. As you listen, be as objective as possible. Assess the validity and usefulness of the criticism by asking yourself:

- **How accurate is it?** Does the issue touch on my performance, health, or safety, or that of others? For example, if your husband says you drive too fast, you have gotten two speeding tickets in the past year—which you had to pay with money you were saving for a weekend getaway—and you have had some frightening near-misses on the road, maybe you should listen.
- **How often have I heard it?** If it is an isolated criticism that deviates from what you normally hear, maybe you can discount it. But if different sources express the same criticism, it may be wise to consider a change.
- **Who is the source?** Is the person qualified to criticize you? Just because you like someone does not mean she is in a good position to evaluate you. Nor is disliking someone a good reason to invalidate her criticisms. Assess the critic's motives. Do they truly want you to grow, or are they criticizing merely out of anger or resentment?
- **Is the energy required to make the change worth the benefit?** Evaluate what you have to gain—how doing what is suggested will help you personally or benefit others.

Giving Constructive Criticism

Sometimes we can criticize without any effort, and other times—when we need to give feedback on key problems—we feel overwhelmed. Some simple steps can help make giving criticism a more comfortable and productive experience:

- **Target the behavior to criticize.** Think it out carefully ahead of time, even writing it down if need be. State specifically what needs changing. Vague statements like "your work needs to improve" are not helpful. Give at least one specific example of the behavior in question.
- **Acknowledge that your criticism is subjective.** Say "This is the way I see things" or "In my opinion," which paves the way for the recipient to express her views. Wording your criticism this way avoids "you" statements, which are often interpreted as "you are to blame" and "you are bad."
- **Ask for feedback about what you are saying.** This gets the recipient involved and helps you determine whether or not she understands your point of view.
- **Explain how you think the problem can be resolved.** Give specific examples. For example, you might say, "Being on time for meetings, listening to the discussion instead of making jokes, and meeting deadlines for the tasks you're assigned would all help you contribute more effectively to the committee."
- **State the incentive.** Let the recipient know how she will benefit. "I'd like to give you more opportunities for direct client contact. If you can show me that you can address client needs more calmly, I would be happy to give you that responsibility."

The Power of Forgiveness

Everyone suffers injustices in life. A boyfriend breaks your heart. Your boss fires you. A close colleague is promoted over you, though you have more experience. Maybe your best friend no longer spends her free time with you, and you are hurt.

Upsetting things happen, and with time, people usually get over them. Sometimes, however, bitterness lingers and grows, becoming a seething hostility.

Resentment can gnaw at you, harming your performance at work, interfering with relationships, sapping your energy, and affecting your happiness. If left unchecked, this resentment, emotional upset, repressed emotion, and anger can be extremely destructive. Some health consequences of longstanding resentments are depression, anxiety, and a higher risk of heart problems. One of the most damaging aspects is that it can keep you from taking responsibility for your choices and prevent you from changing your life in positive ways. It is often easier to remain an angry victim than to risk admission that your behavior or attitude may have contributed to the problem.

Honestly explore the reason for your resentment. Are you using it as an excuse to avoid pursuing a goal or to avoid being more responsible for your actions? Are your feelings of resentment based on the actual circumstances or do they stem from jealousy, feelings of inadequacy, or unconscious conflicts from earlier times in your life? Figuring out what is really bothering you may help you let go of your negative feelings. If you are feeling sorry for yourself, what prompts those feelings? If you feel you were wronged by someone, discuss it with them calmly, directly, and honestly. Usually you find that people do things for their own innocent reasons, not to hurt you. Realize that you can take responsibility for your response to a situation and change your attitude.

Letting go of resentment and forgiving the party that hurt you is healthy and liberating. It does not mean pretending the situation did not happen, however. It means accepting it and deciding that it will not destroy your life. Why waste precious time feeling bad and fantasizing about revenge? In his book *The Art of Forgiving,* psychologist Lewis Smedes says, "Unless we forgive, we give another person the power to hurt us again and again for the rest of our lives." Forgiveness is not the same as reconciliation, in which you both work to rebuild the relationship. Forgiveness is for yourself. With forgiveness, you try to understand the situation from the other person's point of view. For example, in the case of a cold and distant father, perhaps he was dealing with financial pressures while you were growing up that forced him to work long hours and left him preoccupied with worry. Once you understand this, you may be able to release your negative feelings and start healing. It is much easier not to forgive, but in the end, it is you who loses.

Apologizing Effectively

People's feelings are hurt in all kinds of situations. Human interactions are complex, and we all tread on someone else's sensibilities at times—sometimes intentionally, but often by mistake. When people feel humiliated, ignored, betrayed, or offended in some way, it is because something has injured their self-concept. They feel that you do not value them or see them the way they want to be perceived.

Apology is a powerful interpersonal skill that can soothe feelings and restore damaged relationships. But most people are not taught how to apologize skillfully. Botched apologies can spark longstanding grudges or strain relationships beyond repair. Psychologist Aaron Lazare, who has studied the power of apology, explains that what makes an apology work is "the exchange of shame and power between the offender and the offended. By apologizing, you take the shame off your offense and redirect it to yourself. You admit to hurting or diminishing someone." In effect, you are telling the other party that you are actually the one

How to Forgive

Forgiving another person is perhaps one of the hardest aspects of repairing relationships. Here are some points to consider to help you forgive:

- Choose to be happy rather than right. Holding on to unforgiving thoughts is essentially a decision to suffer.

- Decide that you are willing to let go of the past and forgive. This does not mean that you have to condone your own or someone else's behavior. Sometimes, when you plan to forgive another person it is not even necessary to tell that person.

- Figure out what is really bothering you. If your anger is far out of proportion to the offense, perhaps something else is involved. Ask yourself what is at the root of your anger and figure out how to let it go.

- Write down your feelings to help you understand them and figure out how to manage them. You could do this as a daily journal or one long letter. Some people pour everything into a letter and then tear it up as a symbol of release.

who is diminished—you were wrong, insensitive, thoughtless. In this way, you hand the person the power to forgive you.

The art of apology requires you to state the offense or negative behavior specifically and take responsibility for breaking some moral code or mutual understanding in your relationship. Saying "I'm sorry for what I did" is too vague. Much better is "I know I hurt you by missing your wedding, and I'm so sorry." In an effective apology, you also explain why you committed the offense without making excuses for it. This lets you preserve your self-concept: you did something wrong, but you are not a terrible person at heart. Maybe you were sick, overloaded at work, or out of money. Admit that you were wrong and vow sincerely that you will not repeat the wrong. It is important to communicate the distress and guilt you feel, which lets the other person know how much the relationship matters to you.

In unsuccessful apologies, the offender fails to take responsibility for her actions. If you say to someone "I'm sorry you were hurt," you are not acknowledging that the hurt occurred because of you. The most common cause of failed apologies is pride and the unwillingness to own up to a mistake. By saying you are sorry, you may think you are admitting weakness, when in fact you are demonstrating your courage. If you are too egocentric, you may be unable to appreciate another person's suffering and thus find it difficult to apologize effectively. What you regret is that the other person does not like you anymore, not that you hurt her. Timing is an important factor: waiting too long to offer an apology may kill its effectiveness.

When you apologize for hurting someone, you are expressing a commitment to work on the relationship. This sends a strong signal to the other person that things will get better if she can forgive you. Both of you come away with the understanding that you are not perfect, but you are still a good person.

Getting Help

When relationships in your life go wrong, there is much that you can do to set them right. But sometimes you may feel overwhelmed, out of control, or too emotionally exhausted to address problems on your own. Reaching out to others for help is the best thing you can do. Friends and family may be able to offer the support needed to work through interpersonal challenges. Their insights and advice may help you look at a situation in a new way. There are also numerous sources of self-help as well as professional services. The sources of information, training, and support for improving interpersonal skills and communication are limitless. Here are some places to start:

- Community colleges and universities offer communications and interpersonal skills training programs, often through their continuing education offices.
- Check your local library. Many libraries post notices and have racks for brochures about programs useful to people in the community. You can find a wide range of self-help books and tapes at the library as well, and your reference librarian can point you to community resources and books. For example, check the *Encyclopedia of Associations* in your local library. Call or write organizations that deal with family issues, interpersonal dynamics, communi-

cation, marriage—whichever is relevant to your problem—and ask what programs or brochures they offer that might help you.

- Regarding a serious interpersonal issue affecting your health, you may want to call your health insurance company. They can tell you what counseling services are covered by your health plan.
- Look into offerings at your local hospital, clinic, or health maintenance organization. Recognizing the significance of the body-mind connection on health, many of these organizations offer workshops on interpersonal skills, stress management, conflict resolution, and other related topics.
- Check with professional or women's organizations with which you are associated. Many offer lectures, workshops, or printed matter on topics related to interpersonal skills. Some examples are the National Association of Female Executives, Women in Communications, and the YWCA.
- Talk to your doctor. She is likely to be plugged into local sources of assistance or will be able to suggest places to start. If it sounds like you need marital counseling, for example, your doctor can probably refer you to a qualified professional.

What *You* Can Do

Good interpersonal skills and the ability to establish and maintain strong relationships and social support systems are a key part of health. Cultivating good communication skills can help ensure that you send and receive accurate messages and avoid conflict. Certain key principles can be a guide to developing good relationships with family, friends, and coworkers:

- Be alert to negative signals you may be sending, consciously and subconsciously.
- Use effective communication skills for conveying information as well as resolving conflict.
- Be honest, direct, and open with people who are important to you.
- If conflicts arise, try to work them out; if you cannot, seek help.

Chapter 12

Maintaining Your Mental *and* Emotional Health

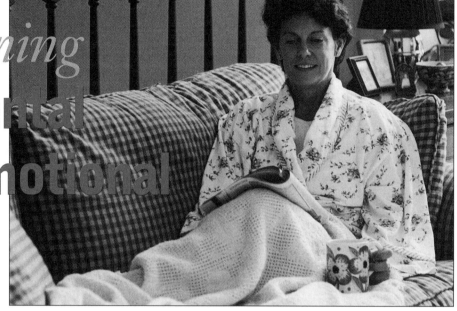

What does it mean to be mentally healthy? Does it mean having no problems? Does it mean never feeling sad, or angry, or upset? Being mentally healthy is not the absence of hardship or unpleasant feelings. It has more to do with the way in which a woman confronts, reacts to, and copes with life's ups and downs. How well women cope impacts their daily lives as well as how they handle major emotional transitions or trauma.

You can take charge of staying mentally healthy by taking care of yourself emotionally. Just as you care for your body by eating nutritious food and getting adequate rest and regular exercise, you can also do things that help you feel mentally fit and happy. Everyone has imperfections, weaknesses, and limitations. The key to emotional wellness is to recognize how your behaviors influence the way you live your life and interact with others.

Emotional wellness also means knowing when to ask for help and understanding that asking for professional help is not a fault or weakness. Counseling and psychotherapy techniques vary widely. The underlying aspect, however, is that a trained professional can help you examine the areas of your life that cause you stress, pain, or unhappiness. A trained professional can also help you find ways to grow and become a mentally healthier—and happier—person.

The Building Blocks *of* Mental Health

There are many elements to mental health and many characteristics that contribute to making you a mentally healthy person. Not everyone agrees on what these characteristics are, but they include such factors as dealing with stress successfully, cultivating self-esteem, caring for others, and reaching out for help when needed.

Dealing with Stress

Everyone experiences stress. Without it, people would find it hard to get motivated to do anything. Stress is a necessary fact of life stemming from negative, as well as positive, sources. You may experience it during an argument with your spouse, but you also experience stress during positive life-events that make you excited and happy, such as getting married, buying a home, or starting a new job.

Although you hear people speak in terms of "getting rid" of stress, the healthiest approach to handling stress is to find ways—called coping mechanisms—to come to terms with it directly. A mentally healthy person may get upset when things go wrong; she may even feel overwhelmed sometimes. But when things threaten to get out of control, she finds ways to preserve her mental balance.

Meditation and Stress Management

Would you believe that taking 20 or 30 minutes for meditation in the morning can help reduce stress throughout the entire day? Meditation produces measurable changes in brain waves, calms the mind, and reduces the stress response. The effect on your physical and emotional health can be remarkable.

Many minor health complaints are triggered by stress. Stress lowers your body's immune responses, making you more susceptible to colds, minor infections, stomach disorders, headaches, and muscle weakness. Some doctors routinely recommend meditation for patients whose physical and emotional health has been affected by stress.

How do you meditate? To begin, you sit or lie comfortably in a quiet place and focus on your breathing. By deepening and regulating the breath—paying close attention to each inhalation and exhalation—you can take your mind off all other thoughts, and gradually your mind seems to "empty" of the regrets, worries, and anxiety that induce stress. At the same time, you find that your muscles relax and your heart slows, giving you a feeling of overall calm and well-being. Later, when the inevitable stresses of the day intrude, you can "remember" that sense of well-being and almost every situation can be dealt with calmly and thoughtfully.

Cultivating Self-Esteem

Acknowledging your strengths and accepting praise from others can build your self-esteem and improve your mental state. Unfortunately, women have traditionally been given the message that taking credit for a job well done is immodest or self-centered. Take pride in your accomplishments and don't underrate them. Learn to accept compliments. During inevitable moments of self-doubt, remind yourself that you are, indeed, a capable woman.

Caring for Others

Compassion for others comes from being able to understand other points of view and to identify with the feelings of others. A mentally healthy person is able to respond to the needs of others without dismissing or ignoring her own needs.

Elements of Emotional Maturity

- The ability to function in a socially acceptable manner
- The capacity to adapt to change
- A relative freedom from tension and anxiety
- The capacity to find more satisfaction in giving than receiving
- The capacity to relate to other people in a consistent manner with mutual satisfaction and helpfulness
- The capacity to direct one's hostile energy into creative and constructive outlets
- The capacity to love

Source: The Menninger Clinic, Topeka, KS.

Recognizing When You Need Help

It is not always easy for people to admit to themselves that they are having problems. In our society, some people still equate seeing a mental health professional with being "crazy" or irrational. Women may have an especially hard time finding and getting help. Studies show that problems such as depression are much more common in women than men, but that men seek help sooner and more often. Learning how to get help with your problems, whether that means taking time out for yourself, writing in a journal, talking with a close friend, or seeking professional help, is an essential component of mental and emotional health.

Risk Factors for Mental Health Problems *Among* Women

Overall in the United States, women are diagnosed with mental problems more often than men. They are also admitted to mental health facilities in greater numbers. No one is exactly sure why, but several factors probably contribute.

Women's Social Roles and Self-Esteem

Most experts agree that women as a whole have made many social and professional advances over the past three decades. More women than ever are working in high-level, well-paying jobs traditionally held by men. More men are sharing household and childcare responsibilities traditionally handled by women. Unfortunately, other traditional ideals have changed more slowly, with the result that many women still feel pressure to be the primary caretaker in the home while pursuing modern careers. These changes have created a "role strain" for many women. They feel that they have to "do it all" in order to meet with success in life. Emotional overload is common among women who have dual roles in society.

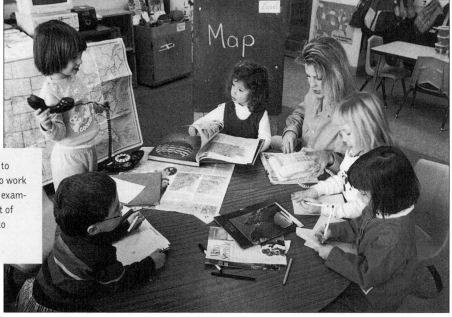

In the professional arena, it is important to identify ways to manage stress in order to work well with others. A preschool teacher, for example, influences the emotional development of children and therefore has an obligation to leave her negative emotions at the door.

Even with all the advances women have made, however, more women than men live in poverty in the United States, more are in lower-paying jobs, and more women than men are single-parent heads of households. A woman who lacks an adequate education and a reasonable income with a job that suitably challenges her skills and talents is at increased risk for emotional instability and depression.

Violence and Victimization

Physical and emotional abuse can have devastating effects on a person's mental health. As many as 2 million women are physically battered by their male partners each year. The number who are abused psychologically is no doubt even greater.

Often the result of chronic abuse is "learned helplessness." A woman's self-esteem plummets with repeated abuse from her partner. At the same time, her feelings of inadequacy, fear, and powerlessness grow. Her abusive partner convinces her that she is to blame and deserves the abuse. And she then feels that there is nothing she can do to improve her circumstances, which puts her at risk for further abuse. Only when this vicious circle is broken can the survivor of domestic violence find ways to change her situation. (See Chapter 14 for more information about domestic violence and abuse.)

Other Risk Factors

Substance abuse and mental illness are known to be closely connected. In some women, chronic substance abuse causes mental disorders, but in other cases women who are depressed or mentally ill seek relief through "self-medication." It is estimated that half of all people who have a substance abuse problem also have a mental illness. (See Chapter 13 for more information on this topic.)

Having a parent or sibling with a mental illness may also increase a woman's risk. Depression, in particular, seems to run in families.

Common Mental Health Problems *in* Women

Mental health problems are common among adults in the United States. About 27 percent of people between the ages of 15 and 54 are diagnosed with psychological disorders each year. The most common psychological disorders in adults fall into two major categories: depressive (or mood) disorders and anxiety disorders. Both groups have multiple subgroups that are commonly recognized.

Depressive Disorders

Depressive (or mood) disorders are the second most common types of mental disorders in the United States, occurring in almost 20 percent of adults. Major depression is the most common of these disorders. Bipolar disorder (sometimes called manic-depressive disorder) is also a type of depressive disorder.

Major Depression. Virtually no one goes through life without sometimes feeling sad, discouraged, or "down in the dumps." It is normal to have these feelings from time to time and normal for them to pass. When they do not go away, however, it may be an indicator of something more than just a passing case of "the

wellness **tip**

If you have a problem with depression, one of the most important things you can do for yourself is establish a regular schedule of being awake, asleep, working, and playing.

Seasonal Affective Disorder (SAD)

People with SAD have recurrent bouts of depression during a particular time of year. Fall and winter are the most common times for seasonal affective changes, although some people experience recurrent episodes of depression in the other seasons. Symptoms of SAD are similar to those experienced by persons with major depression. Medication may be required and psychotherapy may be helpful. The symptoms will ordinarily disappear with the passage of that season.

Recent research has indicated that SAD may be linked to the body's biological clock. This theory suggests that body temperature and hormone production may fluctuate according to the season in response to the waxing and waning of daylight hours. A form of therapy to treat SAD has been developed in which the patient is exposed to light from a specially designed fluorescent tube for a prescribed number of hours throughout the day. This approach seems to diminish the symptoms in some people.

blues." When such feelings persist and make it difficult for a woman to function normally or to enjoy life, she may be experiencing major depression.

Depression and Women. About twice as many women as men are clinically depressed at some point in their lives. Older data indicated that women's biology may put them at higher risk for depression. Current research, however, implies that both biology and social roles play an important role in the development of depression in women.

Symptoms of Depression. Depression is different from being in a bad mood, experiencing grief, or feeling disappointed. It is a persistent and all-encompassing feeling of worthlessness, hopelessness, and despair. Clinically, depression is diagnosed when at least five of the following symptoms have been present for at least two weeks:

- Feeling sad, empty, tearful, and down most of the day
- Loss of interest and pleasure in things that were once enjoyed
- Marked weight loss (when not dieting) and/or greatly decreased appetite
- Weight gain with compulsive eating
- Trouble falling or staying asleep, or sleeping much more than usual
- Feeling either restless, jittery, and irritable or slow and lethargic
- Fatigue and loss of energy
- Feeling worthless and/or extremely guilty
- Trouble concentrating on tasks
- Thinking about or planning for suicide

Because the known risk factors for depression are of special concern for so many women, it is important to be alert to the early warning signs. Any one of the criteria listed could signal the onset of depression, even if it has been present for only a day or two. Do not ignore these signs—and if you feel you need help, by all means seek it.

People who have experienced major depression frequently describe physical aspects to the disorder. A woman in the midst of severe depression may feel that her arms and legs are tired and heavy and that it seems like a great effort to perform even the simplest task. She may want to sleep all the time, yet be unable to sleep through the night. She may feel that nothing is worthwhile and may want to close out the rest of the world, to close herself down emotionally, and consequently she has trouble even moving.

The nature of depression, like many mental disorders, is such that the disorder itself makes it difficult for the person to grasp the state she is in. It may be difficult for a depressed person to get out of bed, to concentrate at work, or to listen to what a loved one is saying. She may occasionally be on the verge of tears for no reason that she can identify. Many women may explain these debilitating feelings as being their own fault or the result of laziness or inadequacy. These thoughts and feelings serve only to deepen the depression.

Triggers for Depression. Most researchers think that some people are born predisposed to depression—that there is, in fact, a hereditary component. In a person who is biologically at risk for depression, childhood trauma—especially molestation or incest—can trigger feelings of guilt, self-blame, and worthlessness that are linked to depression. But trauma does not have to be as obvious as physical or emotional abuse. If a child does not receive the kind of emotional nurturing that is needed for her to become a self-assured, confident person, she is more likely to develop persistent symptoms of depression into adulthood.

Depression can occur for the first time at any age, although it most commonly begins in the mid-twenties. Some people have only occasional bouts of depression separated by years without any signs of the disorder. Others tend to have "clusters" of more frequent episodes over time. In still others, depressive episodes become more frequent and more severe with age. Stress plays an important role in the course of this disorder. A loved one's death, divorce, getting or losing a job, moving to a new place, the birth of a baby, or a serious accident or illness are all examples of stressors that can trigger an initial or recurrent depression.

Depression and the Reproductive Cycle. About 65 percent of women who have a history of depression experience premenstrual syndrome (PMS), which manifests as serious depression before their menstrual cycle begins each month. For many, these feelings resolve with the onset of menstruation. In the worst cases of PMS, symptoms of depression begin immediately after ovulation and continue until the end of menstruation, leaving only about ten days during the cycle when the woman feels well.

Depression following the birth of a baby is also very common; about 80 percent of women report some period of "postpartum blues." Usually starting three to four days after delivery and resolving a few days later, postpartum blues are marked by outbursts of crying, anger, and sadness. Women who experience postpartum blues have an increased risk of experiencing a true postpartum depression.

Postpartum depression is more intense and lingering than postpartum blues, and it occurs in about ten percent of women after delivery. Postpartum depression is a serious depressive illness that affects a women's ability to bond with her infant and the infant's ability to bond with the mother. Estimates about the frequency of this condition vary, and doctors are becoming more sensitive to the potential for the disorder in the women they serve. If you or someone you know experiences depressive symptoms after delivery, then evaluation by a mental health professional may be necessary.

Postpartum psychosis is a fairly rare, serious mental illness, occurring in 0.2 percent of postpartum women. Postpartum psychosis is a serious, life-threatening condition that may require hospitalization for the mother. A few mother-baby postpartum psychiatric units are currently available in this country.

Menopause is another period in women's lives that is often cited as causing depression. While it is true that women who have experienced a major depressive disorder earlier in their lives may experience a recurrence in the perimenopausal period, new onset depression is less common during this time than it is when women are in their twenties. (See Chapter 19 for further discussion of depression during perimenopause.)

Bipolar Disorder. Bipolar disorder (BPD), sometimes called manic-depressive illness, occurs about as often in women as in men. A person with BPD has periods of depression that alternate with manic episodes. Research has determined that the disorder is the result of a chemical imbalance and is most effectively treated with medication.

Risk Factors for Depressive Illness

- **History of depression in one's past**
- **Prior or current depression in a family member**
- **Prior suicide attempts**
- **Being female**
- **Onset of symptoms under age 40 years**
- **Having given birth within the past year**
- **Having a medical illness**
- **Lack of social supports**
- **Stressful life events**
- **Current alcohol or other drug abuse**

Grief and Depression

Grief is very much linked to depression, and its "symptoms" mimic those of major depression: tightness in the chest or throat; trouble sleeping, or sleeping much more than usual; eating more or less than usual; lack of interest in things once enjoyed; trouble concentrating; tiring easily; irritability; and mood swings.

Grief is not only a reaction to death. The loss of one's health or physical ability or those of a loved one; the loss of a sense of safety after violence or victimization; the loss of the family from a divorce; or when a child experiences serious difficulty—all can lead to symptoms of grief.

During a manic episode, a woman's mood is abnormally elevated. She may feel exuberant or irritable or both. People who know her usually notice the change and describe her as being "high." Other features of a manic episode include:

- An inflated sense of self-esteem or grandiosity.
- Feeling the need for much less sleep than usual.
- Extreme talkativeness, with racing thoughts and ideas.
- Being easily distracted and "scattered."

Someone in the midst of a manic episode often seems driven to engage in certain activities without letup. She may start conversations with strangers when normally she would not dare; she may call friends in the middle of the night to talk about trivial matters; or she may go out and buy 20 pairs of shoes. Her speech may be unusually loud, fast, and hard to understand, and she may jump from topic to topic with no clear connection. If not treated, her manic behavior can extend to activities that are clearly harmful: impractical business ventures, reckless driving, or indiscriminate sexual relations, for example.

A woman in the midst of a manic episode is rarely aware of a problem. In fact, she is likely to report feeling "great," and she will probably resist attempts to help her.

More than 90 percent of people who have had one manic episode go on to have another one. Most manic episodes (60 to 70 percent) occur just before or right after a bout of depression. Most people with BPD return to normal between episodes of depression or mania, but some (20 to 30 percent) continue to have mood swings and problems in their business and social interactions. Over time, the period between episodes may grow shorter. The manic and depressive episodes tend to recur in a particular pattern that is characteristic for each person.

Treating Depressive Disorders. In the past, depressive disorders were not well-understood, and there were limited treatment options available. Psychotherapy is the oldest and most consistently successful treatment for depression. The early antidepressant medications were slow to take effect and had numerous side effects that many patients found difficult to tolerate.

Newer antidepressant medications, which seem to work faster and have fewer side effects, are now available. These antidepressant drugs act on specific chemicals in the brain called neurotransmitters. Two types of neurotransmitters that have an important role in depression are norepinephrine and serotonin. Medications that increase norepinephrine and/or serotonin levels have been found to be effective in the treatment of depression. Psychotherapy, with or without antidepressant medication, is also recommended to treat depression and help prevent recurrence.

Antidepressants can cause a number of side effects. In general, the newer medications—called SSRI (selective serotonin reuptake inhibitors)—cause fewer side effects than the tricyclic antidepressants that were previously available. The most common side effects among the newer medications include restlessness, gastrointestinal distress, and occasional dizziness. These side effects usually pass within a few weeks as the body becomes accustomed to the medication. Side effects in sexual function, on the other hand, tend to occur after the medication has been in use for a while. Both men and women may experience decreased sexual desire or difficulty reaching orgasm. This side effect may not be noticed at first, since depression itself often decreases sexual interest. These side effects can often be relieved or lessened by switching to another type of antidepressant medication.

Anxiety Disorders

Everyone knows what it feels like to be anxious: the dry mouth, sweaty palms, and tension in your stomach that precede making a speech, waiting for medical test results, asking your boss for a raise, or taking an important exam. Anxiety is the body's way of preparing you to confront perceived danger. Normal anxiety can be useful. It helps you stay alert when coping with any number of stress-provoking situations. When anxiety becomes excessive, however, it can cause serious mental problems.

Anxiety disorders are more common in women than in men. About 30 percent of women have an anxiety disorder at some time in their lives; for men the rate is about 19 percent.

Anxiety disorders are often successfully treated with some form of psychotherapy or counseling that helps a woman understand the anxiety reaction itself and what causes it to occur. When she cannot function normally because of anxiety symptoms, medication can help control the anxiety and allow her to explore the cause or causes of the anxiety.

Phobias. The word phobia comes from a Greek word meaning fear. As its name indicates, a phobia is marked by extreme or even irrational anxiety. People with phobias usually realize that their fear is excessive, but even thinking about their phobia causes them extreme anxiety.

Specific Phobia. When excessive fear is in response to a particular object or situation, it is termed a specific phobia. Some common specific phobias include a fear of dogs, cats, spiders, snakes, or other animals. Also commonly noted are fears about heights, air travel, or closed-in places, such as elevators and tunnels (called claustrophobia). A person with a phobia will often go to great lengths to avoid the object or situation that causes anxiety. She might, for example, refuse a job offer because it would require frequent air travel or a ride in an elevator each day. The same woman might have no problem riding trains or skiing in high altitudes. It is the irrational nature of the fear that distinguishes this discomfort as a phobia.

If a phobia causes dysfunction, then help is needed. For example, the woman who turns down a much-desired job promotion because it would require air travel has reached a point where her phobia interferes with her life. Professional counseling can help "desensitize" her to her fear so that she can accomplish her goals in life.

Social Phobia. The fear of being in certain types of social settings or performance situations is called social phobia. People who are nervous about speaking in public, or even about asking a question in class, may have a very mild form of social phobia. However, social phobia differs from simple "stage fright" in that social phobia can seriously interfere with a person's ability to function. Someone

Recognizing the Stages of Grief

- **Denial, sometimes described as numbness, is often the initial reaction to learning of a death or other loss. The grieving person may think, "This is not really happening," or may experience a sense of being unable to feel anything. This numbness has a protective element.**

- **Searching and yearning may begin after the initial shock wears off. The grieving person may search for reasons to explain the loss, may lash out in anger at those around her, or blame herself for what has happened.**

- **Depression and loneliness set in after the most intense feelings of grief begin to let up.**

- **Acceptance and resolution eventually allow a woman to come to terms with the loss. Feelings of sorrow, though still a feature of daily life, no longer crowd out everything else. At this time she is ready once again to look toward the future and go on with her life.**

with serious social phobia, for example, may feel extreme anxiety about being humiliated—or even just being looked at—by others in a social situation, which may make it impossible to eat in a restaurant, use a public restroom, speak on the telephone, or sign a check in front of others.

Generalized Anxiety Disorder. About five percent of people in the United States have generalized anxiety disorder (GAD). This disorder is characterized by relentless anxiety and worry that goes on for months or longer. Unlike phobias, GAD appears to have no specific cause and is marked by excessive worry throughout the day.

A woman with GAD may become so impaired that she is unable to make even minor decisions or perform simple tasks, such as driving a car. A woman may find it impossible to be on time for appointments, for example, because of her excessive worry over what to wear. She may be unable to concentrate, to sleep well, or to relax. She may always be expecting a disaster. Like people with phobias, people with GAD may realize that their anxiety is baseless, but they are unable to make it go away.

Panic Disorder. Panic disorder affects about 3.5 percent of people in the United States. The disorder affects twice as many women as men. Panic disorder is marked by repeated episodes of intense fear and anxiety—called panic attacks—that occur without warning and for no apparent reason. These panic attacks are accompanied by physical signs, which may include shortness of breath, a racing or irregular heartbeat, chest pain, sweating, chills or hot flashes, dizziness, and nausea. Often in the midst of a panic attack, a person has an overwhelming sense of impending doom. She may feel as though she is about to die, is losing control, or is going crazy and must escape from whatever situation she happens to be in. Also common is a feeling of unreality and of being detached from oneself and one's surroundings. These panic attacks come without warning and quickly intensify, building to a peak in ten minutes or less. They usually last only a few minutes, although this time seems endless to the person experiencing them. In rare cases, they can last as long as an hour.

Many people with panic disorder become fearful that the attacks indicate some undiscovered health problem, such as heart problems or epilepsy. Medical tests that reveal no physical abnormality are usually not reassurance enough that no problem exists. Some have exaggerated fears about even minor physical symptoms, thinking, for instance, that a single headache may signal a brain tumor.

The frequency of attacks in people with panic disorder varies widely. Some have attacks fairly often, such as once a week. Others may have short bursts of more frequent attacks, followed by weeks or months without any attacks. The attacks can occur over a period of months or years. One particularly insidious characteristic of panic disorder is that fear about the possibility of an attack may become as incapacitating as the attacks themselves.

A person who has repeated panic attacks may develop phobias related to situations in which the attacks have occurred in the past. For example, a person who has had a panic attack in an elevator may develop a specific phobia of elevators and may start avoiding them. More often, a person with panic disorder becomes increasingly fearful about having an attack in public or social situations. She may then begin avoiding public places where it would be difficult or embarrassing to escape in the event of an attack. This fear is referred to as agoraphobia, which literally translates to "fear of the marketplace."

As many as 50 to 65 percent of people with panic disorder also have depression and/or substance abuse problems. It is not uncommon for a person with panic disorder to self-medicate herself with drugs or alcohol, which briefly relieves the uncomfortable symptoms but often creates related problems with substance abuse.

Posttraumatic Stress Disorder. Posttraumatic stress disorder (PTSD) is a syndrome that occurs as a result of severe stress, such as that experienced during military combat, physical or sexual assault, or a natural disaster. At one time this disorder was referred to as shell shock or battle fatigue because it was seen so often in combat veterans. However, it is also extremely common in women who have been the victims of rape or other abuse.

The symptoms of PTSD usually arise within a few months after the traumatic event; in rare instances it may not occur until years later. Symptoms take the form of recurrent memories about the trauma; these memories intrude the person's thoughts and cause her extreme distress. These memories are so vivid that she feels as though she is actually reliving the event. During these relived moments, sometimes called "flashbacks," her pulse and temperature rise. She may enter a "dissociative state," where she becomes completely unaware of her present surroundings and becomes lost in reliving the traumatic experience.

A variety of everyday sights and sounds act as potential triggers that cause flashbacks in a person with PTSD. The case of the combat veteran who falls to the ground at the sound of a car backfiring is just one example. The anniversary of the date on which the trauma occurred, seeing a place or object like those associated with the original trauma, or hearing similar noises can act as triggers for a person to re-experience the traumatic memories.

The extreme nature of PTSD symptoms can keep a person from functioning normally. It is common for someone with PTSD to try to avoid all thoughts, feelings, and conversations about the trauma, as well as the people, places, or activities that remind her of it. A woman who has been raped in a hotel room, for instance, may avoid all hotels as a result. She may feel suspicious of others and be unable to have caring or loving feelings toward anyone. She may also have trouble planning for the future because she feels that her life will be short, that she will not live long enough to achieve personal or professional goals.

Rape, war, torture, and earthquakes are all examples of experiences that can lead to PTSD, although more subtle experiences may also cause the disorder. The primary factor these experiences have in common is that the victim has a profound sense of powerlessness, helplessness, horror, and fear. PTSD can also develop, for example, in a person who has witnessed or even heard reports of traumatic events, such as the violent assault of another person or the news of a loved one's terminal illness. If a person is depressed at the time the traumatic event occurs, the event may be more likely to result in PTSD.

PTSD is often the result of physical and sexual assault by someone close to the victim. This kind of violence and abuse by an intimate partner occurs ten times more often in women at the hands of men than vice versa. Not surprisingly, *wellness* **warning**

If you have been the victim of sexual assault or abuse, you are at risk for PTSD. It is important to get counseling early on, in order to keep this event from causing long standing emotional difficulties. Many women feel—irrationally— that they are to blame for being assaulted or abused. Remember that the assault is not your fault. You deserve help in dealing with the things that have happened to you.

PTSD also affects women more often than men—about one-third more women than men develop the disorder after any type of traumatic event. This is true even though many more men experience active military combat. The higher rate of PTSD among women, mostly as a result of physical and sexual abuse, is testimony to the devastating effects of this type of violence on women. PTSD is also common in people who were molested or assaulted as children. It occurs in about one-third of victims of child molestation and two-thirds of child rape victims.

People with PTSD usually feel shame, despair, and hopelessness. They may feel that they have been permanently damaged, even when this is not the case in a physical sense. During episodes of PTSD, victims may have difficulty sleeping, may startle easily, and usually feel agitated, anxious, and "on guard" much or most of the time. In about half of cases of PTSD, the symptoms resolve within a few months after they began. In other cases the symptoms may persist for more than a year.

Obsessive-Compulsive Disorder. Often when we describe someone as being "obsessed" or "compulsive," we mean that she spends a lot of time thinking about one aspect of her life or that she is rigid about doing tasks in a certain way. With obsessive-compulsive disorder (OCD), these common terms take on a slightly different meaning. OCD can be a debilitating disorder that prevents a woman from being able to function normally. It affects women and men at about the same rate.

A woman who has an obsessive personality has persistent, unwelcome thoughts, ideas, and images that occupy her for much of every day. These obsessions are felt to be intrusive and not within the woman's control, and they cause her great discomfort and distress. An example is the woman who cannot stop thinking about germs in her home, who continually cleans surfaces that are already clean, and who still fears contamination. Another example is the woman who leaves home, only to return time and again to check on the stove or to relock the door. Still other forms of obsession include the need to have objects always in a particular order or arrangement and the constant fear of harming others or of doing something highly inappropriate (such as shouting obscenities in public).

A person with OCD often knows that the intrusive thoughts and images are inappropriate, but she cannot stop them. In response to the obsessions, she engages in ritual-like behaviors—called compulsions—in an attempt to ease her anxiety. She may be unable to concentrate at work because she must wash her hands dozens of times after touching a doorknob or shaking hands. She may be unable to sleep because she must repeatedly get up to check that she has locked the door. Or it may take her hours to leave the house because she is compelled to go back inside over and over to be sure she has turned off the lights. All of these actions could be considered normal in moderation—nearly everyone has, at one time or another, checked that the door is locked or worried about keeping one's hands clean during the cold and flu season. What sets compulsive behaviors apart is that they impair normal functioning and are coupled with extreme anxiety.

Other types of compulsions take the form of activities that have no real connection to the obsessive thoughts. A person with OCD may count to a number over and over or repeat words silently to herself; she may incessantly perform hand or finger movements; or she may repeatedly arrange and rearrange objects in a certain order. Such actions do not give her pleasure—they are an unconscious attempt to suppress or ignore her obsessions. In extreme cases, such repetitive actions leave no time in a woman's life for anything else.

Most people with OCD have obsessions and compulsions that come and go, getting better and worse over time. Stress can trigger symptoms. In some people, symptoms may gradually worsen with age; in others, symptoms occur only in short bouts, with few or no problems in between.

Treating Anxiety Disorders. Treatment of an anxiety disorder takes into account the type of anxiety, the degree to which it interferes with functioning, and the factors that are contributing to the problem.

In most cases, a woman with anxiety disorder needs therapy to help her find ways to overcome her anxiety. Sometimes, however, these symptoms are so severe that she cannot approach her problems effectively in therapy without medication to ease her symptoms. In these cases, an antianxiety drug, also called "anxiolytic," may be prescribed. Some of these drugs pose the risk of physical dependence or psychological addiction. Physical dependence will occur in just a few weeks of use, but such addiction simply requires that the medication be tapered off gradually, rather than stopped all at once.

Psychological addiction, on the other hand, is more serious and difficult to overcome. In general, the antianxiety drugs in the benzodiazapine class with the shortest "half-life," such as Xanax and Valium, are the more potentially addictive. Long-term use of these medications is best managed by scheduled doses (two to three times daily) and should be monitored by a physician. Drugs that are used to treat depression are also quite useful in treating anxiety disorders.

As is true of most psychiatric disorders, medication to treat anxiety disorders works best in conjunction with some type of psychotherapy. This may consist of behavioral therapy, in which the therapist works with the patient to develop strategies to head off a panic attack or helps the patient learn relaxation techniques. For phobias, an approach sometimes called desensitization can be effective. In this treatment, the therapist helps the patient create mental images of the object or situation that causes anxiety. As she holds this image in her mind, the patient's anxiety eventually passes and she feels more relaxed. Over time, anxiety-provoking images are used increasingly, until the patient begins to "retrain" her response and learns that she can overcome her anxiety. She can then begin to apply this technique to real objects and situations, gradually increasing her exposure to them until she can more easily bring her anxiety under control.

Other Mental Disorders

Other types of mental disorders are less common than the ones just described, although they can be more debilitating. Among these are personality disorders and schizophrenia. Some of these disorders are more common among women, whereas others are found more often among men.

Personality Disorders

A person's personality can be described as a set of traits and behaviors that is partly shaped by her life experiences and is partly present from birth. Personality

wellness **tip**

Taking care of yourself—physically and emotionally—is the first line of defense against stress. Taking the time and space you need to care for your body, mind, and spirit is the most important thing you can do for your overall well-being.

disorders share a common pattern—thought patterns, feelings, and behavior cause significant problems in a woman's interactions with others.

A woman with personality disorder sees and responds to the world in a rigid and unchanging manner, regardless of the circumstances she finds herself in. Personality disorders usually surface in adolescence or early adulthood. Intensive psychotherapy, sometimes combined with medication, is necessary to successfully treat these disorders.

Most people with personality disorders do not possess all of the traits of a particular disorder. It is common, in fact, to see traits of more than one personality disorder. The descriptions that follow present examples of more severe cases. In reality, the lines between these disorders are somewhat blurred, and symptoms vary from person to person.

Borderline Personality Disorder. Among people being treated for any type of personality disorder, about 30 to 60 percent have been diagnosed with borderline personality disorder. This disorder is far more common in women than in men: an estimated three-fourths of diagnoses of are made in women.

People with this disorder have an intense fear of being abandoned. They are highly sensitive to changes in their external circumstances, even when these changes are minor or have been planned. For example, they may become furious with someone who is just a few minutes late, or express despair when someone must leave at an agreed-upon time. Their views of people and situations tend to be black and white—all one way or completely the opposite. For example, they may idolize someone until they perceive that person has let them down in some way, and then reject them permanently.

In extreme cases of borderline personality disorder, a woman may engage in self-mutilation or suicidal behavior. About eight to ten percent of people with this disorder succeed in killing themselves. They may also engage in reckless behavior that is likely to bring them harm, such as excessive gambling, binge eating, or sexual promiscuity.

Dependent Personality Disorder. People with this disorder have an excessive need to be taken care of and a marked lack of confidence in their own abilities. They tend to allow others to take over major areas in their lives and make decisions for them. They also have an overwhelming fear of being separated from or abandoned by people who are important to them. This fear can lead them to volunteer for undesirable tasks in order to ensure someone's support in return.

People with dependent personality disorder often "cling" to family members and close friends. They may find it difficult to express disagreement with important people in their lives for fear of disapproval. And when a relationship ends, they may feel incapable and alone, which leads them to enter into a new relationship with the first person they can find.

Histrionic Personality Disorder. More prevalent among women than men, this disorder is characterized by an intense need for attention and approval. People with this disorder feel uncomfortable when they are not the center of attention. Overly concerned with their physical appearance, they often dress flamboyantly, seductively, or provocatively to gain attention. Their desire to be accepted also makes them highly impressionable and very sensitive to criticism and disapproval.

People with histrionic personality disorder are also excessively emotional. They may overreact to everyday situations in ways that often come across as shallow or theatrical to others. They are also prone to rapid changes of emotions. People with this disorder are often very manipulative, using their emotional displays to get what they want.

Avoidant Personality Disorder. Avoidant personality disorder is characterized by social inhibition, feelings of inadequacy, and sensitivity to negative evaluation. People with this disorder often avoid social events for fear of criticism, disapproval, or rejection. They also avoid occupations that involve significant contact with people. Yet, despite their fear of social settings, people with this disorder usually crave social relationships. In fact, when they do enter into a relationship, they exhibit "clingy" behavior common to people with dependent personality disorder.

People with avoidant personality disorder may feel inadequate and undesirable to others. Although they have a desperate need to be accepted, their low self-esteem typically prevents them from interacting with others unless they are absolutely certain they will be accepted. This negative self-image also causes them to fear embarrassment or criticism. As a result, people with this disorder may not trust others and are extremely paranoid, thinking that others are always watching and judging them.

Paranoid Personality Disorder. Paranoid personality disorder (PPD) is marked by extreme distrust and suspicion of others. A woman with this disorder may be convinced that others are "out to get her," although there is no real evidence that this is the case. Some people with PPD become convinced that they are constantly being followed or spied upon.

A woman with PPD is likely to interpret another's remarks and actions as a criticism of herself. She may scrutinize every aspect of others' behavior for evidence that they are plotting against her. If she perceives the slightest sign of another person's disloyalty, she takes this as evidence that her suspicions are correct. She is likely to be quick to react with anger and hostility to what she perceives to be others' slights and insults.

Antisocial Personality Disorder. The chief characteristic of antisocial personality disorder (APD) is a person's blatant disregard for the rights, feelings, and welfare of other people. Although such traits may be present in children, APD is not diagnosed as such in people under the age of 18.

People with APD are highly aggressive and often have a criminal history. They tend to disregard the consequences of their actions, not only for others, but for themselves as well. They rarely are able to hold a job or to function well in society because they are highly irresponsible.

Although APD is far more common in men than in women, it is thought that the diagnosis may be sometimes missed or overlooked in women because women with this disorder tend to be less aggressive than men. The symptoms of APD tend to become less pronounced with age.

Narcissistic Personality Disorder. In Greek mythology, the beautiful, young Narcissus fell in love with his own reflection in a pool of water and became oblivious to everyone and everything around him. Narcissistic personality disorder takes its name from this story. As the name implies, the chief feature of narcissistic personality disorder is a belief in one's own uniqueness and a complete lack of recognition for the needs of others. About 50 to 75 percent of cases of this disorder are found in men.

People with this disorder quite literally think of themselves as the center of the universe. They greatly exaggerate their own worth and accomplishments while belittling and begrudging those of other people. They expect to receive special treatment in most situations because they believe themselves special or unique. But despite their appearance to others as haughty, arrogant, and mean-spirited, their self-esteem is actually extremely fragile. They demand constant attention and praise from others and become puzzled or angry when they do not receive it. Consequently, they are likely to feel humiliated and empty when they are criticized.

Schizophrenia

Although schizophrenia is sometimes referred to as "split personality," it actually has nothing to do with the presence of two or more personalities in the same person, which describes a feature of dissociative identity disorder, once known as multiple personality disorder. Schizophrenia is, instead, a form of psychosis that occurs when a person loses contact with reality.

About 75 percent of people with schizophrenia have delusions—false beliefs that persist despite any logical argument that they are wrong. A common delusion in schizophrenia is the belief that one's thoughts are being controlled by an outside force. About 90 percent of schizophrenics also have hallucinations—sensory perceptions (seeing, hearing, feeling, tasting, or smelling) that do not exist in reality. A schizophrenic person may, for example, "hear" voices telling her that she is a bad person or to harm herself. She is unable to tell the difference between what is real and what is the product of these delusions and hallucinations.

As a result of her lack of contact with reality, the schizophrenic often has trouble speaking in a way that can be understood. She may respond to questions with statements that appear to make no sense or to be unrelated to what was asked. In more severe cases, she may repeat the words and phrases of others or speak in an incoherent jumble of words rather than in sentences. She may also become suicidal or, in some cases, violent toward others.

Until antipsychotic drugs began to be developed in the 1950s, the outlook for people with this disorder was poor. Today, people with schizophrenia have a much better chance for leading a more normal life. Still, hospitalization and drug therapy are often required to stabilize victims and to treat recurrent episodes.

Staying Mentally *Healthy*

One key to mental wellness is heading off problems before they occur. Another is knowing how to handle problems constructively when they do occur. Since no one is immune to problems such as depression and anxiety, women who anticipate events in their lives that might trigger these disorders, and those who plan strategies for handling the accompanying stress, are more likely to avert serious problems.

In planning for a mentally healthy life, however, it is always important to keep in mind that life events can prove overwhelming even for the best prepared women, and bouts of depression and anxiety do not indicate personal failure. The strategies for a healthy future include recognizing the point when coping strategies no longer work, meaning it is time to seek help.

Taking Care of Yourself: Body and Mind

Any event in a woman's life that forces her to adjust to new circumstances can be a significant source of stress. The death of a spouse or family member, divorce, personal injury or loss, and getting fired from a job are all devastating examples that cause anxiety and stress. But stress also occurs when you plan a wedding, begin a new job, move, or learn you are pregnant.

Different women perceive these events differently. One woman, for example, may feel blissfully happy upon learning that she is pregnant, whereas another may be filled with anxiety and doubt. Either way, pregnancy marks a significant lifestyle change for all women, and stress is inevitable.

Physical Health. Coping with life's challenges and hardships is hard enough without the added burden of fatigue or illness. No one can be at her best mentally if she neglects herself physically. Doctors and researchers now recognize that physical and mental health are closely connected. Physical stress, caused by fatigue, illness, or injury, also causes some degree of mental and emotional stress. It is much more difficult to think clearly or to come up with solutions to problems when the body is tired, sick, or hurt. A body that is not completely healthy in more subtle ways, because of poor nutrition or lack of exercise or rest, is also at risk for mental distress.

Taking care of your body includes paying attention to signals about your energy level: do not wear yourself out trying to be all things to all people. "Listen" to your body's need for food, rest, and exercise and learn to recognize the signs of eating disorders, discussed in Chapter 8. Also, learn to recognize the warning signs of illness, such as an oncoming cold, so you can allow more time for resting and healing. If you have a chronic or long-standing illness, you are at greater risk for depression. Consultation with a mental health professional can help you find coping strategies or determine if antidepressant medication is right for you.

Personal Boundaries. The expanded roles of women today have helped them enjoy increased freedom, power, and self-determination. An unfortunate side effect, however, has been that women are often simply expected to do more. In addition to maintaining their traditional roles as mothers and homemakers, many women today fill the multiple roles of employee, spouse, and mother. Between caring for children, working full-time or part-time, and doing household chores, it is not surprising that women often feel overburdened.

Many women find it hard to say no when asked to do something. However, maintaining mental balance sometimes means knowing how to politely but firmly say no to additional duties. Drawing personal boundaries for yourself in this

wellness **tip**

Forgiveness is good for your health. Studies conducted at the National Institute of Healthcare Research, in Rockville, Md., show that the act of forgiving someone can lower your risk of depression and anxiety. It also lowers your hostility level, a major risk factor for cardiovascular disease.

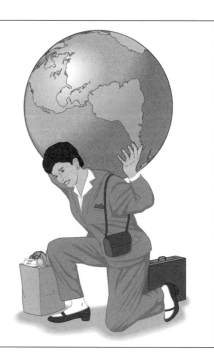

Plan ahead. Work, family, and social schedules are all responsible for unwanted stress. Planning now will help alleviate stress in the future.

Talk things out with a friend, family member, or another person. People who are not directly involved often have meaningful insights into your problems that you might have overlooked.

Spend more time laughing. Laughter has been proven to relieve stress. Surround yourself with friends who laugh and who make you laugh.

Redirect extra energy caused by stress. Since your body reacts to stress by creating adrenaline, put that extra energy to something worthwhile.

Take time to relax. If you cannot actually go somewhere quiet and peaceful, try to imagine that you are there. Or simply try to clear your mind of all troubling thoughts.

FIGURE 12.1

Managing Stress

Stress is an increasing health risk among women today, whose multiple roles may include spouse, mother, homemaker, and breadwinner. Here are some useful tips to help you manage stress.

way is not the same as refusing to be supportive and caring. Rather, it is a way to preserve your own mental and physical energy so that you are able to complete the tasks you undertake to your satisfaction.

Taking Time for Yourself. Do you ever feel you are most valued when you devote yourself to others? You are not alone. Many women find themselves doing things for others for much of the day, and, while they may feel they are valued by others, they sometimes feel that what is valuable to them is not getting done. Women care for others best when they first care for themselves.

Take time to recharge your energies on a regular basis. Whether you read a book, meditate, take a walk, or soak in a hot bath, do something that feels good to you. Often it is best to be alone during part of your day or week. Being in solitude does not mean being lonely. Rather, private time can renew your energy and refresh your perspective. Find some time each day to do something just for yourself, even if only for a few minutes. The difference in your mental outlook may surprise you.

Getting Help When You Need It

When you are in emotional pain and nothing seems to make you feel better, when life seems too much to handle, when troubles increase at home or at work, or when it just seems too difficult to get through the day—it is time to seek help. Contrary to many traditional beliefs, getting help for mental or emotional problems—whether that help comes from support groups, psychotherapy, or medication prescribed by a doctor—is not a sign of weakness, but of strength. It means that you know yourself well enough to understand when you need to take care of yourself. It means that you are wise enough to use whatever resources are available to improve and maintain your well-being and happiness.

Mental disorders can be treated with some form of psychotherapy, with medication, or with both. Psychotherapy involves forming a relationship with a trained professional who can help you sort through your feelings, thoughts, and experiences. Medication for mental disorders alters the biochemistry of the brain to relieve symptoms of, for example, anxiety and depression.

Psychotherapy. Psychotherapy can take place through individual, couples, or group therapy. Individual therapy allows you to meet one-on-one with a therapist and to speak in complete confidence. Couples therapy focuses on the dynamics in a relationship between two partners and on ways to improve communication. Group therapy is led by a psychotherapist who helps members of the group share their experiences with others while exploring their own issues.

Whatever its mode or setting, therapy is designed to help you examine your feelings, experiences, and attitudes, and how you interact with the world. Through this intensive "sifting" process, you can examine the areas of your life that cause you distress and find ways to effect change.

What Happens in Therapy? The relationship that a woman forms with her therapist is unlike any other in her life. In no other relationship—with a friend, a

Types of Psychotherapy

- **Psychoanalysis** was once commonly used when the patient's problems appeared to be related mostly to past experiences. Psychoanalysis is a lengthy process; often patients are seen four hours per week for three to five years. During therapy, the patient is asked to lie on a couch with the analyst sitting outside her field of view. The patient uses a technique of "free association," wherein she says everything that comes to mind without censoring any material that she believes to be unacceptable, unimportant, or embarrassing.

- **Psychoanalytic psychotherapy** is more commonly used today than classic psychoanalysis. This therapy is characterized by interview and discussion between the patient and therapist, and focuses primarily on current issues. There are two main types of psychoanalytic psychotherapy: insight-oriented psychotherapy and supportive psychotherapy. Insight-oriented psychotherapy helps a patient gain new insight into her feelings, responses, and behavior, especially as they relate to interacting with other people. Supportive psychotherapy provides assistance during a period of illness or overwhelming crisis. It uses techniques that help the patient feel more secure, accepted, and safe, and less anxious.

- **Dynamic psychotherapy and crisis intervention therapy** are two psychotherapy techniques that have recently gained popularity. These techniques attempt to repair traumatic events from the past and help the patient believe that

new ways of thinking, feeling, and behaving are possible. The therapeutic experience is brief (20 to 30 sessions) and very focused. Crisis intervention therapy may be even shorter with sessions scheduled over a three to four month period. Crisis work is designed to assist patients during a period of turmoil. It not only helps people through a current crisis but also makes them better equipped to avoid future crises.

- **Behavioral therapy** (also called behavior modification) attempts to change patterns of behavior that have been causing distress. Techniques may include assertiveness training, aversion therapy, or desensitization. Assertiveness training attempts to improve interpersonal relationships by focusing on direct and honest communication with others. Aversion therapy uses unpleasant stimuli to deter undesirable behaviors; it has commonly been used to treat alcohol, drug, or nicotine addiction. Systematic desensitization is used to treat specific phobias. Behavioral therapy is often combined with cognitive therapy in a process called cognitive-behavioral therapy.

- **Cognitive therapy** focuses on changing a person's attitudes, perceptions, and patterns of negative or destructive thinking (such as "I'm worthless") in order to treat mental and emotional disorders. It often incorporates behavioral therapy, and is then termed cognitive-behavioral therapy.

lover, or a parent—is the focus so intensely and constantly on you. This one-sidedness is necessary in order for you to identify your problems and goals.

Therapy is hard work. It can even be scary, especially when exploring uncharted emotional territory, such as past traumas or unresolved issues. It can be unsettling to consider the prospect of changing the way you approach life and interact with the world, even if you know that some of the approaches you now use are counterproductive for you. The discomfort you may experience, though, is usually a sign of progress. Like exercising unused muscles, changing your mental outlook may cause short-term pain, but it usually results in long-term gain.

Finding the Right Therapist. The most productive relationship between client and therapist is based on trust and understanding. Finding a therapist who is well matched to your needs, goals, attitudes, and beliefs may take some time. The process is much like finding a doctor who suits you. It is not unusual for a person beginning therapy to have one or two sessions with two or three therapists before finding one who is a good match. The time spent in finding the right professional is a valuable investment in your happiness and well-being.

Mental health professionals come from a variety of academic and clinical backgrounds. Whatever her background, a good therapist is able to act like a mirror, reflecting you back to you. By asking questions, she can help you probe more deeply the sources of your unhappiness and pain. You may need to look closely at how you felt as a child growing up. You may need to focus on an important event in your adult life. You may be trying to move on with your life after divorce or the death of someone you love. You may want to understand

Therapists and Therapies

When it comes to psychotherapeutic approaches, there are so many schools of thought and so many styles of individual therapists that it is impossible to describe them all here. If you are searching for a therapist, however, it helps to know the background and qualifications of the mental health professionals who are available. Following is a description of some common professions and the types of therapy they may practice.

Types of Professional Therapists

- **Psychiatrists** are medical doctors (M.D.) who have training and experience in diagnosing, treating, and preventing mental disorders. As physicians, they can offer psychotherapy as well as prescribe medication for psychiatric conditions.
- **Clinical psychologists** have a doctoral degree (Ph.D.) in clinical psychology and provide testing and counseling services for people with mental and emotional disorders. Many clinical psychologists have private practices and provide psychotherapy in a variety of forms. They cannot prescribe medications, though they can refer you to a psychiatrist if medication is needed.

- **Psychiatric social workers** have a degree in social work and may work in hospitals, clinics, or private practices, providing care and support to the mentally ill. A licensed certified social worker (L.C.S.W.) may also have a master's degree in social work (M.S.W.) and provide psychotherapy in a private practice.
- **Psychiatric nurse practitioners** have an advanced nursing degree (often a master's degree, M.S.N.) in caring for mental disorders. They may work in general hospitals, mental hospitals, public clinics, or in their own private practices.
- **Psychiatric** (or mental health) **nurses** work in many settings, including hospitals, clinics, and private practices. Their responsibilities, training, and expertise vary widely. They conduct psychotherapy; provide care for the physical aspects of patients' problems, including drug reactions; and assume responsibilities for patients in various recreational, occupational, and social situations.

why you cannot get along with people at your workplace or why you keep falling in love with the wrong type of person. You may want to improve your ability to handle stressful situations. Whatever your goals, a good therapist can be an important ally in helping you find the best way to achieve them.

Treating Mental Disorders with Medication. Anxiety and depressive disorders are usually treatable with medication. Medical treatment for schizophrenia and other psychoses can also be effective. Only a medical doctor (M.D.) can prescribe these medications. If a therapist does not have an M.D. degree, she can refer a client to a psychiatrist who can evaluate the client's condition and assess the need for medication. The client will need to meet periodically with the psychiatrist to check on how well the drug is working, whether the dose needs to be increased or decreased, and so on.

Someone who is taking an antidepressant or antianxiety drug must keep her appointments with the doctor who prescribed it. It may be necessary to increase or decrease the dosage over time. Decisions about how long medication should be used is also an important consideration. Even after medication has been discontinued, follow-up visits with the psychiatrist may be important if you are under extra stress or going through particularly difficult life changes.

How to Find Help. An abundance of services exist to help people with mental health problems. Whether you are seeking care for yourself or a loved one, a good first step is to ask your primary health care provider for referrals to one or two local therapists. You can also check the Yellow Pages for the telephone numbers of community mental health centers, mental health associations, consumer groups, and mutual help groups. Listings to check in your Yellow Pages include "Health," "Hospitals," "Mental Health," "Physicians" (these are often listed in a separate section by specialty—look under "Psychiatry" or "Psychotherapy"), "Social Services," and specific sections, such as "Suicide Prevention" or "Substance Abuse."

State or local chapters of professional associations, such as state psychiatric and psychologists' associations, can help you find professional therapists in your community. Other possible sources of help include:

- Family service agencies.
- State and local departments of social services.
- City or county health departments.
- County medical associations.
- Community mental health centers.
- Private and public medical hospitals and state mental hospitals.

In a crisis situation, mental health or crisis hot lines may be available. These are staffed around the clock with people who are trained and ready to listen and offer help. Look in the Yellow Pages for suicide prevention centers or other mental health hot lines. In cases where violence is involved or you fear you may hurt or be hurt by someone, call the National Domestic Violence Hotline at 800-799-SAFE. (See Chapter 14 for more information on domestic violence.)

wellness
warning

Medications to treat psychological problems must be used carefully and strictly according to the doctor's instructions. Do not adjust the dosage or stop taking these medications without first consulting the doctor who prescribed them.

Self-Help and Support Groups

Self-help and support groups differ from group therapy in that they are usually led by someone who shares the problem with the group, instead of by a trained mental health professional. Such groups may focus on specific issues that the members have in common, such as alcohol or drug abuse, the loss of a child or spouse, or a serious illness. These groups can be extremely helpful at providing a setting in which you can share your experiences and concerns with others, learn that you are not alone, and receive emotional support.

Other groups may have a more general focus. Whatever your main area of concern, there is likely a group that addresses it. There are groups that focus on women's issues, groups for people with AIDS, groups for parents of gay children, groups for women with breast cancer, and groups for people planning retirement, just to name a few. Times and places for self-help and support groups can be found in your local paper's community calendar.

Remember, the first therapist you see or group you join may not end up working out for you. Different therapists have different styles of conducting sessions, and you may need to "test the waters" once or twice to find one with whom you can feel comfortable. Do not give up. Once you find the right form of therapy, stick with it. There is no need to live with anxiety, despair, or any other type of emotional pain when there are so many avenues for getting help.

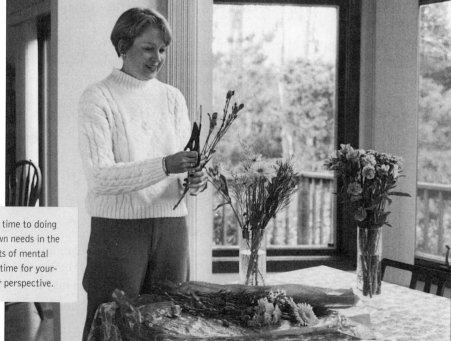

Many women devote the majority of their time to doing things for others, often neglecting their own needs in the process. One of the most important aspects of mental and emotional wellness is making private time for yourself to renew your energy and refresh your perspective.

What *You* Can Do

As with all wellness issues, your mental health is sometimes at the mercy of forces outside yourself; there is always potential for the stresses of life to overwhelm you. At the same time, as with other aspects of wellness, you can take steps to ensure a sense of calm and well-being even in the face of life's crises:

- Recognize that stress is a natural part of life. The goal is not to avoid stressful situations, but to learn to accept them and work through them with a minimum of mental distress.
- Practice meditation and relaxation techniques. Many resources are available—books, audio and video tapes, and classes in meditation—that can help you find the power to remain calm in the face of life's inevitable stresses.
- Exercise, eat well, and get plenty of rest. An inability to "handle" a stressful situation can often be traced to fatigue.
- Assess your mental wellness. You may be the victim of a serious mental disorder. Most serious disorders require medical help to resolve them. If you think you are at risk for anxiety disorder, depressive disorder, or personality disorder, seek the advice of a physician in locating an appropriate therapist.
- Remain open to the possibility of change through mental health counseling. Women are sometimes tempted to believe that their problems are common to everyone and therefore don't warrant the expense and time therapy may require. But mild depression can be treated fairly quickly, and such treatment can mean the difference between mental wellness and a lifetime of distress.

Controlling the Use of Harmful Substances

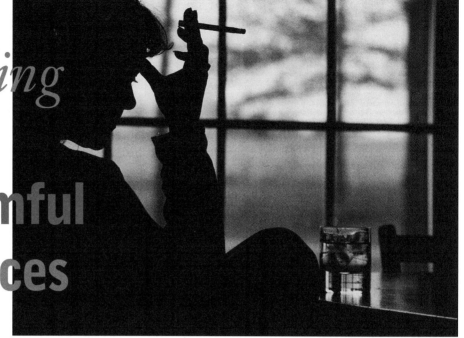

Each year, millions of women in the United States use substances that alter their mood, mental state, or behavior. Nearly half of all women between the ages of 15 and 44 have tried drugs at least once in their lives. Most commonly these "first try" substances are alcohol and tobacco (cigarettes). However, some women use heroin, cocaine, and marijuana first. Other substances, including prescription and nonprescription medicines, are widely used by women and can be harmful if used improperly. In fact, studies estimate that over 4 million women need treatment for drug abuse. From a wellness standpoint, substance abuse may constitute the most promising area of preventable illness and death. Because deaths from all forms of substance abuse (alcohol, cigarettes, and drugs) number half a million a year, it is important that everyone learn to recognize and address the early signs of substance abuse.

Look at the staggering health effects of substance abuse. Used in excess, alcohol causes liver disease and death. Cigarette smoke contains more than 40 chemicals known to cause cancer and heart disease. Injectable "street" drugs, such as heroin, are extremely addictive. Shared needles pose other serious health consequences, including contracting the hepatitis B virus and HIV, the virus that causes AIDS. Drugs such as amphetamines, or speed, can cause a sudden heart attack, even when used only once. Misuse of prescribed medications, such as sleeping pills, tranquilizers, and painkillers, often leads to dependence and addiction. Overdoses can be fatal. The treatment of health problems related to substance abuse costs billions of dollars each year.

In addition to physical problems, substance abuse also has serious consequences for a woman's work and home life, for her relationships with family and friends, and for her children. Substance abuse can also lead to psychological problems, including depression and low self-esteem.

Many women simply do not realize how quickly and easily substance use and abuse can affect their physical, mental, and social health. Although the use of alcohol and tobacco is legal for anyone over the age of 21, these substances can and often do lead to addiction. As well, many drugs, especially alcohol, affect women differently than men, and women have the additional concern of the effect of these substances on the fetus during pregnancy. All women need to familiarize themselves with how these substances work in the body in order to ensure their own wellness and to help identify the early signs of abuse in themselves, their children, or others close to them.

Women *and* Substance **Use**

Although the rate of substance use is generally lower for women than for men, it has been rising since 1992. In 1994 more than one-quarter of the U.S. population had at least one major problem related to alcohol use. Almost as many people reported problems with cigarette use.

Defining Use Versus Abuse

How much use equals abuse? For each woman, the level of substance use that constitutes abuse varies. Substance use can be defined as any consumption of alcohol, tobacco, or other drugs. Having a beer at a baseball game or taking a sleeping pill occasionally can both be thought of as substance use.

Substance use becomes abuse when it creates problems in a woman's life, whether these problems are related to her physical or mental health or her relationships with others. Relying on alcohol to get you through the day or taking more than your prescribed number of sleeping pills every night are examples of substance abuse. Experts describe alcohol use and abuse in women in this way: moderate drinking means no more than one drink a day (a beer, a cocktail, or a glass of wine); heavy drinking, or alcohol abuse, has been defined both as consuming more than two drinks a day (more than 60 drinks a month) or as having five or more drinks on one occasion five or more times within the past month.

With time, substance abuse can lead to dependence or addiction. How does this happen? When used very often over a long period, many drugs—including alcohol, sleeping pills, marijuana, and cocaine—are needed in greater and greater amounts in order to produce the same result. A woman who has one drink every day, for example, will eventually find that one drink no longer produces the same effect it once did. Eventually she will find that, whereas she once felt tipsy after two drinks, she now has to have three or four in order to feel the same level of inebriation. This phenomenon is called increasing your tolerance. Increased tolerance is a "red flag" signalling physical dependence. With continued drinking, many women who become dependent will become addicted.

Although there is no agreement on exactly what level of substance abuse constitutes addiction, most experts agree that it is characterized by four key factors:

wellness
warning

The life expectancy of a woman who abuses alcohol is 15 years shorter than a woman who does not have a drinking problem. She is more likely to die from alcohol-related accidents or crime, or organ damage.

- **Craving and compulsion.** A woman who is addicted usually has a strong—even overwhelming—desire and craving for the substance. She spends a great deal of time thinking about the next time she will use the substance or about how she will obtain more of it.
- **Loss of control.** An addicted person usually has lost control over her substance use. She uses more of the substance more often than she intends. She may also behave in unaccustomed ways while she is using the substance. She may become angry or violent or shirk responsibilities at home or at work, for example.
- **Continued use despite adverse consequences.** Addiction to alcohol or other drugs is typified by a person's continuing to use the substance despite obvious problems with health and her relationships. An addicted person may continue to drink or use drugs even if doing so has caused the loss of money and employment, the breakup of her marriage, problems with her children, or the development of physical problems or serious illness.
- **Distorted thinking.** Despite the hold that addiction has over a woman, she usually continues to think she can control her use. She denies—both to herself and to others—that she has a problem, that the problem is serious, or that she needs help. Even in the face of obvious difficulties in her personal and social life, she may deny that these problems have anything to do with her substance use. She may actually tell herself the opposite—that she drinks or uses drugs because of these problems.

Risk Factors for Substance Abuse

There is no sure way to tell who will and who will not develop a substance abuse problem. The events and circumstances that lead a person to abuse alcohol or other drugs are complex and interrelated. However, experts on substance abuse prevention and treatment have been able to identify a number of factors that seem to make it more likely that a woman will engage in substance abuse.

It is important to understand that none of the following factors "causes" substance abuse by itself. Nor does the presence of these risk factors predict that a woman will abuse drugs. They merely increase the chances that this will happen.

Stress. As is true of so many mental and physical problems, stress plays a key role in the development of substance abuse. In particular, women who have experienced trauma, such as rape, sexual assault, physical abuse, financial difficulty, the loss of a loved one through death or divorce, or job loss, are at higher risk for developing substance abuse problems.

Family History and Environment. In general, women who have a parent, spouse, or sibling with a drug or alcohol problem are more likely to develop such a problem themselves, especially in the case of alcohol abuse. The children of an alcoholic parent seem to be more likely to have a drinking problem themselves by the

Tracking Drug Use

Using any type of drug, including tobacco and alcohol—whether it is prescribed for you by a doctor, bought over-the-counter (nonprescription), or consumed socially and legally—should be a matter you consider carefully. Many women are surprised when they take stock of their substance use. To track your own use, make a list of all the drugs you have used in the past month, including how much and how often you used each one, especially during times of stress. At your next doctor's visit, review the list with your doctor and talk about any concerns you may have. Staying aware of the drugs you use is a good way to keep from developing a drug problem.

time they reach adulthood. It is thought that there may be a genetic factor that predisposes people to alcoholism. Also, many women who abuse drugs have been raised in abusive environments. Studies indicate that 70 percent of women who report using hard drugs were abused sexually before the age of 16.

Mental Illness. When substance abuse and mental illness are both present in the same individual, that person is said to have a "dual diagnosis." This is not to say, however, that one of these problems causes the other. A woman who abuses cocaine, for example, may also have a mental illness, but it would be inaccurate to say that mental illness is the cause of the abuse. The relationship between addiction and mental illness is complex and is the subject of much ongoing research. It is known, however, that some mental problems, in particular depression and anxiety, which are more common in women than in men, increase a woman's risk of turning to alcohol or drug use in order to ease the symptoms of these disorders.

Low Socioeconomic Status. Low income and poor education are important social risk factors in the development of substance abuse. Again, while this does not mean that being paid minimum wage or being unemployed will cause a woman to abuse alcohol or other drugs, it is true that more people in lower than in higher income groups have substance abuse problems.

Alcohol *Use*

Alcohol is by far the most widely used "psychoactive" substance (affecting a person's feelings and thought processes) in the United States. In 1995, more than 110 million people—more than half the population aged 12 and older—reported having used alcohol within the past month. Used in moderation, alcohol is not necessarily harmful to your health. Many people consume alcohol in moderation without harmful effects. But for many others, drinking has serious, adverse consequences for themselves and their families.

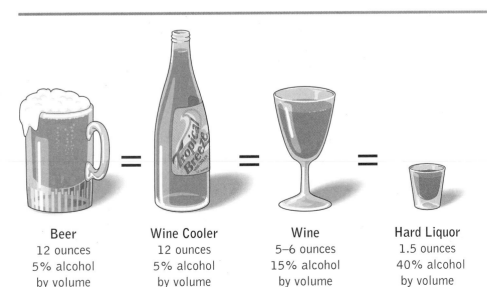

Beer
12 ounces
5% alcohol
by volume

Wine Cooler
12 ounces
5% alcohol
by volume

Wine
5–6 ounces
15% alcohol
by volume

Hard Liquor
1.5 ounces
40% alcohol
by volume

FIGURE 13.1
Alcohol Content
Make sure you know the alcohol content of what you drink—the alcohol in a small cocktail is as potent as a bottle of beer.

Women's Use of Alcohol

Although women tend to drink less than men do, the rate of heavy drinking among women has been rising since the late 1980s. According to the American Psychiatric Association, about 4.5 million women in the United States abuse or are dependent on alcohol today. In fact, women make up about one-third of all alcoholics. Of particular concern is that the rate of drinking is highest among women between the ages of 18 and 34, the prime childbearing years. Furthermore, although drinking is illegal under the age of 21, in a recent survey nearly 30 percent of women under 21 reported having used alcohol in the past month.

Recognizing Alcohol Abuse in Women

There is no clear portrait of the alcoholic woman. In fact, alcoholism in women may be difficult to detect, even by doctors. Many women who drink may function perfectly normally throughout the day, in public, and at work, but then come home and literally drink themselves to sleep. Other women may drink moderately in social situations, but excessively in secret, stashing bottles of vodka (which is undetectable on the breath) in their purses or dresser drawers. Some general factors that put women at risk for alcohol abuse are depression, low self-esteem, being unmarried or unemployed, or having experienced sexual or psychological abuse.

If you are unsure whether you or a friend has a drinking problem, it may be helpful to answer the following questions, issued by the National Council on Alcoholism and Drug Dependence:

- Do you drink when you feel depressed, hoping that it will make you feel better?
- Do you regularly use alcohol as medicine to relieve menstrual cramps, help you sleep, or calm your nerves?
- Do you talk a lot about drinking?
- Do you feel sociable only when you drink?
- Do you drink when you are under pressure or after an argument?
- Do you try to get someone to buy liquor for you because you are too ashamed to buy it yourself?
- Do you hide the empty bottles and dispose of them secretly?
- Do you buy liquor at different places so no one will know how much you purchase?
- Do you plan in advance to reward yourself with several drinks after you've worked hard in the house or on the job?
- Do you have blackouts—periods about which you remember nothing?
- Do you ever wonder if anyone knows how much you drink?
- Do you ever carry liquor in your purse?
- Do you worry about hurting your child when you have been drinking?
- Do you drink to make your partner less angry at you?
- If you drink occasionally, do you have a lot of drinks at one time?
- Do you drink more when you have been emotionally or physically abused?
- Do you feel panicky when faced with nondrinking days or when you are without money to buy alcohol?
- Do you become defensive when anyone mentions your drinking?
- Do you try to cover up when you can't remember promises and feel ashamed when you misplace or lose things?

- Do you drive your car or operate machinery after you've been drinking?
- Do you take sleeping pills or tranquilizers together with alcohol?
- Do you use alcohol to have or to avoid sexual activity?
- Do you think that drinks at home are okay but drinks in a bar are not?
- Have you fallen down or hurt yourself as a result of drinking?
- Are you absent or late for work more often after you drink?
- Do you suffer from indigestion, nausea, or diarrhea due to drinking?

If you or a friend answer yes to five or more questions, you may have a drinking problem. Some experts feel that answering yes to even fewer of these questions may also indicate a problem. A shorter quiz appears in the sidebar on page 260.

Health Effects of Drinking

The effects of drinking alcohol vary from person to person and depend on the amount consumed. Four points of concern for women are that alcohol is a depressant, alcohol poses serious health risks, women's bodies react more quickly to alcohol than men's do, and alcohol poses risks to unborn fetuses in pregnant women.

Alcohol Is a Depressant. Alcohol is absorbed mainly through the small intestine. There it is quickly transported throughout the rest of the body. Although people who drink commonly describe a feeling of euphoria with alcohol consumption, in fact alcohol depresses the central nervous system and thus has a sedative effect.

Small or moderate amounts of alcohol commonly produce sensations of warmth (although in reality, heat loss through the skin is increased with alcohol) and often make a person feel relaxed and less inhibited. With increasing amounts of alcohol, these sedative effects increase. Taken in very large quantities, alcohol can actually be poisonous, hindering vital brain functions, such as breathing and heartbeat, and causing death.

Alcohol Poses Serious Health Risks. Over time, steady, heavy drinking takes a tremendous toll on the body. Thyroid problems, diabetes, liver disease, and circulatory problems are just some of the health effects of heavy and prolonged drinking. In addition to these physical effects, heavy alcohol use can and often does lead to both psychological and physical dependence and addiction. Short-term memory loss occurs in many heavy drinkers, as does liver damage that can be permanent and even life-threatening.

Heavy alcohol use also increases women's risk of stroke. Women who drink heavily are nearly six times more likely to have a stroke than those who do not. Alcohol abuse also increases a woman's risk of developing breast cancer.

Alcohol Affects Women Differently Than Men. In addition to the amount a woman drinks, her body weight and metabolism also determine how alcohol affects her. In general, the same amount of alcohol produces different effects in women and men. The reason for these differences is mainly that alcohol is absorbed into the bloodstream faster in women than in men. This means that when a man and a woman of roughly equal size and body weight drink the same amount of alcohol, the woman will be more greatly and more quickly affected

wellness **warning**

Some women, including adolescents, who may not like the taste of hard liquor, often choose to drink fruity wine coolers or breezers. They may also think they are consuming less alcohol this way. Not so. A typical wine cooler contains as much alcohol as a bottle of beer.

wellness **tip**

Keep in mind that alcohol affects your body more quickly than a man's. At social occasions, limit your alcohol consumption. Two drinks is the recommended limit. Especially if you are at risk for alcohol problems, it is important to have such personal guideposts to monitor your drinking.

than the man. Women generally have more body fat and less total body water than men do. Less water in a woman's body means that alcohol is diluted more slowly.

Women also have less alcohol dehydrogenase, the enzyme that breaks down alcohol in the liver, than men. For example, women have been found to develop severe liver disease with shorter periods of drinking and lower amounts of alcohol than those needed to produce the same effects in men.

Heavy alcohol use may increase a woman's risk of developing osteoporosis (a condition in which the bones become weakened and more prone to fracture). Heavy drinking can also cause reproductive problems, including infertility, failure to ovulate, premenstrual syndrome, and early menopause. Women who chronically drink have also been shown to have more problems in sexual functioning, including inability to reach orgasm.

The decrease in inhibitions caused by alcohol can make it more likely that a woman will do things that she would not normally do when sober. Women are more vulnerable to sexual assault and rape, including date rape, when under the influence of alcohol.

Alcohol Can Have Serious Consequences During Pregnancy. Alcohol consumed by a pregnant woman crosses the placenta and can have serious effects on the fetus, during all three trimesters. It is not known how much alcohol has to be consumed to pose a risk to the fetus, so it is best to avoid drinking if you are planning to become or could be pregnant and to avoid alcohol throughout your pregnancy.

Excessive alcohol consumption by a pregnant woman can lead to a condition called fetal alcohol syndrome (FAS). Babies with FAS are born smaller and lighter than normal babies and do not catch up, even with special care. They also have smaller heads, abnormally thin lips, smaller eyes, and a deep nasal bridge. Children with FAS are usually mentally retarded and have a short attention span and behavioral problems. A more mild condition, known as fetal alcohol effects (FAE), is marked by some but not all of the characteristics of FAS.

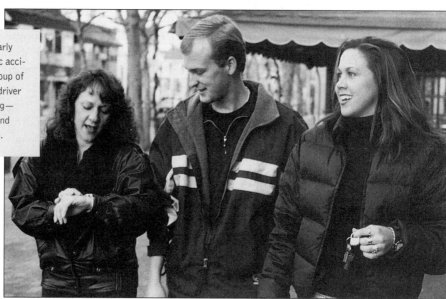

Drinking plays a factor in nearly one-quarter of all fatal traffic accidents. If you go out with a group of friends, choose a designated driver at the beginning of the evening— someone who will not drink and who will drive everyone home.

Tobacco *Use*

The use of tobacco, usually in the form of cigarette smoking, is widespread among Americans. More than 150 million men and women in the United States have smoked at some time in their lives, and about 61 million—more than one-quarter of the population over age 12—are currently smokers. Smokeless, or chewing, tobacco is used much less often—by almost 7 million people—but its use is disturbingly common among young people.

The rates of illness and death related to tobacco use are overwhelming. Each year, there are more deaths from smoking-related illnesses than from cocaine, heroin, and alcohol abuse; automobile accidents; homicide and suicide; and AIDS combined. Tobacco use is the single greatest cause of preventable death in the United States. Lung cancer, most commonly caused by cigarette smoking, kills more women each year than any other type of cancer, including breast cancer.

Smoking Among Women

With cigarettes, especially those that are "slim" or "ultra lite," being marketed directly toward women, the number of female smokers (including female teens) continues to grow. On average, American women now smoke more cigarettes, inhale them more deeply, and begin smoking at an earlier age than they did 40 years ago. As a result, mortality rates related to smoking are now considerably higher. Despite the fact that approximately 150,000 women die from smoking-related diseases each year, over 22 million women aged 19 or over still smoke. Although women still smoke less than men, the difference between the sexes is narrowing: about 27 percent of women and 29 percent of men are estimated to be current smokers. Overall, smoking rates have been declining in recent years for both women and men, but this decrease is less each year for women. The rate of smoking among young girls is particularly alarming: nearly 20 percent of girls ages 12 to 17 currently smoke, and more teenage girls than teenage boys smoke.

Despite the highly publicized health risks of smoking and recent confirmation that nicotine is addictive, many women (and men) continue to smoke. On the flip side, however, people are also quitting smoking in increasing numbers each year.

Health Effects of Tobacco Use

Cigarette smoke contains more than 4,700 chemical compounds, including trace amounts of poisons like formaldehyde, arsenic, DDT, and cyanide. Over 40 of these chemicals are known to cause cancer. The carbon monoxide in cigarette smoke displaces the oxygen in red blood cells, robbing the body's tissues of oxygen.

Doctors and scientists have known for some time that tobacco use, particularly cigarette smoking, leads to illness and death. In fact, according to the Centers for Disease Control and Prevention, smoking kills approximately 150,000 women a year.

The vast list of illnesses caused by or linked to tobacco use is headed by heart disease, lung cancer, and lung diseases, such as emphysema. Many other types of cancer are now known to be linked to smoking. These include cancers of the mouth, throat, esophagus, bladder, and pancreas. In addition, smokers are more likely to get cancer of the kidney, cervix, liver, urinary tract, breast, and rectum.

wellness **warning**

Smoking shortens your life expectancy by an average of five to eight years, compared to non-smokers.

For example, women who smoke are three to four times more likely to develop cervical cancer than those who do not.

Smoking is the cause of over half of the deaths from cardiovascular disease in women under age 65. Women who smoke are almost three times as likely to have a stroke than nonsmokers and are almost four times as likely to have a heart attack. Women smokers who use oral contraceptives increase their risk of having a heart attack by tenfold; for smokers aged 35 years and older on oral contraceptives, the risk is 39 times as great. Of all women who have heart attacks, those who smoke have their first attack an average of 19 years earlier than those who do not smoke.

The list of tobacco-related diseases and conditions goes on and on. In women, smoking also increases the risk of osteoporosis, early menopause, impaired fertility, menstrual problems, and problems with breastfeeding.

Smoking During Pregnancy. Like alcohol, the chemicals in cigarette smoke cross the placenta and reach the fetus, increasing the risks of miscarriage, stillbirth, premature birth, and low birth weight. Infants of mothers who smoked during pregnancy are considered at increased risk for sudden infant death syndrome (SIDS), in which an apparently healthy baby dies during sleep.

Secondhand Smoke. "Passive" smokers—those who do not smoke but who are exposed to others' cigarette smoke—also are at increased risk for health problems. For example, children of parents who smoke are more likely to get bronchitis, pneumonia, asthma and allergies, colds, and ear infections. In fact, it is estimated that each year over 50,000 people die from complications caused by

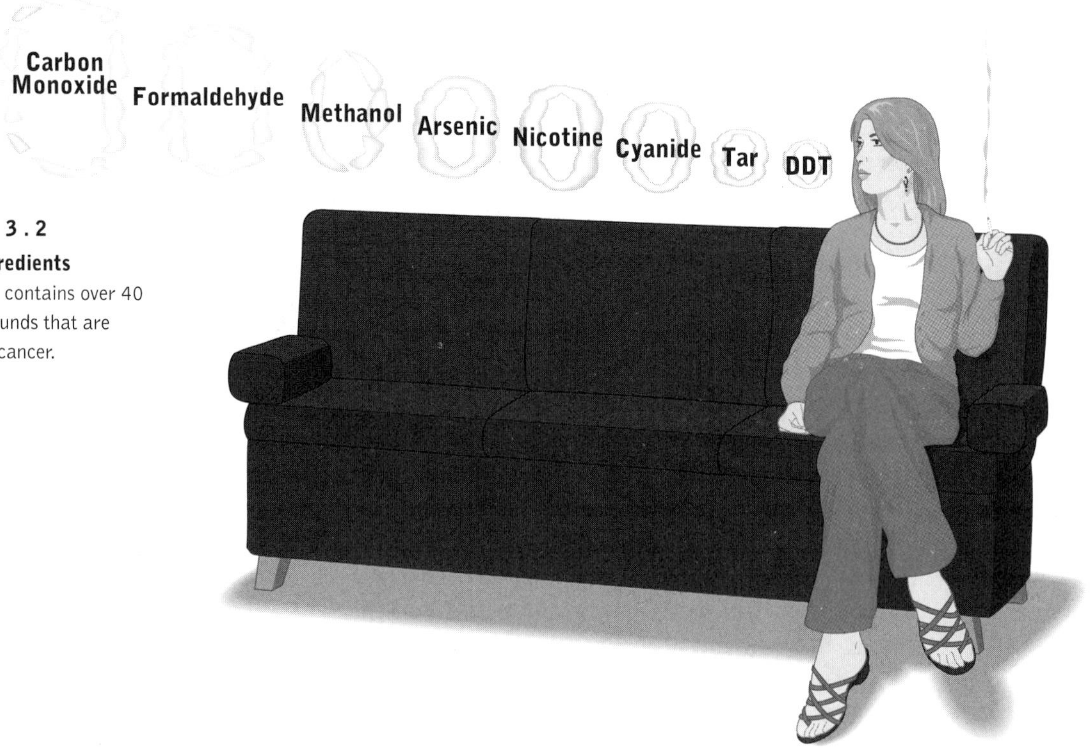
Carbon Monoxide
Formaldehyde
Methanol
Arsenic
Nicotine
Cyanide
Tar
DDT

FIGURE 13.2
Dangerous Ingredients
Cigarette smoke contains over 40 chemical compounds that are known to cause cancer.

inhaling secondhand smoke. Passive smokers are also more likely to become smokers themselves, thereby placing themselves at risk for all of the illnesses linked to smoking.

Smokeless Tobacco. Eliminating the smoke from tobacco use does not eliminate the health risks. The use of smokeless tobacco—chewing tobacco and snuff—carries with it the risks of tooth and gum disease and cancer of the mouth. Smokeless tobacco can be just as addicting as cigarettes.

Quitting Successfully

Most women who smoke are aware that it is bad for their health, yet they persist in their habit. The very fact that they continue to smoke despite adverse consequences is evidence of how addicting tobacco can be. In fact, many researchers consider tobacco to be at least as addicting as heroin, cocaine, or alcohol.

The Four Principles of Quitting. Once they have decided to quit smoking, some women are able quit on their own just using their own willpower. Most women, though, need extended support from family, friends, and physicians. Smoking-cessation programs, counseling, and such methods as nicotine gum or patches are also helpful. There is no one method that will work for everyone, but there are some basic principles behind quitting successfully that are helpful to keep in mind:

- **Make a commitment.** Quitting smoking—or the use of any other addicting drug—is not only a matter of changing a behavior. It also involves changing your outlook. Quitting for good will not be possible until you have made a commitment to stop. Although you should realize that it probably will not be easy, try not to focus only on negative thoughts about how hard it will be. Rather, think about all the benefits of quitting: your improved health and outlook, boosted self-confidence, and the sense of control you will regain over your life.
- **Set a quit date.** Once you have "primed" yourself mentally to quit smoking, pick a date on which you will stop. Try to cut down, tapering off your smoking,

Acupuncture: One Antidote to Addiction

Acupuncture is the ancient Chinese practice of curing disorders and relieving painful chronic conditions by stimulating vital areas in the body using specialized needles that are inserted into the skin. The needles used are so fine that most people describe the procedure as painless. Because the benefits of acupuncture are often immediate and measurable, the practice has steadily gained the respect of medical practitioners in the United States. Now patients interested in acupuncture treatments are regularly referred to certified acupuncturists who work in private clinics and even in some hospitals.

Compelling evidence suggests that acupuncture can help women overcome addiction to cigarettes, alcohol, and other drugs. After receiving treatment for 30 minutes a day, some cigarette smokers have reported kicking the habit in as few as ten days. Some drug and alcohol treatment centers have described a 50 to 75 percent success rate for addicts using acupuncture, as opposed to a 3 percent success rate for those who did not try acupuncture or were given placebo treatments.

There are virtually no risks or side effects with acupuncture. However, if you decide to seek treatment, be sure that the acupuncturist you see has a state license or has been certified by the National Commission for the Certification of Acupuncturists.

wellness **tip**

If you think that quitting smoking will be impossible, do not try to stop all at once. Set realistic and gradual goals for yourself. Do not give up if you give in and have a cigarette—just renew your commitment to quit, starting right then.

until you reach that date. When it comes, throw away all your cigarettes, ashtrays, matches, and lighters. Wash or dry-clean all your clothes to get rid of the stale-smoke smell. Do something that makes it difficult or impossible to smoke at the times of day when you would normally be smoking: wash the car, work in the garden, or do something that requires both hands, like cooking.

- **Get support.** Tell your family, friends, and coworkers that you are trying to stop smoking, and ask for their support. Ask your doctor about support groups, smoking-cessation programs, and using nicotine patches or gum—these are very effective for many people. Above all, do not be afraid to ask for help. It is almost impossible to quit smoking on your own.
- **Stick with it.** Do not punish yourself or give up if you slip and have a cigarette. Do not use the relapse as an excuse to go back to your former levels of smoking. Mistakes are to be expected. Many smokers have to try several times before they quit for good. If you find yourself lighting a cigarette, make yourself put it out. Throw out any other cigarettes you have. If you proceed to smoke it, remember that you do not have to finish it. It is better to smoke half a cigarette than a whole one.

What Does Quitting Feel Like? Withdrawal from nicotine has symptoms, just as withdrawal from other drugs. Women in the process of quitting smoking, whether "cold turkey" (all at once) or gradually, may experience one or more of the following symptoms:

- Anxiety
- Restlessness
- Drowsiness or fatigue
- Lack of concentration
- Indigestion or constipation
- Hunger
- Irritability

Fortunately, these symptoms abate quickly. Once you stop smoking, your body rids itself of nicotine in two to three days. Withdrawal symptoms usually do not last more than three weeks. It is helpful to focus on the positive outcomes of quitting. You will feel better physically and you will have more energy. You will feel better psychologically, because you have succeeded in meeting a very important and very difficult goal. Compliments from others will no doubt build your self-esteem. Your house and clothes will smell better. Nonsmoking friends and family members may be more receptive to you. Most important, you will be taking charge of your wellness.

Use of **Illicit Drugs**

Illicit drugs are sometimes called "street" drugs because they are often literally bought and sold on the street in every type of neighborhood—urban, suburban, and rural. Illicit drugs are highly addictive and include illegal drugs, such as marijuana, cocaine, and heroin, and legal drugs, such as prescription sedatives and tranquilizers, that are used for nonmedical purposes. The use of illicit drugs by American adults aged 26 and over has been increasing steadily since the late 1970s: about 38 percent report having used an illicit drug at some time in their lives. Of special concern is the growing rate of current use (defined as use within the past month) among the young, which has risen steadily since 1992. The age group with the highest current use of illicit drugs are people between the ages of 18 and 25, 13 percent of whom reported current use in 1995. Nearly 5 million American women aged 12 and older currently use some type of illicit drug.

Marijuana and Hashish

By far the most popular illicit drug, marijuana is derived from the dried leaves and flowers of the plant *Cannabis sativa*. It contains numerous chemicals, most notably THC (tetrahydrocannabinol), which is responsible for the drug's psychoactive effects. Marijuana can be smoked in a pipe or as cigarettes or can be eaten (usually in baked goods, such as brownies or cookies). A highly concentrated form of marijuana, known as hashish, or hash, is especially potent.

The effects of marijuana include distorted thoughts, perceptions, and feelings. The experience of being high on marijuana is complex, heightening the user's self-perception and inner awareness.

Chronic and prolonged use of marijuana leads to increased tolerance and the need for increasing amounts of the drug to achieve the same desired effects. Chronic users may become passive and lethargic, apathetic, and uninterested in doing anything except getting high. Chronic depression, impaired intellect and concentration, memory loss, and problems with motor coordination are also common among long-time users.

More than half of people who use marijuana, even on a "casual" basis—at least once a year—develop some aspect of dependence on the drug (such as using it more than they intended or wanting to cut down). Among women, it is used most often by those aged 18 to 25. In women, marijuana has been linked to irregular menstrual cycles.

Cocaine and Crack

Cocaine is a white, water-soluble powder extracted from the dried leaves of the coca plant. It can be inhaled ("snorted") through the nose, injected into the bloodstream, or mixed with solvents to extract a purer form of the drug, which is then smoked—a practice known as "freebasing." Crack is cocaine that has been converted to a more potent, smokeable form that is sold on the street in smaller and cheaper amounts.

Cocaine produces an intense euphoria that peaks about 15 to 20 minutes after the drug is taken and lasts about an hour. Crack's effects are even more rapid, peaking within seconds and lasting only minutes. The effects of cocaine in any of its forms are

How to Tell If You May Have a Drug Problem

Although this questionnaire is not a substitute for a thorough evaluation by your doctor or other health professional, it may help you decide whether you need to get help for a drug problem. Answer yes or no:

1. On many occasions, I have used alcohol or other drugs in greater amounts or for longer periods than I intended to.
2. I have tried, or wanted to try, to cut down or control my alcohol or other drug use.
3. I have spent a great deal of time using, recovering from, or trying to obtain alcohol or other drugs.
4. During times when I should have been somewhere else, I have often been using alcohol or other drugs or having symptoms of withdrawal.
5. Because of my alcohol or other drug use, I have given up or cut down on important social or work activities, either to spend time with others using alcohol or other drugs or to use them by myself.
6. I have continued to use alcohol or other drugs in spite of realizing that it was causing or worsening problems with my health, relationships, or work.
7. Sometimes I have had to use about twice the amount of alcohol or other drugs to get the same effect as before.
8. There have been times when I have had withdrawal symptoms after I stopped using alcohol or other drugs.
9. There have been times when I used alcohol or other drugs in order to avoid having withdrawal symptoms.

If you answered yes to three or more of these questions, you may have a problem, and you should talk to your doctor about your alcohol or other drug use.

Source: American Psychiatric Association.

Drug Use and AIDS

Women who use drugs increase their risk of contracting HIV, the virus that causes AIDS, in two ways. First, women who inject drugs and share syringes and other drug paraphernalia run a high risk of contracting HIV. HIV is easily transmitted through shared needles or syringes. Second, women who are under the influence of illicit drugs or alcohol may also engage in unprotected sex, which further increases their risk for contracting HIV.

Although the number of new AIDS cases among women decreased by 17 percent between 1993 and 1994, AIDS is still the fourth leading cause of death among women of childbearing age in the United States. In addition, in 1995 the Centers for Disease Control and Prevention reported nearly 65,000 cases of AIDS among adolescent and adult women in the United States. Nearly 66 percent of these reported cases were related to women who injected drugs or to women who had sex with someone who used injected drugs.

Source: National Institute on Drug Abuse.

followed by an extreme low that leaves the user feeling despondent and wanting more. As with other drugs, tolerance to cocaine's effects requires the use of larger amounts to produce the same effect. Not surprisingly, the drug causes intense psychological craving.

Long-term users are often restless and agitated. Repeated snorting can cause sores and damage to the nasal septum. Cocaine psychosis, characterized by paranoid hallucinations, develops in heavy users. The drug can also cause sudden spasms of the arteries that lead to the heart, resulting in a heart attack or death. This serious side effect can occur even with the first use of the drug. Cocaine is often laced with amphetamines, such as speed, which increase the heart rate and the chances that serious heart damage, such as a heart attack, will occur.

Cocaine can cause serious complications during pregnancy, increasing the risk of miscarriage, fetal death, and preterm birth. Infants born to cocaine-using women are often addicted themselves, have difficulties with motor coordination, can be unusually irritable and fussy, and are at increased risk for SIDS.

Hallucinogens

Hallucinogens produce vivid and profound changes in a person's senses and mental state. This class of drugs includes LSD (lysergic acid diethylamide) and PCP (phencyclidine), which are the most widely used hallucinogens. Others include the peyote cactus, from which mescaline is derived; psilocybin mushrooms; and Ecstasy, a synthetic compound. Some of the hallucinogens, especially peyote and psilocybin, have traditionally been used for spiritual purposes in the religious rites of some North and South American Indians.

Hallucinogens are usually taken by mouth, although they can also be mixed with tobacco or marijuana and smoked. LSD, which produces its effects in extremely small amounts, is often spread onto thin sheets that are then cut up into tiny squares, each of which contains one dose or "hit," and swallowed.

Under the influence of hallucinogens, a person may have intense sensory experiences—seeing, hearing, tasting, smelling, and feeling things that do not exist. Sometimes the senses seem to "cross over"—such that the user seems to "hear" colors or "see" sounds. The altered mental state induced by hallucinogens can change a person's perceptions of their surroundings and cause them to have accidents if they are operating a motor vehicle.

PCP is a potent drug that was once used to sedate large livestock, such as horses and cows. Its use was stopped by veterinarians because of the confusion and disorientation it caused in the animals. The effects of PCP are highly unpredictable. They may range from euphoria and loss of inhibition to seizures, delirium, and psychotic symptoms that can erupt into violence.

Roughly 1.5 million people are thought to be current users of hallucinogens in the United States. As with most drugs that are abused, the rates are higher in men than in women. Although the effects of hallucinogens in women during pregnancy are not well known, it is thought that LSD use during pregnancy may lead to birth defects.

Heroin and Other Opiates

Heroin, methadone, morphine, and opium belong to the class of drugs known as opiates, all of which are derived from the opium poppy. Opiates are sometimes used to relieve severe pain in hospitalized patients but are often used illegally as well. All are highly addictive when used in large doses over time.

Opiates can be smoked, prepared as a tea, or injected under the skin or directly into the bloodstream through a vein (called "mainlining"). Some hard-core users actually inject the drug through the back of the neck and into the spinal cord in order to intensify its effects. Accidental and permanent paralysis can easily result from such an injection.

A euphoric high quickly follows the injection of an opiate as the drug depresses the central nervous system. The user generally feels tranquil, calm, and even somewhat drowsy. This state may last a few minutes to an hour, depending on the amount of drug and the person's tolerance. After this initial high, the user typically experiences a period of apathy during which reactions are slowed, concentration is impaired, and speech may be slurred.

Over time, the continued use of opiates leads to physical dependence. Stopping use results in highly unpleasant and painful withdrawal symptoms, including nausea, vomiting, achiness, tremors, fever, and intense drug craving. For this reason, people who are addicted to opiates often become desperate to obtain more of the drug after its effects wear off.

Opiates cross the placenta during pregnancy and reach the fetus. As many as two-thirds of babies born to opiate-addicted mothers have a severe and potentially fatal withdrawal syndrome. Symptoms of withdrawal in these babies usually appear within a few days after birth and include a high-pitched cry, poor feeding, tremors, diarrhea, and sometimes seizures.

Abuse of Prescription Drugs

Many people think only of illegal drugs when they think about substance abuse, but drug addiction and dependence also can occur with a host of legal prescription drugs. The most commonly abused of these drugs are the so-called psychotherapeutic drugs. These are medications, such as tranquilizers, that can be legally obtained only with a doctor's prescription. When these drugs are used by someone for whom they were not prescribed or for nonmedical purposes—that is, only for the experience or feeling they cause—this is considered abuse.

Painkillers. Some types of prescription analgesics, or painkillers, can be addicting when used for long periods. This is especially true of narcotic drugs—opiates and opioids (synthetic drugs with properties similar to those of opiates). Analgesics are the only class of psychotherapeutic drugs that are abused by more women than men.

Some of the more commonly used analgesics include hydromorphone (Dilaudid), codeine, and meperidine (Demerol). Used appropriately, these drugs can be very helpful in managing pain. Some are also used to treat disorders of the digestive tract and as supplements to general anesthesia during surgery. Used unwisely, however, they are highly addictive. When an addicted person stops taking an analgesic with narcotic ingredients, withdrawal symptoms include extreme agitation and restlessness, profuse sweating, and anxiety.

Stimulants. The stimulant drugs include amphetamines, which are sometimes prescribed to treat narcolepsy (a sleep disorder in which a person falls asleep

Heroin Chic

According to the Drug Enforcement Administration (DEA), heroin use has never been higher in the United States than it is today. It is becoming increasingly popular in small towns and rural areas. Usage is also up in major cities, as well as on college campuses and in the workplace.

Why the sudden rise? Some experts point to the fact that heroin can now be snorted or smoked, rather than injected. People no longer have to worry about contracting HIV from dirty needles or hiding the track marks caused by injection. Indeed, heroin use has become much more "civilized."

The media is also blamed. Some advertisers use models wearing "the heroin look"— blank expressions, dirty hair, red eyes, and sweaty skin. Movies, like *Trainspotting*, portray the lives of heroin users, making cultural anti-heroes out of their characters. The heroin-related deaths of celebrities Kurt Cobain and River Phoenix drew widespread media attention. Over 4,000 people die from heroin use each year.

Misuse and Abuse of Over-the-Counter Medicines

Without realizing it, many people misuse legal drugs sold without a prescription and become physically dependent on them. A common example of over-the-counter drug abuse is the excessive use of nasal sprays. These contain drugs that shrink the mucous membranes inside the nose, making it easier to breathe. Overuse leads to a "rebound effect," when the medication wears off and actually causes the nasal passageways to become more swollen than before the drug was first used. As a result, a person may use more and more of the drug until she cannot breathe comfortably without it. The only way to break this cycle is to stop using the medication.

After an uncomfortable period of stuffiness, about a week or two, the rebound effect wears off.

Constipation sufferers are prone to overusing laxatives, which can eventually interfere with colon function. As with overuse of nasal sprays, the original condition for which the drug was used—in this case, constipation—can become even worse. Laxatives are also abused by some people with eating disorders, who use the preparations to quickly empty food through and out of their system in order to avoid gaining weight.

Painkillers, cough medicines (many of which contain alcohol), and diet aids are also misused. Drugs sold over the counter should always be used with caution, according to the manufacturer's directions, and with the advice of your physician.

uncontrollably at irregular times) and certain seizure disorders, such as Parkinson's disease. Occasionally they are prescribed to suppress the appetite in people with extreme obesity.

Stimulants produce feelings of energy and elation by activating certain chemicals normally found in the brain. Used in excess, they cause extreme agitation, compulsive behavior, nervousness and anxiety, and physical symptoms, such as rapid heartbeat, sweating, nausea and vomiting, and tinnitus (ringing in the ears).

Tranquilizers. The most commonly prescribed tranquilizers belong to a group of drugs called benzodiazepines. These include diazepam (Valium), chlordiazepoxide (Librium), alprazolam (Xanax), and lorazepam (Ativan). These drugs are used for short-term treatment of anxiety disorders.

Benzodiazepines depress the central nervous system. Used wisely, they have a soothing, calming effect and can reduce excessive anxiety and control dangerously aggressive behavior in mentally ill patients. However, taken in moderate to high doses over a long period, they can also be highly addictive. Women who are addicted to these drugs usually use them in combination with alcohol or other drugs, such as barbiturates (see the next section, "Sedatives"). Used in this way, benzodiazepines can produce effects ranging from mild relaxation to dizziness, weakness, slurred speech, lack of muscle coordination, and breathing difficulties.

Sedatives (Sleeping Pills). Sedatives are usually prescribed for insomnia. Some of the sedatives, like triazolam (Halcion), are classified as benzodiazepines, whereas others, like pentobarbital (Nembutol), phenobarbital, and secobarbital (Seconal), are barbiturates.

Sedatives are abused about equally by men and women. They produce euphoria and loss of inhibition, as well as slurred speech, clumsiness, and impaired judgment and memory. Strangely, long-term, heavy use can result in an effect opposite to sedation; the user becomes aggressive, agitated, and even violent.

Addiction to sedatives, such as sleeping pills, can happen quickly; many users falsely believe that if one pill helps them relax or sleep, two will do an even better job. Once a woman becomes addicted, withdrawal from heavy sedative use can be severe and life-threatening. Symptoms may begin as soon as two hours after the drug is stopped and may last up to two weeks. They generally begin with rapid heartbeat, muscle pain and weakness, anxiety, insomnia or nightmares, nausea and vomiting, and shaking. Within a few days, depending on the degree of the person's addiction, severe withdrawal symptoms may emerge. These may consist of delirium, seizures, psychosis, and possibly death.

Inhalants. Although inhalants are among the least abused substances in the United States, they are used more often than heroin or crack, and their effects can be just as damaging and deadly. Close to 1 million people abuse inhalants, most of them males 12 to 17 years old. In 1995, though, 200,000 girls in this age range reported their use of inhalants. The reason for the high use of inhalants by younger people may be that they have easier access to inhalants than to other drugs.

The most commonly abused inhalants are paint, paint thinner, varnish, correction fluid, and glues that contain solvents. The very ingredients that cause the "high" from these substances are also what make them so deadly.

Other types of inhalants are nitrites, such as amyl nitrite, which is used to treat chest pain; and anesthetics, such as ether and nitrous oxide. Nitrous oxide is used as an anesthetic in doctors' and dentists' offices and is also found in some spray cans, such as those containing whipped cream or nonstick cooking sprays.

Inhalants are inhaled through the nose and mouth. Some are inhaled directly from the container. Others, like amyl nitrite, are supplied for medical use in small glass ampules that are broken (called "poppers") and inhaled from gauze or other absorbent material. Still others, like the anesthetic gases, are inhaled through a hose or mask attached to a pressurized tank.

The long list of effects produced by inhalants includes both short- and long-term responses to the chemicals they contain. The immediate "rush" that accompanies inhalation is short-lived. The user may have a sensation of fullness in the head, stimulation, and reduced inhibitions. Prolonged use can result in loss of coordination, sluggishness, impaired thinking, nausea and vomiting, persistent headache, and weakness. High doses can cause stupor and coma. The inhalants can have depressant effects on the central nervous system, which can eventually result in permanent brain damage and death.

Toward Wellness:
Treatment *for* Substance Abuse

Addiction has long been viewed by many as a weakness of will on the part of the substance abuser. Once a source of shame and secrecy, substance abuse is becoming increasingly understood and recognized as a disease that can be effectively treated. In the past few decades, a whole new field of medicine—the area of addiction medicine—has begun to flourish as researchers and clinicians learn more and more about the processes of substance abuse prevention, treatment, and recovery.

To view substance abuse as a disease, however, is not to say that a woman who abuses drugs bears no responsibility for her actions. On the contrary, modern methods of substance abuse treatment emphasize the importance of learning to take control of one's life and to make wise and healthy choices for physical,

Caffeine Is a Drug, Too

One of the most widely used drugs is also one of the least recognized as having psychoactive effects: caffeine. Caffeine alters mood and mental functioning.

There are about 100 milligrams (mg) of caffeine in a 6-ounce cup of coffee. Tea and soda contain less than half that amount—about 40 mg in 6 ounces of tea and 45 mg in a 12-ounce soda. A chocolate bar contains about 5 mg of caffeine.

Many people like to joke about their love of and dependence on coffee to get them going in the morning, but like any drug, caffeine can be overused and lead to health problems. Overconsumption of caffeine is linked to fibrocystic, or lumpy, breasts and breast soreness in women. Excessive caffeine can also cause digestive tract problems, nervousness, insomnia, and fast heartbeat. It is also linked to some types of anxiety disorders.

Stopping or cutting down can result in a temporary withdrawal syndrome characterized by headache and fatigue, but this should pass in a few days or a week.

mental, emotional, and spiritual well-being. They also focus on personal responsibility. Many people with substance abuse problems tend to blame people and things outside of themselves for their addiction. One of the first steps of treatment is to learn that your addiction is not caused by bad relationships or negative events in your life. Rather than finding excuses for using drugs, it is important to recognize that you yourself are responsible for your substance abuse.

The decision to get treatment for an alcohol or other drug problem is seldom easy and often accompanied by feelings of fear and confusion. It is natural to be afraid of the unknown, even if your present circumstances are dark indeed. Breaking a substance abuse habit involves making big changes in your outlook, behavior, and lifestyle. However, you will not be alone in the treatment process. This is important for anyone under stress to remember, but especially someone trying to make major changes in her life. A first step toward treatment is understanding the nature of substance abuse problems and what to expect from the treatment process.

The Nature of Substance Abuse

Substance abuse is now understood as a condition that affects a person's whole life and that requires long-term, ongoing treatment. Ridding one's body of an abused drug, or detoxification, is just the first step in this process. This is why people who have successfully conquered their substance abuse and have remained drug-free, even for many decades, are said to be "recovering"—not recovered or cured. Both the people who provide and those who undergo substance abuse treatment recognize that remaining drug-free is an ongoing, lifelong process.

A Relapsing and Remitting Disease. Substance abuse is widely seen by experts as a relapsing and remitting disease. This means that over time most people in treatment go through periods of remission—during which they are able to abstain from drugs—interrupted by times of relapse—when they weaken and resume their drug use. Relapses may range from a single episode to a long period of resumed drug use, and they are an expected part of the treatment process. In fact, most people who have successfully overcome their substance abuse problems have had to reenter treatment many times after a series of relapses.

Approaches to Treatment. Today there are numerous schools of thought on how to treat substance abuse. A holistic approach is gaining the respect of increasing numbers of substance abuse treatment practitioners. Most experts agree that treating a person's addiction problems in isolation, without looking at all facets of her life, has little, if any, chance of success in the long run. For this reason, modern treatment methods do not focus only on a person's drug use, but rather look at the context in which the drug use occurs—the events and circumstances that precede and accompany a person's drug abuse.

Addiction is a biopsychosocial disorder. That is, many spheres of an individual's life affect and are affected by her substance abuse. Biologically, substance abuse clearly affects a person's physical health. Psychologically, it influences her mental and emotional state. And socially, it has a bearing on her relationships with others—family, friends, and coworkers. A large part of addiction treatment focuses on counseling and therapy to help a woman look at these areas of her life.

Most current theories of treating substance abuse are based on the idea that healing and recovery can begin only when a person has begun to examine all of these areas. Upon entering a treatment program, a person may be asked about any or all of the following:

- Past treatment she has received for physical or mental problems
- Her family background—what life was like in her family as she was growing up, including any substance abuse by her parents or siblings
- Her history of drug use—what substances she has used/abused, at what times in her life, and for how long
- Past treatment or counseling she has received for substance abuse problems
- Her relationships with her family, her intimate partner, and her friends
- Her past and current sexual relationships
- Whether she has experienced violence, as a child or as an adult, from parents, siblings, an intimate partner, or others, including incest, molestation, and rape, as well as emotional and psychological abuse (see Chapter 12)
- Her work history and her relationships with employers and coworkers
- Her performance in school and at work
- Any other significant areas or events of her past or present life

The Components of Treatment

Many communities have local and state treatment centers where individuals can seek professional help for addiction problems. Private facilities, hospitals, and centers also

FIGURE 13.3
Treatment Settings
Treatment for substance abuse takes place in many types of settings and facilities, including shelters, crisis centers, and hospitals.

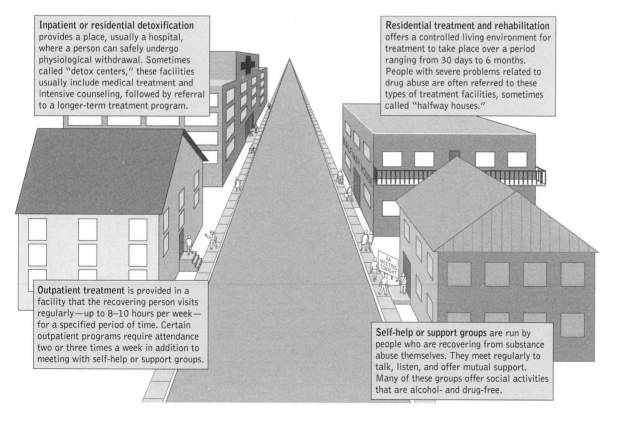

Inpatient or residential detoxification provides a place, usually a hospital, where a person can safely undergo physiological withdrawal. Sometimes called "detox centers," these facilities usually include medical treatment and intensive counseling, followed by referral to a longer-term treatment program.

Residential treatment and rehabilitation offers a controlled living environment for treatment to take place over a period ranging from 30 days to 6 months. People with severe problems related to drug abuse are often referred to these types of treatment facilities, sometimes called "halfway houses."

Outpatient treatment is provided in a facility that the recovering person visits regularly—up to 8–10 hours per week—for a specified period of time. Certain outpatient programs require attendance two or three times a week in addition to meeting with self-help or support groups.

Self-help or support groups are run by people who are recovering from substance abuse themselves. They meet regularly to talk, listen, and offer mutual support. Many of these groups offer social activities that are alcohol- and drug-free.

Finding Treatment Programs

- **Ask your doctor.**
- **Look in your local Yellow Pages under "Drug Abuse Treatment" or in the white pages for local chapters of self-help groups, such as Alcoholics Anonymous and Narcotics Anonymous.**
- **Call your state health department—all 50 states have alcohol and drug abuse treatment programs and 24-hour hot lines, as do many local hospitals.**

offer a variety of treatment approaches in many types of settings (see Figure 13.3). Your doctor can tell you about programs and resources in your community.

There are nearly as many ways of structuring treatment for substance abuse as there are treatment programs. What works for one person, however, may not be suitable for someone else. Despite the variations in how treatment services are offered, though, most treatment and recovery programs encompass the components described here.

Detoxification. The first step in treating addiction is ridding a person's body of the substance abused. Until a woman is free from the immediate physical effects of alcohol or other drugs, she cannot begin to focus on the issues she will need to face during recovery.

Symptoms of withdrawal from some substances can threaten an individual's health or life; therefore detoxification should only be carried out under the supervision of medical professionals in a professional detoxification setting. In addition to the physical effects of withdrawal, most people also experience distressing psychological symptoms, including intense drug craving. Sometimes medication is used to ease the physical and psychological aspects of the withdrawal process. One example is the use of disulfiram (Antabuse) for alcohol detoxification. This drug produces a highly unpleasant reaction when a person consumes even a small amount of alcohol. Another is the use of methadone, which was developed as an alternative to morphine by the Germans during World War II. It eases the withdrawal symptoms from heroin without the feelings of euphoria heroin provides.

Assessment. After detoxification and before treatment is begun, a treatment counselor usually conducts an interview in order to get an overall picture of the person's life. Some of the areas explored during this interview might be:

- Current living arrangements
- Any past or current legal or criminal involvement
- Financial situation
- Intimate relationships and sexual orientation
- Country of origin, citizenship status, and primary language
- Recent death or current serious illness of loved ones
- Pregnancies and number of children

With this information, treatment can be targeted to a woman's specific concerns and needs through a plan designed especially for her. At this time, she will also be acquainted with the treatment program's overall philosophy and goals, her rights and privileges, and how much treatment will cost.

Treatment Planning. The next step in most substance abuse treatment programs is developing a treatment plan. The treatment plan devised by the treatment staff working with the person, is a sort of "recipe" that is flexible and can be changed as the need arises. It may specify, for example, the number and type of therapy sessions the person will attend, education and counseling about substance abuse, and sometimes also larger concerns, such as transportation to the program, housing, medical care, legal assistance, childcare, and employment.

A person undergoing a treatment program is also usually assigned a case manager who has special training in working with people with substance abuse problems and may be, for example, a psychiatric social worker or nurse. The case manager will track the patient's progress throughout treatment and will meet with her periodically to determine whether the treatment plan is meeting her needs or if the plan needs to be adjusted.

The Treatment Process. Treatment for substance abuse does not consist merely of a set of services that a person passively receives. Rather, it is a dynamic process for which the substance abuser must assume responsibility. This is done by communicating with her counselors and other treatment providers about her concerns and needs and by following the treatment plan to which she has agreed (for example, attending counseling and education sessions). Treatment will not work unless there is a sincere effort to change.

Much of substance abuse treatment consists of psychological counseling for the addicted person and her family. This counseling can be provided in a variety of ways—through individual, one-on-one sessions with a mental health professional; group sessions with others who have similar problems or are from similar backgrounds; or family counseling that involves the person's parents, siblings, or children. For most people undergoing substance abuse treatment, these various types of therapy are combined in a treatment plan that has been designed specifically for them.

Preventing Relapse. Making the transition from treatment back to everyday life can be as difficult as the original decision to get treatment. People usually need a lot of support to leave treatment as they try to go forward with their lives without relying on drugs or alcohol.

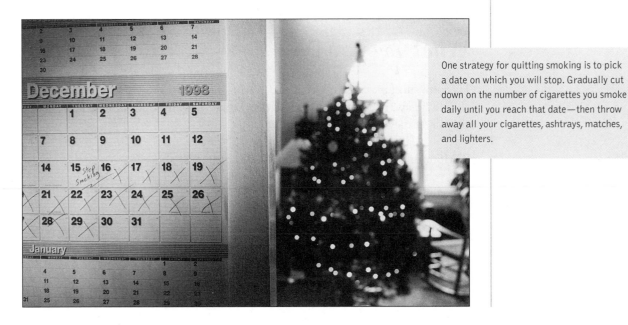

One strategy for quitting smoking is to pick a date on which you will stop. Gradually cut down on the number of cigarettes you smoke daily until you reach that date—then throw away all your cigarettes, ashtrays, matches, and lighters.

Sources of stress—emotional, physical, and environmental—in a recovering woman's life that make her more likely to resume using drugs are called "relapse triggers." One of the skills learned during substance abuse treatment is relapse prevention—how to avoid relapse triggers or, when that is not possible, to manage these stressors without resorting to drug use.

Handling relapse triggers begins with learning how to recognize the people, places, and events or situations that act as triggers for relapse. A woman recovering from alcoholism, for instance, may find that she needs to avoid old "drinking buddies"—relationships based primarily on drinking together. Building new friendships with people who do not use drugs or alcohol is an important part of preventing relapse.

Stress is another important relapse trigger—and one that cannot be as easily avoided as people or places. Stress can come in many forms—emotional and physical, external and internal. The loss or serious illness of a loved one, a change in one's living situation, financial difficulties, or a physical illness or injury are all examples of stressors that can lead to relapse in a recovering person. Even after years of remaining drug-free, stresses can sometimes make a person prone to relapse. Strange as it may seem, stress can also be caused by positive, welcomed events, such as becoming a parent or getting a new job.

Stress management techniques are effective ways of dealing with relapse triggers. These methods vary but generally involve ways to take care of oneself physically, emotionally, and spiritually. They include good hygiene, nutrition, relaxation, and engaging in a favorite sport or hobby. (Chapter 12 contains information about stress management techniques.)

A Lifelong Process

Recovery from substance abuse does not have a defined endpoint. It is a lifelong process. The goal is not just to keep from using drugs; it is to regain control over one's life and to become a whole person again—one who is free to make choices, to love and be loved, to grow and find meaning in life, and to enjoy all that life has to offer—free from drug addiction and dependence.

What *You* Can Do

Harmful substances—both legal and illegal—are a part of today's society. Women should be aware of the health risks drug abuse presents and know what to do if they think they have a problem:

- Monitor your alcohol consumption and be honest about it.
- If you cannot quit smoking, at least try to cut back and think about using a nicotine replacement, like a patch or gum.
- Talk with your doctor if you think you have a drug problem.
- If you have a drug problem, call a hot line and learn about your options for treatment. Investigate self-help and support groups, too.

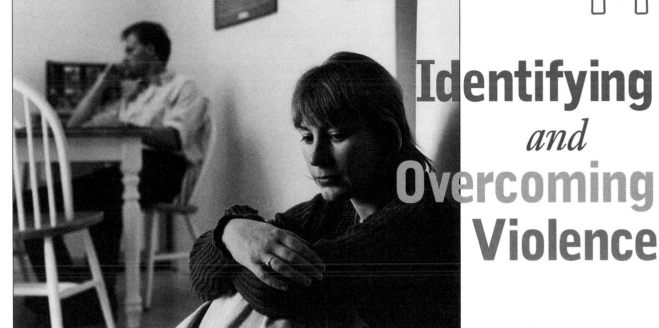

Identifying *and* Overcoming Violence

Millions of American women are embroiled in some form of violence on a daily basis. Sometimes women commit violence, but far more often they are the victims. In fact, while some women live closer to violence than others, all are potential victims. Every woman needs to think clearly about the extent to which violence touches her life. An important aspect of wellness for women is learning how to recognize and avoid potentially violent situations that can injure them physically and scar them emotionally. And, since no protection against violence is one hundred percent certain, women can benefit from learning what support is available if they do fall victim to violence.

Domestic **Violence**

Historical records relate incidences of wife battering from as far back as 2000 B.C. In many societies, including Roman and European civilizations, wife battering was legal and socially accepted. The expression "rule of thumb" is thought to derive from British common law, which described the diameter of the rod with which a man could legally beat his wife.

Although today's society is less overtly barbaric, violence continues to plague millions of women. And, most violence against a woman continues to be committed by a male partner with whom she is or has been intimate. Violence from a woman's partner threatens not only her own life and safety—it threatens the lives and safety of her children as well. Studies show that in families where the woman is being abused, the children are also likely to become victims.

Abuse of the Elderly

The abuse and mistreatment of elderly people is not often discussed but is a widespread problem. It is estimated that as many as 2.5 million elderly persons are abused each year, and the rate seems to be rising. The forms of abuse run the gamut from neglect and abandonment, to physical and sexual abuse, to emotional abuse and financial exploitation. The abuser is usually the elderly person's caregiver, often a son or daughter, but may also be a grandchild, spouse, sibling, or other family member.

Elder abuse is a special problem for women because they live longer than men do. About two-thirds of abused elderly persons are female. The large majority are white, and most are in their mid-70s and older.

Elder abuse can be stopped—if it is reported. Many state and federal agencies exist to address this problem. Some examples are state Adult Protective Services, area Agencies on Aging, and county Departments of Social Services. To find the agency closest to you and to report suspected elder abuse, call the national Eldercare Locator number, 800-677-1116.

How Widespread Is Domestic Violence?

The scope of domestic violence in this country is startling:

- Of all women who are murdered each year in the United States, 42 percent are killed by their male partners.
- Nearly 4 million women in the United States were physically abused by their husbands or boyfriends in 1996.
- A woman is physically abused every 15 seconds in this country.
- More women are the victims of domestic violence than of all other types of physical crimes combined.
- An estimated 22 to 35 percent of women admitted to hospital emergency rooms have suffered injuries from their partners.
- It is estimated that more than one-third of Americans have experienced or witnessed an instance of domestic violence.

Awareness of domestic violence—who is most likely to be abused, what forms the abuse takes, and why it happens—is growing among lawmakers, human service organizations, and women's advocacy groups. As studies in women's psychology have expanded, the public has gained deeper insight into the complexity of the problem. Although we tend to think of violence as a physical threat that leads to visible injury, there are, in fact, many other forms of abuse against women. Verbal, emotional, psychological, and economic abuse are prevalent forms of violence and are all equally damaging to a woman's health, well-being, and self-esteem. Insults, threats, criticism, and withholding financial resources are all abusive acts that are destructive to the women who endure them.

Who Are the Victims?

Domestic violence affects women of all races, all ages, and in every economic situation and living environment. The myth that the only victims of domestic violence are poor women who have no resources to escape has been debunked in recent years. Furthermore, research shows that white, African American, Hispanic, and non-Hispanic women are equally likely to be the victims of abuse from a male partner. Although women in the 20 to 34 age range are more often abused than any other group, younger and older women are frequently physically and emotionally abused by partners. Also, women experience similar rates of partner violence whether they live in an inner city, suburban area, or rural setting.

A common thread among many victims of domestic violence is that they have a hard time recognizing the behavior of their violent mates as abusive. Some women do not realize that it is not normal behavior because, as children, they witnessed the same interactions between their parents. Some women refuse to believe that their partners, whom they love, are capable of abuse, and they make excuses for them. And some women become convinced that they bring the violence on themselves; that the abuse is justified because they are somehow "failing" their partners and are deserving of the punishment. The first step to achieving wellness when a relationship is causing emotional or physical pain is to look honestly at a partner's behavior and decide rationally whether it is violent or abusive.

Is Your Relationship Safe? A Warning Checklist

Abusive people are usually seeking to control the lives of others beyond their right to do so. This list identifies a series of behaviors that are typical of batterers and abusive people. The list can help you recognize if you or someone you know is in an abusive relationship. Check off those behaviors that apply to the relationship. The more checks on the page, the more dangerous the situation may be.

Emotional and Economic Tactics of Abuse

Does your partner or someone you know use any of the following techniques to gain power over you?

☐ **Destructive criticism/verbal abuse.** Name-calling; mocking; accusing; blaming; yelling; swearing; making humiliating remarks or gestures

☐ **Pressure tactics.** Rushing you to make decisions by "guilt-tripping" and other forms of intimidation; sulking; threatening to withhold money; manipulating the children; telling you what to do; threatening to report you to welfare or other social service agencies

☐ **Abusing authority.** Always claiming to be right (insisting statements are "the truth"); making big decisions without your approval

☐ **Disrespect.** Interrupting; changing topics; not listening or responding; twisting your words; putting you down in front of other people; insulting your friends and family

☐ **Abusing trust.** Lying; withholding information; seeing other women; being overly jealous

☐ **Breaking promises.** Not following through on agreements; not taking a fair share of responsibility; refusing to participate in childcare or housework

☐ **Emotional withholding.** Not expressing feelings; not giving support, attention, or compliments; not respecting feelings, rights, or opinions

☐ **Minimizing, denying, and blaming.** Making light of bad behavior; not taking your concerns seriously; saying the abuse didn't happen; shifting responsibility for abusive behavior, saying you caused it

☐ **Economic control.** Interfering with your work or not letting you work; refusing to give you money or taking your money from you; taking your car keys or otherwise preventing you from using the car

☐ **Self-destructive behavior.** Abusing drugs or alcohol; threatening suicide or other forms of self-harm; deliberately saying or doing things that will have negative consequences (e.g., telling off your boss)

☐ **Isolation.** Preventing or making it difficult for you to see friends or relatives; monitoring telephone calls; telling you where you can and cannot go; belittling your friends

☐ **Harassment.** Making uninvited visits or calls; following you; checking up on you; embarrassing you in public; refusing to leave when asked

Acts of Violence

☐ **Intimidation.** Making angry or threatening gestures; using physical size to intimidate; standing in a doorway during arguments to block your exit; out-shouting you; driving recklessly

☐ **Destruction.** Destroying your possessions; punching walls; throwing and/or breaking things

☐ **Threats.** Making and/or carrying out threats to hurt you or others close to you

☐ **Sexual violence.** Degrading treatment based on your sex or sexual orientation; using force or coercion to obtain sex or perform sexual acts

☐ **Overt physical violence.** Being violent to you, your children, your household pets, or others; slapping; punching; grabbing; kicking; choking; pushing; biting; burning; stabbing; shooting

☐ **Weapons.** Keeping weapons around that frighten you and using them to threaten you or those you love

Source: Adapted from *Domestic Violence: The Facts: A Handbook to STOP Violence*, courtesy of Peace at Home (formerly Battered Women Fighting Back), Boston, MA.

The Nature of Domestic Violence

Contrary to what many people might think, battering is not the result of the abuser's losing control of his temper. It is also not caused by his or the victim's use of alcohol or other drugs, although substance abuse often accompanies the violence. Rather, abuse is a way for the abuser to manipulate his victim, to gain control over her, and to make her fearful of him. For whatever reason, an abuser

Domestic Violence and Substance Abuse

Abuse is often linked to the abuse of alcohol and other drugs—by the abuser, the victim, or both. It is thought that up to 80 percent of cases of spouse abuse, for example, may involve alcohol.

In many abusive relationships, both partners are likely to blame the abuse on drinking or drug use. It is a mistake, however, to think that an abuser's alcohol or drug habit "causes" his abusive behavior. This merely gives him an excuse for his actions, so that he will not be forced to take responsibility for them.

Health professionals who treat batterers who have alcohol or drug problems know that getting rid of one problem will not eliminate the other. Rather, it is necessary to look at the underlying causes of violent behavior and substance abuse and treat both problems.

has come to believe that he can resolve conflicts through the use of force and intimidation. Although it is typical for a violent partner to blame stress, drugs, or the victim herself, in reality he alone is responsible for his abusive behavior.

A common characteristic of abuse is its unpredictability. Living with chronic abuse is like being in a land mine field. The victim never knows when the attacks will come. Often there is very little, if any, warning of their approach. Any minor action or comment can spark an angry response from her partner that builds into a full-fledged attack. Many abused women have learned to read subtle signs and cues in their partners' behaviors and moods in order to stave off the violence. They are under constant stress as they try to avoid "stepping on land mines" hidden in their own homes.

Sadly, abuse rarely stops when a woman becomes pregnant. In fact, 45 percent of abused women continue to be abused during their pregnancies. And some men who previously did not abuse their partners begin abuse during a pregnancy.

Physical Abuse. Physical abuse ranges from bullying and intimidation to life-threatening acts. It can take the form of shoving, slapping, kicking, beating, or attacks with a knife or a gun. These attacks can end in death for the victim. In 1992, for example, an estimated 1,500 women in the United States were killed by their partners.

Sexual Abuse. Battering and other forms of abuse by a partner are often accompanied by sexual abuse. Many times, a battered woman does not think of coerced sex with her husband or boyfriend as sexual abuse or rape. However, whenever sex is forced, by either physical or nonphysical means, it is rape or sexual assault. (See the section "Rape and Sexual Assault" later in this chapter.)

A woman who has been repeatedly victimized by her partner may go along with sex in order to appease her abuser. She may fear that he will become violent if she does not consent and be worried for her own safety and that of her children. Or she may not realize that rape is a crime, even when it is committed by her husband.

Nonphysical Forms of Abuse. Most abuse targets the victim's sense of independence and her feelings of self-worth. Nonphysical types of abuse often accompany physical violence as a means to prevent a woman from doing anything on her own, such as leaving her attacker. But even when they are not accompanied by physical injury, emotional and psychological abuse are devastating for the victim.

Emotional and Psychological Abuse. Emotional abuse involves putting down, shaming, ridiculing, or criticizing the victim and otherwise trying to damage or destroy her self-esteem. Psychological abuse can be defined as behavior intended to control the victim's actions and functioning in everyday life. It may take the form of isolating her from her friends, family, and other sources of support or keeping her from having money to pay bills and other expenses. It can also be manifested by the perpetrator's giving his partner the "silent treatment." He may refuse to speak directly to her for long periods, such as days or weeks, leaving her guessing as to how she has displeased or offended him.

Economic Abuse. An abuser may extend his attempts to control his partner by refusing to let her have money or by strictly controlling her "allowance." Typical forms of this type of abuse include:

- Interfering with her work, or not letting her work
- Taking her money or refusing to give her money
- Taking her car keys or otherwise preventing her from using the car

Why Do Women Stay in Abusive Relationships?

A victim of domestic violence may go to great lengths to keep the abuse a secret from her friends and family. In such a case, she might lie about the causes of her injuries. If she needs medical attention, she may rotate among two or more hospital emergency rooms to avoid being identified as a victim of repeated abuse.

For someone who has never been abused, it can be hard to understand why anyone would stay with an abusive partner. Why don't these women leave their partners at the very first sign of abuse? The answer is complex. One explanation is that most victims love their abusive partners, and, while they want the violence to stop, they want the relationship to continue. Another reason has to do with the helplessness and powerlessness that abuse victims feel. Chronic abuse destroys a woman's self-esteem and creates an enormous sense of shame. In fact, it is very common for an abused woman to feel that she deserves the abuse. She may explain away her abuser's behavior by blaming it on his alcohol or drug use

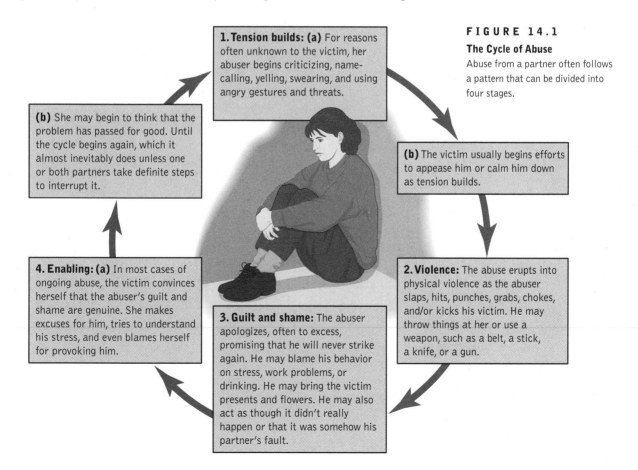

FIGURE 14.1

The Cycle of Abuse

Abuse from a partner often follows a pattern that can be divided into four stages.

1. Tension builds: (a) For reasons often unknown to the victim, her abuser begins criticizing, name-calling, yelling, swearing, and using angry gestures and threats.

(b) The victim usually begins efforts to appease him or calm him down as tension builds.

2. Violence: The abuse erupts into physical violence as the abuser slaps, hits, punches, grabs, chokes, and/or kicks his victim. He may throw things at her or use a weapon, such as a belt, a stick, a knife, or a gun.

3. Guilt and shame: The abuser apologizes, often to excess, promising that he will never strike again. He may blame his behavior on stress, work problems, or drinking. He may bring the victim presents and flowers. He may also act as though it didn't really happen or that it was somehow his partner's fault.

4. Enabling: (a) In most cases of ongoing abuse, the victim convinces herself that the abuser's guilt and shame are genuine. She makes excuses for him, tries to understand his stress, and even blames herself for provoking him.

(b) She may begin to think that the problem has passed for good. Until the cycle begins again, which it almost inevitably does unless one or both partners take definite steps to interrupt it.

Leaving Violence Behind: A Safety Plan

If you or your children may be in danger from an abuser, you can take steps to plan for a quick exit in a potentially violent situation. Making plans ahead of time can boost your self-confidence as you realize that you have the power to take action. If you are not in an abusive situation, but someone you know is, showing her the following list might be a way to begin a dialogue with her that will let her know you are available to help.

Here are some suggestions for putting a plan in place that will give you a safe place to go, someone to call, and reassurance that your important papers and belongings are in a secure place. Fill in the items in these lists and talk to someone you trust about it. Make as many copies of the completed forms as you need and give one to someone you trust. If you feel completely alone in your situation, locate a local battered women's shelter and call their hot line. There you will find help in making your plans, and someone who knows what you are going through will be available if or when you need her.

Increasing a Sense of Safety in an Abusive Relationship

- I will have important phone numbers available to my children and myself.
- I can tell _____ and _____ about the violence and ask them to call the police if they hear suspicious noises coming from my home.
- If I leave my home, I can go (list four places):
  _____, _____, _____, or _____.
- I can leave extra money, car keys, clothes, and copies of documents with _____.
- If I leave, I will bring _____ (see checklist later in this box).
- To ensure my safety and independence, I can: keep change for phone calls with me at all times; open my own savings account; rehearse my escape route with a support person; and review safety plan on _____ (date).

Increasing a Sense of Safety When the Relationship Is Over

- I can change the locks, install steel/metal doors, a security system, smoke detectors, and an outside lighting system.
- I will inform _____ and _____ that my partner no longer lives with me and ask them to call the police if he is observed near my home or my children.

- I will tell my children's caregivers/day care providers the names of those who have permission to pick them up. The people who have permission are: _____, _____, and _____.
- I can tell _____ at work about my situation and ask _____ to screen my calls.
- I can avoid stores, banks, and _____ that I used when living with my battering partner.
- I can obtain a protective order from _____ [local civil court]. I can keep it on or near me at all times, as well as leave a copy with _____.
- If I feel down and ready to return to a potentially abusive situation, I can call _____ for support or attend workshops and support groups to gain support and strengthen my relationships with other people.

Important Phone Numbers

Police _____
Hot line _____
Shelter _____
Friends _____
_____

Checklist of Items to Take

- Identification
- Birth certificates for me and my children
- Social Security card(s)
- School and medical records
- Money, bank books, credit cards
- Keys: house, car, office
- Driver's license and registration
- Medications
- Change of clothes
- Welfare identification
- Passport(s), Green Card(s), work permits
- Divorce papers
- Lease/rental agreement, house deed
- Mortgage payment book, current unpaid bills
- Insurance papers
- Address book
- Pictures, jewelry, items of sentimental value
- Children's favorite toys and/or blankets

Source: Adapted from *Domestic Violence: The Facts: A Handbook to STOP Violence*, courtesy of Peace at Home (formerly Battered Women Fighting Back), Boston, MA.

or on something she did to "provoke" him. Each episode of violence makes her feel more powerless, which in turn assures that she will be further victimized. The literally vicious cycle of abuse continues because the victim believes that she cannot change it.

Breaking this cycle can be an enormous challenge for the victim, especially if she has children. She may be financially dependent on her partner, or she may believe that it is best for the children if the family is kept together, no matter what the cost to her own well-being. Often it is only when the abuser turns his attacks on her children that a woman finally finds the courage to seek help in leaving him.

Child **Abuse**

The effects of violence and abuse are by no means limited to adults. Children who live in households where one partner is abused by the other are at risk for being abused themselves. In a national survey of 6,000 American families, for example, half of the men who abused their wives also abused their children.

Clearly, child abuse is a major national problem. In 1995 alone, more than 1 million children were found to be the victims of abuse. The number of cases of child abuse has been rising each year. From 1986 to 1993, it increased by 67 percent. Much of the reason for this documented rise is probably due to increased efforts by government and private organizations to identify and document child abuse and to raise public awareness of the problem. The number of actual cases of child abuse is widely believed to be far higher than these estimates. And the sad fact remains that many instances of child abuse end in the death of the child.

Who Are the Victims?

Boys and girls have about equal risk for abuse. In reported cases of child abuse, approximately 52 percent of the victims are girls and 48 percent are boys. The majority of the children in these reported cases are under the age of eight. Children aged 12 and older are victims in about 20 percent of reported cases. The highest rate of abuse occurs in children from birth to three years of age.

Although girls may be slightly more likely to be abused, boys are more often killed by their abusers. The highest rate of death from abuse occurs in boys from newborn to three years old.

Child abuse happens to children of all races and ethnic backgrounds. Surveys show that a little more than half (55 percent) of all victims are white, a little more than one-quarter (27 percent) are African American, and about 10 percent are Hispanic. The rest are American Indian, Asian, or of other racial/ethnic origin.

In most cases of child abuse, the attacker is a parent—usually a birth parent. Fewer cases of abuse are perpetuated by adoptive parents, step-parents, foster parents, separated or divorced parents, or the biological parent's new boyfriend or girlfriend. On the other hand, the factor most predictive of a child's *death* by abuse appears to be the presence in the home of a male who is not the biological father.

The ways in which children are mistreated differ depending on whether the abuser is a man or woman. A national survey showed that children were more often neglected by females; they were more often physically abused by males.

wellness tip

Abuse and maltreatment of children takes many forms. A child may or may not be physically injured by an abuser, but *any kind of abuse or maltreatment of a child, whether physical, sexual, or emotional—and including neglect and abandonment—has profound and lifelong effects on the child.*

The Nature of Child Abuse

Most child abuse, whether physical, sexual, or emotional, is accompanied by threats from the attacker that "bad things will happen" if the child tells anyone about the abuse. It is common, for example, for children to be told that they will be separated from the family if they tell. Or they are told that they will go to jail if they tell. Child abusers know that children are easy to intimidate. These threats usually have the desired effect, instilling fear in the victim so that she is afraid to tell anyone. Even children who are abused love their parents and do not want to get them in trouble or risk separation from them.

Neglect. Neglect is the most common form of child abuse, comprising more than half of reported cases. Neglect occurs when the people on whom the child depends ignore basic needs. It can take many forms.

- **Physical neglect.** Children who are physically neglected do not receive the care and attention needed to keep them healthy and out of danger—
  - ➤ They may not be fed properly or may be left to their own devices to find food.
  - ➤ They may not receive needed health care, to the point that their health or their lives are endangered.
  - ➤ They may be abandoned—simply left in a public place or an abandoned apartment—to fend for themselves.
  - ➤ They may be thrown out of their homes before they are old enough to take care of themselves, or if they have left or run away, they may not be allowed to return.
  - ➤ They may not be given adequate supervision, leading to exposure to danger (for example, leaving a young child at home or in a public place by herself for hours at a time).
- **Emotional neglect.** Children need positive attention from adults in order to develop intellectually, socially, and emotionally. Children are at risk when they
  - ➤ receive very little or no attention and affection. This is especially crucial for infants and very young children.
  - ➤ are deprived of care for a serious mental health problem.
  - ➤ frequently witness the battering of a parent.
  - ➤ are allowed, or even encouraged, to use alcohol or other drugs.
- **Educational neglect.** Parents or guardians who fail to attend to children's educational needs deprive them of a basic right and leave them unprepared to compete for jobs later in life. Children are victims of educational neglect when they:
  - ➤ are allowed to be absent from school most or all of the time.
  - ➤ are not enrolled in school when they reach the age required by law.
  - ➤ have special educational needs (a physical or mental disability) that are not addressed by caregivers.

Cases of neglect present a dilemma for the authorities who investigate them. In a country as culturally and economically diverse as America, many factors can lead to neglect. Among some cultures represented in America, for example, leaving children alone is not considered unusual, and adults are not always aware of the danger. For such families, authorities must be sensitive to the need for education as opposed to punishment. Some families do not value education as highly as others and are quick to have older children stay home with younger children so the parents can work. And some families cannot afford special educational or psychological services for their children and may be unaware of how to obtain them. These families are not guilty of neglect; rather, they need information and support so that they can meet the special needs of their children.

Physical Abuse. The second most common way in which children are abused is by being punched, kicked, beaten, bitten, burned, shaken, or otherwise physically harmed. Often this kind of abuse is the result of a parent's losing her temper while caring for or disciplining a child. But physical abuse can also be a genuinely aggressive act of violence. No matter what the cause, however, physical violence, in addition to presenting physical harm, is emotionally devastating for children. Nearly 40,000 children are believed to be the victims of physical violence each year.

Sexual Abuse. Many experts believe that sexual abuse may be the least reported type of child abuse because of the shame and secrecy that surrounds this problem. Sexual abuse may consist of touching, fondling, or oral, anal, or vaginal sex. An adult's exposing his or her genitals, prostituting a child, and producing pornographic materials featuring children are also considered forms of child sexual abuse.

Girls are far more often the victims of sexual abuse than are boys. Government surveys have found that sexual abuse makes up about 13 percent of all cases of child abuse and that three-quarters of sexual abuse cases occur in children under age seven.

Records show that most child sexual abuse is committed by a friend or relative of the child's family, or by someone else known to the child. If a woman has

---

What to Do When a Baby Cries

Physical abuse can start when a new parent becomes frustrated at not being able to console her crying infant. Babies cry for a variety of reasons—such as when they are hungry or need to be changed. Crying also exercises a baby's lungs. Sometimes, though, babies cry because they are having a hard time adjusting to life outside the womb. This is not unusual. Crying is the only way babies can communicate with their parents and caregivers. If your baby is fed, warm, dry, and rested and if there is no medical reason for the crying, the best thing to do is to let your baby "cry it out" and keep your frustration under control.

When faced with a baby who will not stop crying, it is easy to think that the baby is crying just to irritate you. *That is never the case.* Rather, the baby is just responding to an internal need to cry. No matter how frustrated you get, it is important to remember: *Never shake a baby.* Shaking will not stop the crying. In fact, the crying will most likely intensify. Severe shaking can cause brain damage and even death (see sidebar titled "Shaken Baby Syndrome").

Here are some things you can do when a baby cries:

- Feed her slowly and burp often.
- Offer a pacifier.
- Hold her against your chest and walk or rock.
- Put on soft music or sing.
- Take the baby for a ride in a stroller or car, or put her in a baby swing.
- Sometimes babies just have to cry it out. If you have met all the baby's basic needs, but she continues to cry, it is recommended that you put the baby down in a crib or other safe place and walk out of the room. It is okay to go to another part of the house for a while, checking on her every 5 to 10 minutes. If, however, the crying continues for a very long time, and the baby can't seem to fall asleep, then call someone who can come and give you a break.

Source: The Shaken Baby Campaign, California Department of Social Services.

Shaken Baby Syndrome

Shaken baby syndrome (SBS) is a very serious problem that results when an infant or young child is violently shaken, usually by an adult caregiver to stop the child's crying. Because a baby's neck muscles are not yet strong enough to support her head, forceful shaking causes the fragile brain to bounce against the skull. The result can be blindness from a detached retina, brain damage, or death.

No one is certain how many babies suffer from SBS. This is because external injuries are rarely apparent in babies who are shaken. In about one-third of SBS cases, evidence is found that the child has been shaken previously. This suggests that the problem is not an isolated event, but rather occurs repeatedly.

It is remarkably easy for a new parent to become frustrated with a crying baby and feel at a complete loss about what to do. The temptation to shake a baby can happen unconsciously, even to an adult who is normally calm and rational. (See the box on page 285 for tips on calming a crying baby.)

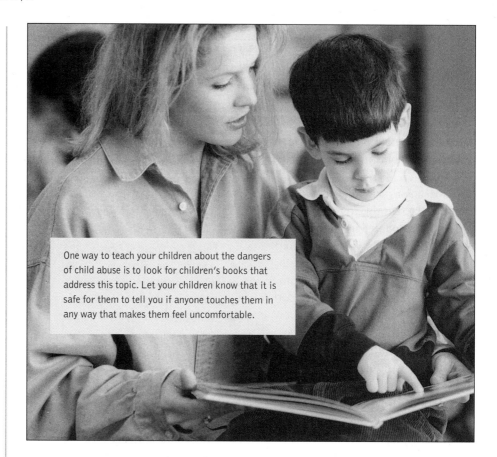

One way to teach your children about the dangers of child abuse is to look for children's books that address this topic. Let your children know that it is safe for them to tell you if anyone touches them in any way that makes them feel uncomfortable.

any reason to suspect a friend or relative, she is wise to watch carefully the behavior of that person around her children until she is reassured that there is no reason for alarm. It is difficult to explain to a child that a loved one or relative might be a threat. It is best to make sure a child knows she can come directly to you if she ever feels uncomfortable around anyone. With older children, it is possible to discuss real-life stories from newspapers or magazines that objectively introduce to them the idea that, though most people are trustworthy, threats and sexual advances from loved ones can sometimes happen.

Emotional Abuse. Children can be deeply hurt by emotional abuse, even though they suffer no physical injury. Emotional neglect is considered a passive form of abuse where children's needs are not met. Emotional *abuse* occurs when an adult intentionally rejects a child, punishes a child with extreme measures, or mistreats a child in any way that causes serious problems in behavior or mental health.

Because of its hidden nature, it is difficult to say how often emotional abuse occurs in children. Older children (aged 12 and over) seem to suffer emotional abuse more often than younger children, and it seems to be more common in girls than in boys. About 6,000 cases of emotional abuse are reported each year, but the true number of cases is almost certainly much higher.

This kind of abuse may take the form of extreme or bizarre forms of punishment, such as locking a child in a dark closet. More often, emotional abuse is less obvious. An emotional abuser may criticize, belittle, mock, or reject the child.

She may call the child names, swear at the child, or tell her that she is stupid, incompetent, or worthless. The abuser may switch back and forth from being loving and affectionate toward the child to being angry or indifferent.

This type of treatment, especially from a parent or caregiver, devastates children. A child who is abused may not understand what is going on, and blame herself. At the very least, emotionally abused children suffer damaged self-esteem. At worst, they may develop serious mental and emotional problems. Symptoms of emotional abuse include aggressive and violent behavior, withdrawal, fear of all people, difficulty connecting with friends, and difficulty concentrating. Anxiety and depressive mental disorders are thought to occur more often in people who were emotionally abused as children. Like the effects of more obvious forms of abuse, the effects of emotional abuse in childhood can last throughout a person's lifetime.

Long-Term Effects of Child Abuse

No matter what form child abuse takes, its victims are deeply affected by it physically, mentally, and emotionally. Many abused children have nightmares, for example, which interfere with getting proper rest, and then have trouble paying attention in school. The effects are usually long lasting, and people who were abused often require treatment by mental health professionals in order to form adequate relationships and achieve productive adult lives.

Abused children live in perpetual fear. They are at the mercy of their parents and are unable to leave the abusive situation. They are physically outmatched by their abusers and cannot defend themselves against the abuse. Furthermore, they have not yet developed the inner resources to protect themselves mentally and emotionally. So they react to their plight in any number of ways that are destructive to themselves and to others.

Taking Action to Prevent Child Abuse

Child abuse is a problem with far-reaching effects in society, but the situation is not hopeless. Being aware of the problem and helping to raise others' awareness is an important first step in stopping and preventing child abuse in all of its forms.

If You Suspect Child Abuse. The abuse of a child is a crime. In certain professions, especially health care, teaching, and counseling, it is required by law that any suspected or known instance of child abuse be reported to authorities.

Even if you are not legally bound to do so, it is important to take action if you know, or have reason to believe, that a child is being abused. It is not recommended that you attempt to confront an adult whom you suspect of abusing a child. If you are right, then the situation for the child may worsen, while you are helpless to act. It is best to enlist the aid of authorities.

If you suspect child abuse, call the National Child Abuse Hotline at 800-4-A-CHILD (800-422-4453). Counselors there can talk to you about the situation, give you more information about child abuse, and take steps to look into the matter themselves if necessary.

If You Are a Survivor of Abuse. Some statistics hold that as many as 30 percent of adult women have a history of having been abused as children. Because the

Talking to Your Child About Sexual Abuse

Child sexual abuse is a difficult subject for adults to talk about with children. It is crucial, though, for children to understand that no one has the right to touch them in the genital area or in any way that they don't like. In talking with children about sexual abuse, the point is not to frighten them but to make sure they know that adults who make sexual advances to children are doing a bad thing.

In many cases, the abuser threatens to harm or kill the child or someone she loves, such as her mother or sibling, if she "tells." So even if you ask a child if she is being abused, she may deny it to protect herself or her family from danger. Children must understand that it is safe to tell you if any adult approaches them in a sexual way, even if the abuser threatens them, and that you will never blame them for what has happened.

The Warning Signs of Child Abuse

If you work in a profession where you have contact with children, such as in a school or a childcare setting, it is important to be aware of the following indicators of possible child abuse or neglect. Most states have a specific reporting procedure.

Physical Indicators

- Unexplained bruises, welts, lacerations, or burns
- Unattended physical problems or medical needs
- Consistent hunger, poor hygiene, or inappropriate dress
- Torn, stained, or bloody underclothing
- Bruises or bleeding in the genital area

Behavioral Indicators

- Wary of adult contact
- Behavioral extremes— aggressiveness or withdrawal
- Afraid to go home
- Extended stays at school —arrives early and leaves late with no reason
- Constant fatigue, listlessness, or falling asleep in class
- Delinquent behavior

Source: National Committee for Prevention of Child Abuse, Raleigh, NC.

events were traumatic, the memories of abuse, especially sexual abuse, can be deeply buried or even "forgotten" for long periods. Survivors of childhood abuse are at risk for a number of physical, mental, and emotional problems. A large number of abused children overeat. Approximately one-third of women who were abused in childhood are depressed or have gynecological disorders. About one-fifth are in fair or poor health or have seriously thought about suicide.

Women who were abused as children are also at risk for a mental disorder known as posttraumatic stress disorder (PTSD). About one-third of child molestation victims and two-thirds of child rape victims develop PTSD. The disorder is marked by recurrent and frequent memories of the trauma that intrude on the person's thoughts, causing her extreme distress. These memories are so vivid that she feels as though she is actually reliving the event. The symptoms of PTSD can be so severe that the woman is unable to function normally. (See Chapter 12 for more information on PTSD.)

If you remember being abused, it is likely that the experience has left its mark. Fortunately, there are many sources that you can turn to for help. Chapter 12 and Resources at the end of the book provide information on seeking help for the emotional effects of trauma.

If You Are Tempted to Abuse. A surprisingly large number of parents report that they have been tempted to strike or shake their children, especially their babies, at times. Those who are successful at resisting the temptation are often those who can talk to friends, family members, or professional counselors about it. Such discussions do not have to be formal. Merely mentioning to a friend how difficult your child can be often alleviates the feelings of loneliness, isolation, or lack of control that parents of small children often feel.

Rape *and* **Sexual** Assault

Sexual crimes against women have occurred throughout history and have always been accompanied by shame and secrecy. Ironically the ones who feel shamed are generally not those who commit these acts, but their victims.

Until fairly recently, our society responded to rape and sexual assault with silence. Consequently, few rape victims pursued legal recourse against their attackers. When a woman did report an assault, thus bringing the subject out into the open, she was often treated with mistrust and suspicion. In court, her sexual history was scrutinized by the defense in an effort to discredit her. The circumstances surrounding the attack focused on her and her actions—what she was wearing and what she was doing out in the first place—with the implication that she had somehow invited the assault. Men, after all, have strong, even overpowering, sexual drives, the theory went, and cannot be expected to control themselves in the face of temptation.

Another prevalent attitude toward rape victims was that some women want to be assaulted, that "any woman who is raped is asking for it." No wonder so few women were willing to report that they had been raped.

The legal situation for women is slowly changing. Laws have been put into place that protect victims of rape from this "blame the victim" mentality. But real attitudes are slower to change. Women are still challenged, sometimes even by lawyers and judges, to prove that they did not want to be raped or did not somehow bring it on themselves. As recently as two years ago, a judge in a United States courtroom announced that a woman could not become pregnant while being raped, because for her to become pregnant, she would have to be sexually aroused. His statement was scientifically inaccurate, but was intending to convey that he believed she had consented to sex instead of being forced to have sex against her will.

Who Are the Victims?

Rape and sexual assault can and do happen to women of all ages, races, and ethnic backgrounds. There is no "typical" rape victim, but data show the crime to be more common among women aged 20 to 24, those who have never been married, and women with some college education. The very young, the mentally or physically handicapped, and the elderly are also susceptible. Rates of sexual crimes, like all other violent crimes, are higher in urban areas.

About three-quarters of rapes and sexual assaults are committed by someone the victim knows. In about half of cases, this is a "friend" or other acquaintance. Intimate partners are responsible for about one-quarter of these crimes.

The Nature of Sexual Violence

It is now understood that rapists are men who are usually driven not by sexual desire, but by violence and a desire for power and control. Like battering and other forms of chronic abuse, rape terrorizes women. Men who assault women often have a need to punish, humiliate, and terrify their victims in order to make themselves feel powerful and in control.

Legally, rape is defined as forced sexual intercourse—vaginal or anal—by another person who penetrates the victim with his penis or with an object. Sexual assault is defined as the forcing of sexual behavior on another person, but without completed or attempted sexual intercourse, such as oral sex.

Nearly half a million women reported being raped or sexually assaulted in 1994 alone, which translates to about four assaults for every 1,000 females aged 12 and over. Because of the shame and secrecy that still surrounds sexual violence, many victims fail to report these crimes, so the actual rate of these crimes against women is difficult to assess. It is widely believed that the actual number of victims each year is closer to 2 million.

Marital Rape. Can a woman be raped by her husband? Historically, in many societies, sex was considered a married man's due, and he had the right to demand it. Forcing his wife to have intercourse with him, then, was not considered a crime, and the idea that rape could occur within a marriage was an almost impossible notion.

Marital rape remains one of the least studied and least often reported forms of rape, and it is difficult to find reliable statistics on the subject. Women who have been raped by their husbands may not necessarily consider the incident as rape. Surveys suggest, however, that at least ten percent of all married women have been raped or sexually assaulted by their husbands. Since rape is primarily a violence-driven act, marital rape is believed to be more common among women who are also abused by their husbands in other ways.

wellness **tip**

Don't be a victim. Be street savvy when you are out, especially at night. Avoid dark streets and buildings. Stay in populated areas—the more people around, the safer you are. If you are often in a high-risk neighborhood, consider carrying mace or pepper spray, but be sure you know how to use it against an attacker without harming yourself. Your local police department, YWCA, or community center may give classes in how to protect yourself. A loud whistle can be effective in warding off a possible assault.

Date Rape. A woman who is raped or sexually assaulted by a boyfriend, a casual date, or an acquaintance is the victim of date rape (sometimes called "acquaintance rape"). Like marital rape, the rate of date rape is difficult to estimate because the crime is so rarely reported. One survey of college women found that 12 to 15 percent had experienced date rape.

As stated earlier, the majority of assaults on women are made by men they know. So it is important for women, and especially for young women, to realize that, just because they have agreed to go out with a boy or a man, he does not have the right to force sexual activity on her. Date rape is still rape.

Even if a woman engages in sexual play of her own free will, she has the right to limit the extent of the activity. If she is forced to submit to intercourse and accuses her attacker of rape, the man may try to use the argument that she "led him on," or she "asked for it." But, in fact, unless she actually did ask for it, or gave clear consent, then his forcing her to have sex constitutes rape. Women and girls need constant reminders that *any sexual act that is not freely consented to is a form of sexual assault. This includes acts that a woman feels pressured to perform, even if she is not threatened physically.*

The Aftermath of Rape

Any type of sexual violence or coercion can be an overwhelming experience for the victim. Sexual crimes are a gross violation of a woman's personal integrity, and victims often suffer profound emotional effects, sometimes along with severe physical injuries. Both physical and emotional effects are equally damaging to a woman's health, and women need treatment for both in order to heal.

Physical Effects. The most apparent effects of rape are physical injuries, unintended pregnancy, and transmission of sexually transmitted diseases (STDs). Injuries from a rape are often doubly painful because of the way in which they occurred. Suffering physical pain from injuries, having to decide what to do about an unintended pregnancy, and dealing with discomfort and health threats from STDs are all constant reminders to a woman that she has been raped.

Injuries. As many as 40 percent of rape victims sustain physical injuries. Whether or not a woman is physically injured during a rape mostly depends on whether she tried to defend herself or fight off her attacker. Almost all women—up to 85 percent—do try to protect themselves from being raped. Those who do not—usually for fear of being more seriously hurt—are less likely to be injured, but are also more likely to be the victims of a completed rape.

Injuries from a rape may be minor and need minimal care, or they may be severe enough to put the victim in the hospital. A small number are fatal.

HIV and Other Sexually Transmitted Diseases. A tragic consequence of rape for some women is infection with HIV, the virus that causes AIDS. It is not known how many women with AIDS were infected from sexual assault. Chlamydia and gonorrhea may be the most common STDs acquired during rape. These are genital infections that can be cured with treatment. If untreated, however, they can have serious consequences. (See Chapter 22 for more information on STDs.)

Women who seek care after having been raped are given antibiotics to prevent the development of chlamydia, gonorrhea, syphilis, pelvic inflammatory disease, and other problems. They are also advised to be tested for HIV at intervals over the next year.

Pregnancy. It is estimated that two to four percent of rape victims who are not using a continuous form of birth control (such as an IUD or the pill) become pregnant as a result of the attack. For those who see a doctor soon afterward, pregnancy can be prevented by taking the "morning-after" pill—a high dose of oral contraceptive—which prevents the fertilized egg from attaching to the inside of the uterus. Often this treatment is given whether or not a rape victim thinks she may have a chance of becoming pregnant.

If a woman does become pregnant as a result of rape, the decision about what to do can be a difficult and painful one. Some women decide to continue the pregnancy and either raise the child or offer it for adoption. Others decide on abortion. Counseling and therapy can be enormously helpful for a woman trying to decide how to respond to this unwanted pregnancy.

Emotional Effects. A woman who has been raped or otherwise sexually assaulted has had her integrity, her dignity, and her sense of self damaged on a profound level. The emotional trauma that follows a sexual attack may be less obvious to the eye than the physical effects, but it can be even more painful and long-lasting. Injuries heal, and most STDs can be cured, but emotional pain and the memory of the event can take many years to overcome.

Posttraumatic Stress Disorder. Rape and sexual assault are common causes of PTSD in women. This disorder, described earlier in the chapter, occurs in one-third more women than men after any type of trauma. The effects of PTSD can seriously interfere with a woman's ability to function. Therapy—and sometimes medication—is needed to help a woman overcome this disorder. (See Chapter 12 for information about PTSD.)

Rape Trauma Syndrome. The intense anxiety and fear that many women feel after being raped can lead to a condition known as rape trauma syndrome. This condition usually begins when a woman loses her ability to cope with everyday life. She may feel "paralyzed" and unable to function. Some women lose all emotional control and others appear calm and almost unaffected by the incident. Such outward demeanor, however, almost always conceals deep emotional pain and turmoil.

The Date Rape Drug

Rohypnol (generic name, flunitrazem) is a powerful sedative made in Europe and Latin America. Sometimes called "roofies," the drug has been implicated in date rape cases. Rohypnol relaxes the muscles and lowers inhibitions. Taken in high doses or combined with alcohol, it acts quickly—within 15 to 30 minutes—and causes complete blackouts and memory loss for up to 12 hours. It is illegal in the United States.

Recent reports suggest that the drug can be dropped into a woman's drink at a party or a bar. It has no odor or taste and dissolves quickly, making the unsuspecting woman feel ill or dizzy. She may then be "helped home" by a man who subsequently rapes her. Women have reported waking in an unfamiliar place, with bruises that clearly indicate they have been raped but with no memory of the incident.

Always keep a close eye on what you eat and drink in social situations, especially when you are among strangers. (Manufacturers of Rohypnol are now adding color and making it less soluble so particles float to the top.) Go out with one or more friends so that you can keep an eye on one another if someone becomes ill. If a friend seems to be having symptoms of Rohypnol intoxication, do not under any circumstances allow her to leave with an untrustworthy escort.

wellness **tip**

If you have been assaulted, whether you plan to press charges or not, call a rape crisis hot line and discuss the incident and your emotions. Remember, the people who staff rape-crisis centers are professionally trained and familiar with the emotional effects of sexual assault.

This first phase of rape trauma syndrome may be followed by other signs and symptoms, which can surface months or even years after the rape. The woman may have trouble eating and sleeping. She may feel she is going crazy or may have nonspecific pain throughout her body. She may have symptoms, such as vaginal or rectal itching or discharge, for which no cause can be found. She may develop phobias or begin to have flashbacks or nightmares.

Counseling and therapy are needed to overcome rape trauma syndrome. A therapist who is skilled in working with rape and trauma victims can help a woman come to terms with the emotional aftermath of rape so that she can move on with her life.

Should You Report an Assault? As stated earlier, it is estimated that only about half of all rapes are reported to the police. Many women feel that they will not be believed if they report the crime. Others may simply feel unable to talk about it.

If you have been raped, you do not have to report the crime in order to get an appropriate medical examination and preventative care, but you *should* be examined by a physician. If more than a day has passed since your rape, you may have missed the chance to collect evidence of the rape, but you should still receive an evaluation of your STD and pregnancy risk.

The Post-Rape Examination: What to Expect. Though it is extremely difficult for most women, it is best not to shower or clean up after an attack. All your instincts may be directing you to rid yourself of your clothes and submerse yourself in a hot tub or shower. But if you do, you will wash away valuable evidence that can help authorities catch and punish your attacker.

Even if you do not want to report the assault, call someone you trust who will accompany you to the hospital emergency room. Take a change of clothes. You need to be examined and treated, if necessary. They can also collect evidence in case you later decide to press charges. Many women decide to report the rape days after their physical examination, and they are grateful that evidence has been collected that can convict the rapist.

At the hospital, doctors and nurses will perform a thorough examination. Many hospitals have access to rape crisis workers who will come and stay with you through this examination. The procedures used may vary from state to state, but the following are standard:

- You will be told what to expect during the examination and asked to sign a consent form.
- In order to record and retrieve evidence of the crime, doctors and nurses will:
  - ➤ Inspect the surface of your entire body to look for bruises or scratches.
  - ➤ Examine the genital area.
  - ➤ Comb the pubic hair to find pubic hair of the attacker.
  - ➤ Collect fingernail scrapings in case you scratched your attacker.
  - ➤ Collect clothing that might reveal additional evidence.
- Any physical injuries will be documented and treated.
- A pelvic examination will be performed to find whether you have been injured externally or have any internal injuries to your vagina or lower abdomen. Specimens will also be taken from your vagina and cervix to test for STDs.

- Blood will be drawn to check your baseline syphilis, HIV, and pregnancy status. (Follow-up testing will also be required—especially for HIV.)
- You will be asked to give a detailed account of what happened, including the identity of your attacker if you know him, or a physical description if you do not. Examination and treatment will not be withheld if you choose not to identify your attacker for any reason.
- You will be asked detailed questions about your last menstrual period, your birth control methods, and when you last had consensual sex. This helps to interpret the findings of your examination and make appropriate recommendation for treatment.

After the examination and other procedures are completed, you can bathe and change into fresh clothes.

Your Legal Options and Rights. If you decide to pursue your legal rights, you may be asked to give an account of events to the police or other authorities. It helps to have a support person with you to help you through this difficult process.

There are many local rape crisis centers across the nation that can help you find legal services and support. A national network, the Rape, Abuse, and Incest National Network (RAINN), has a 24-hour hot line that will direct you to the crisis center nearest you. RAINN can be reached at 800-656-HOPE (800-656-4673).

Youth **Violence**

Violence affects the lives of many young people in the United States. Statistics show that teenagers and young adults are more likely than older persons to be the victims of violence:

- Young people aged 12 to 24 are the victims of almost half of all violent crimes, though they make up less than one-quarter of the U.S. population.
- Violence is the second most common cause of death in young people ages 15 to 24.
- Violence is the third leading cause of death in all African American males.

Women need to be aware of the factors that are linked to youth violence so that they can protect themselves and their families and head off violent behavior before it begins in older children and teenagers. They can also lend their voices to the support of prevention programs and legislation that address the causes of youth violence.

High-Risk Factors

Teenagers and young adults are more likely to commit violent acts against others. In fact, the number of youthful violent offenders has risen sharply in recent years. The causes of violent behavior in young people are complex. Experts believe that personal characteristics, life experience, social influences, and genetics may all contribute to a young person's tendency toward violence. No one can say for sure what leads a particular person to commit violent acts, but some personal characteristics and environmental influences have been associated with a high probability of violent behavior.

- Personal factors predisposing toward violent behavior:
  - ➤ Low self-esteem; impulsiveness; an inclination to take risks
  - ➤ A history of family or neighborhood violence or abuse
  - ➤ Indifference to disapproval and punishment
  - ➤ Lack of empathy for the feelings of others

- Environmental factors predisposing toward violent behavior:
  - ➤ Poverty, unemployment, and poor education
  - ➤ Easy access to weapons
  - ➤ The presence of violent role models in daily life, on TV, and in books, movies, and popular music
  - ➤ Pressure from peers or gangs
  - ➤ Access to alcohol or other drugs

None of these variables can be said to directly cause violent behavior in a young person, but they do increase the risk. Many young people who resort to violent behavior feel that they have few prospects for leading lives that society deems successful. In some neighborhoods where violence, drug dealing, poverty, and unemployment are prevalent, it is relatively easy for a young person to conclude that joining a gang or dealing drugs is the best available option for winning some measure of esteem, security, and financial gain.

Protective Factors

Social scientists have also identified traits in young people that indicate a low risk for violent behavior. Sometimes called protective factors, they help a child resist the stresses that could otherwise lead to violence:

Youth Gang Violence

In major cities across the United States, youth gangs raise the level of daily violence. Youth gangs are structured, organized groups of young people with strict codes of conduct and extensive involvement in drug-dealing and violence. Wars between rival gangs lead to injury and death for many members each year, and untold numbers of innocent bystanders are also injured or killed.

Young people join gangs out of a need for acceptance, support, and a sense of belonging and commitment. In an environment where these needs are not met by adults and positive youth movements, gangs provide a way for many youths to endow their lives with meaning and purpose, however destructive the consequences may be.

Other reasons for joining youth gangs may include:
- Desire for recognition and power
- Need for companionship and friendship
- Love of excitement
- Need for physical safety and protection
- Tradition set by older siblings

Many parents feel helpless in preventing their children from joining gangs. Solutions include becoming involved in youth centers where meaningful community activities are encouraged, finding mentors, and focusing on establishing strong, extended family where positive role models are a continual positive influence on the lives of young people.

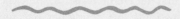

- A thoughtful approach to decision making and an awareness of times when they may be prone to impulsive acts of violence
- A sense of self-worth and a belief that one can change one's circumstances and environment for the better
- Personal strategies for coping with stress and avoiding conflict
- Good interpersonal skills with friends, parents, and teachers

Young people who successfully emerge from adverse circumstances and become nonviolent, caring adults have many of these traits in common. They also have parents, mentors, and peers who have helped them establish these positive habits.

Preventing Violence *at Home* and in *Your* Community

Across the country, women are finding ways to stop or prevent violence and abuse and to support the victims of violence. Many public and private groups are running programs to curb the violence in their communities. More parents are realizing the importance of raising their children in a strong and supportive environment in which parental involvement is high. More women than ever before are speaking out about the violence and abuse they have experienced throughout their lives.

Guns and Drugs

Drug abuse and access to a gun are closely linked to violent crime. Alcohol use is found to be a factor in more than half of all the murders that occur each year in the United States. Alcohol is a depressant; it impairs thinking and judgment and decreases inhibitions, sparking rash and impulsive behavior. Narcotic drugs,

FIGURE 14.2
Teaching Kids About Guns
Parents can play a vital role in preventing gun violence in their homes and communities. Here are seven things parents can do to make a difference.

1. Teach all children—from preschoolers to teenagers—that guns can hurt and kill.

2. Encourage children to report any weapon they know about at school or on the street to the police or an adult they trust. Tell them not to touch the weapon for any reason.

3. Explain to children that gun violence in the movies, on TV shows, and in video games is not real. Stress that in real life guns hurt and kill people.

4. Show children how to settle arguments without resorting to words or actions that hurt. Talk openly with your children about their problems. Set a good example in how you handle anger, disagreements, and sadness.

5. Support school staff in their efforts to keep guns, knives, and other weapons out of schools.

6. Because handguns are more likely to be used in suicide, homicide, or fatal accidents than in self-defense, it's safest not to keep a gun in the home.

7. If you choose to own firearms—handguns, rifles, or shotguns—make sure they are unloaded and securely stored. Invest in trigger locks, gun cabinets with a lock, or pistol lock boxes. Lock up ammunition separately.

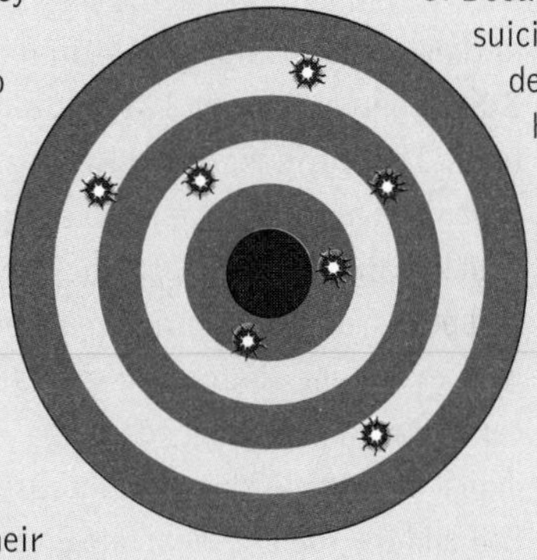

Source: Adapted from materials from Handgun Control, Inc.

such as heroin and cocaine, are also strongly linked to violent behavior. Street drugs are highly addictive, and addicts often commit violent crimes in order to obtain money to buy drugs. In the illegal drug market, violence is also used routinely to protect or expand a dealer's territory.

It is estimated that well over 200 million guns are privately owned in the United States. This number reflects only registered guns, with large numbers of unregistered and illegal weapons suspected. Many of the guns used to commit violent crimes are sold illegally or obtained from family members or friends.

Women Who Have Made a Difference

Many women feel so overwhelmed by the widespread gun violence in the United States that they believe they cannot possibly influence change on their own. The following three stories illustrate that individuals can make a difference and will hopefully encourage you to take action. Looked at collectively, the efforts of individual women in their own families, neighborhoods, or towns add up to positive changes that benefit everyone.

Tina Johnson, whose husband was shot in the back on a business trip to San Francisco in 1992, initiated the Silent March, a national memorial demonstration against gun violence. Pairs of shoes representing the 40,000 people who are killed by guns each year are donated by family members, relatives, and friends of the victims, and displayed in Washington, D.C. This event, held every other year, brings together gun control activists and concerned individuals from across the country. Johnson is currently involved in a class action suit against every firearm manufacturer in the country, suing them for negligence in marketing and advertising their products.

In December 1993, Arlene and Jacob Locicero lost their daughter Amy in the Long Island Railroad massacre, in which a man opened fire on the passengers of a crowded railroad car. In response to their daughter's death, Arlene and Jacob have lobbied vigorously in Washington,

speaking before senatorial hearings to support the Brady Bill, the Assault Weapons Ban, and other gun control measures. They have also worked on the campaigns of state legislators who pledge to eradicate gun violence.

On October 31, 1992, a Japanese exchange student named Yoshi Hatori, who was staying with Holley Galland Haymaker and her husband, Dick, in Baton Rouge, La., went to the wrong address for a Halloween party. Instead of simply asking Yoshi who he was, the man who lived there pulled out a gun and yelled "freeze!" Yoshi didn't understand and took a step forward saying he was lost. The man shot him in cold blood.

Sparking international outrage, Yoshi's murder had broad ramifications. Yoshi's parents took their son's body back to Japan and initiated a petition, gathering over one million signatures of Japanese citizens, asking President Clinton to do something about the easy availability of guns in the United States. Holley and Dick Haymaker launched a similar nationwide campaign in the United States, gathering over 125,000 signatures. The Haymakers and Hatoris then organized a conference in Washington, which featured all the petitions signed and boxed, and were granted a meeting with President Clinton. These and other related activities influenced the President's decision to sign both the Brady Bill and the Assault Weapons Ban.

Handguns can be bought for $100 or less.

The fact that guns are so easy to obtain is a major factor in ongoing violence across many areas of the country. Organizations, such as the Center to Prevent Handgun Violence, are working hard to pass legislation that makes it more difficult for people to acquire weapons. They are also working on safety regulations, such as childproof gun locks, and safe storage legislation. Another national organization, the Coalition to Stop Gun Violence, serves as a clearinghouse for information, ideas, and advice to help citizens have more of an impact in reducing gun violence in their communities. The Violence Policy Center in Washington, D.C., which has conducted research on women and guns, also works to prevent handgun violence and promote greater regulation of the firearms industry. Their statistics, for example, have debunked the gun industry's promotional efforts toward women ("You'll be safer with a gun" and "A gun will protect you from strangers") by documenting that women are more likely to get shot by husbands or lovers (or ex-husbands or ex-lovers) than by strangers.

Other organizations, such as the National Rifle Association, work to counter such efforts, arguing that the right to bear arms should not be compromised for any reason. They also argue that if laws are changed to make the purchase of legal firearms more difficult, only the criminals will have access to weapons, leaving the law-abiding population defenseless.

The controversy rages on, but it is important to know that women can mount an eloquent argument for the reduction of firearms. Many have already been instrumental in creating concrete solutions. Sarah Brady, for example, whose husband was rendered handicapped by the gunman who attempted to assassinate President Reagan, worked tirelessly to pass the Brady Bill, which specifies a five-day waiting period so that a background check can be made on anyone buying firearms in this country.

Another way women can help prevent gun violence is to insist that firearms be handled safely by their partners. Although women do own guns, by far the majority of gun owners are men. Research shows that having a gun in the house greatly increases the chances that either accidental or intentional violence will occur. Women can influence their partners in the safe storage of weapons in the home and can educate children about the dangers of handling firearms.

Community Solutions

Programs to reduce violence in neighborhoods and communities have been found to work best when they address the roots of the problem. Job and vocational skills training, counseling, educational assistance and tutoring, and social and recreational activities provide people with a sense of community and purpose. These programs offer alternatives to violent behavior for increasing numbers of adults and instill in young people a sense of hope for the future.

To stop domestic violence and child abuse, many community centers offer classes in parenting skills and family counseling. Public information campaigns continue to help raise awareness of the problem of violence. In many schools, peers are learning to help resolve disputes, reshaping students' thinking about violent behavior. Youth programs, such as the Center to Prevent Handgun Violence's STAR (Straight Talk About Risks) program, teach anger management, peer mediation, conflict resolution, and life and social skills to young people so that they can confront the problems and challenges of daily life without the use of violence or drugs.

These and other efforts are vital to violence prevention at all levels of society. The most effective initiatives start at the level of the individual, helping her to see the available options for confronting life's challenges. When they know what

wellness **warning**

If you have children, talk to them about the dangers of playing with guns, or even handling them. Many mothers now ask first if a gun is kept in the home of their children's friends before allowing them to play there. The best way to set an example for your children is never to have a handgun in your house.

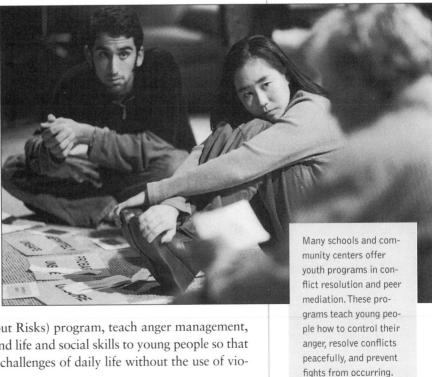

Many schools and community centers offer youth programs in conflict resolution and peer mediation. These programs teach young people how to control their anger, resolve conflicts peacefully, and prevent fights from occurring.

resources are available to them, women can increase their own as well as their children's safety and health.

What *You* Can Do

It is essential that you learn to recognize and protect yourself and your family from violence. Whether you live in a relatively dangerous environment or in a relatively safe one, you are at risk. The following guidelines can help make your community safer for women and children:

- Make a commitment to raise your children in an atmosphere of love, respect, and trust, which can go a long way toward preventing them from becoming involved in violence as they grow older.
- Bring other trustworthy adults into your children's lives to serve as role models who can help them see the rewards of a life without violence. Research suggests that the more interactions children have with caring adults who are not their parents, the more likely they will be to resist violence, drugs, and other threats to their health and safety.
- If you suspect child or partner abuse, or if you yourself are a victim, seek help and advice from domestic violence hot lines or social workers, or from the resources provided in this book.
- If you know someone who is a victim, try to be a source of support and strength for her. Let her know that your home can be a safe haven for her and her children in an emergency, and let her know about organizations that can help with support and information.
- Protect yourself by being street smart: be aware of who is around you in public, and avoid unlit and sparsely populated places after dark.
- Get involved in supporting efforts to prevent violence, both in your community and across the nation. Support legislation that increases positive police presence in violence-prone neighborhoods and that decreases access to firearms.
- Volunteer for a community program, or start a Neighborhood Watch on your street. You just might make the difference that can break the cycle of violence.

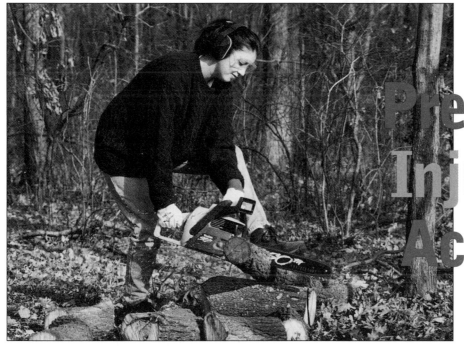

Chapter 15

Preventing Injury *and* Accidents

According to the U.S. Public Health Service, unintentional injuries are the fourth leading cause of death in the United States, and the leading cause of death for those aged 5 to 34 years. Many injuries are directly tied to common, everyday activities, such as driving, bicycling, or making household repairs. They are, for the most part, both predictable and preventable. Behaving within sensible limits, making time for appropriate and thorough preparation, and using appropriate protective equipment can drastically reduce your risk of causing or having an accident, and therefore, an injury—no matter what the activity.

At home it makes good sense to examine your house and yard for potential hazards and plan for safety by taking simple steps to avoid fire, falls, electric shock, and other "accidents waiting to happen." Basic safety and accident prevention are neither time-consuming nor expensive—especially when you weigh the benefits against the pain, damage, and cost of an injury. Thinking safety means taking simple precautions around the house and during activities away from home to protect you and your family.

Safety is also an important consideration in the workplace. Apart from risks of accidents and repetitive injury, you need to be concerned about any potentially toxic substances with which you might come into contact—especially if you are pregnant or planning a pregnancy in the near future.

This chapter offers suggestions for preventing common accidents in and outside the home and in the workplace. For specific suggestions on preventing injuries in age-related accidents—among infants, children, adults, and older adults—consult Part II of this book.

preview

▶ **Preventing Motor Vehicle Injuries**

▶ **Safety at Home**

▶ **Safety at Work**

▶ **Preventing Recreational Accidents**

▶ **First Aid and Cardiopulmonary Resuscitation**

▶ **What You Can Do**

Preventing Motor
Vehicle Injuries

"Don't Drink and Drive!" "Buckle Up for Safety!" We've all heard these slogans countless times. Far too often, however, these warnings go unheeded or are disregarded. According to the U.S. Public Health Service, most motor vehicle crashes and injuries can be linked to alcohol use, failure to wear safety belts, or both. Motor vehicle accidents are the leading cause of deaths due to preventable injury, accounting for nearly half of all such fatalities.

Most automobile injuries can be avoided by the proper placement and use of seat belts and shoulder harnesses, car seats for infants and toddlers, and air bags. In addition to avoiding drinking and driving, driving defensively instead of aggressively—including not driving over the speed limit and watching out for others—can help keep you and others on the road out of danger.

Understanding Blood Alcohol Levels

According to the National Highway Traffic Safety Administration (NHTSA), 41 percent of all traffic fatalities in 1995 involved alcohol. Clearly, not enough drivers understand that it takes surprisingly little alcohol to impair judgment, coordination, vision, and responsiveness. For most people, a blood alcohol content level of between .04 and .08 percent will dim their faculties. However, the *legal* blood alcohol content for driving is higher. Depending on what state you live in, the legal limit ranges from .05 to .10 percent.

Most people become legally intoxicated when they consume up to three drinks in an hour. (A "drink" equals one 12-ounce beer, a 4-ounce glass of wine, or a 1 1/4 ounce shot of hard liquor.) It may take less for women, because they have lower levels of alcohol dehydrogenase in their bodies, the enzyme that breaks down alcohol. Lower body weight, medications (especially antihistamines or sedatives), drinking on an empty stomach, and lack of sleep can also lead to quicker intoxication. Many people think they can safely drive after a couple of drinks and refuse to recognize that they are intoxicated.

Passenger Restraints

Passenger restraints (safety belts and air bags) have been proven to save lives in car collisions. In a crash, unrestrained drivers and passengers can be thrown against the front or side of their vehicle's passenger compartment, causing fractures, internal bleeding, organ damage, and too often, death. Such injuries can even occur in low-speed crashes. Most accidents happen within a 20 mile radius of one's home, so it is important for *everyone* riding in a car to buckle up *every time,* no matter how short the trip.

Safety Belts. All car passengers need to wear both lap and shoulder restraints. The shoulder strap must be snug and positioned over the collarbone—not behind the back, under the arm, or over the abdomen. The lap belt should fit low and tight across the hips. Check the condition of safety belts yearly, and have them replaced if they are frayed or worn. When you bring your car in for service, have the safety belt mechanisms checked as well.

In cars with air bags, seat and shoulder restraints must also be worn. Air bags were not developed to replace seat belts, but rather to work with them. Injury or even death may result from not wearing a safety belt when an air bag is deployed.

Air Bags. Air bags are designed to buffer the head, neck, and upper body in the event of a front-end collision. They deploy instantaneously on impact, using compressed air, and deflate quickly thereafter. Air bags have been proven to save hundreds of lives every year.

Air bags deploy with an explosive velocity (up to 200 miles per hour). For passengers and drivers who are not seated in the proper position (upright in their seat) or are not restrained by a seat belt, an inflating air bag can deal a sharp blow to the head and body. That is why it is essential for drivers and front seat passengers to wear their seat belts. It is also wise to sit in a normal, upright position (with your back fully against the seat).

Child Car Seats. By law, infants and toddlers must ride in specially designed car seats. (It is illegal in the United States for a newborn to leave the hospital by car without being placed in a car seat.) To work properly, the seat must be appropriately sized and anchored securely, using the car's safety belts. Infant seats should face the rear of the car and be used from birth until the child weighs more than 20 pounds.

Convertible car seats provide rear-facing protection for infants and forward-facing protection when children have reached sufficient size (over 20 pounds). Among convertible seats there are different types of harness systems, as well as some with tray shields that flip down over the child's chest and waist. When children have outgrown convertible seats, they should ride in booster seats, which come in styles designed to fit cars with rear seat shoulder-lap restraints, and those with only lap belts. Some newer model vehicles feature built-in child seats for toddlers. These are also considered to be safe.

The American Academy of Pediatrics recommends that parents keep car seat instructions attached to the car seat, and that they check to see that the child seat is securely attached to the vehicle with seat belts every time they put their child in the car.

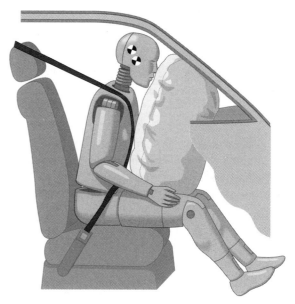

FIGURE 15.1
Airbag Watch
While airbags save hundreds of lives each year, they can also be dangerous if not used in conjunction with seat belts, since they deploy with an explosive force of up to 200 miles per hour. For maximum safety, wear your lap and shoulder belts every time you ride in a car, whether it is equipped with airbags or not.

Driving Safely

Nothing can help you avoid motor vehicle accidents and maintain the well-being of your passengers better than driving safely. Following are some tips for safe motoring.

Defensive Driving. Good driving includes, of course, obeying all traffic rules and being courteous to other drivers. Defensive driving means being alert at every moment for irresponsible driving on the part of others. It also means identifying dangerous situations in plenty of time to avoid them. For example, a defensive

Safety Tips and Air Bag Precautions

The NHTSA and the National Safety Council urge drivers and passengers to follow a few simple but important steps in order to prevent injury from air bags while also enhancing protection:

- For maximum safety protection in all types of crashes, always wear your safety belt.
- Do not sit or lean unnecessarily close to air bag panels (in the steering wheel and dashboard).
- Move driver and front passenger seats as far back as possible.
- Do not place any objects over the dashboard air bag panel or between the panel and yourself.
- Do not install rear-facing child car seats in the front passenger seat.
- Place children aged 12 and under in the back seat, in proper restraints.

Source: National Highway Transportation Safety Administration, Proposal for Air Bag Safety Warning Labels. Notice #103.

driver slows down and looks both ways at an intersection even when she has a green light, just in case another driver runs the red light.

Other defensive driving techniques you can practice include giving yourself ample time to reach your destination, paying attention to road conditions, and keeping your vehicle in safe working order.

Medications and Other Substances. Apart from alcohol, other substances can hamper your ability to drive. It is important to avoid driving when you are taking any medications that can make you drowsy, including antihistamines, antinausea medications, and sedatives. It is a good idea not to drive after taking a new medication, just in case it makes you drowsy. Marijuana and other illicit substances are not only illegal but also impair your judgment, coordination, vision (especially in dim light or at night), and responsiveness.

Sleepiness. Many car accidents occur when a driver falls asleep at the wheel. If you are significantly fatigued, it is best not to drive at all. If sleepiness overcomes you while you are driving, do not try to fight it and keep going. Pull over and rest. If you are traveling with another licensed driver, let her know of the problem and ask her to drive. Do not rely on caffeine and other stimulants to counteract the effects of sleepiness.

Even with ample sleep, driving for long periods can make you less alert. To prevent becoming sleepy on the road, avoid driving for long stretches. Stop every 100 miles or so and take a brisk walk. Play music and keep fresh air circulating throughout the car. Also try to limit the bulk of your driving to daylight hours, when possible.

Carbon monoxide from a damaged car exhaust can leak into a car's interior and cause drowsiness or even death. If you find yourself feeling drowsy without good reason, open the windows at once and stop the car. Have the exhaust system inspected as soon as possible.

Personal Upset. Try to avoid driving if you are experiencing any type of emotional upset. Anger, anxiety, depression, grief, nervousness, and fear can spawn erratic behavior and impair your faculties, raising your risk of having an accident. If you have an argument with a loved one, are given bad news, or experience an attack of anxiety, be sure you have calmed down before you drive, or ask someone else to take you where you need to go.

Distractions. Although it should go without saying, it is important that drivers concentrate on driving when behind the wheel, and nothing else. Disregard the distractions of passengers, poor radio reception, the desire to smoke, eat, drink, or change radio stations, and any inclination to check your appearance in the rearview mirror while the car is moving. If something really must be dealt with, such as an argument between children in the back seat, pull over, or wait until you are stopped at a traffic light.

One relatively new distraction to safe driving are car or cellular phones. A study conducted in Canada found that drivers are 4.3 times more likely to have an auto accident when driving while using a phone (both the handheld and speaker varieties), than they would be without using a phone. If you own a car or cellular phone, limit use to when you are at a stop light or parked.

Safety *at* Home

The home, if not carefully checked and maintained, can be full of health hazards. Fire, poisoning, falls, cuts, electric shock, and other unforeseen accidents and injuries are all largely avoidable. They tend to occur in homes where the occupants have not taken simple precautions.

Fire Prevention and Escape Planning

Carelessness with cigarettes and matches, improper storage of flammable liquids, candles left unattended, incautious use of wood-burning stoves and space heaters, and worn out or faulty wiring are common causes of housefires. Homeowners can greatly reduce the risk of a blaze by taking the time to conduct a careful search for fire hazards and practicing caution with cooking, candles, fireplaces, and wood-burning stoves. Planning an escape route and training family members are essential to avoiding injury in case there is a fire. And no home should be without smoke detectors and fire extinguishers.

Prevention. The best way to protect yourself from fire injury is to prevent fire altogether. Conduct a careful inspection of your house on a yearly basis. You might also want to call your local fire department for assistance. Free fire safety checklists and brochures are often available, as are home fire safety inspections. It can never hurt to have your house checked by a professional.

Care with Flames and Combustible Materials. A significant number of household fires are caused by such flammable solvents as paint thinner and turpentine, and by such fuels as kerosene, charcoal lighter fluid, and gasoline. Always use flammable materials outdoors or in well-ventilated spaces. These compounds emit strong vapors and should be kept away from flames or sparks. Store them in well-sealed, metal safety containers. If you can, avoid storing flammable liquids inside your home.

Fires often stem from errant flames or sparks from such common sources as matches, candles, and cigarettes. Always keep matches well out of the reach of children. Teach your children about the dangers of fire and the risks posed by playing with matches. Some parents teach their older children how to strike matches safely.

Smoking is a leading cause of household fires. If you or someone in your household must smoke indoors, provide ashtrays made of glass, metal, or some other fireproof material. Do not empty ashtrays into the trash until all embers are out and the ashes have *cooled completely.* Never smoke in bed or when drowsy.

Teaching Your Children to Be Fire-Savvy

Children are especially vulnerable to fire. A lack of knowledge about the dangers posed by flames and matches (combined with natural, youthful curiosity) can often lead to burns and household blazes. Here are some tips for educating your children about avoiding fire and about the steps they should take when fire strikes. By teaching fire safety, you will protect not only your children, but the rest of your family and your home as well.

- Make sure your children understand the seriousness of fires.
- Show your children the location of fire extinguishers. Teach them how to use them.
- Plan fire escape routes and plans, and rehearse them as a family.
- Teach children to keep flammable materials away from heaters.
- Teach children how to extinguish burning clothes by dropping and rolling.
- Ensure that your children know how to call for help by dialing 911.

Safety Items to Keep in the Home

As part of accident and emergency preparation, it is advisable to keep certain items accessible in a central location in the home (in the bathroom or near the telephone). Store a first-aid kit, working flashlight and extra batteries, and a list of telephone numbers to call in an emergency. The American Red Cross recommends that you also keep a first-aid kit in each car and one near you at sporting events or on camping trips. A first-aid kit should include the following items:

- **A small flashlight and batteries**
- **Scissors and tweezers**
- **Triangular bandages**
- **Antiseptic towelettes and ointment**
- **Adhesive bandages in assorted sizes**
- **Gauze pads and rolled gauze**
- **First-aid adhesive tape**
- **Disposable latex gloves**
- **Cold pack**
- **Ipecac syrup**
- **Activated charcoal**

Cooking. According to the U.S. Consumer Product Safety Commission (CPSC), cooking equipment is associated with more than 100,000 fires annually and almost 400 deaths and 5,000 injuries. The CPSC offers the following recommendations for avoiding cooking-related fires:

- Never place or store pot holders, plastic utensils, towels, and other noncooking equipment on or near the range since these items can ignite.
- Avoid wearing long, loose sleeves since they may catch fire while one is cooking. They may also catch on a pot's handle, overturning the pot and causing scalds. If you do wear long, loose sleeves roll them up or fasten them with pins or elastic bands while cooking.
- Always keep an eye on what you are cooking on the stove. Untended pots and pans can ignite into grease fires or can boil over.
- Keep cookware handles turned toward the back of the range top, out of reach of grasping children. Also, do not put cookies or other treats on the stove. Children might be tempted to reach up to or even climb on the stove.

If a fire does break out on the stove or in the oven, use a fire extinguisher or douse the flames with baking soda. Never use water on a cooking fire. If there is burning grease, water can actually cause the flames to flare up and spread. Never mix water and hot grease. Add foods to hot oil very carefully, because splashed or spattering grease can cause severe burns. Allow greasy pots and pans to cool before you wash them.

Supplemental Heat. According to the CPSC, wood- and coal-burning stoves and space heaters (fueled by gas, kerosene, or electricity) have been linked to roughly 22 percent of all household fires annually, as well as to thousands of contact burns and carbon monoxide poisonings. Through faulty installation or improper use, they can easily cause injury and destruction.

If you have a fireplace in your home, use a proper spark screen or glass fire doors. Burn only wood, never highly flammable materials, such as trash or plastic, and never use gasoline or lighter fluids to light indoor fires. Also, be sure to have your fireplace, flue, and chimney inspected and cleaned to ensure proper functioning and to guard against creosote buildup, which can cause chimney fires. Keep rugs and other flammable materials well away from the hearth; a flame retardant hearth rug is a good idea. Never leave a child alone with a fire unless she has been properly educated about fire safety.

Most supplemental heat mishaps have to do with faulty installation and improper use. Coal- and wood-burning stoves must be installed by a professional, following manufacturers' instructions and fire and building code restrictions. They need to be cleaned regularly and should be used to burn approved materials only.

When using space heaters that burn gas or kerosene, make sure to follow the manufacturer's instructions for operation, and use only approved fuels. Never use gasoline in a kerosene heater. Use such devices only in rooms that are properly ventilated, as they can emit toxic or volatile fumes. Although they do not require special installation, electric space heaters also pose a significant fire risk. According to the CPSC, half the deaths and one-third of the injuries resulting from these heaters occur at night when users are asleep. It is recommended that electric heaters be operated away from combustible materials, that they not be used to dry out clothes, towels, or shoes, and that they not be placed atop cabinets, tables, or other furniture.

Wiring and Appliances. For wiring to be safe, it must be sufficient to handle the load required by each appliance it powers. Otherwise, fuses and circuit breakers will shut down conduction. If, as often happens, such safeguards are absent or malfunctioning, an excess of power will cause wires to overheat or short out, either of which could lead to a fire.

Many electrical fires can be traced to old wiring, installed before the advent of volt-hungry electrical appliances. If your home is old, or if your wiring shows signs of age, have your entire system inspected by a licensed electrical contractor. Signs of aging include wiring insulated with fabric (knob-and-tube wiring), dead electrical outlets, outlets and appliances that produce smoke, and exposed wires.

As part of your fire safety inspection, make sure that your appliances are powered by wiring and circuit breakers certified to handle heavy electric loads. Such systems should meet standards set by local coding authorities, as well as national standards (set by certified laboratories, such as Underwriters' Laboratories—indicated by the "UL" label). Before installing additional lighting or plugging in a powerful appliance, be sure that you have adequate wiring. This applies to extension cords as well. Like house wiring, extension cords must be able to handle the load required by the given appliance. Overloading outlets with extra adapters and extension cords that drive multiple appliances is another invitation to fire.

Smoke Detectors. These simple, inexpensive devices save thousands of lives each year. When properly installed and maintained, a smoke detector will sound a loud buzz or beep at the first hint of smoke. If properly heeded, this alarm should provide you with sufficient time to escape flames and the noxious smoke and gases they often produce. Household fires often occur at night, and many victims succumb to smoke inhalation in their sleep. Smoke inhalation is the leading direct cause of deaths due to fire.

Install smoke detectors in all living and sleeping areas. Test them regularly (every month) and change the batteries every six months. Many needless deaths occur each year in homes with smoke detectors that do not function because the batteries are dead or have been borrowed and never replaced.

Fire Extinguishers. Every home should have at least one fire extinguisher. A logical storage place is in the kitchen, where many household blazes are triggered by cooking and malfunctioning appliances. It is also recommended that one be installed on each floor of a multistory house, near a wood-burning stove, and in the garage. Check fire extinguishers regularly to ensure that they are charged.

Use a fire extinguisher only when you are sure it will put out the fire. Otherwise, evacuate the house immediately. Be sure that all members of your household learn how and when to use a fire extinguisher.

Planning Your Escape. In order to escape fire, it is critical that you have a clearly devised and rehearsed plan. Following are some basic guidelines:

Determine a meeting place that is a safe distance from the house, such as the mailbox at the end of the driveway. In the case of a fire, every family member should go to the meeting place, and once everyone is safely gathered, someone should call 911 from a neighbor's house. Under no circumstances should anyone reenter the burning building.

Make a floor diagram of the house, showing all doors and windows and clearly marking a primary and alternate escape route.

Practice the escape routes by turning off all lights and having each member sit in their rooms. Activate the fire alarm; family members should attempt to wake up the others and exit their rooms according to the plan, crawling low (under smoke), feeling doors (for heat), and meeting at the designated area. Practice the plan until you can do it quickly.

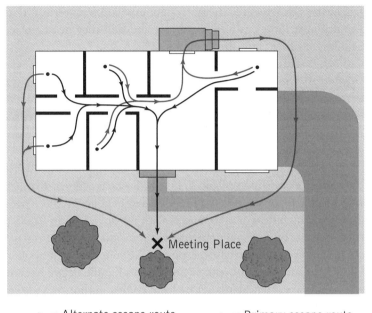

✕ Meeting Place

⟶ = Alternate escape route   ⟶ = Primary escape route

FIGURE 15.2

Fire Escape Plan

For quick and safe evacuation in case of a fire, devise a fire escape plan for your home. Draw up a sample plan, following the basic tips listed here, and make sure everyone in your home practices the escape routine.

- Establish at least two escape routes for each room in the home.
- Ensure that windows can be opened easily. Make sure safety grills can be removed from the inside.
- Provide escape ladders for upper-story windows. Be sure that everyone in the house can use them.
- Choose a place outside the house where the family can meet and you can quickly determine that everyone got out safely.
- Include all family members in fire escape planning. Practice escaping through all planned routes.

In the event of a fire, follow these tips and teach your entire family these important skills:

- Test a door for fire by touching the bottom. If it is hot, find another way out.
- When moving through a burning structure, stay below smoke and fumes. Crawl to safety.
- Get yourself and your family out of the house as quickly as possible. Do not try to save favorite objects or pets.
- Once you are out, stay out. Never reenter a burning building.

The fire department can also provide valuable information for preventing fires and mapping out escape routes for you and your family.

Avoiding Electric Shock

Electric shock can be caused by contact with exposed live wiring or the use of improperly grounded appliances. Depending on the amount of electricity you come into contact with, a shock can merely cause a quick buzzing in your finger-tips, knock you over, or kill you. Electrical shock can also cause burns.

If you have any questions or are unfamiliar with the status of your home's wiring system, have it inspected by a licensed professional. Also, when using appliances, be sure to follow manufacturer's recommendations regarding power supply, outlets, and extension cords.

Wiring. The electricity that powers household appliances runs on a system known as alternating current (AC). One "hot" wire brings power to the motor, light bulb, or heating element, and the other "neutral" wire completes that circuit. When this circuit is broken, the power is lost. Electricity cannot always be fully harnessed. Stray current sometimes runs out of wires and appliances and seeks the quickest possible route to the ground, where it naturally dissipates. In these cases, the power finds the nearest conductive material to get it there, such as metal, water, or moist materials—including skin.

Electric shocks occur when a person comes in contact with stray current seeking ground, either directly or by touching charged metal or water. To help prevent such stray current, household electric systems should be properly grounded, using a special contact wire that runs into the earth, usually through the basement. Three-holed outlets include a grounding plug and are used to ground high-voltage appliances and equipment, such as refrigerators, air-conditioners, hair dryers, computers, and power tools.

All home wiring should meet or exceed code standards. Look out for exposed or frayed wires or cables, but never touch them. Call an electrician or other professional who will inspect your home's electrical system to make sure that it is properly grounded, and that the wiring and fuse/switch mechanisms are all up-to-date.

Careful Use of Appliances. When using any appliance, whether it is a refrigerator or a hair dryer, look to see that it is certified by a federal agency or testing laboratory (look for the "UL" imprint or sticker). Make sure that the power cord is well insulated and securely attached. Also check to see that the plug is secure. Only use three-pronged plugs in outlets designed with the third grounding prong. Make sure to plug appliances all the way in. Never use appliances in wet areas or when you yourself are wet. Also, be careful not to touch metal or water when using an appliance.

Take special care with small appliances, such as hair dryers and electric razors in the bathroom, and hand mixers or toasters in the kitchen. Do not use electricity near sinks or tubs full of water. When using small appliances in the bathroom, it is best to make sure that the moisture from a recent bath or shower has been mopped up or allowed to dry and that the sink and tub have been drained dry. If the size of your bathroom requires that you dry your hair or shave near the toilet, close the lid first. In the kitchen, be careful not to use appliances when your hands are wet. Also, do not use them on wet floors.

If an appliance malfunctions, smokes, sparks, or does not work at all, switch it off, then take care to unplug it, or switch the power off at the circuit breaker. Simply turning the appliance off will not solve the problem. Then have the device repaired or replaced.

Carbon Monoxide Poisoning

Carbon monoxide (CO) is a silent killer. The gas is colorless, odorless, and tasteless and is produced during the incomplete combustion of various fuels, including gas, oil, kerosene, and gasoline. When inhaled, carbon monoxide hampers the flow of oxygen through the body. In small amounts, it can cause flu-like symptoms, sleepiness, disorientation, headaches, and unconsciousness. Long-term exposure—especially in houses, garages, and other structures with limited ventilation—can lead to death. Carbon monoxide is a common threat in the home because furnaces, stoves, water heaters, and certain space heaters emit the gas when they do not function properly. Automobile exhaust also contains carbon monoxide. Approximately 200 deaths each year can be attributed to this gas.

Carbon monoxide poisoning is entirely avoidable with proper prevention and detection. Checking your home for carbon monoxide emissions and proper ventilation, properly installing carbon monoxide detectors, and learning how to identify and respond to early symptoms of carbon monoxide poisoning can help you eliminate or reduce the risk of serious illness or death.

Prevention. The first—and most important—step in preventing carbon monoxide poisoning is ensuring that furnaces and other fuel-fired appliances work properly. The National Safety Council recommends that homeowners have a professional inspector check and clean furnaces, flues, and chimneys once a year. Follow the manufacturer's recommendations for changing furnace air filters. Also, if you have a gas-fired water heater, have it checked regularly. Your local gas or utility company should be able to answer questions about carbon monoxide prevention. In some communities, these same companies conduct home inspections.

If you use supplemental fuel-burning space heaters, be sure that they are working properly. Use them only in well-ventilated spaces.

Never run your car, such as to warm it up in cold weather, in an enclosed garage—especially if it is attached to your house. Pull the car outside first.

Detection. Carbon monoxide detectors are widely available and highly effective. Equipped with a loud alarm, a CO detector will alert residents to the presence of the gas before it reaches dangerous levels. The CPSC and the National Safety Council both recommend the installation of at least one carbon monoxide detector in each home, near bedrooms. Most carbon monoxide detectors cost around $100, a worthwhile investment in your family's safety.

Another important means of detecting the presence of carbon monoxide is watching for the physical signs of poisoning. Because its symptoms often mimic those seen with the flu or food poisoning, many people don't recognize carbon monoxide intoxication in time. If a family member exhibits such symptoms, think seriously about the possibility of carbon monoxide poisoning, especially if symptoms arise after a long time spent in a house or other structure where fuel-fired appliances are used and ventilation is poor. Pets are frequently affected first, becoming agitated then sleepy, often with bright red noses. Be especially wary of carbon monoxide poisoning during the winter, a time when furnaces are working and houses are sealed up tight against the cold. The National Safety Council recommends that if somebody in your household shows any carbon monoxide poisoning symptoms, evacuate your home and get the victim to a hospital. If you suspect the presence of carbon monoxide and no one appears to be ill, open the doors and windows and call the fire department's nonemergency telephone number to request a carbon monoxide reading.

Avoiding Falls

Falls are a major health hazard. In 1991, for instance, they caused the second highest number of unintentional deaths after automobile accidents. Falls account for a high percentage of injuries around the home, yet they are very easy to avoid. Keeping pathways clear, ensuring that you and your family can see where you are walking at all times, and providing stable climbing structures and slip-free walking surfaces help you avoid falls. Following are some simple, common sense tips:

- **Strive for basic neatness.** Keep floors, stairways, and hallways clear of objects and debris that may cause someone to trip. Secure electrical cords out of the way behind furniture.
- **Install handrails on both sides of staircases.** In many cases, one railing is not adequate. A second rail ensures steady climbing and descending when two people pass on a stairway, or when someone carrying an object is unable to grasp a single rail. If someone is ill, frail, or otherwise unsteady on her feet, she will need that added stability.
- **Install adequate illumination in hallways and stairwells.** It is a good idea to install switches at both ends of these passageways. In some locations, motion detector lights may be helpful.
- **Avoid skids and slips.** Wipe up water or spills on floors as soon as they occur. Secure loose rugs to the floor (which will also help prevent tripping). Apply nonskid pads under loose rugs, or tape to steps and slick floors. Don't walk around the house in socks.
- **Watch your step.** When you are ill, tired, or under the influence of alcohol or other substances, your agility will be hampered, raising your risk of tripping. Move slowly, especially on stairs. Install grab bars and nonskid pads in bath tubs and showers.
- **Take care when using ladders.** Always use a stable ladder or stepladder. With folding foot ladders, be sure that locking devices are set and secure. Place the ladder on level ground. Do not use the top step.

Use and Storage of Knives and Tools

Knives, tools, and other useful implements are a common source of household injury. Proper maintenance, storage, and use will help prevent most cuts and other injuries.

Knives. Keep knives sharp—a dull knife requires more pressure to work and is therefore more likely to slip and cause cuts. Always use a cutting board. Make sure your work surface is clear before you begin cutting. To avoid losing your grip, ensure that both your hands and the knife handle are clean and dry. Always keep your hands and fingers away from the knife blade. When chopping or mincing, fold your fingers and rest your knuckles against the side of the blade to act as

wellness
warning

Do not use stairs for storage. Though it may seem handy to set shoes or clothing on a step, it is also an invitation to a fall. Keep stairs clear at all times. Teach your children to keep toys, clothes, and shoes out from underfoot. Be sure to check that their favorite stuffed animals and toys make it all the way up the stairs at bedtime.

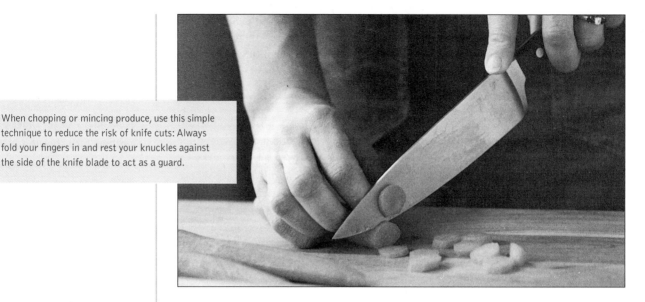

When chopping or mincing produce, use this simple technique to reduce the risk of knife cuts: Always fold your fingers in and rest your knuckles against the side of the knife blade to act as a guard.

a guard. Avoid wiping your knife on your apron; you could easily cut yourself. Warn children (and adults) not to startle you or reach for samples when you are cutting something. Teach your children the basics of proper knife use.

People often cut themselves on loose knives in drawers or sinks. Avoid storing sharp knives loosely in drawers. Place them in a knife tray or rack (preferably with guards over the blades). Also, never leave a knife in a sink or dishwasher. When you are done using the knife, clean and dry it carefully by hand and store it properly. If you have small children, be sure to keep sharp knives locked up.

Tools. Before you use a manual or power tool, make sure it is in good condition and proper working order. It is important to use the right tool for the job and to know how to use it properly. An implement too large or small for a job could cause injury. Keep blades and bits sharp. Do not use too much force on sharp tools—you could slip and cut yourself. As you would with any electrical appliance, make sure that your power tools are functioning properly, that cords and plugs are intact, and that you have an ample, well-grounded power source.

When using power tools, always practice basic safety. Focus on what you are doing, and never use tools when fatigued or under the influence of alcohol or medications. Following are some tips for safe tool use:

- Do not use electric tools near water.
- Wear protective eye goggles.
- Use requisite blade guards and safety aids.
- Maintain a clean work area.
- Store tools properly, and lock them up if you have children in your household.

Poisoning

Accidental poisoning is a preventable but all too common source of serious injury in the home. Pesticides, cleaning fluids, polishes, medicines, and disinfectants are among the most common sources of poisoning, but there are others. Learn to identify potential poisons. Read labels carefully. Make an inventory of potentially harmful substances, and take precautions to use them properly and store them securely.

General Precautions. Check your kitchen, basement, garage, and bathroom for potentially poisonous chemical substances (all should have clearly visible warning labels). Be sure to look outside and in the shed as well (charcoal lighter fluid and insecticides are highly toxic). Store all poisonous or caustic substances (and all medicines) well out of children's reach, preferably in cabinets that are locked or secured with child safety latches. Store all poisonous substances and medicines in their original containers with childproof lids. Also, be sure to store—and use—poisonous substances away from food and food preparation areas.

What to Do When Someone Is Poisoned. Keep the telephone number of the local poison control center posted by the telephone. If you suspect that someone in your household has ingested poison, try to determine what she consumed. If you see the poison container, grab it and go to the telephone. If the victim is unconscious or experiencing convulsions, dial 911 immediately. Otherwise, call the poison control center. Follow the telephone instructions of the emergency personnel. Be prepared to tell them the weight of the person, what substance they took, how much they ingested, and any symptoms.

To be adequately prepared in the event of a poisoning, keep on hand two remedies: activated charcoal (which neutralizes many poisons) and ipecac syrup (which induces vomiting). Most prepackaged first-aid kits include these compounds. They are also available at pharmacies. The poison control center may advise you to use one of these. Be sure, however, not to use either substance until directed to do so by emergency personnel.

Lead Poisoning. Lead-based paint, found mostly in older homes, poses a significant health threat to both adults and children. In adults, lead poisoning can cause irritability, poor muscle coordination, nerve damage, and problems with reproduction. In pregnant women, low levels of lead can retard fetal development. Children exposed to lead can experience irreversible brain damage, impaired mental functioning, and retarded development. Exposure generally occurs when individuals inhale the dust created by sanding or scraping or by eating flakes of lead-based paint.

If your home was constructed before 1980, the CPSC recommends that you have the paint tested for lead—especially if you plan to renovate the house. Although there are some home-based testing kits available, the CPSC recommends using a professional laboratory. If lead-based paint is detected, you can cover it with a sealant or another layer of paint or have it removed by painters trained in proper paint-removal procedures.

Guns in the Home

Former Surgeon General C. Everett Koop declared violence, including gun violence, a public health epidemic. An alarming number of shootings are caused each year by firearms that are improperly stored—quite often in the home. Nearly half of U.S. homes contain some type of gun. One in four has a handgun.

wellness
warning

When using cleaning fluids, be careful never to mix ammonia and bleach. This combination creates highly noxious fumes that can make you sick.

Adults who own and store a gun in their home often underestimate a child's ability (their own child or a visiting child) to gain access to and fire a gun, to make good judgments about handling a gun, and to follow rules about gun safety. Children are likely to have accidents when they handle a loaded gun, thinking it is a toy.

According to the Educational Fund to End Handgun Violence, in 1991, 1,441 unintentional shooting fatalities occurred, and 551 of the victims were children aged 19 or younger. One survey has revealed that 59 percent of parents who said they had a gun in the home admitted to not locking it away from their children. In the United States, more than 1.2 million elementary-aged children have access to guns in their homes.

Given these statistics, it is recommended that guns not be kept in homes, and certainly not in homes where children live or visit. If families must own guns, the U.S. Public Health Service recommends that they be kept unloaded and locked up securely, with ammunition stored in a separate location. Childproof trigger locks are available for between $2 and $15 at large discount stores, as well as through various health organizations. (In 1997, President Clinton proposed that every handgun sold by a federally registered gun dealer have a mandatory built-in, childproof trigger lock and in the same year, 80 gun manufacturers agreed to do so.) Parents who own firearms (for hunting, target shooting, or personal protection) need to educate their children about gun hazards—before they notice the presence of weapons in the home.

Safety *at* Work

Accidents and injuries occur regularly in the workplace. Heavy machinery, manual labor, and the repetitive stresses of many assembly line jobs and trades all pose a risk of injury. Jobs requiring less physical exertion can also be hazardous. When simple ergonomic considerations are not met, simply sitting and keyboarding on a computer, for example, can lead to lower back injury or carpal tunnel syndrome.

The U.S. Department of Labor's Occupational Safety and Health Administration (OSHA) and other groups have established regulations and guidelines to ensure worker safety. Nevertheless, many employees sustain injuries every year—largely because they have not followed simple steps for prevention. It is important that all employees, no matter what their occupation, learn how they can enhance safety and avoid injury on the job.

Avoiding Harmful Substances

There are a number of workplace substances considered to be toxic, many of which are used in manufacturing and printing. If you work in a factory, printing plant, medical office or hospital, or other site where chemicals or other harmful substances are used, be sure to find out if you are being exposed to any toxic or potentially toxic substances. If you are about to start a new job, make a similar inquiry. By law, employers must inform you about harmful substances and train you in safe handling techniques or procedures.

Office products can also be hazardous; glues, correction fluid, and copier toner may be harmful if sufficient fumes are inhaled. Try to work with these substances in well-ventilated areas and for short periods of time.

Women who are pregnant, who may be pregnant, or who are planning a pregnancy need to be especially diligent about substances that can affect fertility or harm a growing fetus. These include lead and other heavy metals, such as mercury. High levels of radiation and materials used out of sight, such as rat poison, can also be harmful. Ask your doctor about substances that may have an effect on your fertility or pregnancy. Then find out if any of these are used in or around your worksite.

Accident Prevention

Accidents on the job involving vehicles or machinery are fairly common but highly preventable. Proper precautions, adequate safety training, and common sense are the keys. If you operate any equipment or machinery on the job, do not begin until you feel absolutely confident that you have been thoroughly trained. Never operate equipment when fatigued or under the influence of alcohol or medications likely to cause drowsiness.

Injury Prevention

In the seventeenth and eighteenth centuries, workers were expected to accept injury and disability as the normal part of working. As a matter of course, miners got black lung disease, textile mill workers went deaf from long hours spent operating loud machines, and domestic workers suffered from a form of bursitis called "housemaid's knee." Although modern reforms have created laws and precautions aimed at protecting employees from workplace hazards, many workers still sustain injuries because they rarely heed, or they disregard altogether, safety and injury prevention guidelines, including warnings to wear basic protective equipment. Following are some common workplace injuries and ways to avoid them. As you will see, injury prevention depends largely on your own consistent efforts.

FIGURE 15.3 **Injury-free Computing**
Remember these tips to prevent stress and strain while working at a computer terminal.

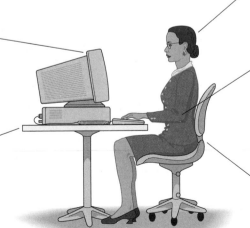

Your head should not be bent forward toward the monitor. Your shoulders should be relaxed and comfortable. Do not slouch.

Adjust the monitor angle to minimize glare and reflections from windows and lights. Make sure your monitor is clean and that the brightness and contrast settings are to your liking.

Keep your elbows in a position parallel to the keyboard and your wrists in a neutral position. Organize frequently-used desk equipment and supplies so that you do not need to stretch or twist your body to reach them.

Your computer table should be between 25 and 30 inches high. At this height, the top of your monitor will be at or a little below eye level.

Adjust your chair height so that your thighs are horizontal and your feet are flat on the floor. Make sure the backrest supports your lower back.

Protective Equipment on the Job

A number of simple, widely available devices protect workers from on-the-job injuries. Hard hats, goggles, steel-toed shoes, ear plugs, and other equipment are effective tools for safety. Nevertheless, Labor Department statistics paint a troubling picture of injuries incurred despite the existence of protective equipment. In one series of studies of workers who have sustained head injuries, data indicate only 16 percent wore hard hats. Only 1 percent of approximately 770 workers suffering facial injuries were wearing face protection. Only 23 percent of workers with foot injuries wore safety boots. About 40 percent of workers with eye injuries failed to wear goggles.

Employers in many types of businesses are required by law to furnish protective gear. If such protection is not required or provided, and you feel you need it, request it from your employer or purchase it yourself. You can request reimbursement from your employer.

Lower Back Injuries. Lower back pain is the leading cause of disability for workers under age 45. Although many back injuries can be linked to job responsibilities (especially if duties include frequent lifting), such complaints usually stem from a combination of factors: poor posture, improper lifting technique, weak and underused stomach and back muscles, stress, physical inactivity, and obesity. Virtually all of these risk factors can be reduced or eliminated.

If your job involves frequent carrying and lifting, even if it is not "heavy" lifting—if you are a day care provider, for example, who picks up infants and young children regularly—it is important to practice proper lifting technique. If you spend all day sitting at a desk, sit up straight in a chair with ample low back support. (For more information on lower back injuries, treatment, and prevention—including tips for safe lifting and office ergonomics—see Chapter 25.)

Repetitive Stress Injuries. Many workplace injuries can be linked to activities that involve moving one part of the body repeatedly over long periods of time. Two of the most common repetitive stress injuries are tendinitis in the elbows and knees, and carpal tunnel syndrome, which affects the hands and wrists. These and other repetitive stress conditions can be avoided or improved by taking steps to reduce excessive motion and the level of stress placed on the joint. Frequent resting, stretching, use of braces, and making modifications to the ergonomics of one's workspace (such as using a wrist pad or an ergonomic keyboard for computer use) are all very helpful. (Chapter 25 discusses repetitive stress injuries and steps you can take to avoid them.)

Preventing
Recreational **Accidents**

A sensible person would not take a car out on the highway without ever having driven before. The risk of accident and injury would be too great. The same common sense applies to recreational activities. Yet, many people are injured in recreational activities because they are not adequately trained, do not know what they are doing, and are not aware of the hazards involved. A common story is that of the inexperienced hiker found cold and frightened after a night spent lost on a mountainside without the proper equipment or supplies.

Before you undertake a new activity, think carefully about your abilities. If you are physically inactive or afraid of heights, for instance, rock climbing may not be for you. If you are unfamiliar with the procedures and necessary precautions to take on long hikes, think twice about undertaking anything more than a brief hike in your local nature preserve.

Unfamiliarity need not limit you from trying something new, however. The key to accident-free recreation is preparation. Read up on a given activity. Look into classes, clubs, or private instruction. If you know someone who is an avid mountain biker or boater or is involved in some other sport you would like to try, ask her to show you what it is like and then ease into it .

Acting Within Your Limits

Before undertaking activities that are strenuous for you, make sure that your body is appropriately conditioned. You can prevent many activity-related injuries simply by warming up and stretching. (For more information on proper preparation and conditioning for recreational activities, see Chapter 9.)

Using the Right Protective Gear and Equipment

Using appropriate protective gear and proper equipment reduces recreational risks. Familiarize yourself with the equipment needed for any particular sport or recreational activity you are interested in, and then gear up appropriately.

Shoes. Many foot and leg injuries are caused by a poor choice of footwear. Make sure that the shoe fits the activity and provides adequate foot and ankle support. If you plan a hike, for instance, invest in a good quality, well-fitting pair of hiking boots. Flat, casual shoes or sneakers are not appropriate because they do not protect against slips or twisted ankles.

Jogging, long-distance running, basketball, tennis, and aerobics all require shoes constructed for proper shock absorption and support according to the particular demands of the sport. Ask at the shoe store of your choice which shoe is most appropriate for the activity you choose.

Helmets. Head trauma is a significant risk in recreation. Helmets are recommended for several sports and recreational activities, including rock climbing, batting (in baseball and softball), football, inline skating, ice hockey, biking, and of course, motorcycling.

Head trauma is common in bicycling. According to the CPSC, it is estimated that helmets are worn by fewer than one out of 10 bicyclists. Furthermore, the CPSC reports that about 1,200 bicyclists are killed each year, and more than half a million bicycle-related injuries are treated in hospital emergency rooms. Three out of four of the deaths are due to head trauma and about one-third of the injuries are to the head or face. Many of these injuries and deaths can be prevented if riders wear helmets.

Safety helmets are widely available and inexpensive. Generally made of crushable, expanded polystyrene foam, they absorb the force of an impact, thereby minimizing or preventing most head injuries. Many helmets are encased in a hard outer shell, which provides additional protection (and sporty designs and colors). When buying a helmet, make sure that it fits snugly but comfortably and learn how to wear it properly.

If you have children, see that they also wear safety helmets. About one-third of the above-cited deaths and two-thirds of the injuries involved children under the age of 15.

Safety in the Water

Swimming and boating accidents account for most water-related deaths. To a large degree, both types of accidents result from lack of experience or underestimating the risk of drowning. Water hazards can be avoided by gaining proper instruction and behaving within sensible limits.

wellness **warning**

Never dive into a pool, lake, or river unless you are sure the depth is adequate for the dive. Diving accidents, caused by rocks or deceptively shallow water, are a common cause of severe head and neck injury.

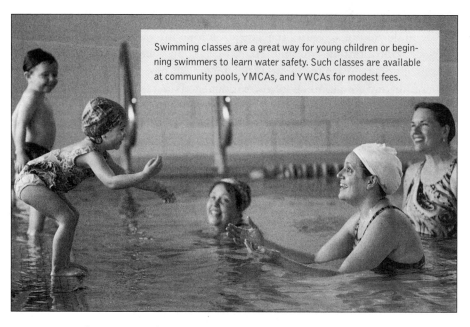

Swimming classes are a great way for young children or beginning swimmers to learn water safety. Such classes are available at community pools, YMCAs, and YWCAs for modest fees.

Swimming. If you are only a beginning or moderately experienced swimmer, swim only in lifeguard-attended swimming pools and beaches. At the ocean or lake, be careful to avoid swimming too far from shore, where it would take a long time for a lifeguard to reach you in an emergency. Avoid swimming alone, and stay in sight of lifeguards or friends on the beach. Know where safety and rescue equipment is kept at all swimming locations. Listen to your body for signs of fatigue and be sure to get yourself back to shallow water or land before wearing yourself out.

Even if you are a veteran swimmer you need to be wary of ocean and river currents and lake mud and vegetation that can pull you down under the water. If you are in the water and someone you are with is in distress, do not go near her unless you yourself are trained and certified in life saving. In her panic and flailing about, she could pull you under the water. Summon help from someone on shore.

Swimming skill improves with practice and instruction. Many local chapters of the American Red Cross, YMCA, and YWCA offer a wide range of swimming and water safety classes, all for modest fees. Instruction is a great way to improve your technique, enjoyment, and level of safety.

Life Jackets Save Lives

According to the National Safety Council and the U.S. Coast Guard, three out of four drowning victims in recreational boating accidents were not wearing life jackets. Most accidents occur when a person falls overboard or their boat capsizes. Cold water and fatigue cause even the most experienced swimmers to tire and lose coordination quickly, so it is imperative that all boat passengers wear an approved life jacket. Use the following tips for proper life jacket selection and use:

- If you can, buy your own personal life jacket.
- When buying or selecting a life jacket, make sure that it is rated for someone of your weight and size. Check the fit to ensure that, when buckled, the life jacket does not slip over your head or come above your ears.
- Never use water toys in place of a life jacket approved by the U.S. Coast Guard.
- Check your life jacket yearly for flotation and fit.
- If you detect air leakage, mildew, or rot, throw the life jacket away.
- Set an example for children by wearing your life jacket.

Boating. Failure to use life jackets, the use of drugs or alcohol, excessive speed, and inattentiveness account for most fatal boating accidents. Boating, like swimming, requires adequate instruction and common sense. A high percentage of boating accidents involve an operator with no boating instruction. If you have spent little time on the water, do not take a speedboat or sailboat out on your own. Seek instruction from a veteran, either a friend or an instructor at the local marina or yacht club.

Once you are able to handle watercraft, be sure to practice the same kind of common sense and "safe driving" that you would on the road:

- Learn and obey all boating rules and laws.
- Be alert to changing weather conditions and other watercraft.
- Don't drink or use drugs while boating.
- Ensure that you and your passengers wear adequate and proper flotation devices.
- Have a functioning radio to summon help if needed.

First Aid *and* Cardiopulmonary Resuscitation

Unfortunately, no matter how diligent you are or how many preventive steps you take, you or someone you know will probably one day suffer some kind of mishap. Short of prevention, a quick and effective response is the best means of protecting health in emergencies both great and small. First aid, cardiopulmonary resuscitation (CPR), the Heimlich maneuver, and rescue breathing are simple and effective emergency techniques.

Basic First Aid — Getting and Giving Help

When someone has been injured, your first responsibility is to see that she gets the help she needs. If she has sustained a nonserious injury (such as a simple cut or sprain), or if you are skilled in the first-aid concepts required to provide primary treatment (and are equipped to do so), give aid promptly. Otherwise, it is important that you get the person to a medical facility or summon help immediately. Dial 911 if the person is unconscious, is bleeding severely, has possible broken bones or head or neck injury, is experiencing severe chest pains, or appears to have been poisoned.

Cuts and Scrapes. Most cuts and scrapes can be treated with simple first-aid techniques. First, stop the bleeding by applying pressure, using a clean cloth or gauze. If the wound is on a hand, arm, foot, or leg, try to elevate the affected limb to reduce blood flow. Then make sure that the wound is clean and stays clean. Swab the affected area with a wet cloth, or place it under running cold water. Finally, apply a sterile dressing (such as an adhesive bandage). Most simple wounds will heal on their own if they are kept clean and dry. You generally do not need to apply antibiotic ointments or sterilizing agents (alcohol, hydrogen peroxide, or iodine).

Seek medical attention if the wound is deep (and its edges spread open) or if the bleeding cannot be stopped. Deep puncture wounds should also be treated by a medical professional, especially if they were caused by a dirty nail or other implement. In that case, the victim may need a shot to prevent a tetanus infection.

Burns. Primary care of most burns is simple. The first step is to extinguish any flames or remove the victim from the burn source. Second, cool the burn with cold water. Third, cover the burn with a dry, clean dressing to prevent infection. The use of ice or burn ointments is not recommended. If blisters appear, avoid breaking the skin. If the blisters have opened, clean the burn gently with soap and water and apply antibiotic ointment.

Less serious burns (a first-degree burn, which causes only redness, and some second-degree burns with slight blistering) can usually be treated without medical assistance. People suffering from more severe burns (those that cause heavy blistering and discoloration of the skin) must be taken to see a physician promptly after the administration of primary treatment. Critical burns, those that cause charring and bleeding and show underlying skin tissues (which appear white), can be life-threatening and require immediate medical assistance. Call 911. If you can, cover the burn with sterile gauze. Otherwise, leave it alone until help arrives.

Sprains and Strains. Mild sprains and strains are common and are often fairly simple to treat. However, it is important to seek medical help promptly if the injury was accompanied by a snapping sensation or popping sound, if the pain and swelling are severe, or if there is bruising at the wound site. These could be signs of a severe sprain, a torn muscle, joint dislocation, or a fractured bone.

If the pain is not severe, you can treat most injuries with rest, ice, compression, and elevation (RICE): Ice the injury promptly and elevate it (if possible) to reduce swelling. Then apply compression (with a brace or elastic bandage), and make sure the limb is not used for the first 24 to 48 hours after the injury.

Choking

If someone is choking or has stopped breathing, a quick response is essential. In either event, the first goal of a caregiver is to clear the airway. Choking is usually indicated by a clutching of the throat with one or both hands or an inability to speak, breathe, or cough. In such instances, the Heimlich maneuver is a simple, highly effective emergency technique. If a person is unconscious, you must remove the airway obstruction (if there is one, such as food or dentures) and then get her breathing, using a technique called rescue breathing.

The Heimlich Maneuver. The Heimlich maneuver helps force food or foreign objects from a victim's windpipe using the air already in the person's lungs. Follow the steps in Figure 15.4 when you see someone choking.

Rescue Breathing. The following steps are used to resuscitate an unconscious victim:

- Lay the person down. Tilt her head back. Lift her chin.
- Pinch the victim's nose shut and, placing your mouth over hers, give two slow

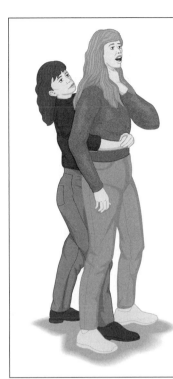

1. Send someone to call for help.

2. Stand behind the victim with your arms around her waist (or around her chest if she is pregnant or obese) and your thigh between her legs to help hold her upright.

3. Make a fist with one hand and place the thumb-side in the middle of the victim's abdomen, about an inch above the navel (or in the middle of the victim's breastbone if she is pregnant or obese).

4. Grasp your fist with your other hand and, keeping your elbows out, quickly pull your fist upward and inward.

5. Repeat the abdominal thrusts until the object is dislodged. If the object remains stuck or if the person loses consciousness, begin rescue breathing.

FIGURE 15.4
Heimlich Maneuver
A person with a partially obstructed airway can usually cough to remove the object from her airway. But if the airway is completely blocked, the person is choking—having difficulty speaking, coughing, and breathing—and immediate first aid is necessary.

breaths. Breath into the victim until her chest rises. If air won't go in, try two more breaths.

If the victim still cannot breathe:

- Place the heel of one hand on the middle of the abdomen, just above the navel. Place the other hand on top of the first.
- Give as many as five quick, upward thrusts.
- Use your finger to try and sweep any object out of the victim's mouth (remembering to check under the tongue).
- Repeat all of the above steps until the victim's lungs can fill with air.
- If the victim remains unconscious, check her pulse. If you cannot find it, administer cardiopulmonary resuscitation or find someone who can.

Cardiopulmonary Resuscitation

CPR is designed to restart the heart and lungs of an unconscious victim with no pulse. It also serves the important function of pumping blood and oxygen through the victim's body, preventing brain damage. If someone's heart has stopped because of a heart attack or injury, quick, steady administration of CPR until professional help arrives can mean the difference between life and death.

If someone is unconscious, lacks a pulse, and is not breathing, call 911 or send someone to call an ambulance immediately. Only someone who is properly trained should administer CPR to the victim.

Learning More About First Aid

Courses and other instruction in first aid and emergency response are highly recommended. They are inexpensive and widely available from local chapters of the American Red Cross, as well as from local agencies and community colleges. If you are a parent, teacher, counselor, or other person whose regular daily activities bring you into contact with lots of people, consider some instruction. You will feel better knowing you are able to provide help in an emergency situation.

What *You* Can Do

Even the most careful person will fall victim to accidental injury from time to time. But doing all you can to protect yourself and your loved ones minimizes the risk and helps give you peace of mind. Accident prevention is mainly a matter of common sense, and taking a few basic precautions can go a long way toward keeping you free from injury:

- Avoid driving even after drinking a small amount of alcohol. Never get into a car with someone who has been drinking.
- Follow all traffic laws and the rules of courtesy on the road; drive defensively; and use safety restraints properly and consistently.
- Examine your home for hazards and take steps to remove them. Be sure smoke detectors are properly installed and have fresh batteries. Purchase a fire extinguisher for each floor of your home.
- Make a family plan for escaping a fire. Have a different plan for day and night. Practice until you are sure everyone in the family understands what to do and can follow the plan in an emergency.
- Install a carbon monoxide detection device in your home.
- Remove weapons from your home, or, if you must have them, lock them away and store ammunition separately.
- Research your work environment to determine whether there are harmful substances present and whether there is risk of accidents. Take the necessary steps to solve any problems you find.
- Choose recreational activities according to your level of fitness. Acquire the necessary equipment to make the activities safe for you. Be sure you get the instruction you need before starting a new activity.
- Consider taking courses in basic first aid and CPR. Familiarize yourself with techniques that can save lives in the event of an accident or illness.

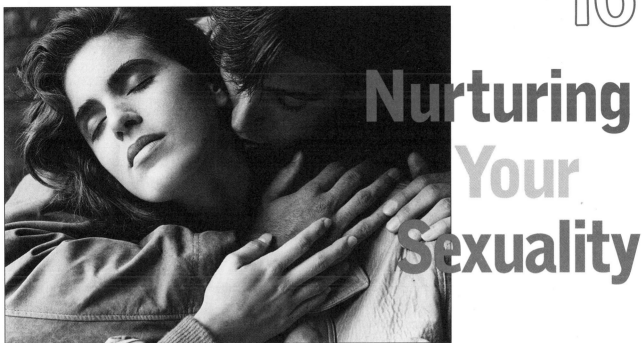

Chapter 16

Nurturing Your Sexuality

S exuality is an ongoing process of recognizing, accepting, and expressing one's self as a sexual being. It is a key part of an individual's identity. As women grow and change throughout their lives, their sexuality changes also.

Sexuality can be a source of great pleasure and of great pain. Concern about sexuality and sexual function is a universal phenomenon for most women and men at some point in their lives. In a recent survey almost two-thirds of the women surveyed expressed concerns about their sexuality. Yet many women are not comfortable talking with a doctor, a counselor, or even their partner about sexual issues.

Understanding sexuality and ensuring sexual health are important parts of women's wellness. Sexual health is the physical and emotional state of well-being that enriches and enhances sexual expression in all its many forms and allows women to lead fuller, more satisfying lives.

The **Many Facets** *of* Sexuality

The process of sexual development begins at birth and continues throughout life. Biological, psychological, and social factors mingle to form an individual's sexuality. These factors are further influenced by gender, roles and identities, self-image and self-esteem, and cultural values. Although your gender is determined at conception, your sexuality is learned through exposure to outside influences and is not a force or instinct imparted at birth. Social conditioning begins at birth with the exclamation "it's a boy" or "it's a girl."

Biological Factors

Your genetic makeup determines whether you will be male or female and which organs and hormones you will need for sexual function. Biological factors control sexual development and the ability to reproduce after puberty. These factors play a much broader role, however, in sexual function. Healthy sexual function relies on the ability of certain parts of the body—the sex organs, hormones, and centers of the brain—to respond to stimuli. The response triggers a biological reaction called the sexual response cycle, discussed later in this chapter. A healthy sexual response cycle is a key component of sexual satisfaction.

Psychological Factors

Your emotions and personality, combined with interpersonal skills, have a major impact on your sexuality. Psychological factors that contribute to your sexual identity are the basis for normal function but can also have negative effects on sexual behavior. For example, low self-esteem can create an obstacle to a woman's sexual pleasure.

Sexual and Gender Identity. Sexual identity is biologically determined—you are chromosomally male or female. Gender identity, on the other hand, is almost entirely a function of how the parents perceive the child's biological sex and raise the child in the context of culturally determined social expectations. Seemingly unimportant comments from parents or other trusted adults like "isn't she beautiful" or "big boys don't cry" constitute an important part of gender imprinting, as do the influence of toys given to the child and the type of play the child is encouraged to engage in. Gender imprinting is usually irreversibly established by age two and a half. Sexual and gender identity do not necessarily predict sexual orientation.

Sexual Orientation. Sexual orientation addresses sexual practice in terms of whom a person has sex with or finds sexually attractive. The extensive research of Alfred Kinsey, which began in the 1940s, attempted to define sexual practices in the United States. He devised a scale for ranking a person's level of attraction to a member of the opposite sex (heterosexual), attraction to certain characteristics in either the opposite sex or the same sex (bisexual), and attraction to members of the same sex only (homosexual). He concluded that most people exhibit some form of mixed behavior, even though most adults identify themselves as either heterosexual or homosexual.

Sexual behavior is the result of very complex biological and psychological interactions. Most cultures and religions have their own rules about sexual orientation and practices—with deeply held beliefs about what is allowed or forbidden. The need to assure continuation of the reproductive family has been the driving force in most cultures. Whether those cultures accepted or condemned homosexual behavior, every civilization throughout history has included homosexual men and women.

Social Factors

Social values regarding sexuality strongly influence the expression of sexual behavior. As Masters and Johnson pointed out in *Sex and Human Loving*, there is no sexual value system that is right for everyone and no single moral code that is indisputably correct and universally applicable. Any behavior is acceptable if it is consistent with a person's personal and cultural value system, is mutually satisfying, and is not harmful to individuals and society.

Views on sexual behavior in this country were initially established by the early Puritan settlers, who equated sexual interest with sin. Later, the Victorians continued to equate sex with immorality and set strict religious standards to control sexual behavior. That stern code was eased somewhat by Sigmund Freud, whose writings in the early twentieth century focused on the powerful influence of sexuality on people's lives. His pioneering work was followed by research that increased understanding of sexuality and sexual practices.

Today, sexual behavior is affected by a number of social changes that have swept the nation during the past 50 years. Gender roles, once rigidly defined as masculine or feminine, have softened and merged. No longer are men perceived only as the aggressors or women only as the pursued. Instead, a model of mutual participation, communication, and satisfaction is emerging. There is an ever-broadening openness about sexual activity in our current culture. Sexual intimacy is seen as a source of comfort and pleasure, as a form of self-expression, and as an important component of healthy adult function. Modern society is more honest about sexual activity than those puritanical ancestors. A number of factors were important in bringing about these changes, but the most powerful change was probably the introduction of reliable birth control in the 1960s. Within one generation after the introduction of birth control pills, the responsibility for pregnancy prevention rapidly shifted from men to women. Once they could be sexual without being pregnant, women found their lives changing in other ways.

A **Lifetime** of **Learning** *About* Sexuality

Sexual intimacy is the result of a complex series of learned behaviors that change throughout a woman's life cycle.

What We Learn in Childhood

Sexual attitudes are formed early in infancy and often last into adulthood. From birth, children learn about touching, holding, and caressing from their parents and caregivers. This warm, close bonding aids in forming close relations later in life. Children also form attitudes by watching their parents show (or withhold) affection with each other and seeing how they react to and interact with people of the same and opposite sex, to nudity, and to other expressions of affection. Children ultimately learn about sexuality from their family as well as from their peers.

Genital Touching. Babies begin to touch and fondle their genitals early in life, although they do not derive any sexual sensation from this touching. Even at this early age, however, parents send messages to their children that such behavior is acceptable or unacceptable. It is not helpful for parents to scold toddlers and young children or show disapproval for genital touching. The behavior is only

Mixed Messages

Parents need to be aware that children learn from spoken and unspoken forms of communication. They watch, listen, and imitate. They can form attitudes on a subject, sometimes without a word being spoken. Parents can unknowingly send mixed messages to children by saying one thing and doing another. It can be confusing to children when parents encourage them to be aware of their body and learn the names of the parts of the body, but exclude the genitals.

Scolding a child for touching her genitals can communicate the message that sex is "dirty." This message can also be imparted by early toilet training and its emphasis on cleanliness. Toilet training can be used as an opportunity to teach a child about body parts and functions in a positive way. Also, by seeing parents enjoy loving behavior, such as kissing and hugging, children get a positive message about sexuality.

discovery-oriented, and not sexual at all. Parents do, however, need to explain to their children what is correct behavior in public as well as outline their own rules for acceptable behavior in the home.

Gender Issues. A child's sense of her own gender identity develops in infancy and is fully formed by age two and a half. Between ages three and six children show a strong awareness of and interest in the differences between boys and girls. They often are curious about where babies come from. Parents need to answer their questions openly and honestly in clear, direct terms.

Influences Outside the Family. As children grow older they are exposed to other views about sex from their friends, school, church, and the media. Sometimes

Talking to Children About Sex

Begin teaching your children about sex at an early age with basic information, building on it bit by bit as your child is ready for more details. The earlier this dialogue takes place, the better. Some parents worry that talking about sex increases the chance that their child will have sex at an early age. This is not true. Lack of knowledge creates problems with sexual understanding and increases the likelihood of unsafe sex. Not discussing sex also suggests that sex is bad or should not be talked about. If your child does not raise questions by about age 5 or 6, look for ways to raise the subject. Children know when a topic is uncomfortable for a parent and may not bring it up for that reason.

Both mothers and fathers play a role in developing the healthy sexuality of their sons and daughters. Children learn from both parents, together and singly, and both parents should feel comfortable discussing sexual matters with their male and female children. It is important that boys be aware of girls' sexual and biological functions and anatomy and vice versa. For example, boys need to learn about menstruation and girls about erections. Both need to learn the meaning of the terms heterosexuality, homosexuality, bisexuality, and abstinence.

Following are some basic principles to follow in talking to children about sexuality:

DO

- Use correct terms for genital organs and functions, not slang or "cute" names.
- Discuss sex in a matter-of-fact manner.
- Discuss values, emotions, and decision making when relating biological facts.

- Encourage your child to come to you with questions and answer all of them openly and honestly. If you do not know the answer, be honest about it.
- Be aware of nonverbal as well as verbal messages.
- Explain how to recognize sexual abuse and protect against it.
- Take every opportunity to reinforce positive attitudes about sexuality.

DON'T

- Don't lecture; a casual give-and-take dialogue with plenty of time for questions is more suited to the attention span of a child.
- Don't worry that you are giving the child too much information; there will always be a chance to revisit the subject.
- Don't encourage a child's use of profanity by laughing or joking about it; instead, explain the exact meaning of the words she is using and that profanity should not be used.
- Don't embarrass a child by telling her "you're too young to understand that now."
- Don't wait until adolescence to discuss sexuality and birth control.

Listening is just as important as talking. Maintain eye contact while talking to your child, and repeat key concepts or statements your child makes. After answering a child's question, check to make sure the answer is understood and give your child a chance to ask more questions. Communication with children, as with anyone, is a two-way process.

they may get mixed messages. Much of a child's exposure to sex may come from television, music, movies, magazines, advertising, and even the Internet. These forms of entertainment may give distorted views of reality and create false impressions. Because peers and other influences have such a strong bearing on forming a child's sexual behavior, it is important for parents to be aware of their children's activities and whereabouts and to keep the lines of communication open. Parents need to know their children's friends, what they are watching or listening to, and how they are forming their views about sexuality. It is recommended that a child have basic information about the facts of life and a sense of sexual values by the time she reaches adolescence.

Preventing Child Abuse. Parents need to explain to their children that every child is in charge of her own body and that it is OK to say no to an adult who tries to touch them in a "private place." Sexual abuse in childhood can have a long-lasting negative impact on a person's mental health, sexuality, and sexual function, as well as causing other lifelong health problems. Parents and caregivers can instruct children to recognize inappropriate behavior and advances from others and to report it to a parent or authority figure right away.

What We Learn in Adolescence

Puberty usually occurs between ages 11 and 13, when hormone levels are in a state of constant change in both girls' and boys' bodies. Coupled with these physical changes, adolescents are also trying to master social skills, improve intellectual performance, and form personal values. This passage into adulthood can be a time of turmoil as well as joy.

FIGURE 16.1
How Children Learn About Sex
Children's and teenagers' ideas about sex are heavily influenced by their friends and the media. It is important to discuss sex with your children to help them form balanced, accurate viewpoints.

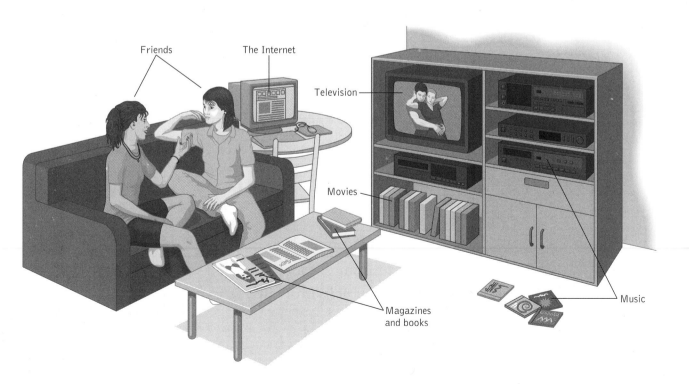

Friends The Internet Television Movies Magazines and books Music

During puberty, interest in sex increases as sex organs develop. Sex hormones are produced at adult levels. In girls, increased levels of the hormone estrogen cause breasts to develop, pubic hair to grow, and menstruation to begin. Girls often mature about two years ahead of boys—a source of concern to both genders. In boys, the hormone testosterone increases, triggering growth of the penis and other sex organs that allow ejaculation. Nocturnal emissions, known as "wet dreams," occur in an estimated one-fourth of 14-year-old boys. Growth of pubic hair is followed by facial hair and a deepening voice.

Adolescents struggle with the powerful emotions surrounding sexual feelings. For many, their emotional maturity has not kept pace with the rapid growth of their bodies, resulting in difficulty dealing with decision making about sexual behavior.

Learning About Sexual Expression. Adolescents should be taught that there are different forms of sexual expression. When they are given the definitions for heterosexual, homosexual, gay, lesbian, and bisexual, they are less likely to become confused about these terms. Children and adolescents also need to be taught the definition of abstinence and the benefits of abstaining from sexual activity. It is important that they learn about the risks of pregnancy and sexually transmitted diseases (STDs). Most unintended pregnancies among teens occur during the first six months of sexual activity. If teens do decide to experiment with sex, they need to be encouraged to practice safer sex. (Sex is never 100 percent "safe"—condoms can break and increase the risk of pregnancy and STDs—so experts and educators have adopted the term "safer" sex.)

Sex and Relationships. Experts agree that teens who are encouraged to think about sexual activity in terms of a meaningful relationship are more likely to find sexual satisfaction and stability. Open discussion with trusted adults will help them learn strategies to resist being pressured into sexual relations before they are ready. Adolescents can learn to make decisions about sexual behavior within the context of their own value systems and to decide about responsible sexuality.

Homosexual experiences are not uncommon in adolescence, and do not necessarily translate into adult homosexual behavior. Such incidents can be a source of concern to adolescents, resulting in guilt and emotional upset. Adolescents who have been given information and taught to respect different choices tend to weather such episodes well.

About five to ten percent of adolescents are gay. These teens often feel lonely and different. They struggle with their sexual identity as well as their "secret." These adolescents have higher rates of depression and risk for suicide. Children who are homosexual need the love and support of their parents as well as their peers.

What We Learn in Adulthood

As individuals pass through adolescence and grow into adulthood, they make important life choices about relationships, marriage, and lifestyles, and they continue to learn from their partners and their friends. Following are several current trends that reflect the issue of adult sexuality:

- Young adults are single longer and are making personal decisions about sexual behavior outside marriage. While new standards of sexual freedom allow more options, they can also make it difficult to establish and maintain meaningful relationships.
- Many couples live together without being married. In the past few decades, cohabitation before or without marrying has become quite common. Today, the first union of a couple is usually living together, not marriage—as in the past. The age of the first union has not changed, however, and remains steady at around age 22 for men and 20 for women.
- Many couples who do marry are making the decision to have children later in life.

Young Adulthood. The average number of partners that people have during their adult years has increased. One reason is that adults are staying single longer. Also, couples that live together tend to break up within a short period of time and seek new partners. The divorce rate has climbed as well, putting more adults out into the singles marketplace. Views toward sex outside of marriage have relaxed. In short, people now have more sexual partners over their lifetimes because they are spending a longer period being sexually active but unmarried.

Middle Adulthood. Middle adulthood is a time in which energy is focused on productivity—work, family, recreation, creative endeavors, and social responsibilities. It can also be a time when attention is distracted from sexuality, leaving some in what they consider a sexual "rut." Confronting one's mortality can sometimes shift a person's goals and identity, leading to what is commonly referred to as a midlife crisis. This period can be especially hard for women, who have higher rates of depression than men and are more sensitive to the biological effects of aging on their sexuality and self-image. Contrary to popular view, however, there is not an increase in divorce in midlife, and most women actually find their sexuality improves in midlife. While there are many variables in the midlife changes that both men and women undergo, both men and women have the same need for love, affection, and a sense of belonging.

Older Adulthood. Women are living longer, and most can enjoy a satisfying sexual life throughout their lives. The effects of aging alone do not inhibit a person's ability to have sex, although it may require a change in approach. Both men and women experience some changes in how they respond sexually as they age. For example, sexual arousal may take longer than before and may not be as dramatic as during young and middle adulthood.

Negative views toward aging—personal as well as societal—may be the greatest obstacle to sexual satisfaction in older women. Older women who maintain their health, vigor, and independence are also more likely to maintain their sexuality. Viewing the effects of aging as natural can enhance sexuality. For example, women may find that it takes them longer to become aroused—but that the arousal lasts longer. For healthy older adults, sexual desire, physical love, and sex continue to be basic parts of their lives. Intimacy is expressed through closeness, touching, and body warmth, as well as through intercourse. Caring and gentleness in loving activities may be as important or more important than intercourse in older men and women.

wellness **tip**

Take time for romance with your partner and talk often and openly about your feelings. Healthy sexuality relies on a healthy relationship. Healthy relationships require "maintenance" and good communication.

The **Biology** of Sex

The response to sexual stimuli is physical and emotional. Sexual response can be triggered by an event—a thought, a look, a kiss, a touch, a smell—that launches a series of reactions. These reactions are called the sexual response cycle, which calls into play both the sexual organs and the nervous system. Your understanding of the parts of the body involved in and the events that occur during the sexual response cycle can heighten your awareness of what provides pleasure and how your sexual satisfaction may be enhanced.

Anatomy

In order to understand the sexual response cycle, it is important to have a basic understanding of human sexual anatomy. (Believe it or not, many adults do not have this basic understanding, usually as a result of inadequate sexual education in childhood.) In both men and women, some reproductive organs are located inside the body and some outside the body. In general, those inside the body are equipped for reproduction whereas those outside the body function more for physical pleasure. These organs play a key role in sexual activity.

Male. The penis, scrotum, and testes are outside the body; the prostate gland, seminal vesicles, and bulbourethral glands are inside the body.

- **Penis.** There are two parts to the penis: the shaft and the glans, which is the rounded portion at the tip. The glans is a highly sensitive area richly supplied with nerves. In uncircumcised males, the foreskin covers the glans and is retracted during sex. The penis is made up of an internal network of spaces that are connected to arteries and veins. When the penis is stimulated, these spaces fill with blood and cause the penis to grow and become firm (an erection).
- **Scrotum.** A thin sac that forms a pouch to hold the testes, the scrotum contains muscle tissue that contracts with exercise, cold, or sexual excitement. These actions protect sperm, which are produced in the scrotum and are sensitive to changes in temperature.

FIGURE 16.2

Male Sexual Anatomy

In circumcised males, the foreskin is surgically removed at an early age so that the glans is exposed.

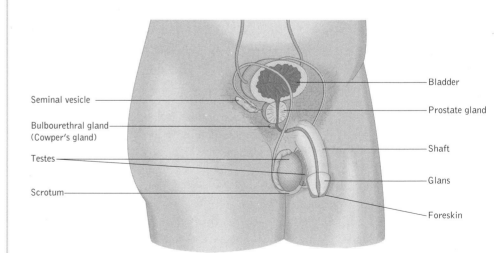

Seminal vesicle

Bulbourethral gland (Cowper's gland)

Testes

Scrotum

Bladder

Prostate gland

Shaft

Glans

Foreskin

- **Testes.** There are two testes contained in two chambers of the scrotum. The testes produce sperm as well as the male hormone, testosterone.
- **Prostate gland.** Located just below the bladder, this gland produces fluid that makes up about 20 percent of semen, the fluid that is ejaculated during orgasm.
- **Seminal vesicles.** Forming part of the duct through which a male ejaculates, these vesicles produce about 60 percent of semen. The fluid contains agents that help preserve sperm and keep them active.
- **Bulbourethral glands.** Also known as Cowper's glands, these glands secrete a small amount of fluid just before ejaculation. This fluid helps protect sperm and may contain some sperm, which could cause pregnancy.

Female. A woman's external organs are collectively known as the vulva, which includes the mons pubis, the labia majora and minora, the vaginal orifice, and the clitoris; the internal organs are the ovaries, fallopian tubes, uterus, and vagina.

- **Mons pubis.** This fatty tissue covers the pubic bone and is covered in pubic hair during and after puberty.
- **Labia majora.** These two outer lips surround the entrance to the vagina.
- **Labia minora.** The inner lips of the vagina form a hood to cover the clitoris and enclose the vaginal orifice, or opening.
- **Clitoris.** This extremely sensitive area is the source of a woman's most intense sexual pleasure. It has two parts—the body and the glans, or head—and contains nerves and blood vessels that cause it to swell when stimulated.
- **Ovaries.** Inside a woman, on either side of her abdomen, the ovaries produce eggs that are released each month to be fertilized. If the egg is not fertilized, a woman has a menstrual period. The ovaries also produce the hormones estrogen and progesterone, which are needed for reproduction.
- **Fallopian tubes.** Situated between the ovaries and the uterus, the fallopian tubes contain fingerlike projections that carry the egg from the ovary into the uterus and often are the site of fertilization.
- **Uterus.** Also known as the womb, the uterus is a hollow muscular organ that holds the fertilized egg, which develops into a fetus. If the egg is not fertilized, the lining of the uterus is shed each month as a menstrual period.

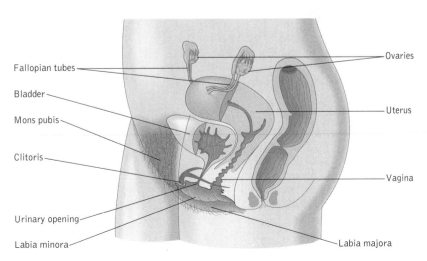

Fallopian tubes

Bladder

Mons pubis

Clitoris

Urinary opening

Labia minora

Ovaries

Uterus

Vagina

Labia majora

FIGURE 16.3

Female Sexual Anatomy

A woman's external sexual organs—mons pubis, labia, vaginal opening, and clitoris—are collectively termed the vulva. The labia include the labia majora (outer lips), which cover the entrance to the vagina, and the labia minora (inner lips), which cover the clitoris and enclose the vaginal opening.

- **Vagina.** Connecting the uterus with the outside genital orifice, the walls of the vagina are very elastic and serve as a source of lubrication during intercourse. The vagina also plays a role in orgasm.

A woman's breasts are not strictly considered genital organs, but they do play a role in sexual expression. The breasts are made up of glands, fibers, and fatty tissue. The nipples contain a rich supply of nerves. They respond to sexual excitement, stimulation, cold, or friction by becoming hard and more prominent.

The Sexual Response Cycle

Sexual stimulation triggers a series of events known as the sexual response cycle. The stages of the cycle in both men and women follow a similar pattern, but can vary considerably. The stages are not clearly separated from one another, and may be felt in different ways from one time to another, and one person to another.

The sexual response cycle has been described in various ways. The concept was introduced by Masters and Johnson, who divided the cycle into four stages: excitement, plateau, orgasm, and resolution. Later, Helen Singer Kaplan presented a different classification that began with an initial stage of desire, also called the appetitive stage. In general, these classifications describe a response that begins with a resting state, proceeds to one of sexual arousal and satisfaction, and returns to a resting state.

FIGURE 16.4

The Sexual Response Cycle

While each person's sexual response cycle is different, most people experience the stages of arousal, plateau, orgasm, and resolution. This graph shows the general pattern of sexual response in women and men.

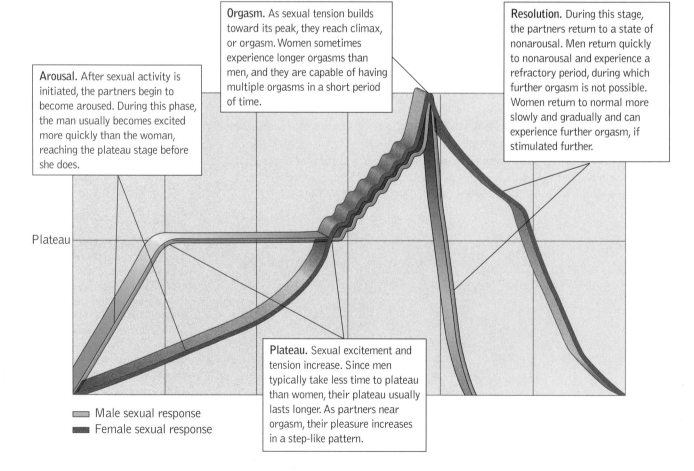

Orgasm. As sexual tension builds toward its peak, they reach climax, or orgasm. Women sometimes experience longer orgasms than men, and they are capable of having multiple orgasms in a short period of time.

Resolution. During this stage, the partners return to a state of nonarousal. Men return quickly to nonarousal and experience a refractory period, during which further orgasm is not possible. Women return to normal more slowly and gradually and can experience further orgasm, if stimulated further.

Arousal. After sexual activity is initiated, the partners begin to become aroused. During this phase, the man usually becomes excited more quickly than the woman, reaching the plateau stage before she does.

Plateau

Plateau. Sexual excitement and tension increase. Since men typically take less time to plateau than women, their plateau usually lasts longer. As partners near orgasm, their pleasure increases in a step-like pattern.

Male sexual response
Female sexual response

Two basic physiological reactions play a key role in sexual response. The first is vasocongestion—an increased amount of blood in the genitals and female breasts, causing them to become engorged and to swell. The second is increased neuromuscular tension and tone, which refers to a buildup of energy in the nerves and muscles. In response to sexual arousal, muscle tension builds throughout the body in both men and women. The response is the same during both homosexual and heterosexual behavior.

The Phases of the Sexual Response Cycle. The phases (also called events or stages) of the sexual response cycle need to be considered within the context of the thoughts and feelings that are a part of the sexual experience itself:

- **Desire.** Sexual desire causes one to begin to be open to sexual activity. Factors that can influence desire are sexual fantasy, sexually explicit visual images and sounds, and sexual acts.
- **Excitement or arousal.** Touch, warmth, and pressure combined with a mental state that is receptive to sexual activity can lead to excitement. During this phase, the genital organs become filled with blood, causing an erection in the man and increased vaginal lubrication in the woman. This stage is easily interrupted, prolonged, or ended by mental or physical distractions.
- **Plateau.** This phase is a continuation of the excitement phase in which sexual tension increases. Vasocongestion of the genital organs continues, and the

wellness **tip**

Sexual response can be affected by sights, sounds, and visual perceptions, as well as feelings. The proper setting is important to sexual satisfaction. To create a romantic atmosphere, couples may light candles, have a fire in the fireplace, play soft music, use room fragrance, and so on.

The Sexual Response Cycle

PHASE	CHANGES IN WOMEN	CHANGES IN MEN
AROUSAL	· Vagina becomes lubricated · Labia thicken · Lower vagina expands · Nipples become erect · Clitoris swells	· Penis becomes erect · Scrotum thickens · Testes elevate
PLATEAU	· Orgasmic platform occurs · Labia swell · Clitoris pulls back · Labia color intensifies · Sex flush appears · The uterus expands and rises · Nipples and breasts enlarge	· Head of the penis enlarges · Testes swell · Testes elevate and rotate · Penis color deepens · Penis secretes clear fluid
ORGASM	· Vagina, uterus, and other muscles contract	· Penis ejaculates · Muscles contract
RESOLUTION	· Sex flush subsides · Organs return to normal state	· Erection subsides · Refractory period begins

outer third of the woman's vagina swells to grip the penis to create what is called the "orgasmic platform." Heart rate, breathing, and blood pressure increase, and the woman's skin may become flushed, especially on her chest, in what is sometimes referred to as the "sex flush."

- **Orgasm.** During this phase, excitement and pleasure build, leading to a release of sexual tension in pleasurable contractions. The man ejaculates semen in rhythmic contractions. The woman's lower vagina, uterus, and the muscle surrounding the rectum also contract. Women's orgasms may be longer then men's, and they can have multiple orgasms close together. The experiences of these orgasms can vary greatly, however.
- **Resolution.** This phase is the return to a state of nonarousal. It includes the refractory period in men, a recovery time during which further orgasm or ejaculation is not possible. Women do not have a similar refractory period and can have multiple orgasms if sexual stimulation is continued.

Personal Differences in the Sexual Response Cycle. The way in which a person goes through the sexual response cycle varies greatly from one person to another and from one sexual encounter to another. There is no set standard for what is "normal." Reaching and passing through each stage is key to sexual satisfaction, however; disruption in any stage can interfere with that satisfaction.

Sexual **Practices**

While sexual behavior is made up of a deeply personal set of attitudes, actions, and responses, staying informed about research findings in the area of sexual practice can give you a perspective on your own ideas about sex and sexuality. Most research in this area looks at the number of sexual partners people have, how often couples have sex, and how sexual preferences vary between both genders and among different populations.

Recent findings reveal some surprising and not so surprising results. Sexual activity among adolescents and the number of sexual partners have increased dramatically. Other findings indicate that Americans are more traditional than was previously thought; for example, one study confirmed that most married couples are monogamous and that the most favored form of heterosexual sexual activity remains vaginal intercourse. Following are several more trends in sexual behavior in the United States.

Frequency of Sex

Overall, the average man has sex seven times per month and the average woman six times per month. Following is a breakdown of how often American women reported having sex with a partner:

Four or more times a week	7 percent
Two to three times a week	32 percent
A few times a month	47 percent
A few times a year	12 percent
Never	3 percent

Homosexuality

There may be fewer men and women who are homosexual than previously thought. Although earlier estimates were that 10 percent of the population is homosexual, in a recent survey only about 1.3 percent of women reported having sex only with women over the previous year. The number of gay and lesbian individuals is very hard to project with accuracy, however.

Heterosexual Sex

Research indicates that heterosexual couples follow a familiar pattern when having sex. The couple starts with hugging and moves into kissing and bodily caressing, followed by intercourse. Vaginal intercourse is the most common sexual activity, followed by oral sex. Many women also enjoy masturbation, fantasizing, and watching their partner undress.

Solitary Sex

Masturbation is sexual self-stimulation through rubbing, stroking, fondling, squeezing, or otherwise stimulating the genitals or other parts of the body. It often begins during childhood, as children explore their genitals and learn about sexual response. While masturbation was once considered taboo, today it is thought to be a normal, healthy part of sexual development. Among individuals aged 18 to 59 years who participated in a survey, 60 percent of men and 40 percent of women said they masturbated in the past year. About one woman in ten reported masturbating at least once a week. These techniques can also be used by couples as a means of enhancing mutual satisfaction and learning more about each other.

There are a variety of techniques for female masturbation. Often several techniques will be used together. Women may combine genital stroking with the use of a vibrator, or dildo. A vibrator can produce an intense sexual response. Other forms of solitary sex can come from reading or looking at sexually explicit materials. Such materials are widely available and can produce arousal by triggering the imagination in a non-threatening setting. Erotic materials can also aid in sexual fantasy.

Sexual Fantasy

Sexual fantasy can be a means of expressing or provoking sexual desire. It is an important creative process that allows people to escape from everyday life and be transported into a dream world filled with excitement and pleasure. Sexual fantasies can be used to induce or enhance sexual arousal and may be combined with other forms of stimulation. They provide a safe environment for engaging the imagination to explore new and exciting forms of expression without any risk. Most women who have fantasies about unusual

Favorite Sexual Activities

A survey of sexual practices in the United States disclosed that the following activities were ranked "very appealing" by men and women aged 18 to 44:

ACTIVITY	WOMEN	MEN
Vaginal intercourse	78%	83%
Receiving oral sex	33%	50%
Watching partner undress	30%	50%
Giving oral sex	19%	37%
Group sex	1%	14%
Using dildo/vibrator	3%	5%
Watching others do sexual things	2%	6%
Same gender sex partner	3%	4%
Sex with a stranger	1%	5%

Source: Adapted from *Sex in America* by Laumann, E.O., Michael, Robert T., and Kolata, G. (Boston: Little, Brown) 1994.

or "kinky" sexual activity have no interest in actually participating in such activity. Men, however, may be more inclined to act out their fantasies.

Common sexual fantasies include having sex in a public place, conquest fantasies with an element of power, and fantasies about switching partners. Other themes include group sex, watching others engage in sex, or forced sex. Although there may be some gender differences in the theme, overall men and women are fairly similar in their sexual fantasy patterns and their use of fantasy to enhance sexual arousal.

Sexual **Fulfillment**

Having a fulfilling sexual experience depends on a number of complex emotional and physical factors. Many women are juggling work, family, and home obligations, and they struggle to find time for relaxation and intimacy with their partners. It is not surprising that a woman who is troubled by problems with school, work, and/or family might have difficulty escaping into her sexual fantasies or enabling herself to let go long enough or completely enough to attain sexual fulfillment. Many women are single parents and faced with financial and childrearing obligations, compounded by the lack of a partner.

It is important that women not lose sight of their sexuality as a key aspect of their broader experience of living and wellness. Setting priorities for intimacy, finding time for personal fulfillment, keeping the lines of communication open with their partner, and using relaxation techniques to help enjoy sexual experiences add to the fullness of life as well as sexuality.

Factors That Affect Sexual Fulfillment

Stress, fatigue, and a general state of anxiety are occupational hazards of today's fast-paced lifestyles. They can upset the delicate balance of women's lives and result in obstacles to sexual satisfaction and fulfillment. Other factors, such as aging, chronic illness, and relationship problems can also cause problems.

Aging. Both men and women experience changes in their sexual response as they age. Some of these changes have to do with the natural changes of aging, whereas others may be related to illness or losing one's partner.

The changes in the production of the hormone estrogen that accompany menopause can affect the sexual response cycle in women. Sexual desire and frequency of intercourse decrease as women age, although women remain interested in sex and continue to have the capability to enjoy sex for their entire lives. Much of a woman's sex life after menopause is related to her sexuality before menopause. The more sexually active a woman was, the more likely she is to maintain that level of activity.

Physiological changes associated with estrogen depletion include thinning and dryness of the vaginal walls. Women require more time to become sexually aroused and produce lubrication. Inadequate lubrication can cause discomfort during intercourse at any age, but may be more problematic after menopause, due to changes in the vaginal mucus membranes. Adequate lubrication may be enhanced with any one of the many over-the-counter products now available.

Spending a longer time in foreplay before intercourse can also be helpful.

Men often experience a decrease in sexual desire and have sex less often as they age. They have fewer nocturnal and morning erections and may require more intense stimulation for erection and ejaculation. When the erection occurs, it often is not as firm. The refractory period, the length of time until a man can have intercourse again, is longer in older men. Most men appreciate their partner's sensitivity to these changes.

Illnesses that accompany age, as well as the medication used to treat those illnesses, can affect sexual function in both men and women. Circulatory problems can decrease blood flow to genital organs and reduce arousal, vaginal lubrication, and the intensity of an orgasm. Chronic obstructive pulmonary disease can lower testosterone levels and impair sexual desire. Pain from arthritis may make it difficult to find a comfortable position during intercourse. Couples may find that they have difficulty adapting to new ways to function sexually that do not include intercourse. They may be further hindered by privacy issues if they are living in a nursing home or with their children.

Many of the problems confronting older people can be overcome by a change in technique. Taking a warm bath before lovemaking can loosen stiff joints. Couples may have more energy for making love in the morning, when they are less fatigued. Couples can consider using other means of stimulating each other to orgasm without intercourse. Feeling comfortable with changes in approaches to their lovemaking is important; neither partner should feel forced into doing something. Men and women can enjoy a warm, close relationship in a variety of ways.

Illness. Illness, whether in young, middle, or older adulthood, can affect all aspects of functioning, including sexuality. Short-term or acute illnesses usually have limited or temporary negative effects. Chronic diseases, however, can have a major impact on a person's self-image and her ability to respond sexually. Illness and disease can create pain, fatigue, depression, or directly interfere with the normal mechanisms required for sexual functioning. The following chronic conditions can impair sexual function:

- Multiple sclerosis
- Arthritis
- Spinal cord injury
- Diabetes
- Thyroid disease
- Heart disease

Everyone experiences natural changes in their sexuality during long-term relationships, including marriage. You can make periods of transition more smooth by maintaining a warm, close relationship with your partner.

wellness **tip**

Water-based lubricants, available as gel, liquid, or suppositories, can be used to increase vaginal moisture at the time of intercourse. Some water-based lubricants contain a spermicide for an added measure of birth control protection. There are also "bioadhesive" products available that deliver small amounts of lubricant and only have to be used two or three times weekly. Never use petroleum-based lubricants. These products introduce foreign material into the vagina and may increase vaginal infections. They also break down the latex in condoms.

A chronic illness may require a major change in a person's life, including her sexuality. Most chronically ill individuals can and do develop new forms of sexual activity, especially if they have a history of satisfying sexual relationships before their illness.

Drugs and Medications. Both recreational drugs and prescription medications can interfere with sexual function. Alcohol, for example, is a depressant. It depresses the central nervous system and can interfere with messages that trigger sexual response. Although alcohol may lower a person's inhibitions and make her more likely to engage in sexual activity, alcohol does not enhance satisfaction and in some cases may even limit performance.

Sexual response is also altered by recreational drugs, such as cocaine and marijuana. Cocaine may make the user feel more comfortable socially, but it tends to divert her attention away from sexual interest. Marijuana can reduce production of vaginal lubrication and cause irritation or pain unless lubrication is replaced with over-the-counter products.

Medications that interfere with sexual function can do so by decreasing desire, delaying or preventing orgasm, or causing painful swelling of the clitoris. The most commonly used medications that cause sexual problems are antihypertensive agents, diuretics, antipsychotic agents, antidepressants, antihistamines, barbiturates, and narcotics. Some antidepressants in the category called selective serotonin reuptake inhibitors (SSRIs) can depress sexual interest as well as interfere with a woman's ability to function sexually or have an orgasm. Medications can also cause men to be unable to get or hold an erection.

Psychosocial Problems. Stressors in a world that is increasingly complicated can have a dramatic impact on physical intimacy and other quality of life issues. Basic needs for income, food, shelter, or childcare may limit a woman's time and energy for sexual interest. Achieving these basic needs may also be a source of conflict between partners that decreases the desire for physical contact. The onset of mental or physical disability may directly affect basic needs as well as sexual ability.

The use or inappropriate use of tobacco, alcohol, or other drugs can be a source of conflict between partners or may directly affect sexual desire and performance. Cultural or religious differences between partners and their families may result in unmet expectations for abstinence, for sexual activity, or for childbearing.

Unplanned or mistimed pregnancy, inadequate readiness for parenting, and the presence of children in the home are often distracting to sexual intimacy. Increasing demands from outside the partnership—aging parents, stepchildren, or work responsibilities, for example—are a common source of conflict and disruption.

Some couples encounter problems because they have differing views on how physically and emotionally close each would like to be to the other. One partner may want to be very close whereas the other wants some distance. Other couples may have different levels of desire. Many factors can affect a couple's sexual function and lead to anger, fear, and frustration. These include: spouse abuse, financial disagreements, poor communication, work-related stress, day-to-day childcare responsibilities, and marital power or control issues. (See Chapter 14 for a discussion of domestic violence.)

Psychological problems that affect sexual function can stem from inappropriate learning or conditioning earlier in life. Sexual abuse can be traumatic and have a lasting emotional impact. Some women who have been abused as children feel that their sense of trust has been violated and may have difficulties relating in an intimate and sensual way to their partners. Other women may lose their sexual desire or ability to have an orgasm.

Problems that have a psychological basis—either from a past event or ongoing conflict—may respond to counseling. If candid and honest dialogue does not improve the situation for the couple, they need to consider seeking the help of a marriage counselor or sex therapist.

Pregnancy and Childbirth. Patterns of sexual behavior may change during pregnancy, but in most cases they do not need to change. Some of the discomforts of early pregnancy, such as morning sickness and fatigue, may make a woman less interested in sex. As the pregnancy progresses, however, these symptoms ease and many women have renewed interest in sex. Sexual activity usually decreases in late pregnancy because of discomfort.

Sexual intercourse does not harm the fetus, which is protected inside the uterus. There are certain conditions, however, under which the couple may be advised to avoid intercourse. The most common reasons are bleeding or cervical changes at any stage of pregnancy. Couples with threatened preterm labor or a history of preterm delivery should get advice from their physicians about all forms of sexual intimacy, since the strong uterine contractions associated with orgasm in women may initiate labor.

wellness **tip**

Depression itself often results in a lack of interest in sex. Certain drugs to treat depression can add to the problem. If you are being treated for depression and do not regain interest in sex, ask your doctor if your medication has that side effect. If it does, another medication can often be substituted.

Unplanned Pregnancy

More than half of the 6 million pregnancies conceived in this country each year are mistimed or unintended. Women who carry these pregnancies begin prenatal care later and receive less adequate prenatal care than women with planned pregnancies. The fetuses are more likely to be exposed to harmful substances, like tobacco and alcohol. The child produced by an unplanned pregnancy is at greater risk of being born at a low birth weight and dying within its first year.

The mother is at a greater risk for depression and physical abuse. The relationship with her partner is at greater risk for breakup. Both parents may suffer economic hardship and may fail to achieve their educational and career potentials. This is especially striking among teens who become pregnant accidentally.

The children that result from these pregnancies have higher rates of physical abuse and neglect. They are more likely to be impoverished. They are more likely to be raised by a single parent—usually the mother. They themselves are more likely to drop out of school. All of which means that these children absorb a disproportionate share of the federal and state financial resources allocated for physical and mental health, as well as resources allocated for social interventions. Consider these alarming statistics:

- 56 percent of the 6.4 million pregnancies in the United States are unplanned.
- More than 75 percent of young women and 85 percent of young men have had sexual intercourse by age 20.
- Each year one out of ten sexually active women under age 20 becomes pregnant.
- An estimated 85 percent of teen pregnancies are unintended.

Planned or unplanned pregnancy among teens is higher in the United States than in any other country in the developed world. U.S. teens are not more sexually active than European teens, but they are much less likely to use contraception and much more likely to become pregnant and to contract sexually transmitted diseases. Recent public policies and consumer education efforts focusing on abstinence have had little effect and must be modified to promote the use of contraception in those teens who choose to be sexually active.

wellness **tip**

A side entry position, with the woman in front of the man ("spoon" fashion), puts less pressure on a woman's abdomen and may be more comfortable during pregnancy.

Sexual satisfaction in pregnancy is closely related to feeling happy about the pregnancy, feeling attractive, and achieving orgasm. A couple may choose to try different forms of expressing their sexuality during pregnancy. Forms of sexual activity that may be enjoyable include genital and oral-genital stimulation. Most women have an increased desire to be held while they are pregnant. The need for closeness, emotional support, and nurturing during late pregnancy can be met with touching, caressing, and holding.

Normally, a woman can resume sexual activity after birth as soon as she feels comfortable. She may, however, find herself tired and overcome by the demands of a new baby. As demands from the infant settle into a routine, most women resume sexual relations at the same level as before pregnancy.

Infertility. Infertility can affect a woman's feelings about her self-worth, her self-esteem, and her body image. It can cause her to feel depressed, hopeless, unattractive, and sexually undesirable. The need for scheduled intercourse while trying to get pregnant disrupts sexual spontaneity, puts enormous performance pressure on both partners, and often dulls sexual satisfaction even during unscheduled intercourse. There are many options available these days to couples who need assistance with fertility issues. Many centers that specialize in this kind of care routinely recommend counseling to help couples through this difficult time. (See Chapter 17 for more information on infertility.)

Gynecological Conditions. Alteration of a woman's sexual organs by disease or surgery may affect her sexuality directly, indirectly, or both ways.

When there is surgical alteration of the vulva or vagina, intercourse may temporarily be prohibited. Once intercourse is resumed, experiences of painful intercourse or concern about the condition may cause it to be less pleasurable than before surgery. With some cancer diagnoses, radical surgery or radiation damage may permanently alter a woman's ability to have vaginal intercourse. Counseling for the patient and her partner will help them learn other sexual techniques and retain the physical intimacy that has been important to them at other times in their lives.

Most women cope well with breast cancer treatment and do not develop sexual problems as a result of it. In a study comparing women who had a breast removed (mastectomy) versus those who had a lump removed (lumpectomy), researchers found there was no difference in marital satisfaction, psychological adjustment, frequency of sex, and sexual problems. Women with mastectomies may have problems with self-image, however. The best indicator of sexual satisfaction after surgery is a good mental outlook, a secure relationship, and a satisfying sex life before surgery.

Many women worry about a change in their sexual response after a hysterectomy, but most women report no permanent effects. In the period following a hysterectomy, some women report feeling "different," some note a slow return to normal vaginal lubrication, and some express concerns about their partners' response to them. Again, the advice of the surgeon may be helpful.

Removal of the ovaries in a premenopausal woman will result in marked alterations in her hormonal status, which causes significant changes in many areas. Vaginal changes include decreased lubrication, increased fragility of the mucous membranes, and loss of support for the bladder and urethra. Alterations in mood, memory, sleep, and libido are often more intense than those experienced by women who go through natural menopause. These symptoms can be relieved by hormone replacement therapy, unless there is a medical reason not to use this type of therapy.

Improving Sexual Fulfillment

Wellness includes achieving and maintaining sexual fulfillment. There are many ways you can take a proactive role in improving your sexual relationships and experiences.

Communication. Keep the lines of communication between you and your partner open. Try to pinpoint any obstacles to sexual satisfaction. If you have a delicate issue to talk about related to sex, choose a neutral setting outside the bedroom, such as over a quiet dinner when you are both rested and relaxed.

New Approaches. Experiment with new approaches, such as making love in different settings and trying different positions for intercourse, to promote better understanding between you and your partner. Consider using sexual aids, such as lubricants, sensual clothing and lingerie, sexually explicit literature and videos, as well as vibrators and other devices.

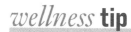
wellness **tip**

If you have had a mastectomy and are concerned about your appearance, consider surgical breast reconstruction. Familiarize yourself with the types of implants available to be sure you understand any risks or restrictions.

Keeping the Lines of Communication Open

Lack of knowledge is one of the major obstacles couples face in achieving sexual satisfaction. In many cases, simply not sharing information about wants and needs can close the door of communication. Both partners have a responsibility to tell the other what they want, what pleases them, and what does not give pleasure.

If the problem is a new one, talk with your partner about it to clear up any misunderstandings or disagreements. If that doesn't work, try talking to a doctor or counselor. There are techniques you can learn to help you relax, communicate better, and discover what gives you pleasure. There are also many good books and videos to provide guidance about new forms of communication and expression.

Women who learn how to tell their partners about their sexual needs have a better chance of having a satisfying sex life. Here are some tips for good communication:

- Think over in advance what you want to say and how you want to say it.
- Stick to key points and be concise.
- Give your partner a chance to respond and interact.
- Do not be critical or put your partner on the defensive.
- Ask for feedback.
- Be aware of your nonverbal messages—make sure they are consistent with verbal ones.

wellness **tip**

A woman may not be aroused because of a lack of foreplay. Take time to go through the stages of sexual response, but try not to focus too much on performance.

Mutual Pleasure. Focus on giving each other mutual pleasure. Understand that both partners deserve to enjoy giving and receiving pleasure. Do not rush sex.

Sensate Focusing Exercises. Sensate focusing exercises were introduced by Masters and Johnson as a way to reduce sexual anxiety, improve communication, and overcome a lack of sexual experience and knowledge. Pressures to perform are removed by banning direct sexual contact during the initial stages of therapy. The counselor then helps the couple discover the sensual pleasures of touching and being touched without the goal of a particular sexual response. Following are the stages of sensate focusing exercises, which take place over an extended time under the direction of a therapist:

- The partners take turns touching one another, with breasts and genitals being off limits.
- Touching is expanded to include the breasts and genitals.
- The couple engages in mutual touching.
- Touching is continued with the female shifting to the top position without attempting intercourse.
- The couple can proceed with intercourse if they wish and stop if either partner becomes goal-oriented or anxious.

Sexual **Disorders**

A sexual problem can stem from biological factors, such as vaginismus, or psychological factors, such as prior sexual or emotional abuse. More likely, a combination of factors is involved. Sexual problems can arise at any stage of the sexual response cycle. Many of these disorders can be treated with therapy.

For some the problem stems from lack of desire. Others can suffer from performance anxiety, low self-esteem, depression, fear of intimacy, or guilt about sex and pleasure. Some individuals are so afraid that they will lose control of their sexual feelings they may suppress them altogether. Others may work so hard at their performance that they cannot enjoy the experience.

Sexual disorders can be classified as situational or generalized; they can also be divided into lifelong or acquired:

- Situational disorders occur in some situations and not others.
- Generalized disorders occur regardless of the situation.
- Lifelong disorders have been present from onset of sexual behavior.
- Acquired disorders arise at some point after a person has had unimpaired sexual function.

Disorders that relate to women include sexual arousal disorders, orgasmic disorders, and vaginismus. Those that relate to men include erectile dysfunction, orgasmic disorders, and premature ejaculation. Inhibited sexual desire can occur in both men and women.

Lack of Desire

Lack of desire is the most common sexual problem in women, although it also affects men. In a recent survey, over 30 percent of women and 15 percent of men reported a lack of interest in sex for at least one month in the previous year. Lack of desire is considered a disorder only if it is perceived as a source of distress to a person or a relationship.

Lack of desire can be caused by both physical and psychological factors. For example, some women on birth control pills (which regulate hormones) find that their level of sexual desire is lowered. They may not attribute those feelings to being on the pill, simply because their doctor never explained that this is a potential side effect.

Women who experience a lack of desire usually avoid all forms of genital sexual contact with a sexual partner. They do not experience sexual fantasies, notice attractive potential partners, or feel frustrated by being deprived of sexual contact. Treatment usually involves psychological counseling to identify the causes of the condition.

Female Sexual Arousal Disorders

Lack of arousal can disrupt sexual response. In women who cannot become aroused, the vagina does not lubricate or expand. Women with a sexual arousal disorder usually have limited erotic sensations. They may have mixed feelings about physical contact or an inability to communicate with a partner about what sensations they find pleasurable.

Lack of arousal can be situational or generalized, lifelong or acquired. Some of the most common causes are guilt and hostility. The guilt may stem from an inner conflict about sexuality. The hostility often involves feelings toward the partner. Counseling can often be helpful in identifying and treating the causes of lack of arousal.

Female Orgasmic Disorder

Female orgasmic disorder is the delay or absence of orgasm in a woman following normal sexual excitement. With this condition, a woman can become aroused, but she has difficulty in reaching the orgasm stage. Some women have never had an orgasm, whereas others require a great deal of stimulation, on the part of themselves or their partner. Some women may think they have this disorder if they are only able to reach orgasm through clitoral stimulation and not intercourse. This is not true; there is no "right" way to have an orgasm. Orgasms are the same, regardless of whether the source is clitoral or vaginal. They may vary in intensity, however, both from one time to another and in one woman to another.

Lack of orgasm can result from setting intercourse and orgasm as the goal for sexual satisfaction. This attitude creates pressure, which often prevents orgasm. "Spectatoring," in which a person becomes overly involved in watching what they are doing and not participating in it, and anxiety about performance can prevent orgasm. Another factor is fear of loss of control, of "letting go." Often lack of orgasm can result from ineffective sexual techniques and can be corrected by learning how to give or receive sexual stimulation.

Becoming Orgasmic

Certain exercises increase a woman's self-awareness by allowing her to explore her genital areas in a nonthreatening way. Once she has identified the most sensitive and pleasurable parts of her body, she can manually stimulate her clitoris and other areas until she reaches orgasm. Sexual fantasy and a vibrator may be useful.

Once a woman has had an orgasm through masturbation, she can teach the technique to her partner, showing him how and where she likes to be touched during lovemaking. The partner can be guided in manual stimulation by the woman placing a hand on top of her partner's hand.

Once a woman has reached a high level of arousal or orgasm, she and her partner may engage in intercourse if they choose to do so. Stimulation of the clitoris by the woman or her partner during intercourse may help her have an orgasm.

wellness **tip**

The "squeeze" technique, in which the man's penis is squeezed either at the base or head before intercourse, can be used to control premature ejaculation.

Vaginismus

Involuntary spasm of the muscle at the entrance of the vagina can make intercourse impossible. This condition may also include difficult or painful intercourse due to such contractions. It has been estimated to affect approximately 20 percent of women at some point in their lives. The cause is often linked to a painful experience, such as sexual assault or abuse, painful intercourse, or pelvic disease. It can often be treated through medical care and exercises.

Erectile Dysfunction

The inability of men to attain or maintain an erection until completion of sex is called erectile dysfunction. It often can be situational. Most men at some point of their lives have difficulty getting and keeping an erection, and this can have many causes. Some men are unable to have an erection during foreplay, while others have difficulty only when it is time to have intercourse. Erectile dysfunction can also occur with certain partners and not with others.

As men get older, erectile dysfunction often has a physical cause. The most common cause is surgery for prostate cancer. It can also be related to drug use (especially alcohol), chronic diseases, and injuries. Anxiety or conflict between partners also can play a role. A thorough physical and psychological evaluation is needed. Treatment options include counseling, medication, or more drastic options, like devices that are implanted in the penis.

Male Orgasmic Disorder

The persistent or recurrent delay in, or absence of, orgasm following normal sexual excitement is called male orgasmic disorder. It is fairly rare and can be confused with retrograde ejaculation, in which the man ejaculates into the bladder instead of out the urethra. The cause often is psychological, related to a traumatic sexual experience, strict religious upbringing, hostility, or lack of trust.

Premature Ejaculation

Ejaculation with minimal sexual stimulation before, upon, or shortly after penetration—and before the man wishes it—is considered premature. The treatment is often a matter of mental training—the man trains himself to detect and avoid particular erotic sensations that lead to ejaculation in an effort to prolong his ability to maintain his erection. Therapy can often help men identify such sensations and learn how to control them.

Seeking **Advice**

Many sexual problems can be treated in a primary care setting or by referral for counseling. It is important to be open and honest with your health care provider and to feel comfortable talking with her. Counseling for sexual problems is often short term and very effective. There are also quite a few sources of self-help information and support groups.

Primary Care

Sexual function is an important part of wellness that needs to be nurtured and maintained just as any other aspect of health. A primary physician should inquire about sexual health and history during routine examinations. If she does not ask, volunteer information yourself, ask questions, and voice concerns. You may need to schedule another visit to discuss these issues. Although some health care plans limit your choice of physician, try to find someone with whom you are comfortable. If you are not comfortable discussing these matters with your primary care physician, or if you feel you are not getting adequate answers, you should see someone else. While you may find that your primary care provider or obstetrician/gynecologist helps you address questions in this area, leave the option for therapy open for later consideration should a problem persist.

In evaluating sexual issues and exploring the need for counseling and therapy, some physicians use the PLISSIT model:

- Permission validates the woman's feelings and gives her permission to address her sexual concerns.
- Limited Information provides information about sexual anatomy, physiology, and behavior.
- Specific Suggestions involve specific reeducation regarding the woman's sexual attitudes and practices.
- Intensive Therapy is reserved for those women who do not respond to the first three levels and may require further individual therapy or treatment as a couple.

Counseling

Your primary care provider or obstetrician/gynecologist may refer you to a counselor. The choice of whether to pursue counseling or not may depend on the nature of the problem. If the problem is of a sexual nature, a sex therapist may be the best choice.

Sex therapists help couples work through their sexual problems, uncovering the cause and relearning behavior patterns. Some forms of therapeutic exercises, such as the sensate focusing exercises mentioned earlier, may be directed toward helping women achieve full sexual satisfaction. These exercises help a woman explore what gives her pleasure and how to show her partner. Other exercises help couples relate to each other without the pressure to perform.

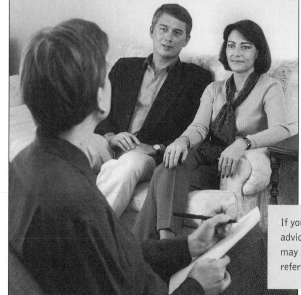

If you have a sexual problem, first seek the advice of your primary care physician. She may be able to help you herself, or she may refer you to a professional counselor.

Sex therapists should have basic training in the field of medicine, psychology, or social work. They should have advanced training in human sexuality and treatment of sexual dysfunction. Most sex therapists are certified by the American Association of Sex Educators, Counselors, and Therapists. Check any therapist's credentials thoroughly in advance.

A good source of self-help information is SIECUS (Sexuality Information and Education Council of the United States), a nonprofit organization that affirms that sexuality is a natural and healthy part of living. It develops, collects, and distributes information on sexuality, including a helpful annotated bibliography. Other sources of information include books, videos, and the Internet. One of the most important sources of information may be your partner.

What *You* Can Do

Sex is a normal, natural part of living. Healthy sexuality is as important as any other component of women's wellness. Sexual problems can arise at any time and in most cases can be worked through to achieve the fullest expression of sexuality:

- Talk with your children openly and honestly about sexuality; be aware that they will learn about it from others whether or not it is discussed at home, so it is best if they know they can talk openly with you about any questions they have.
- Be attuned to your sexuality and to messages being sent from you or your partner.
- Take responsibility for your own sexual pleasure. Don't expect your partner to know what you want without your communicating it.
- Explore new techniques and approaches to sexual fulfillment.
- If you have a concern about your sexuality, discuss it with your partner, doctor, or a friend.

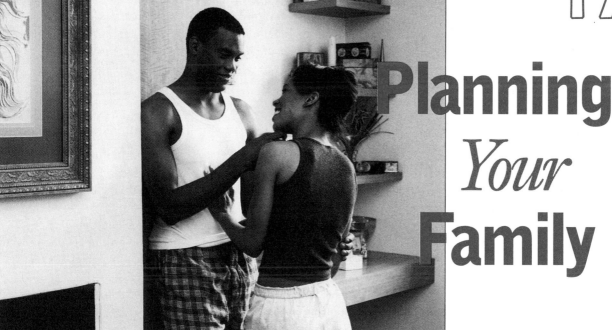

Chapter 17

Planning *Your* Family

The freedom to decide when—or if—a child becomes part of her life empowers a woman in ways not possible before safe and reliable birth control methods became available. Family planning can enable a woman to pursue goals, including higher education and a career. Having control over how many children to have and when to have them has positive effects on many aspects of a woman's life, including her health, her finances, and her sense of independence. Careful family planning is one key to maintaining good physical and emotional health throughout the childbearing years.

Above all, family planning is a choice. Some women prefer not to interfere with conception because of religious beliefs, because they want a large family, or because they simply feel the natural order of things is best. The majority of women in the United States, however, choose a method of birth control that allows them to plan how many children they will have, when they will have them, and under what circumstances.

Throughout her childbearing years, the sexually active woman has a number of choices with respect to family planning. During the time she wants to prevent pregnancy, choosing which birth control method is best for her is the primary decision. When she begins to think about having a child, the important considerations become centered around whether she is physically, emotionally, and financially prepared to raise a child, and whether her partner is prepared to share those responsibilities.

Although some women without partners decide to have a child alone, the decision is usually made with a partner. Communicating openly is the best policy when it comes to family planning. If one partner is not satisfied with the decision to have a child, bitterness about the decision can interfere with the relationship.

preview

► **Choosing Your Birth Control**

► **Hormonal Birth Control Methods**

► **Barrier Methods**

► **The Intrauterine Device**

► **Natural Birth Control Methods**

► **Sterilization**

► **When Birth Control Fails**

► **Coping with Infertility**

► **What You Can Do**

How Reproduction Occurs

A woman's menstrual cycle is about 28 days, beginning on the first day of her period. At around day 14, an egg is released from the woman's ovary. It then moves into the fallopian tube, where it can be fertilized by a man's sperm. If the egg is fertilized, it moves to the woman's uterus, becomes implanted in the lining of the uterus, and begins to grow. If it is not fertilized, the lining of the uterus and the unfertilized egg are shed as the next menstrual period.

The monthly cycle is regulated by hormones. Artificial birth control works by changing hormone levels or by preventing the sperm from meeting the egg. Natural birth control works by partners agreeing to avoid intercourse during the days when ovulation is likely to occur.

Or if one person is unhappy with the birth control method used, the sexual relationship may suffer. Open, ongoing communication about family planning enhances and strengthens relationships. This chapter offers a comprehensive description of birth control methods available to women and men, along with suggestions for deciding when and how to prepare for pregnancy.

Choosing *Your* Birth Control

Most women who use birth control try several methods before settling on the one that seems to work best and feels right to both partners. Before you explore the birth control options available to you, there are several factors to consider:

- **Effectiveness against pregnancy.** For some women, accidental pregnancy is physically, emotionally, or financially disastrous. If you absolutely do not want to become pregnant, then you need to consider birth control methods that have the lowest failure rates. Currently, the most effective methods are birth control pills, the intrauterine device (IUD), contraceptive injections or implants, and sterilization (male or female).
- **Disease protection.** Every woman should think carefully about whether or not she is at risk for sexually transmitted diseases (STDs). Even women who think they are in monogamous relationships can sometimes be surprised. If you think there is any chance you could contract a sexually transmitted infection, you will want to choose a method of birth control that also protects against STDs. The best choice for protection against STDs is the latex male condom. Female condoms are also believed to offer good protection. If a woman needs both excellent effectiveness against pregnancy and STD protection, she may combine methods—i.e., birth control pills and a latex condom.
- **Availability.** Some types of birth control require a prescription or even require medical procedures. Others can be purchased at the local drugstore. If you are interested in a method that does not require you to see a doctor, you should consider the male condom, female condom, spermicides, and natural family planning methods, such as the ovulation method.
- **Cost.** The cost of a birth control method may vary with the number of times you need contraceptive protection. If you have intercourse frequently, then a method that gives you "continuous" coverage—like the pill, implants, or the IUD—may be the most cost-effective. These options may also be covered by your health insurance or may be available at minimal cost through specialized clinics. If you have intercourse less frequently, then a method that provides protection on an "as needed" basis—like condoms, spermicides, or a diaphragm—makes more sense. These options are less often covered by health insurance, but specialized clinics may also provide assistance.
- **Health considerations.** Consider your overall health when choosing a birth control method. Talk with your doctor about your personal medical history, medications you are currently taking, and any previous health issues that might make a particular method more risky or less effective.

- **Personal vs. partner involvement.** Some women like having their partners share the responsibility for birth control. If this is true for you, consider the male condom, natural family planning, or male sterilization (bearing in mind, of course, that sterilization is permanent). Other women prefer to take the responsibility for contraception themselves. Methods that require more responsibility on the part of the woman include the female condom, the diaphragm, the cervical cap, birth control pills, IUDs, and hormonal implants. The last three have the advantage of not requiring a woman to do something at the time of intercourse in order to have protection against pregnancy. Many women find this more "natural" and less disruptive to making love.
- **Personal issues.** Moral issues sometimes dictate the choice of birth control. Some women, for example, do not choose the IUD because it may allow an egg to be fertilized but then prevent its implantation. Women for whom artificial birth control violates religious beliefs usually choose natural family planning.

Hormonal *Birth* Control Methods

A woman's body makes the hormones estrogen and progesterone, which play a major role in ovulation (the monthly release of an egg from the ovaries). When a woman is pregnant, the hormone levels in her body rise, signaling the ovaries to stop producing eggs. Introducing contraceptive hormones into a woman's body essentially "tricks" it into functioning as though she were pregnant. This means that no eggs will be available to be fertilized by sperm.

Hormonal contraception—which includes birth control pills, implants, and injections—is only available by prescription in this country. Birth control pills can be purchased over the counter in Europe and the United Kingdom.

Birth Control Pills

Birth control pills contain synthetic hormones that prevent ovulation. The birth control pills that are available today have low doses of hormones. For effectiveness, it is important that you take a pill each day at about the same time of day. Remembering to take the pill routinely is an important consideration if you choose this method. If you forget to take a pill for even one day, the level of hormones in your blood starts to drop, which may cause breakthrough bleeding and increase the likelihood of getting pregnant. If you forget to take one or more pills, refer to the package insert for appropriate directions. Don't take chances—use a backup method of birth control for the remainder of that cycle.

Benefits of the Birth Control Pill. When used correctly, the pill has a failure rate of less than one percent. There are other health benefits that do not have to do with birth control:

- **Easier periods.** Women who take the pill tend to have less cramping and pain with their menstrual period. Menstrual cycles are more regular, and menstrual bleeding is shorter and lighter.
- **Protection against pelvic inflammatory disease.** Although the pill does not protect against STDs, it seems to afford some protection against a complication

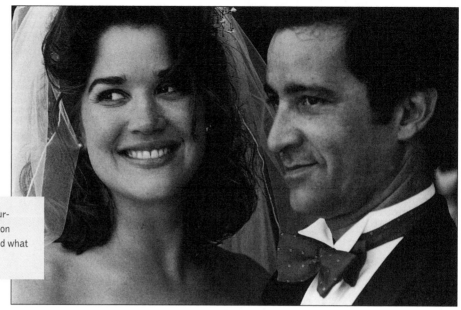

Among the many important decisions surrounding marriage is the couple's decision whether to have children (and when) and what method of birth control they will use.

of these diseases—pelvic inflammatory disease (PID). (See Chapter 22 for a discussion of PID.) Little is known about the reason why, but the prevailing theory is that the presence of less menstrual fluid and the pill's tendency to thicken cervical mucus reduces the chances that an STD will lead to PID.

- **Protection against ovarian cancer and endometriosis.** Taking the pill provides long-term protection from cancers of the ovary and the endometrium. The longer a woman has taken the pill, the greater her protection from these types of cancer.
- **Less fibrocystic breast disease.** Fibrocystic (lumpy) breasts are less likely in women who take the pill.
- **Acne relief.** Most birth control pills also suppress the hormone testosterone, which can cause acne, and thus may help to clear or control acne.
- **Protection against osteoporosis.** Researchers have discovered that taking birth control pills can provide protection against osteoporosis by helping keep bones dense. This is especially important in extremely thin or athletic women who do not have regular menstrual cycles.

Side Effects and Risks. Most side effects that women experience when taking birth control pills are minor, but they can be worrisome if you do not know what to expect. If you have questions about any side effects you are having, be sure to ask your doctor or nurse at your next visit, or call the office for information between visits. Any sudden or severe pain that cannot be explained should be reported to the doctor as soon as possible.

Following are some of the common side effects experienced by women who take birth control pills:

- **Headaches.** Headaches are almost never serious and can be treated with over-the-counter pain relievers. Some women who have migraines, however, find that birth control pills sometimes make their migraines worse. Any severe headache that does not respond to usual pain relievers or is accompanied by changes in vision or sensation should be evaluated by a doctor.

- **Breast tenderness.** Many women report tender breasts when they first begin taking the pill. The condition usually subsides within a few cycles.
- **Stomach upset.** Nausea akin to the morning sickness experienced by pregnant women occurs in some women when they first start taking the pill. The body adjusts rapidly, however, and nausea usually subsides within one or two cycles.

Serious complications linked to birth control pill use are extremely rare. In fact, for most women, the risks of becoming ill or dying from complications of pregnancy are much greater than the risks associated with taking birth control pills:

- **Blood clots.** Venous thrombosis, blood clots in the veins, occurs because estrogen helps the blood to clot. (Most birth control pills contain estrogen.) Blood clots can break apart and move into the brain (causing stroke), into the heart (causing cardiac arrest), or into the lung (causing pulmonary embolism). Women who have had a stroke, heart attack, or thrombosis should not take estrogen. You can talk to your doctor about the possibility of taking the mini-pill, which contains only progestin.
- **Elevated blood pressure.** Birth control pills sometimes cause small increases in blood pressure, but rarely does it rise above the normal range. Your doctor or nurse will check your blood pressure each time you get a new prescription for pills. If your blood pressure is significantly higher and remains high for several visits, your doctor will probably suggest that you stop taking birth control pills and use another type of birth control.
- **Breast cancer.** A few studies have linked pill use with breast cancer, but many other studies have found no link—not even for women who have a family history of breast cancer. Some questions remain, however, so it is recommended that you talk with your doctor if you are concerned.
- **Cervical cancer.** There is good evidence that birth control pills most likely do not increase rates for cervical cancer. Although some studies have shown higher rates of cervical cancer in women who use the pill, the higher rates are probably due to other factors—like smoking, multiple sexual partners, and loss of the protective effect from condom use. Fortunately, the Pap test taken at a woman's annual gynecological examination is a very effective way of detecting early changes in the cervix that could lead to cancer.
- **Liver problems.** Researchers have been concerned that pill users may be at a higher risk for liver cancer, but the actual

---

wellness tip

To remember to take your birth control pills, leave them out where you will see them—on your night table or bathroom counter—and take your pills at the same time you do some daily activity, such as brushing your teeth or putting on your watch. If young children are in the house, you must, of course, keep the pills out of their reach.

Watch Out for Pill Myths

Many women believe things about the pill that just aren't true. Here are some of the myths—and truths—about birth control pills:

Myth: The pill causes cancer.
Truth: The pill provides protection against cancers of the ovary and endometrium.

Myth: I'll gain weight if I take the pill.
Truth: As many women lose weight as gain when taking the pill.

Myth: Taking a break from the pills is a good idea from time to time.
Truth: Stopping pill use increases the chance that you will become pregnant.

Myth: The pill will make me infertile later, when I want to have a baby.
Truth: There is no connection between pill use and a woman's efforts to become pregnant after stopping pill use.

wellness
warning

If you are over age 35
and smoke cigarettes,
birth control pills are not a
good choice for you. The
combination of smoking and
taking the pill has been
shown to increase the risk
of heart attack and stroke.

studies do not reach that conclusion. The pill is broken down by the liver, so women who already have problems with their liver—for example, women with hepatitis—should probably use another method.

- **Drug interactions.** Combining the pill with other medications can cause side effects or may even make the pill less effective. For example, medications that are used to control seizures may make progestin less effective. Other medications that affect progestin include the antibiotics rifampin and griseofulvin, used to treat yeast and other fungal infections. The pill can also change how other medications work. Be sure to let your doctor or nurse know if you are taking other medications so your dosages can be adjusted, if necessary.

Contraceptive Injections and Implants

A contraceptive injection utilizes a progestin called depot medroxyprogesterone acetate, which is commonly injected into the buttock. The injection usually is not painful, but if it is, it is important that you avoid massaging the area where you were injected, which can lower the effectiveness of the injection. If you schedule your first injection for within five days of the start of your menstrual period, you will get full protection against pregnancy right from the start. If you get your first injection at any other time, use a backup method of birth control, such as condoms, for the first two weeks after your shot.

The injection works for at least three months. After you have been on contraceptive injections for a few three-month cycles, the injections will usually provide you with a little more than three months of protection—about an extra two weeks. This gives you a cushion in case you cannot get to the doctor right at three months. Once you have had the injection, there is no way to reverse it—that is, to become fertile again—until the injection wears off at least three months later.

Contraceptive implants are small matchstick-shaped capsules made of soft plastic placed under the skin of the upper arm, using local anesthesia. Implants contain levonorgestrel, a type of progestin. Originally, implants came only in sets of six—all six implants had to be used to provide effective birth control. The Food and Drug Administration (FDA) has recently approved a new type of contraceptive implants that requires only two implants. Ask your doctor or nurse about it.

If you can, schedule your implant placement for within seven days after the start of your menstrual period. You will then be protected right away against pregnancy. If you get your implants later in your cycle, use a backup method for a few days after the insertion. Implants protect against pregnancy for five years, but you can have the implants removed at any time, with the return of fertility within a short period of time.

Benefits of Injections and Implants. Contraceptive injections and implants share the following benefits:

Women Who Should Not Use Contraceptive Injections and Implants:

Contraceptive injections should be avoided by women who:

- Are pregnant or might be pregnant.
- Have had unexplained, abnormal vaginal bleeding in the past three months.

Contraceptive implants should be avoided by women who:

- Are pregnant or might be pregnant.
- Have unexplained, abnormal vaginal bleeding.
- Are taking antiseizure medications or the antibiotic rifampin.
- Have blood clots in the veins or have had pulmonary embolism (blood clot in the lungs).

- **Estrogen free.** One of the special advantages of progestin-only methods is that they do not have estrogen. Women who should not take estrogen may be able to use these methods. Women who want to start hormonal contraception soon after birth are often given progestin-only pills, injections or implants. Contraceptive injections and implants are considered safe for use by women who are breastfeeding, but they are usually started after breastfeeding is established.
- **Easy to use.** Convenience is a major benefit of contraceptive injections and implants. You do not have to remember to take a pill each day, nor do you have to do anything before you have sex, except to protect against STDs.

Side Effects and Risks. Following are the major side effects and risks associated with the use of contraceptive injections and implants:

- **Spotting.** While progestin-only methods may cause bleeding to stop completely (which usually does not cause complaints), they occasionally cause bleeding to occur at unpredictable times. Once bleeding starts, it often is like a normal period—but these unpredictable episodes of bleeding are the main reason women stop using these methods.
- **Headaches.** Headaches are the second most common problem with implants and injections. Women who have migraines or other types of headaches should be aware that they may have more headaches with these methods. If you have headaches, tell your doctor or nurse before you are prescribed either implants or injections.
- **Drug interactions.** There are some medications that interact with progestin-only methods that could make them less effective. As with the pill, the antibiotic rifampin and most types of antiseizure medicines may make progestin-only methods less effective. Contraceptive injections may be less affected to a lesser degree by these other medications, but a thorough discussion with your doctor is advised before you begin these birth control methods. You should also mention the birth control if you see a doctor and get new prescription medications after you have begun one of these methods—to prevent drug interaction and to prevent pregnancy.
- **Loss of HDL.** The hormone used in contraceptive injections reduces the level of high-density lipoprotein (HDL or "good") cholesterol in the body. These changes do not occur in women using contraceptive implants or the minipill. Even with this side effect, progestin-only methods are less likely than the birth control pills to be implicated in cardiovascular disease.
- **Ovarian cysts.** Ovarian cysts are more common in women who use progestin-only birth control methods. Most go away on their own. Sometimes, though, ovarian cysts can be painful. If this is the case, your doctor can switch you to another method. Because pain is also a symptom associated with ectopic pregnancy, you may need to be checked by a doctor if you have severe, unexplained abdominal pain.
- **Skin infection.** Because inserting contraceptive implants involves a minor surgical procedure and placing a foreign object in the arm, there is a small risk (less than one percent) that infection may occur where the implants are placed. Skin irritation is more common, but still occurs in less than five percent of women who get implants.

When to Call Your Doctor

If you are using contraceptive *injections* or *implants* for birth control, call your doctor if you experience excessive weight gain, severe headaches, heavy bleeding, depression, or frequent urination. You should also call your doctor if you experience severe lower abdominal pain (ectopic pregnancy is rare but can occur). If you are using contraceptive *implants,* you should contact your doctor in the case of arm pain, pus or bleeding at the insertion site (these may be signs of infection), expulsion of an implant, or delayed menstrual periods after a long time in which periods were regular.

If you are using the *minipill* (progestin only), call your doctor if you have any abdominal pain. It may be due to an ectopic pregnancy or ovarian cyst. You should not stop taking your pills, but you should call your doctor right away. If you take your pill late, you increase the chance of pregnancy. Even if you take your pill as little as three hours late, you should use a backup method of birth control for the next two days to be sure you are protected against pregnancy.

- **Weight gain.** It does seem that contraceptive injections and implants are more likely to make a woman gain weight than the pill or other types of birth control. Studies have shown that women who use contraceptive injections gain an average of almost 5.5 pounds during the first year of use and about 2 to 2.5 pounds per year thereafter.
- **Breast tenderness.** Tenderness in the breasts may require additional medication to relieve the problem.
- **Mood changes.** Mood changes, especially depressed mood, may be more common in users of progestin-only methods.

Barrier *Methods*

As the name suggests, barrier methods stop the sperm and egg from meeting. They are currently the only type of birth control—other than sterilization—that can be used by men. The barrier methods available today are the condom for men and the condom for women, the diaphragm, the cervical cap, and spermicides, which are usually used along with another type of barrier method for the best protection. Some barrier methods are available over-the-counter (without a prescription) while others require a visit to a doctor.

The most important thing to know about barrier methods is that they must be used *every time* you have intercourse—no exceptions. If you are not comfortable touching your genital area, or if you are extremely modest, the barrier method may seem intrusive to you. In that case, it may not be the best choice. If you are comfortable with whichever method you choose, it is more likely you will keep using it.

In general, barrier methods have two major benefits. First, side effects are minimal and serious risks are uncommon. Second, when used correctly and used every time, they are effective protection against pregnancy.

The Male Condom

The condom is one of the oldest forms of contraception. It is a thin sheath that covers a man's penis and prevents any semen from entering a woman's vagina.

Most condoms are made of latex, a type of rubber. Latex condoms not only prevent pregnancy by trapping sperm and semen, they also help prevent the transmission of STDs, such as gonorrhea and human immunodeficiency virus (HIV), which causes acquired immunodeficiency syndrome (AIDS).

About five percent of the condoms sold in the United States are made of natural animal membranes. These condoms are as effective as latex condoms in preventing pregnancy. However, they are not as effective in preventing STDs. They have small pores that, while small enough to prevent sperm from passing through, are large enough to let viruses, such as the herpes virus and HIV, pass through them.

Both latex and animal-skin condoms are available over-the-counter in many types of stores. They come in a variety of styles. Some have small pouches at the end to collect the semen after ejaculation. Many condoms are lubricated, some with a spermicide. It is a good idea to use spermicide with condoms for added protection against both pregnancy and STDs.

If you would like to use condoms either as your main method of birth control or as a backup method, you will need to talk frankly with your partner, as he is the one who has to use it. Don't depend on your partner to have condoms on hand, however. Keep your own supply so that you will always be prepared. Remember that condoms can be damaged if exposed to too much heat or light. Do not keep condoms in the glove compartment of a car or in pants pockets. Keeping condoms in your wallet is probably safe for a short while—about a month. Do not use condoms that are past their expiration date.

Benefits of the Male Condom. Advantages of the male condom include the following:

- It is the most effective means of preventing STDs (when the latex version is used).
- It is inexpensive and readily available without prescription.
- Some men report it helps them keep an erection longer.
- It can be used easily by those who have sex only occasionally.
- It is the only birth control method that can be used by men except for sterilization, which is not usually reversible.
- It can be used during a woman's menstrual period.

Side Effects and Risks. The only significant health risk associated with condom use is that condoms can rip or slip off, causing pregnancy or the transmission of STDs. Other issues follow:
- Because many male condoms are made of latex, they cannot be used by men—or their female partners—who are allergic to rubber.
- Some men report that condoms reduce their ability to feel sexual sensations, so sex is not as enjoyable.

wellness
warning

Use a new condom every time you have sex, whether your partner has ejaculated or not. Never reuse a condom.

Using the Condom Correctly

When you are ready to have sex, you or your partner will place a condom on his erect penis—before it comes anywhere close to the vagina. (Even before a man ejaculates, he releases some fluid, and sperm is sometimes found in this fluid.) The condom comes out of the package rolled up. If it has been pretreated with lubricant or spermicide, it may be wet or slippery. Rest the rolled-up condom on the head of the erect penis and slowly begin unrolling it down the length of the penis. If you are using the type of condom that does not have a small pouch at the end to collect the semen, leave about a half inch of space at the tip. As you unroll the condom, squeeze the air out of the space at the end of the condom. Unroll the condom the whole way, so that it covers the base of the penis.

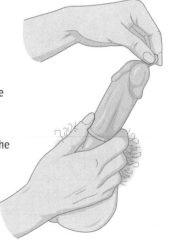

FIGURE 17.1
How to Use the Male Condom

The penis should be withdrawn from the vagina soon after the man has ejaculated and while it is still firm. Hold the condom against the penis as it is withdrawn to help prevent it from slipping. Gently pull the condom off the penis, being careful not to let the semen spill out.

During sex, if either you or your partner think the condom is slipping or has ripped, stop what you are doing. Hold the condom onto the penis and withdraw the penis from the vagina. If the condom is slipping or has ripped, replace it with a new one before you start having sex again. If the condom slips off during sex or appears to have ripped, you need additional protection against pregnancy. If you have not already used a spermicide, use it now. You may also want to use emergency contraception, which is described later in this chapter.

- Some users complain that because the condom must be put on after the penis is erect the romantic mood is broken.

The Female Condom

The female condom is one of the newest methods of birth control available. It is a thin, polyurethane sheath with a ring at both ends. Because it is not made of latex, it can be used by people who are allergic to latex. One end of the female condom is closed, and that end is positioned inside the vagina. The other end is open and remains outside the vagina. The condom lines the vagina, and the part outside the vagina drapes over part of the vulva and covers the base of the penis.

Because the female condom places a barrier between partners, it can protect against STDs. The plastic used in the condom, polyurethane, can stop even small virus particles from passing through. It is thought to provide at least as good protection against STDs as the male condom. Because it is new, however, there are not yet many studies to prove how well it protects against STDs.

The female condom comes packaged with its own lubricant. Spermicides may also be used with the female condom. If a female condom is not pretreated with a spermicide, you will need to purchase a separate spermicide to use. The female condom is available in drug stores and some groceries—wherever the male condom is sold.

The female condom is similar to the male condom in several ways, but one of its biggest advantages is that it puts you in charge of birth control decisions. If your partner does not like using male condoms, you can be prepared.

Benefits of the Female Condom. The female condom offers the following advantages:

- It is not made of latex, so it can be used by those allergic to rubber.
- It can be used by a woman without her partner's involvement.
- It is available without a prescription.

Using the Female Condom Correctly

You can insert the female condom either right before you have sex or up to eight hours before. To insert, squeeze the inner ring between your fingers so that it makes a narrow oval and push it up inside the vagina as far as it will go. It must cover the cervix completely, and the edge should be tucked underneath your pubic bone. If the condom is inserted correctly, it will hang down straight inside the vagina, and the outer ring will be about one inch outside the vagina. The manufacturer includes pictures with the instructions for using the condom that may help you use it correctly.

During sex, the vagina expands, and part of the condom outside your vagina will be drawn into the vagina. Once your partner has ejaculated, the condom should be removed before you get up. Squeeze and twist the outer ring and gently pull out the condom. This will keep the semen inside the condom and away from your body. Use a fresh condom each time you have intercourse.

FIGURE 17.2

How to Use the Female Condom

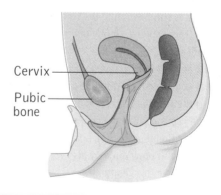

Cervix

Pubic bone

- It can be used easily by those who have sex only occasionally.
- It is considered to protect against STDs as well as the male condom.

Side Effects and Risks. There are no medical side effects or risks associated with using the female condom except for people who are allergic to polyurethane. There are, however, some aspects of the condom that make it less attractive to use:

- Some people find the portion hanging out of the vagina unsightly or a turn-off.
- Some users complain of a squeaking noise during use.
- It costs much more than the male condom.

The Diaphragm

The diaphragm is a dome-shaped rubber cup with a flexible rim. It is inserted high into the vagina before intercourse. Because it covers the cervix, the diaphragm prevents sperm from entering the uterus.

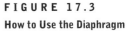

wellness **tip**

Check the fit of your diaphragm at every annual gynecological examination, any time you gain or lose ten pounds or more, after an abortion or miscarriage, and after a full-term pregnancy.

Using the Diaphragm Correctly

Be sure that your doctor or nurse shows you how to insert and remove your diaphragm. If you are not asked to insert and remove it yourself during your visit, tell your practitioner that you want to do it yourself and have her check you afterward to be sure you know how to insert it correctly. With some types of diaphragms, you can use an introducer (a small applicator that holds the diaphragm) to help you insert your diaphragm properly.

You must use spermicide with your diaphragm. When you are planning to have sex, have your diaphragm and a supply of spermicide at hand. You can either insert your diaphragm right before having sex or up to six hours before you have sex. Wash your hands before you insert the diaphragm to help prevent infection. Each time you are preparing to use the diaphragm, check it for holes by either holding it up to the light or filling it with water. *If you think there is even the smallest hole, do not use it.* Instead, use a backup method of birth control until you can replace your diaphragm.

Place about one teaspoon of spermicide inside the dome, and rub a little more on the rim of the diaphragm. To insert the diaphragm, squeeze the sides so that the diaphragm folds, and hold it with the dome down. Insert it inside the vagina and gently push it up and back as far as it will go. Slide the back rim past the cervix, and tuck the front rim under the pubic bone. When the diaphragm is in place correctly, it will cover the cervix and you can feel the cervix through the diaphragm with your finger. If the diaphragm feels uncomfortable, take it out and try again.

If you use tampons, you may find that the same position you use to insert a tampon (for example, sitting on or placing a foot up on the toilet) may be comfortable for inserting your diaphragm. Practice inserting and removing your diaphragm so that you become comfortable with using it.

Leave your diaphragm in place for at least six hours after having sex. This gives the spermicide a chance to work. Douching is not a good idea in general, but if you do want to douche after having sex, wait at least six hours. If you have sex again during the time that your diaphragm is in place, you need to add some more spermicide first. Do not take out your diaphragm; just insert more spermicide with an applicator into the vagina.

When you are ready to remove your diaphragm, reach your finger inside your vagina and find the front rim of the diaphragm. Hook your finger under the rim, and ease the diaphragm out of your vagina.

After each use, wash your diaphragm with plain soap and water and dry it. Check it for any holes or rips. Do not use any powder on it. Place it in its case and keep it somewhere cool and dark. With proper care, you may be able to use the same diaphragm for three years. After that, you should replace it with a new one.

FIGURE 17.3
How to Use the Diaphragm

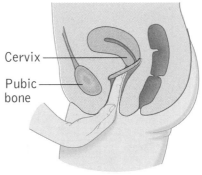

Cervix

Pubic bone

Diaphragms come in different sizes and styles and are available only by prescription. Your doctor or nurse will try different sizes to find the right size for you. For example, women who have recently given birth or who have gained or lost a significant amount of weight may need a larger or smaller size than they used before.

Benefits of the Diaphragm. The diaphragm has the following advantages:

- The same device can be used up to three years.
- It can be used easily by those who have sex only occasionally.
- It can be used by a woman without her partner's involvement.
- When inserted in advance, it does not interrupt lovemaking.

Side Effects and Risks. Problems with the diaphragm usually are the consequence of a poor fit or poor hygiene:

- The diaphragm stays in place partly because it presses into the vaginal walls. If the diaphragm is too large, it might be painful and can lead to sores in the vagina.
- The diaphragm presses against the urethra, which can increase the risks of urinary tract infections.
- The diaphragm must be carefully and thoroughly cleaned after each use to prevent vaginal infections. Toxic shock syndrome (TSS), a serious but rare infection, caused by the bacteria *Staphylococcus aureus,* has been linked infrequently to diaphragm use. Generally, women are at risk of TSS if they forget to remove the diaphragm for more than 24 hours. If you have ever had TSS, you should not use the diaphragm.
- Women with an allergy to rubber cannot use the diaphragm.

The Cervical Cap

The cervical cap is a small, rubber cup that fits over the cervix. It is shaped a bit like a small dome or a thimble and fits snugly against the surface of the cervix. There is just one type of cervical cap available in the United States, the Prentif Cavity Rim Cervical Cap. It is only available by prescription.

Because the cap clings so tightly to the surface of the cervix, any irregularities in the cervix may make the cap a poor choice. About ten percent of women cannot use the cap because they cannot be fitted properly.

Benefits of the Cervical Cap. Among the benefits of the cervical cap are the following:

- The same device can be used up to three years.
- It can be used easily by those who have sex only occasionally.
- It can be used by a woman without her partner's involvement.
- It can be left in place up to 48 hours, and once in place, nothing else need be done for subsequent sex.

Side Effects and Risks. Because it sits on top of the cervix, the cervical cap does not pose the same risk of urinary tract infections that the diaphragm does. However, some problems have been reported:

Using the Cervical Cap Correctly

Have your doctor or nurse show you how to insert and remove your cervical cap. You should also try placing it and removing it during your visit so that you can be sure you are doing it correctly. When the cap is properly in place, it will cover the surface of the cervix completely and may extend past it just a bit.

Wash your hands before you insert the cap to help prevent infection. Each time before you use it, check it for holes by either holding it up to the light or filling it with water. *If you think there is even the smallest hole, do not use it.* Instead, use a backup method of birth control until you can replace it.

Fill the cap about one-third full of spermicide. To insert the cap, squeeze the sides together so that the rim of the cap folds, and push in the dome of the cap. Insert it inside the vagina, along the back wall, and gently push it up until it covers the cervix. Run your finger around the rim of the cap to check that there are no gaps between the cap and the cervix and that you cannot feel the cervix outside the cap.

If the cap is properly in place, the dome will be up against the cervix. In a way, your cap is like a jar of food with a safety button. Before the jar is opened, there is a vacuum inside that keeps the button down. After it is opened, the button pops up. The same is true of the cap. When the dome is up against the cervix, it is because the suction is holding it there. If the dome pops up, suction has been broken, and you need to reinsert the cap.

If you use tampons, you may find that the same position you use to insert a tampon (for example, foot up on the toilet) may be comfortable for inserting your cap. Practice inserting and removing your cap so that you become comfortable with using it.

After you have had sex, you need to leave your cap in place for at least six hours. This gives the spermicide a chance to work. Douching is not a good idea in general, but if you do want to douche after having sex, wait at least six hours. The cap can be left in place for up to 48 hours, so one insertion can provide birth control for a whole weekend. If you have sex again, you can, of course, add more spermicide to the front of the cap, but you do not have to.

To remove the cap, reach your finger inside your vagina and find the rim of the cap. Press on the rim until the seal is broken, hook your finger inside the cap, and pull the cap sideways out of your vagina.

After each use, wash your cap with plain soap and water and dry it. Check it for any holes or rips. Do not use any powder on it. Place it in its case and keep it somewhere cool and dark. With care, you may be able to use the same cap for three years. After that, you should discard it and get a new one.

If you are having your period, do not use your cap. Your menstrual fluid can fill the cap and pop it off. Use a backup method instead.

- In early studies, Pap tests were sometimes abnormal in cap users. For this reason, it is recommended that women make sure they have had a recent, normal Pap test before they start using the method and again after three months. If the result is abnormal, discontinue using the cap and choose another method.
- Like the diaphragm, the cap potentially increases the risk of TSS and should not be used by women who have a history of TSS.
- Women with allergies to latex should not use the cap.

Spermicides

Spermicides come in many forms: gels, creams, foams, suppositories, and films. As their name suggests, spermicides contain chemicals that kill sperm. The main type of chemical used is nonoxynol-9, although some brands use another chemical called octoxynol. Some types, especially spermicidal foam, also produce a physical barrier that helps prevent the sperm from moving through the cervix to the uterus and fallopian tubes. Spermicides are available without a prescription and are usually sold next to condoms.

Some types of spermicides, such as foams, gels, and creams, can be placed inside the vagina right before you plan to have sex. Others, such as the supposi-

Using Spermicides Correctly

You need to use spermicide with each act of intercourse. Because spermicides come in several different forms, read the instructions that come with the package you choose to be sure you know how to use it correctly. Every type of spermicide needs to be placed high in the vagina so that it reaches the cervix. Some types need time after insertion to soften, melt, or otherwise become active. Follow the instructions on the package. If you do not have sex for more than an hour after inserting the spermicide, you may need to reapply it. After intercourse, wash and dry the applicator, if there is one.

~~~~~~~

tories and films, need to be inserted a little bit ahead of time. They need time to melt and cover the cervix to work effectively.

Spermicides can be used either alone or, for added protection, with another method of birth control. Some male condoms come pretreated with a spermicide.

Benefits of Spermicides. Spermicides have the following advantages:

- They are inexpensive and readily available without a prescription.
- They can be used with most other birth control methods to improve effectiveness.
- They can be used easily by those who have sex only occasionally.
- They can be used by a woman without her partner's involvement.

Side Effects and Risks. There are few known or proven risks involved in using spermicides:

- Some users report being allergic to them or find the chemicals irritating to the skin.
- Spermicides may make a woman more prone to yeast infections, since yeast organisms are better able to survive a dose of spermicide than are other organisms that normally live in a healthy vagina. If the normal organisms are killed off, yeast organisms may grow out of balance.
- In the early 1980s, there were a few studies that suggested that if a woman conceived while using spermicides, the fetus might be harmed. Numerous studies have now shown this is not true.

The Intrauterine Device

The IUD is a small device implanted inside the uterus to prevent pregnancy. It is available only by prescription. When the IUD is mentioned today, many people still think of the Dalkon Shield, a type of IUD that gained notoriety in the 1970s for causing serious—sometimes fatal—infections. The Dalkon Shield was withdrawn from the market in 1974.

Because lawsuits forced the Dalkon Shield off the market, safer IUDs that had been developed later were also taken off the market in the United States and the myths about IUDs persisted. By the early 1980s, there was only one type of IUD left on the market, the Progestasert, an IUD that contains the hormone progesterone. The percentage of women using birth control who used an IUD dropped from ten percent in the 1970s to two percent by 1988.

In 1988, another IUD was introduced in the United States along with strict screening requirements to prevent women at risk for IUD problems from getting IUDs. The Cu T 380 A takes its name from its T-shaped body (the "T") and arms (the "A"), which are wrapped with 380 mm^2 of fine copper (the "Cu") wire.

How does the IUD work? There has been some controversy over whether the IUD actually prevents conception or prevents a fertilized egg from implanting on the uterine wall. Most practitioners believe the latter. Women who should not use an IUD include those who:

- Have a pelvic infection now, have had one recently, or have frequent pelvic infections.
- Are pregnant or may be pregnant.
- Have never had children.
- Have cancer of the cervix or uterus, have suspected cancer, or have an abnormal Pap test.
- Have irregular, heavy, or abnormal vaginal bleeding for unknown reasons.
- Are at risk for an STD (have multiple sexual partners or a partner with multiple partners).
- Have blood changes due to a condition called Wilson's disease, wherein copper accumulates in various organs of the body, or an allergy to copper (applies only to copper IUD).

The IUD does not protect against STDs. And, if an IUD user gets an infection, the consequences may be more serious. If you have risk factors for infection, including more than one sexual partner, this method is not recommended.

You can use the acronym PAINS to remember the warning signs of problems with the IUD. If you have any of these signs, get in touch with your doctor right away:

- Period late (possible pregnancy), abnormal spotting or bleeding
- Abdominal pain, pain with intercourse
- Infection exposure (any sexually transmitted disease), abnormal discharge
- Not feeling well, fever, chills
- String missing, shorter, or longer

Benefits of the IUD

About 80 percent of women prescribed the IUD are still using it after a year. Only the contraceptive implants, contraceptive injections, and sterilization methods are more likely to be used after a year. Among women using the IUD, 60 percent are repeat customers. Following are the primary benefits:

- Among methods that are reversible, only contraceptive implants and contraceptive injections are more effective. The IUD can be used by some women who cannot use hormonal methods.
- It is convenient. After doctor's visits for insertion and checkups, you do not have to do anything else to have protected intercourse, although you may wish to use a condom to protect yourself from STDs.
- It is cost-effective. You pay the cost of the IUD once—and every time you have intercourse, your "cost per use" goes down.
- Women who use the IUD that contains progesterone find that they lose less blood each month—which may help women who tend to have problems with anemia or who previously had heavy periods. This type of IUD can also ease the pain and cramping that some women have with their periods.

Why It Is Safer to Use IUDs Today

Two factors make the intrauterine devices (IUDs) available today far safer than the Dalkon Shield (in the early 1970s). The first has to do with the type of string on the Dalkon Shield. All IUDs have a string on the end that users can check to assure themselves that the device is still in place. The Dalkon Shield's string was unusual. Instead of being one fine thread, it was made of several threads. This multifilament string made it easier for bacteria to travel up the string from the vagina into the uterus, where they could cause pelvic inflammatory disease or other serious infection.

Second, doctors came to recognize that infection was the most serious risk with IUDs and that certain women were at greater risk of infection regardless of IUD use. Today, women at risk for infection are not prescribed the IUD.

How the IUD Is Inserted

Before you have an intrauterine device (IUD) inserted, your doctor will review your medical history to be sure that the IUD would be a good choice for you. Among appropriately screened women, the IUD presents no greater hazard than other methods and has many potential benefits.

Some doctors recommend giving antibiotics before an IUD is inserted to help reduce the risks of infection associated with IUD insertion. Studies disagree about whether this is helpful, so you may want to discuss it with your doctor.

Prior to inserting the IUD, your doctor will give you a painkiller or a drug that reduces cramping. You will have a pelvic examination to be sure that you are not pregnant and to check for any signs of infection. Then, your doctor will clean your cervix with an antiseptic solution. If it is used, local anesthesia can be given now.

A small pair of forceps is used to stabilize the cervix, and a thin probe is inserted into your uterus to measure how deep it is so the doctor will be able to place the IUD properly. The IUD is then loaded into a thin tube that keeps the arms of the IUD next to its body. This tube is inserted through the cervix into the uterus. The IUD is released into the uterus as the tube is slowly drawn back and out of the uterus.

When it is properly in place, the arms of your IUD will be at the top of your uterus, each arm near where your fallopian tubes join the uterus. The body of the IUD will be down the center of your uterus, and the device's string will hang outside your cervix. The string can be felt in the vagina. Your doctor may have you check it so that you know how to find it. This is how you will check to be sure that your IUD has not been drawn up into your uterus too far or been expelled from your body. You should return to your doctor's office a month or so after the IUD was inserted—after you have had a period—to be sure that everything is okay.

After the IUD is inserted, your doctor will review with you the warning signs that suggest you may be having a problem with your IUD. Be sure that you understand them or call if questions arise.

Once your IUD has been properly inserted, you do not need to do anything else before having sex in order to prevent pregnancy. You should check for your string at least once a month to be sure that you can still feel it. If you cannot feel it, you may not be protected against pregnancy. Use a backup method until you can have your doctor check your IUD.

The Progestasert IUD can be left in your uterus for one year, and then it needs to be replaced. The Cu T 380 A is effective for a much longer period of time—10 years. When it is time to replace your IUD or you've decided to stop using the method, you return to your doctor's office to have it removed.

Side Effects and Risks

In spite of the new safety standards, there are risks associated with the IUD:

- There is a real risk of infection, especially soon after insertion. To limit the risk of infection, your doctor will use sterilized equipment and may prescribe antibiotics. After the IUD is in place for one month, the risk of infection decreases greatly.
- If you are at risk for any STD, the IUD is not a good choice for you. If you get an infection with your IUD in place, you have an increased risk of pelvic inflammatory disease, which causes infertility. This is especially important for women who may be planning to have another child in the future.
- While the IUD containing progesterone can actually reduce your menstrual flow, other types of IUDs increase it. With other types, your periods tend to be longer and heavier, with more cramping. Too much blood loss can lead to anemia. Let your doctor know if you have any changes in your period after you start the IUD.
- Although the IUD is very effective in preventing pregnancy, there is a chance that pregnancy could occur if you expel your IUD and do not notice. Up to ten percent of IUD users spontaneously expel the device within their first year of use. You are at increased risk of expelling your IUD if you are young, you have

abnormal periods, or you had a lot of cramping with your periods before getting the IUD.

- Ectopic pregnancy occurs when a fertilized egg attaches to the fallopian tube. The overall risk of an ectopic pregnancy with an IUD is about five percent, and IUDs that contain progesterone have a much higher risk. Ectopic pregnancy can become a life-threatening condition. Call your doctor if you have any sense that you might be pregnant.
- If a fertilized egg does succeed in implanting in the uterus, the rate of miscarriage is about 50 percent. If you wish to continue the pregnancy, the IUD should be removed immediately. Removal may result in miscarriage, but if the pregnancy continues, the miscarriage rate decreases to about 25 percent.
- There is a slight risk (1 in 1,000) that the IUD may poke through the walls of the uterus, sometimes migrating to the abdomen. If you suspect perforation, see your doctor as soon as possible.

Natural *Birth* Control Methods

Some women like the idea of planning their families without the use of chemicals or medical devices or they may be opposed to artificial methods of birth control on religious or moral grounds. Recent research on natural family planning (NFP)—also called fertility awareness—has led to greater reliability on these methods than in the past.

NFP requires that a woman be able to know the times when she is most likely to become pregnant. That is, she needs to be able to tell when she is ovulating. After ovulation, an egg must be fertilized within a day or two or it loses viability. After ejaculation, sperm remain alive and can fertilize an egg for 72 hours or more, but probably not longer than five days. With this knowledge, a woman can either avoid having sex around the time she ovulates, or she can have sex at those times if she wants to become pregnant. Women who wish to use NFP to become pregnant may also use ovulation detection kits, which are available in stores without a prescription. These kits detect the presence of hormones that occur in a woman's urine as ovulation occurs.

Women who use NFP need to work closely with their partners. If a couple strictly avoids sexual contact during unsafe times, NFP can be an effective means of birth control. However, if the length of your cycle varies from month to month, natural family planning methods will not work as well for you.

The Rhythm Method

The most familiar form of NFP is the rhythm method, also called the calendar method. A woman must have regular periods to use this method. A woman with an average 28-day cycle can expect to ovulate around day 14 of her cycle. By avoiding sex for the days surrounding day 14, she is likely to avoid pregnancy.

Women who have shorter or longer cycles have to calculate their own safe days and mark them on the calendar. Day 1 of your cycle is the first day you experience bleeding. Cycle length is calculated by counting the number of days from the first day of your menstrual bleeding to the first day of your next period. If you have a long cycle—for example, 35 days—you can calculate ovulation as 35 minus 14, to

Birth Control Methods That Do Not Work

In addition to knowing about the different types of effective birth control you can use, you also need to know what does not work. Do not rely on any of the following to prevent pregnancy:

- **Douching after sex.** Sperm will not be flushed from your system and may actually be forced higher into your uterus.
- **Washing after sex.** Sperm travels rapidly through the cervix and will not be "caught" with washing.
- **Urinating after sex.** The urinary tract and reproductive system are separate in women.
- **Having sex during your period.** It is still possible to get pregnant if you have sex during that time.
- **Withdrawing the penis from the vagina before ejaculation occurs.** Pre-ejaculatory fluid usually contains some sperm. If the penis is near or in the vagina at any time, the sperm can fertilize an egg.

estimate ovulation occurring on day 21. If you have short cycles—for example, 21 days—calculate ovulation as 21 minus 14, to estimate ovulation occurring on day 7.

The Ovulation Method

The rhythm method has been updated by the ovulation method—and it works even for women who have irregular cycles. With the ovulation method, a woman checks for signs in her body that ovulation is about to occur. The main sign is changes in her cervical mucus, which can be seen as a discharge from the vagina and felt as a wet feeling. As a woman approaches ovulation, her cervical mucus becomes wetter, thinner, and more slippery. On the day of ovulation, the mucus is at its wettest and thinnest—it is clear and stretchy and looks a lot like raw egg white.

As soon as ovulation occurs, the mucus begins to dry up and thicken and become more paste-like. Then the mucus becomes thinner and wetter again after ovulation. Women who do not want to become pregnant should avoid having sex from the time the mucus starts to become wet and stretchy until three days after the wettest mucus is seen or felt.

The Basal Body Temperature Method

As a woman's body prepares to release an egg each month, the hormones estrogen and progesterone ready her body to support a pregnancy if one should occur. After ovulation, the hormone progesterone makes her body temperature rise slightly—up to 1°F or so. A woman who uses the basal body temperature (BBT) method takes her temperature with a sensitive thermometer each morning before getting out of bed. If she wishes to avoid pregnancy, she avoids having sex from the time when her period occurs until her temperature goes up at least four-tenths of a degree and stays up for a few days. The BBT method is not very effective for preventing a pregnancy because the temperature rise occurs only after a woman has ovulated—but it is a good way to time intercourse for women who wish to conceive.

The Symptothermal Method

Women who combine the ovulation and BBT methods use a method called the symptothermal method. They check both their body's symptoms ("sympto-") and their temperatures ("-thermal"). In addition to checking their cervical mucus and feelings of wetness, they may check other symptoms, such as breast tenderness and position of their cervix. Women who are using the symptothermal method to avoid pregnancy abstain from sex from the time of their period until after ovulation has occurred.

The Postovulation Method

The lowest pregnancy rates are found when women abstain from sex until *after* ovulation occurs, regardless of how ovulation is determined. This is known as the postovulation method. Some users of this method abstain from sex totally from day one of their period through the third or fourth day after ovulation.

For any NFP method, you will need to keep track of your daily symptoms on a chart. If you use the BBT method, you will need to have a sensitive thermometer that shows temperature by tenths of a degree Fahrenheit. Because you must keep track of your symptoms, and possibly temperature, each day, you need to take your chart and thermometer with you if you travel or are away from home.

TABLE 17.1
Effectiveness of Birth Control Methods

METHOD	FAILURE RATE WITH TYPICAL USE*	FAILURE RATE WITH PERFECT USE*
No Method	85%	85%
Spermicide	26%	6%
Natural Family Planning	25%	–
Calendar		9%
Ovulation method		3%
Symptothermal		2%
Postovulation		1%
Cervical cap		
Women who have had children	40%	26%
Women who have not had children	20%	9%
Diaphragm (when spermicide is also used)	20%	6%
Condom (without spermicide use)		
Female	21%	5%
Male	14%	3%
Birth control pill	5%	
Minipill		0.5%
Combination		0.1%
Intrauterine device		
Containing progesterone	2%	1.5%
Containing copper	0.8%	0.6%
Contraceptive injections	–	0.3%
Contraceptive implants	–	0.05%
Sterilization		
Female	–	0.5%
Male	–	0.1%

*Failure rate is the percentage of women using the method who have an accidental pregnancy within the first year of use

Source: Adapted from Hatcher, R.A., Trussel, J., Stewart, F., Cates, W., Stewart, G.K., Kowal, D., Guest, F. *Contraceptive Technology*, 17th rev ed. New York: Irvington Publishers, 1998.

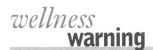

wellness
warning

Couples who use natural family planning for birth control must be dedicated to the method and be very conscientious about its use. Even with perfect use, however, these are not the most effective methods of birth control. If you have a health condition that would make pregnancy dangerous for you or you absolutely do not want to have any children now, it is recommended that you talk with your doctor and your partner about choosing a more effective method.

If You Are Considering Natural Family Planning

If you are considering using natural family planning (NFP) for birth control or to achieve a pregnancy, the first thing you should do is get training. You will need your partner's cooperation to use NFP effectively, so invite him to get training with you. Because these methods rely on your being able to interpret some fairly subtle symptoms, you should have someone experienced with the method teach it to you.

In addition to learning the signs of ovulation, you also need to learn how common events in your life can make these signs less reliable. For example, changes in your cervical mucus will be thrown off if you have a vaginal infection. Douching must be avoided if you are checking your cervical mucus. Your temperature can be affected by illness, getting up in the middle of the night, not taking your temperature at the same time each morning, or using a different thermometer. During certain times of a woman's life, for example, when she nears menopause or has recently had a baby, changes in her body make NFP much harder to use effectively.

Regardless of which type of NFP you use, it will only work if you know how to identify whether you are in a fertile period *and* if you act on that knowledge. You and your partner must both agree to do this. If you are using NFP to prevent pregnancy, you and your partner must be willing to abstain from intercourse frequently throughout your cycle (or use a barrier method then).

Benefits of Natural Family Planning

The benefits of natural methods of birth control are obvious to women who generally wish to avoid the use of chemical treatments and synthetic medications or materials. Many women enjoy the knowledge that there are few side effects or medical risks involved in NFP. In addition, some women like the fact that their partner is involved with NFP. Deciding on periods of abstinence requires open communication that usually strengthens the relationship.

Side Effects and Risks

NFP provides no protection from STDs, including HIV and AIDS. If you have irregular menstrual cycles or an irregular daily schedule or are often up past midnight, the BBT method may not be reliable for you. While NFP has no direct medical risks, it may have emotional risks because of the way it interferes with spontaneous sexual enjoyment. Whether you are using NFP to achieve a pregnancy or to prevent one, you may find that having the chart dictate when you have sex puts a strain on your relationship with your partner.

Sterilization

Sterilization is a permanent method of birth control. For women, sterilization involves surgically blocking or cutting the fallopian tubes so that the sperm and egg cannot meet. For men, sterilization involves cutting the tube through which the sperm travel so that no sperm will be released during ejaculation. Sterilization is one of the most popular ways of preventing pregnancy: about 14 million women in the United States rely on sterilization (of themselves or their partners) for birth control.

The advantage of sterilization is that with one operation, you never again need to worry about contraception. Some people who are sterilized, though, come to regret the decision. Before undertaking sterilization, serious thought must be given to the decision.

Making the Decision

If you are considering being sterilized, the first thing to do is nothing. Take some time to think about this decision. Think about why you are considering sterilization as an option. If you are just tired of using pills and diaphragms and meet the screening requirements, you may want to consider using a long-acting, reversible method of birth control, like the IUD (lasts up to ten years), contraceptive implants (good for five years), or contraceptive injections (good for three months).

If you have decided that sterilization is the best method for you and your partner, the next choice is between tubal ligation for women and vasectomy for men. Bear in mind that while tubal ligation is as effective as vasectomy it requires more surgical intervention and therefore has a slightly greater risk.

Once you have chosen sterilization and selected a procedure, tubal ligation or vasectomy, your doctor will have you sign a form indicating that you are giving your informed consent to have the procedure done. Before you sign any agreement regarding sterilization, be sure that you understand the following:

- What type of operation will be done and its risks and benefits
- That there are other types of birth control you could use instead
- That a successful operation will prevent you from having children but that failure (pregnancy) is possible
- That sterilization is meant to be permanent
- That you may be able to have the operation reversed but that this is expensive, requires another operation, and may not work
- That you do not have to have sterilization done—it is completely up to you

Do not agree to have sterilization done if there is something you do not understand, if you do not feel emotionally ready to make the decision, or if someone else is pressuring you to have it done.

If you have a partner or husband, you do not need to have his approval to be sterilized. However, a lack of communication or agreement on this subject can lead to difficulties in your relationship.

Sterilization for Women

There are three basic types of sterilization procedures that can be done for women:

- **Electrocoagulation** uses electrical energy to cauterize (burn) the walls of the fallopian tubes so that they are fused, blocking the passage of the egg.
- **Mechanical blockages** are clips or bands that mechanically block and crush the fallopian tubes so that the two parts of the tube are blocked.
- **Tubal ligation,** commonly known as "tying the tubes," involves the tying of surgical sutures around the fallopian tubes in two places and removing the section between the ties.

Sterilization for Men

For men, the basic procedure for sterilization is called vasectomy. It is so named because it involves cutting the vas deferens, the tube that carries sperm from the testes, where they are formed, to a "holding area" called the seminal vesicles. The doctor makes a small incision in the scrotum, the sac containing the testes.

wellness **tip**

If you have any doubts at all that sterilization is the right choice for you, do not have it done. There is no rush. You can have the operation done whenever you wish, but reversing it may not be possible or affordable.

The vas deferens is drawn through the small hole and then cut or tied. Vasectomy is a simple operation that is done under local anesthesia in the doctor's office.

A man can have sex within a few days after having a vasectomy, but he can still cause pregnancy, since some mature sperm remain in his reproductive tract. The general rule of thumb is that a man needs to ejaculate at least 15 times before he can assume that he is infertile. It is best to use a backup method of birth control until the doctor verifies that the sperm count is zero.

Benefits of Sterilization

The failure rate for sterilization is extremely low. Once you or your partner has been sterilized, you are well protected from pregnancy for the rest of your reproductive years. When you want to have sex, there will be nothing you need to do before or during sex.

Side Effects and Risks

- Sterilization is meant to be permanent. It is not known exactly how many women and men later regret being sterilized, but it is estimated to be between five and ten percent. Although there are operations that can reconnect the tubes in men and women, they are expensive and are not guaranteed to work.
- Neither tubal ligation nor vasectomy provides protection against STDs. If you are at risk for STDs, you should use a barrier method of birth control even if you have been sterilized.

Emergency Contraception

Emergency contraception is birth control that a woman can use soon after she has had unprotected sex. Sometimes referred to as the "morning-after pill," emergency contraception can be effective when taken within 72 hours after unprotected sex.

TECHNIQUES

The most common technique for emergency contraception requires taking two 50-microgram estrogen birth control pills as soon after sex as possible (within 72 hours) and repeating the dose (two pills) 12 hours later. Other methods include inserting an intrauterine device (IUD) or taking large doses of progestin-only pills. *All these methods should be discussed with your doctor.*

EFFECTIVENESS

Emergency contraception is not perfect, but it reduces the risk of pregnancy by at least 75 percent.

HOW IT WORKS

It is not known exactly how emergency contraception works.

The large doses of hormones may prevent the lining of the uterus from growing thick enough to prepare for a pregnancy and a fertilized egg will not be able to implant successfully. Emergency contraception may also have some effect on fertilization or on the sperm and egg traveling through the fallopian tube.

SIDE EFFECTS

Side effects of the pills used for emergency contraception are similar to, but may be more severe than, ordinary doses of birth control pills. If you feel sick after the first dose, your doctor may give you medication to help prevent nausea when the second dose is taken. If you actually vomit, let your doctor know. She may suggest that you retake the pills. Because emergency contraception affects the menstrual cycle and the lining of the uterus, your next period may be a little late. If it has been more than three weeks since your treatment, though, and you have not had a period, see your doctor to make sure you are not pregnant.

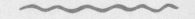

- Although more research is needed, some studies indicate that some women experience changes in their menstrual cycles and have abdominal pain after sterilization. Some women who were sterilized when they were young have seemed more likely to need hysterectomies (removal of the uterus) than are women who have not been sterilized.
- Some studies have suggested that a man who has a vasectomy is later more likely to get prostate cancer than one who has not been sterilized. Although researchers believe that more studies are needed on this issue, they agree that men can continue to have vasectomies and that those who have already had them need not have them reversed.
- If you or your partner later regrets being sterilized and decides to seek reversal of the operation, there will be additional factors to consider. Not every woman or man is a good candidate for reversal. If you are too old, your chances of pregnancy may be lower, and your doctor may not agree to perform a reversal operation because of the risks involved with surgery. If either you or your partner is considering reversal, the other one should be examined for signs of infertility before the reversal operation is done.

When Birth Control *Fails*

Once an unplanned pregnancy is confirmed (or if emergency contraception techniques fail), you have two options: abortion or carrying the fetus to term (birth). The stress caused by the decision-making process surrounding an unwanted or mistimed pregnancy may result in an emotional crisis for you and you partner. The sooner you can begin to make your decision, the more likely you will reach a decision you can live with, and the more protection you can afford yourself and the fetus, if you decide to continue the pregnancy.

If you elect to terminate your pregnancy, you should seek care from an experienced abortion provider who can help you outline your options. Complications from late-term abortions are *much* more dangerous than from early-term abortions. You should begin seeking care as soon as you know you are pregnant.

Although abortion is constitutionally legal, several states have mandatory waiting periods, require parental involvement, and/or require that health care providers show patients graphic materials specifically designed to discourage abortion. If such laws apply in your state, it is all the more important that you seek professional care early and do your best to gain the balanced information you need to make an informed, careful decision.

The Abortion Process

There are two types of abortion. One is surgical and the other is medical, employing the use of drugs.

Surgical Abortion. Surgical abortion is currently the only type available in the United States with FDA approval, and in some states it is obtained only with extreme difficulty. Abortion services are available in some hospitals and in many clinic settings designed to provide complete reproductive services for women. More than half of surgical abortions take place before 8 weeks of gestation, 91

wellness **tip**

If you have an abortion, be
sure the practitioner does
a blood test to determine
your blood type. If you
have Rh negative blood,
you could be at risk for
complications in future
pregnancies. An injection
of Rhogam before leaving
the clinic will protect you
during future pregnancy.

percent before 12 weeks of gestation, and 96 percent before 15 weeks. After 11 to 12 weeks, the complication rate rises markedly.

For early surgical abortion, suction techniques are most commonly used. With the woman in the same position used for Pap tests, the doctor places a speculum into the vagina and examines the cervix. She then scrubs the cervix with an antiseptic solution to prevent infection and injects a local anesthetic. Rods (cervical dilators) are then used to dilate (open) the cervix enough to allow introduction of the suction device. The doctor then inserts the suction "curette" directly into the uterus and the fetus is removed. Once the abortion is completed, the woman usually remains in the clinic for a short observation and recovery period.

When the pregnancy has progressed further than 15 weeks, the procedure is more complicated because the size of the fetus means more cervical dilation is needed. Compressed seaweed or other devices can be placed in the cervix overnight to help it dilate wider. A combination of powerful uterine contractions and other evacuation techniques may be needed for aborting these more advanced pregnancies, and the observation and recovery period may be longer.

After surgical abortion, women will experience light to moderate bleeding over the next five to seven days. Most practitioners recommend abstaining from intercourse until the cervix has closed, about the time the bleeding stops. If a woman develops heavy bleeding or signs of infection—fever and chills—immediate medical attention is necessary.

Medical Abortion. Medical abortions, using mifepristone (previously called RU-486) or methotrexate (a drug used in cancer treatment), are only available in limited settings in the United States at this time, but FDA approval for mifepristone (the "French abortion pill") is expected. Unlike surgical abortion, which is often not done before seven to eight weeks of gestation, medical abortion is used earlier in pregnancy. In fact, it can be used as soon as pregnancy is determined, and the earlier it is used, the more effective it is.

Medical abortion utilizes "antiprogestins," like mifepristone, which fit into progesterone receptors in the uterus and block the action of naturally occurring progesterone. Without the effect of progesterone, the lining of the uterus softens and breaks down, causing the onset of menstruation. The action of antiprogestins is most effective in the first few weeks after fertilization and implantation, a time when naturally occurring progesterone is being produced primarily by the ovaries. As pregnancy progresses, the placenta itself takes over the role of progesterone production and these abortion agents are less effective.

In patients electing medical abortion in Europe, mifepristone can be used from 49 to 63 days after the first day of the last menstrual period. The patient swallows the medication and then remains in the clinic for an hour afterward. Two days later, she returns to the clinic and is given an oral dose of prostaglandin, which increases contractions in the uterus. After she is given the prostaglandin, the woman remains in the clinic for about four hours—wearing a sanitary napkin but remaining in her own clothes. In the majority of patients, the uterine lining sheds, and they pass the fertilized egg or embryo. The process usually continues into the next day.

The patient returns to the clinic for a third visit two weeks later for a follow-up. About four percent of women do not abort and require surgical abortion.

Post-Abortion Syndrome

Before abortion was legalized, case reports suggested that there were psychological concerns related to abortion (extreme pain, fear of dying, fear of rape by the abortion provider). Since abortion was legalized in the United States in 1971, more than 250 studies have looked at psychological effects related to induced abortion. All studies agree that negative emotional effects usually fade rather quickly and that most women who choose abortion feel increasingly relieved and comfortable over time.

Patients are at higher risk for problems when they are pressured or coerced into abortion, when they are unsure about their decision, when they have limited social support, or when they have had prior psychiatric illness. In the rare instances in which patients have severe concerns after induced abortion, early psychological care to resolve the trauma is important.

Deciding to Continue an Unexpected Pregnancy

Although they may feel unprepared to have a baby, many women who become pregnant unexpectedly decide to carry the fetus to full term, often for religious, moral, medical, or psychological reasons. Some women, however, feel ambivalent about caring for a baby they did not expect, but do not want to make the baby

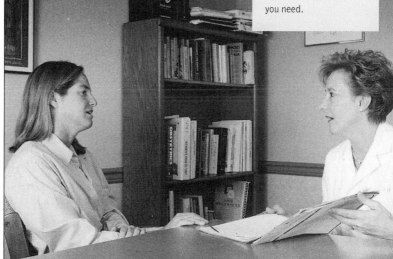

Emotional support is essential when making the decision whether to continue an unexpected pregnancy. If your family members and the baby's father are unable to provide support, contact a trusted physician, midwife, psychologist, or a family planning clinic for the advice and counseling you need.

available for adoption. If you decide to continue your pregnancy but feel ambivalent about it, you still owe it to the baby and yourself to take special care of your health. (Consult Chapter 18 for a full discussion of wellness during pregnancy.)

The key to overcoming ambivalence about delivering an unexpected baby is finding emotional and psychological support. If family members and the baby's father are unavailable for such support, contact a trusted physician, midwife, psychologist, or a family planning clinic for advice and counseling on your options after the baby is born, and for moral support during your pregnancy.

Coping *with*
Infertility

For the majority of women and couples, family planning means using birth control to prevent pregnancy until the decision is made to try to conceive a child. For one couple in ten who are of reproductive age, however, family planning becomes more complicated when they discover that the woman cannot become pregnant.

Infertility is suspected when a woman does not conceive a child after one year of healthy sexual relations using no birth control. No one expects to be infertile, but it is not unusual. More than 5 million Americans of every race and socioeconomic status are coping with infertility. They all face difficult choices, and they often must make those choices while feeling adrift in a sea of conflicting, medically complex information and strong emotions.

Although people of all ages are affected by infertility, it is more difficult to conceive the older a woman becomes. Infertility issues have become more prevalent in recent years as baby boomers and generation Xers—the first two generations of Americans to have access to reliable birth control—have delayed childbearing into their thirties and even into their forties.

Increasingly, researchers and doctors have focused their skills on understanding the causes of infertility and developing treatments. Consequently men and women are more likely than ever before to find out the reason for their infertility, and about 20 to 35 percent of couples treated for infertility will conceive eventually.

What Causes Infertility?

Fundamentally speaking, there are three causes of infertility:

1. The sperm from the male partner or the egg from the female partner is not present or is not healthy enough to achieve fertilization.
2. Viable sperm from the male partner (sperm that would under normal circumstances succeed in fertilizing an egg) never reach an egg from the female partner (thus, fertilization is blocked).
3. There is a condition present in the sperm or egg which prevents a fertilized egg from developing past the embryo stage.

There are almost countless causes for any of these three conditions. For most couples the specific reason they cannot conceive a child is not readily apparent. About 40 percent of the many factors that might be at work are related to men (sometimes called male-factor infertility), and 40 percent are related to women. Up to 20 percent of couples who are infertile never discover the cause.

Infertility in the Male Reproductive System. Following are some of the most common problems in men who are experiencing infertility:

- Men who are impotent or cannot sustain an erection throughout sexual intercourse will not be able to conceive a child unless those difficulties are resolved first.
- An elevated body temperature damages or kills sperm before ejaculation.
- Some men have a low sperm count, which is not discovered until the ejaculatory fluid is tested and observed under a microscope. Normally, one milliliter of semen contains at least 20 million healthy sperm. However, only a few will be strong enough to reach the partner's egg and break through its outer layer. Usually only one actually succeeds. If a man has fewer than the normal number of sperm with each ejaculation, the chance of one being strong enough to fertilize an egg is diminished.
- After laboratory testing of their ejaculatory fluid, some men discover that no sperm are present in their semen at all. In such cases either the testicles are not producing semen, which is rare, or there is an abnormality in the vas deferens, the passageway through which the sperm travel from the testicles to the urethra where it mingles with semen prior to ejaculation.

- Some men produce sperm that are malformed or weak, so that none of the sperm can navigate and reach the partner's fallopian tubes. Sometimes, sperm contain material that causes the fertilized egg to lose viability soon after fertilization.

Infertility in the Female Reproductive System. While men generate sperm on an ongoing basis throughout their sexually active years, women are born with all the eggs they will ever have. The eggs are normally released at regular intervals— every 28 days—during ovulation. Below are some of the common ways in which the normal process of fertilization can be interrupted:

- Women who have trouble conceiving often do not ovulate regularly. Some naturally have longer than normal cycles, making it difficult to plan a pregnancy.
- Eggs are sometimes damaged, either congenitally or through the use of certain drugs or radiation therapies, so that they are not conducive to fertilization.
- As women age, so do their eggs. Older eggs, though they may be fertilized, often cannot sustain a viable embryo for more than a few hours or days, which is why older women have more difficulty becoming pregnant.
- Also as women age their estrogen levels drop, and estrogen is needed in order for the ovaries to release eggs into the fallopian tubes. If estrogen levels are too low, the ovaries will cease to release eggs at all. This can occur in young women who lack sufficient estrogen for any reason.
- Some women discover that they have "hostile" mucus. That is, the mucus present in the vagina, which is meant to facilitate the passage of the sperm into the cervix, instead inhibits movement (for example, it may be too thick) or produces chemicals that destroy the sperm as soon as they enter the vagina. Current research suggests, for example, that women who smoke have high levels of nicotine in their vaginal mucus, which may be poisonous to sperm.
- Women can have a wide range of anatomical abnormalities that lead to infertility. Blockages in the fallopian tubes caused by infections and scarring, congenital defects in the cervix or uterus, or scarring due to surgery are all possible causes of infertility.
- Some women's immune systems malfunction, causing them to produce antibodies against sperm. When sperm are present, the antibodies attack them as foreign agents of disease, and they prevent the sperm from moving freely.

Diagnosing Infertility

The field of infertility medicine has grown extensively in the last two decades. After a year of unsuccessfully trying to conceive, the best place to start looking for medical explanations is with an obstetrician/gynecologist who can recommend a specialist—called a reproductive endocrinologist—and give a referral. If the male partner seeks treatment, he may begin with a urologist, though the woman's gynecologist may also be able to offer him an initial consultation.

Covering the Expenses. The road to a diagnosis of infertility can be long and expensive. However, anxiety over the costs should not prevent women from seeing a specialist. Couples are advised to do all the research necessary to be sure they are getting the maximum insurance coverage allowed through their policy. Even though many insurance companies do not cover costs associated with infertility diagnosis and treatment, the information on this issue is constantly changing, and various companies and managed care systems do offer some degree of coverage.

Finding a Cause. Infertility diagnosis generally starts with a series of tests called the infertility work-up. The work-up may include blood tests, a record of basal body temperature, tests on cervical mucus, semen analysis, a postcoital test to examine sperm after it has been exposed to vaginal mucus, and in some cases, a diagnostic laparoscopy—minor surgery that allows the doctor to examine the woman's fallopian tubes and ovaries for signs of endometriosis, blockages in the tubes, and adhesions. When physiological problems, infection, or immunological disorders are suspected, more specialized diagnostic procedures may be used.

Treatment Options
Depending on the diagnosis for the probable cause of infertility, treatment can be as simple as taking over-the-counter decongestants to thin vaginal mucus or as complicated as major surgery. If it is discovered that a woman is not ovulating, the most common treatment involves drugs and hormones that stimulate ovulation. During this drug therapy, specialists conduct tests to determine when ovulation occurs. In 80 to 90 percent of cases treated with hormones and drugs, women begin ovulating, thus increasing the chance that pregnancy will occur.

Artificial insemination is an option when the female partner ovulates normally, but the male partner appears to have a low sperm count or to produce no sperm at all. If sperm can be collected from the male partner, his sperm is placed in the female partner's vagina by means of a long tube attached to a cup that has been placed over her cervix. If no sperm is available from the partner, some women choose to be inseminated by a donor.

If neither of these methods can be used to boost the potential for fertilization, techniques called assisted reproductive technologies (ART) may be tried. Some of the more common forms of ART include in vitro fertilization, where the female partner is given medication to stimulate the production of multiple eggs. The eggs are then collected and placed in a laboratory dish, mixed with sperm, and incubated for one or two days. The fertilized eggs are then introduced into the woman's cervix with a bulb syringe. If the procedure is successful, one or more of the fertilized eggs will attach to the uterine wall, and the pregnancy usually proceeds normally.

GIFT, or gamete intrafallopian transfer, is often more successful than in vitro fertilization for women with at least one functioning fallopian tube. The sperm and egg are removed from each partner and then injected together directly into the fallopian tube where fertilization takes place, and then the natural movement of the fallopian tube pushes the fertilized egg into the uterus. Different variations on this technique are being tried successfully.

In cases where problems are more physiological or anatomical in nature—requiring repair to reproductive organs or the removal of blockages—surgery is indicated. Some options for women include surgical (as opposed to diagnostic) laparoscopy, minor surgery involving the insertion of a small telescope in a hole in the abdominal wall to repair defects. A newer procedure, called a hysteroscopy, uses a fiber-optic device inserted into the uterus for minor repairs.

Laparotomy is major abdominal surgery, which is required to repair tubes, remove adhesions, or remove diseased or blocked portions of the fallopian tubes.

Surgery for men sometimes involves the dilation of veins that carry blood out of the scrotum (varicocelectomy) to correct a condition that causes scrotal temperature to rise, which damages or kills sperm. If some abnormality is discovered in the vas deferens (the tube that moves the sperm out of the testicles), surgery called vas reversal can sometimes correct the problem.

Infertility and Wellness

Most causes of infertility are not within a woman's control. However, certain lifestyle factors, including smoking and the overuse of alcohol, have been found to impair fertility. Nicotine is present in high concentrations in the vaginal mucus of women who smoke, and it is toxic or deadly to sperm. STDs are also a cause of infertility. Taking every precaution against contracting STDs is a practical step toward wellness for all women, including those who wish to eventually have children.

A healthy body is better prepared to conceive and carry a child than one that is not healthy. While good health includes exercise, researchers and doctors suspect that excessive exercise can block fertility in women. Dieting and exercising to the point of extreme thinness clearly interferes with ovulation, which is often the cause of infertility. Studies also show that extremely obese women have difficulty becoming pregnant.

Beyond these controllable issues—healthy diet, moderate exercise, avoiding nicotine and alcohol, and remaining free of STDs—there are no grounds for a woman to blame herself when she discovers she is infertile. A major part of maintaining wellness when coping with infertility is avoiding feelings of guilt, which interfere with your emotional health. Research shows that the popular myths about stress causing infertility, previous abortions making pregnancy impossible, and other such "wives tales" only add to the emotional burden of infertility.

Some experts in the field recommend that couples begin fertility treatment programs with a clear idea of how long they are willing to work on achieving pregnancy and how much money they will be able to spend. They suggest that couples also think seriously about the emotional energy they will expend. A diagnosis of infertility can stir up deep emotions—fear, self-doubt, anxiety, disappointment, or anger. It is important for women to understand that seeking the cause and cure for infertility indefinitely with poor results can cause a devastating strain on a marriage, a career, and emotional health. Experts recommend that women make sure they have an adequate support system, that they can communicate openly with their partners, and that they are prepared to stop treatment after a reasonable time has passed without success.

Most women experience grief and other emotions associated with loss when fertility treatments do not succeed month after month and year after year. Emotional and moral support are essential. Some women find support with their partners, but many find that depending on their partners for such support places stress on the relationship, which, again, adds to the emotional burden. Most communities offer support seminars and ongoing meetings where women can talk openly about their feelings surrounding infertility. Your fertility specialist can provide information about local groups.

Where to Learn More

Numerous organizations and publications exist that provide up-to-the-minute information on research in the field of infertility medicine, information about support groups, discussions of the ethical questions involved in fertility treatments, and many other services. The following are among the most helpful organizations:

- **The American Society for Reproductive Medicine**
- **The American College of Obstetricians and Gynecologists**
- **RESOLVE, Inc.**

Information about these organizations can be found in Resources at the end of this book.

What *You* Can Do

Family planning involves preventing pregnancy as well as planning when to get pregnant. Women today have many choices and options, including various methods of birth control. By making good use of these options women can take responsibility for their overall health as well as their reproduction health.

- If you do not want to become pregnant now, choose a method of birth control that fits your lifestyle.
- Use birth control each and every time you have intercourse, or make sure your partner does.
- If your birth control method has failed, consider emergency contraception.
- If you are concerned about STDs, use a barrier method every time you have sex.
- If you have tried for a year to become pregnant and have not been successful, speak with your obstetrician/gynecologist about recommending a reproductive endocrinologist. Your partner can seek the advice of a urologist.
- If you or your partner is diagnosed with a condition that causes infertility, be sure to keep yourself well during the treatment process. Eat well, exercise, and find the emotional support you need.

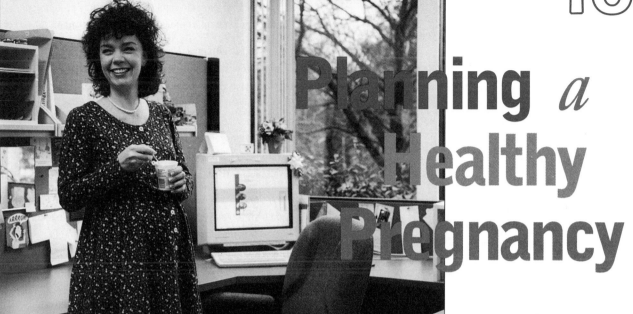

Chapter 18

Planning *a* Healthy Pregnancy

W hen women choose to have children, they find themselves faced with many decisions and options. What type of prenatal care is best for me? Are my diet and lifestyle as healthy as they need to be? In what setting do I want to give birth to my child? What type of care do I and the baby need after the baby is born? Together with her health care provider, a pregnant woman decides what type of care she will receive while pregnant and what type of delivery she can expect to have. The better informed a woman becomes about her options, the smarter her choices will be—and the better they will suit her, her baby, and her family.

The First Questions

During the early part of pregnancy, many questions arise. Some require answers right away, whereas others can be explored throughout pregnancy. Having a health care team working with you can give you the resources you need to make good decisions throughout your pregnancy.

Am I Pregnant?

For women who are seeking to become pregnant, few things bring more joy than the news that a longed-for baby is on its way. Once a woman suspects she is pregnant (because of a skipped or abnormal period, breast tenderness, or nausea), she will want to confirm her pregnancy with a test. Early confirmation of pregnancy means a woman can begin prenatal care right away.

Before You Become Pregnant: Preconception Care

Preconception care refers to the steps you take to care for yourself while you are trying to conceive. An implanted embryo immediately begins to develop its nervous system, digestive system, and cardiovascular system. Therefore, your health and well-being at the time of conception is as important to your baby's health as the care you take after you learn the baby is on the way.

The best thing you can do if you are planning a pregnancy is to act as though you are already pregnant.

Nutrition. Stock up on the nutrients in the five food groups by eating a healthy, well-balanced diet. Start taking a multivitamin containing 0.4 milligrams of folic acid during the month before you plan to get pregnant. Folic acid has been proven to help reduce a group of birth defects called neural tube defects. Folic acid only works to prevent neural tube defects if taken early in pregnancy, when the fetus's organs are beginning to form. Increase your calcium "bank" by drinking lots of milk and eating calcium-rich foods.

Weight. If you are planning a pregnancy and know you are not pregnant yet, you have the opportunity to bring your weight up or down to a more healthy level. If you are underweight, you may have trouble becoming pregnant. If you have very low body fat, your body slows down its production of estrogen. Estrogen is necessary for ovulation to occur. If you have run competitively or have had an eating disorder, you may have found that your periods became irregular or stopped completely. This is a sign that you are not ovulating regularly—or at all. When your weight goes back up to a healthier level, periods and ovulation usually resume.

Pregnant women who are overweight are more likely to have certain problems during pregnancy, such as high blood pressure or diabetes. They may also find that after the pregnancy they are left with additional weight to lose. It is better for you and the fetus if you bring your weight down to a healthy level before you conceive. If you weigh more than you should, plan a healthy, gradual, weight-loss program with your doctor before you conceive.

Avoiding Harmful Substances. Almost everything that enters a pregnant woman's bloodstream also enters the fetus's bloodstream. Substances like alcohol, tobacco, and drugs can harm your health and that of the fetus. Some medications, such as Accutane (used to treat acne), may also be dangerous to your fetus. Discuss these topics with your doctor. If you or your partner smokes, it is strongly recommended that both of you quit before you become pregnant.

Diseases and Pregnancy. If you are planning a baby, you will want to know whether any medical conditions you have will affect your baby. Some women have medical conditions that can worsen when they are pregnant or affect a fetus. These conditions include: diabetes, infections [such as human immunodeficiency virus (HIV), chlamydia, gonorrhea, herpes, and syphilis], epilepsy, heart disease, kidney disease, and phenylketonuria (PKU).

The Preconception Visit. If you decide to make a preconception visit to your doctor, she will review your pregnancy plans and provide you with advice on how you can improve your health. For example, you can get advice on when to stop using birth control in order to become pregnant.

Your doctor will review your medical history with you and ask you questions about your lifestyle in order to determine any factors that could make pregnancy risky for you or a fetus. Some pregnancy problems and birth defects are more common in certain families and ethnic groups. If you have had a miscarriage before, if you have had a baby with a birth defect before, or if someone in your family has a birth defect, you may be at risk for having problems with your next pregnancy.

In some cases, you can take steps to lower your risk before you become pregnant. For example, if you are African American, you may be at risk for sickle cell disease, a blood disorder. Even if you do not have this disease yourself, you could carry one gene for the disease. If your partner also carries one gene, then you could have a fetus with sickle cell disease. You and your partner can be tested before pregnancy to see if you are at risk.

Financial Issues. Aside from verifying your insurance coverage for maternity care, you should also make a financial plan to meet the additional expenses associated with child rearing. If you have not started saving, do it now. You will soon have a lot of new expenses—a crib, car seat, baby clothes, and diapers. If you decide to go back to work or school after having the baby, you will need to pay for childcare. If you decide to leave your job and become a stay-at-home mom, you will need to compensate for the income you will no longer receive. Even if you just take a regular or extended maternity leave, your income will decrease. Putting the equivalent of a few months' income aside can give you a sense of security.

Today, a woman can reliably find out whether she is pregnant in minutes. She may choose a home pregnancy test from the drugstore or make an appointment with her obstetrician/gynecologist or nurse practitioner/midwife. Both home pregnancy tests and pregnancy tests offered in a health care provider's office work the same way, by detecting the presence of human chorionic gonadotropin (hCG), a hormone produced soon after a pregnancy begins. Home kits measure hCG in a woman's urine. Health care providers may choose either a blood or a urine test, depending on the circumstance, but both measure hCG.

There is a variety of home pregnancy test kits on the market. Many are as effective as the tests used by doctors and, in fact, many are the same tests. The answer—yes or no—appears within five minutes. As simple as these tests are, a woman must carefully follow the directions to get a reliable result. In very early pregnancy, the most reliable urine test results are produced by assessing a first morning urine, which is more concentrated.

A woman who discovers she is pregnant through a home pregnancy test may wish to have the results confirmed by a health care professional. When a positive result is revealed in the doctor's office, a pregnant woman can often begin prenatal care at the very same visit and have her first questions answered.

Who Do I Want As a Health Care Provider During My Pregnancy?

The medical and personal support of a trusted health care provider (or a group of providers) is essential for a healthy pregnancy. Three types of health care professionals care for pregnant women:

1. **Obstetrician/gynecologists** (ob/gyns) are doctors who are specially trained in caring for women. In addition to having completed medical school, they have several years of advanced education in women's health care. Ob/gyns can have further specialized training in maternal-fetal medicine, which is highly specialized care for women with high-risk pregnancies.

2. Some **family doctors and general practitioners** choose to provide care for pregnant women as part of their practice. In addition to having completed medical school, physicians certified in family practice have advanced training in all aspects of medical care for both men and women.

3. **Certified nurse–midwives**(CNMs)are trained as nurses and then receive advanced training in caring for pregnant women.

Following are some questions a woman may consider in choosing a health care provider for her pregnancy:

- Do I have any medical concerns or previous problems with pregnancy that could pose a risk during pregnancy?
- Would I feel more comfortable in a "high-tech" clinical setting, or would I prefer a "high-nurturance" health care setting?
- Where would I like to deliver my baby?

wellness **tip**

Save money by purchasing a home test kit that provides two tests in one box. They cost less per test than single tests and allow retesting in a few days to confirm the results. If you have medical insurance, testing in a doctor's office is likely to be covered by your insurance.

Barring unforeseen circumstances, the decision comes down to what makes the mother-to-be and her partner feel most secure and comfortable.

Where Do I Want to Deliver My Baby?

Most pregnant women have their babies in hospitals. Some women prefer to have their babies in a birthing center, which may be part of a hospital or a free-standing center. A few women choose to give birth in their homes. The choice of location depends on the personal comfort level of the mother and her partner, the health of the fetus, pregnancy complications, choice of anesthesia, and availability of the health care provider chosen.

Hospital Birth. A hospital is considered the safest place to give birth. The greatest risk for life-threatening and often unexpected complications occurs during labor and delivery. For women who have particular health problems or those who develop pregnancy complications that could affect the safety of the mother or fetus, a hospital birth is the only choice. Giving birth in a hospital also gives a woman the greatest choice of medical providers, anesthesia, and other services. Depending on the hospital, deliveries can be performed by ob/gyns, family doctors, and CNMs.

In an effort to attract prospective parents, many hospitals have made tremendous strides to offset their reputation as cold and noisy places by offering comfortably decorated rooms where a woman can go through labor, delivery, and recovery after birth all in the same room. Although the rooms look "homelike," the equipment required for an emergency is tucked away out of sight and ready for immediate use should the need arise. A postpartum hospital stay is usually two days following a vaginal delivery and four days following a cesarean delivery.

Birthing Centers. An alternative to a hospital is a birthing center. Birthing centers offer some of the same medical care available at hospitals but in a more relaxed setting. Some birthing centers are in a special wing of the hospital or across the street in proximity to the hospital, should a medical emergency arise. Others are some distance away from the hospital, but all have arrangements to transfer women to a hospital in case of an emergency.

In many birthing centers, midwives direct a woman's prenatal care as well as the labor and delivery. The staff at birthing centers generally take a more natural approach to pregnancy and to labor and delivery. They may be a good choice for women whose goal is to experience childbirth without anesthesia and with a short postpartum stay. Most birthing centers do not have the availability of epidural or regional anesthetic. Postpartum stays are usually quite short, with many women leaving for home within 6 to 12 hours after birth.

Giving birth in a birthing center usually costs less than giving birth in a hospital. Because some insurance plans do not cover births in this setting, however, it is recommended that a pregnant woman check with her health insurance provider before deciding where to give birth, particularly if she is depending on the insurance company to help pay for the delivery.

Home Births. Home births are a rare choice. The home is the riskiest place to give birth, and most doctors and many midwives refuse to attend home deliveries.

Critical medical problems can arise without warning in labor, even in a woman who has had a completely normal, healthy pregnancy or a woman who has had previous uncomplicated deliveries. Because of the risks, home births are less likely to be covered by insurance. Women who are attracted by the idea of birth with all the comforts of home should visit birthing centers and the new birthing suites at hospitals, which combine homelike comforts with appropriate standards of hygiene and cleanliness as well as necessary emergency equipment.

Prenatal Care

Because a tremendous amount of critical growth by the fetus occurs during the first weeks of pregnancy, starting prenatal care as early as possible is one of the best things a pregnant woman can do for herself and her baby. Prenatal care is a program of examinations, tests, and advice that a doctor or midwife offers throughout pregnancy to help a woman ensure a healthy mother and baby.

Prenatal Visits

The first prenatal visit can take place as soon as a woman knows she is pregnant. The first visit is usually longer than the others, because there is a lot of information the doctor needs to know. Some essential information includes age, general health, the health of the parents' families, lifestyle issues (including any alcohol, tobacco, or drug use), and the outcome of any previous pregnancies. This information is confidential but is essential for good prenatal care, since certain conditions are more common in certain ages, ethnic groups, or families. Usually a number of tests are also done at the first visit, including blood tests, urinalysis, and a Pap smear. Depending on the data collected as well as the results of initial tests, further testing may be suggested at a later time.

At the first visit, the health care provider will calculate a woman's due date. This date is based on the first day of her last menstrual period. A normal pregnancy is 40 weeks, counting from the first day of a woman's last menstrual period. Only about 5 percent of babies arrive on their due date.

wellness **tip**

You can figure out your due date from the date of your last menstrual period. Just add seven days to the date and then subtract three months. For example, if the first day of your last period was October 28, add seven days to get November 4, then subtract three months— your due date is the upcoming August 4.

Tests at the First Prenatal Visit

Samples of a woman's blood are taken for the following tests:

- Blood type (A, B, AB, or O) and Rh factor (positive or negative). If mother and baby have different blood types, some problems can arise.
- Sexually transmitted diseases; hepatitis B; HIV (human immunodeficiency virus, which causes AIDS—acquired immunodeficiency syndrome)
- Anemia (not having enough red blood cells to carry oxygen; usually reflects iron-deficiency in reproductive age women)
- Antibodies to rubella (the virus that causes German

measles), which can cause multiple abnormalities if the mother is not immune and catches rubella during early fetal development

A urine specimen is also studied for evidence of problems:
- Urinary tract infections
- Presence of glucose or protein may indicate that further evaluation is needed

During a pelvic examination, other tests are done:
- Pap test (to check for cervical abnormalities)
- Tests for chlamydia and gonorrhea (infections that can harm a woman or her baby)

How a Baby Grows

An average pregnancy lasts 40 weeks. During this time, an amazing amount of growth and development takes place. The illustrations here show how the baby changes over the course of the pregnancy.

Pregnancy is divided into three trimesters of about 14 weeks each. A baby's growth begins at conception, the joining of egg and sperm. Even as the now-fertilized egg slowly moves down the fallopian tube, it is growing and dividing rapidly into new cells. The cells first form a clump and then a hollow ball with a cluster of cells inside that

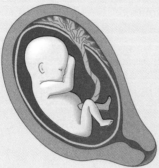

FIGURE 18.1
12 Weeks

will be the baby. About a week after conception, the ball of cells implants in the wall of the uterus. There it will receive the nutrients it needs from the mother's body.

In the first trimester, a baby undergoes the greatest changes. The cells begin to divide by function: the brain and nervous system, the stomach and digestive system, and so on. All the major organs begin forming. As early as 5 weeks after conception the baby's heart begins to beat; although it can be seen on ultrasound, it is not audible by doppler until 10 to 12 weeks. The baby's life support—the placenta— carries nutrients to the baby from the mother's blood system and carries the baby's wastes away through her blood. Early in the first trimester, the baby looks more like a tadpole than a person, complete with a small tail. By the end of the first trimester, though, it has arms, legs, hands, and feet,

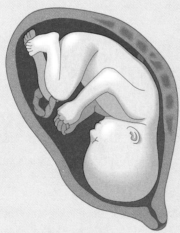

FIGURE 18.2
24 Weeks

and looks more like a person each day. At the end of the trimester, the baby weighs about one ounce and is about four inches long.

In the second trimester, weight gain increases sharply. Fingernails, tastebuds, eyelids, and eyebrows form. The organs continue to develop. Genitals are forming and the baby begins to eliminate urine. If the mother has a sonogram during the second trimester, she may be able to tell whether she is having a boy or a girl. The baby also begins to move and kick, and the mother can feel, and sometimes even see, the baby's movements. At the end of this trimester, the baby weighs 2 to 2$\frac{1}{2}$ pounds and is about 11 to 14 inches long.

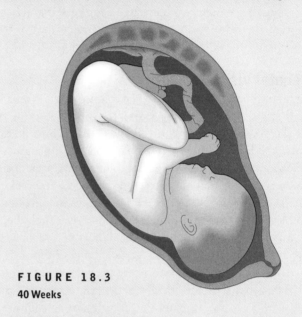

FIGURE 18.3
40 Weeks

In the third trimester, the baby gets ready for life out- side the uterus. Fat cushions the baby's muscles and bones. Bones harden, and lungs firm up so that they will be able to inflate and draw in air. The baby practices the movements needed for life outside—stretching, turning, breathing, kick- ing. In most pregnancies, the baby turns head downward so that its head locks into the bottom part of the uterus. At birth, the average baby weighs between 6 and 9 pounds and is about 20 inches long.

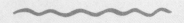

Subsequent routine visits are scheduled about once a month at first and then closer together as the delivery date approaches:

- From the first visit to 28 weeks—every 4 weeks
- From 28 weeks to 36 weeks—every 2 weeks
- From 36 weeks to birth—weekly

At each visit, the woman's weight, blood pressure, and urine will be checked. If there has been any bleeding or vaginal irritation, the doctor or midwife may wish to perform a pelvic examination. After about 10 to 12 weeks, the baby's heartbeat can be heard, and the doctor or midwife will listen for it at each visit. They will also measure to make sure that the fetus is growing at an appropriate rate. In early gestation, growth is checked by palpating the uterus. As pregnancy advances, growth will be measured with a measuring tape or with calipers.

One of the most important parts of every prenatal visit is the opportunity a woman has to talk with her doctor or midwife. She can share new or unusual feelings she is having, get reassurance about normal experiences, and have her questions answered. The prenatal visits allow the health care provider to observe and discuss signs that could warrant special care and to see how the mother is doing in general. It also allows the woman and her partner an opportunity to establish a trusting relationship with the health care provider.

Testing—When and Why?

In addition to the routine tests that are a standard part of prenatal care, other tests are offered in pregnancy. They can help a woman learn whether her baby is healthy, has some birth defect, or is otherwise at risk. Some tests are offered to all women, while others are only offered if the health care provider believes that the testing is necessary.

Testing for Birth Defects. Screening tests for birth defects are offered routinely during prenatal care visits. If a test indicates a problem, more testing may be necessary to verify the results. The three common screening tests discussed below are chorionic villus sampling, amniocentesis, and maternal serum testing.

Chorionic Villus Sampling. In this test, samples are taken from the chorionic villi, tiny threads of tissue that are a part of the placenta. Because the chorionic villi and the baby are both formed from the same fertilized egg, they have the same genes and chromosomes. The chorionic villi are analyzed to study the baby's chromosomes.

Chorionic villus sampling (CVS) can be done in one of two ways. A needle is passed through a woman's abdomen to the placenta, or a thin tube can be passed through her vagina and into the cervical opening to get to the placenta. The advantage of CVS is that it can be done earlier than amniocentesis—as early as ten weeks gestation. The disadvantage is that CVS slightly increases the chance that a woman will miscarry after the procedure.

Amniocentesis. For amniocentesis, a needle is inserted through a woman's abdomen into the sac surrounding the baby, which is filled with amniotic fluid

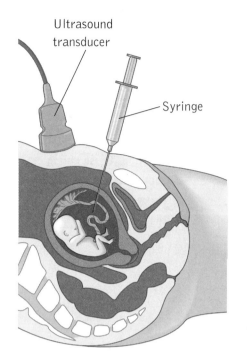

Ultrasound transducer

Syringe

FIGURE 18.4
Amniocentesis
During amniocentesis, the doctor uses an ultrasound transducer to see the position of the fetus in the uterus. This allows her to safely withdraw a sample of amniotic fluid with a syringe.

(see Figure 18.4). The amniotic fluid contains skin cells the baby has naturally shed, and these skin cells can be treated so that the baby's chromosomes can be studied. In addition, the fluid itself can be analyzed for other abnormalities. Early amniocentesis, which is only performed when infants are at high risk for abnormalities or when the earliest possible information about the pregnancy is needed, is usually done between 14 and 15 weeks of pregnancy. Routine amniocentesis is done at 16 to 18 weeks. Like CVS, amniocentesis slightly increases the risk of a miscarriage, but rates are lower than for CVS.

Maternal Serum Testing. Maternal serum testing is used to detect the possible presence of genetic disorders, such as Down syndrome or neural tube defects. Maternal serum screening is recommended between 15 to 18 weeks of pregnancy. It involves taking a sample of blood from a pregnant woman and testing it for substances made by the baby. Because the woman's and baby's blood systems do not mix but are indirectly linked through placental sites, certain substances made by the baby are measurable in the woman's blood stream.

The first substance used for maternal serum testing was alpha-fetoprotein. Women with higher than normal amounts were more likely to have a baby with neural tube defects. Women who had lower than normal amounts of alpha-fetoprotein were more likely to have a baby with Down syndrome. Technical advances in maternal serum screening have improved the likelihood of accurately predicting whether a fetus has Down syndrome. If the screening tests are abnormal, then specific diagnostic procedures can verify if a certain condition exists. The most common diagnostic procedures are ultrasound and amniocentesis. The most common reason for an abnormal screening test result is an incorrect due date, for example, if the gestation period has actually been shorter than originally thought.

Testing for Other Disorders. Some tests are also utilized to detect a medical disorder that can complicate pregnancy. Two such disorders are gestational diabetes and hypertension in pregnancy. Although both diabetes and hypertension can occur in women who are not pregnant, they can both begin during pregnancy and pose a threat to both mother and baby.

Gestational Diabetes. Diabetes occurs when a woman's body either does not make enough insulin (a protein needed to move sugar, also known as glucose, from the bloodstream into the cells, where it can be used for energy) or cannot use the insulin it makes. When this condition occurs for the first time during pregnancy it is called gestational diabetes. If a woman has untreated gestational diabetes, her baby is more likely to be very large (ten pounds or more), more likely to be stillborn, more likely to be injured during birth, and more likely to have problems with low blood sugar after delivery. Gestational diabetes can usually be controlled through diet. A pregnant woman with gestational diabetes will have more frequent prenatal checkups than a pregnant woman without such complications.

All women will be offered testing for diabetes at 24 to 28 weeks of pregnancy; earlier testing may be suggested for a woman who has had gestational diabetes in the past, had a large baby before, or has a family history for diabetes mellitus. For the test, a woman drinks a very sweet glucose solution. An hour later, her blood glucose level is drawn. A higher than normal amount of sugar in her blood suggests a possibility of diabetes. Confirmation is made by the glucose tolerance test. As in the screening test, the woman drinks a very sweet glucose solution and then blood is drawn. For this diagnostic test, however, blood is taken several times—at one hour, two hours, and three hours after the drink. Glucose levels that are too high on two or more of the samples confirm the diagnosis of gestational diabetes. Blood sugars should return to normal after delivery— if they do not, then this is a new diagnosis of diabetes mellitus that was picked up during pregnancy. Management for diabetes mellitus during pregnancy is the same as for gestational diabetes. Many experts also feel that women who have gestational diabetes are at risk of developing diabetes mellitus later in life, especially if they are overweight.

Pregnancy-Induced Hypertension. Pregnancy-induced hypertension, high blood pressure brought on by pregnancy, complicates five to seven percent of pregnancies in otherwise healthy women who are having their first child. It may complicate the pregnancies of a higher percentage of women who already have chronic hypertension, diabetes, or other disorders.

A risk to the fetus associated with pregnancy-induced hypertension is placental abruption, in which the placenta separates from the uterus. Placental abruption, usually signaled by vaginal bleeding, abdominal pain, and uterine tenderness, can decrease or interrupt the flow of oxygen-rich blood to the baby. It is one of the leading causes of fetal death in the third trimester. If placental abruption is suspected, the baby and mother will be closely monitored, and the mother may be hospitalized if she has not yet reached term. If the baby is in true danger, cesarean delivery may be needed.

In certain cases, pregnancy-induced hypertension is an early sign of a more serious condition called preeclampsia. Preeclampsia is characterized by high blood pressure, swelling in the face and hands, and protein in the urine. It develops in the second half of pregnancy, most commonly during the last few weeks of pregnancy. Severe cases of preeclampsia may require complete bed rest or hospitalization, to prevent life-threatening seizures. Sometimes, labor must be induced or a cesarean delivery performed. Following are the warning signs of preeclampsia:

- Blood pressure readings of 140/90 (or a blood pressure reading that is 30/15 greater than baseline blood pressure)
- Sudden weight gain of more than about 1 pound a day
- Swelling (edema), especially of the face
- Severe or constant headaches
- Blurred vision or spots in front of the eyes
- Pain in the upper right part of the abdomen

Checking Up on Baby. Practitioners check up on the baby in many ways. Doctors can learn a great deal by simply measuring the size of the uterus and listening to the heartbeat. If the uterus is growing too quickly or too slowly, an ultrasound may be needed. Once the baby starts moving, the mother can tell a lot about the

Two Common Birth Defects

Two common birth defects that can be detected during pregnancy are Down syndrome and neural tube defects. Screening tests can show whether a woman is at risk for these conditions, and diagnostic tests can show whether her baby is affected.

Down syndrome is caused by having three copies of chromosome 21 instead of the normal two copies. Babies with Down syndrome are mentally retarded and often have heart problems.

Neural tube defects occur very early in pregnancy, when the baby's spine and brain are forming. If the problem occurs where the baby's spine will form, the condition is called spina bifida. A hole is formed in the baby's spine that may or may not be covered with skin. When the problem occurs where the baby's brain will form, the condition is called anencephaly. In anencephaly, the baby's brain fails to form completely. Babies always die from anencephaly, although they may live a short time after birth.

wellness **warning**

Call your doctor if you experience any of the following warnings before your due date:

- Unusual vaginal discharge
- Pelvic or lower abdominal pressure not relieved by rest
- Constant, low, dull backache
- Mild abdominal cramps, with or without diarrhea
- Regular contractions or uterine tightening, even if painless
- Ruptured membranes (water breaks)

baby herself. She becomes accustomed to the ways it moves and can use that information to determine whether or not the baby is well. Sometimes a combination of ultrasound and fetal movement assessment are necessary. Some commonly used techniques are outlined below.

Ultrasound. The technique of ultrasound uses sound waves to create a moving picture of the baby. Although the test does not hurt, it may be uncomfortable in early pregnancy because a woman needs to have a very full bladder in order for the sound waves to create a clear picture. Later in pregnancy, ultrasound is done with the bladder empty.

Many mothers-to-be show their ultrasound pictures (or videos, available in some doctors' offices) with as much pride as they would baby pictures. In England and Europe, ultrasound is routinely used to assess fetal wellness during each trimester. In this country, the ob/gyn community is divided about whether even one "routine" ultrasound should be done in pregnancy. The controversy is more about cost than medicine. Diagnostic (as opposed to routine) ultrasound is commonly used and less controversial. Ultrasound can reveal the following information:

- The presence of one baby or more
- Whether the heart is beating
- The baby's size (and therefore, gestational age)
- The baby's gender
- The presence of some birth defects

Kick Count. The kick count is simple and free, and a woman can do it herself at home. A healthy baby moves around often, and the kick count helps a woman keep track of her baby's movements. It can be done in different ways. Some women count how many times their baby moves in a certain amount of time; others note how long it takes for the baby to move a given number of times. The important thing is for the woman to become familiar with what pattern of movement is normal for her baby. If she notices a sudden lessening of movement, it is important that she inform her doctor or midwife as soon as possible.

Fetal Monitoring. Although fetal monitoring was initially used just during labor, it is now used to assess fetal well-being in high-risk and postdate pregnancies. There are two types of tests commonly used: the nonstress test and the contraction stress test. Both tests involve listening to the baby's heart rate with a special monitor strapped onto the woman's abdomen. In the nonstress test, the baby's heart rate is measured along with her movements. The woman pushes a button whenever she feels the baby move, and a mark is made on a paper monitor strip that is simultaneously recording the heart rate. It is normal for the baby's heart rate to speed up when she moves around. If the baby's heart rate does not speed up, it may indicate that the fetus is not doing well. In such cases, the doctor may then use a contraction stress test to confirm the results.

In the contraction stress test, the baby's heart rate is measured in response to contractions. Just for the test, a few contractions are brought on by giving a medication called oxytocin or by having the woman rub her nipples (this causes her own body to produce contractions). These contractions go away once the test is over and do not cause labor to start. If the baby's heart rate decreases in response to the uterine contraction, the placenta may not be supplying the baby with adequate oxygen and nutrients. The practitioner will often assess this baby very carefully to make sure that it is safe to remain in the uterus. The biophysical profile discussed below may help to determine if the baby is well or if it needs to be delivered.

Biophysical Profile. In the biophysical profile, an ultrasound examination is combined with listening to the baby's heartbeat. The technician or nurse notes the baby's score on five items:

1. Heart rate (including patterns of decreased heart rate, called a deceleration)
2. Body movement
3. Muscle tone
4. Amount of amniotic fluid
5. Breathing movements

A perfect score is 10, but any score above 8 is normal.

A Healthy Lifestyle

There is so much a woman can do to make pregnancy a happy, healthy experience—and increase the chance that her baby will be born healthy. A woman's healthy lifestyle is the cornerstone of a healthy pregnancy and a healthy baby. Elements of a healthy lifestyle during pregnancy include a nutritionally balanced diet, a moderate exercise program, avoidance of harmful substances and behaviors, and a good balance of work and relaxing activities.

Diet

Everyone has heard the saying, "Eating for two," and it is true—to an extent. It is true that a pregnant woman's diet is her baby's sole source of nutrition, but eating for two does not mean eating twice as much. It does mean choosing foods for a varied, well-balanced diet (see Chapter 8 for more information about eating for wellness). Women who eat well before pregnancy only need to make small changes in their diet during pregnancy.

A woman of average weight should gain between 20 and 25 pounds during pregnancy. This is usually enough for a healthy baby and its support system. In general, a pregnant woman needs about 300 more calories per day as well as the following supplements:

• Iron
• Folic acid
• Calcium

It is hard for a pregnant woman in this country to get enough iron solely from her diet. Her body needs extra iron during pregnancy, both to build the red blood cells that increase her own circulating blood volume and to make sure that she has adequate iron storage to replace blood lost during delivery and the postpartum period. The fetus is also building red blood cells and takes its iron supply from the mother. For this reason most pregnant women are prescribed iron supplementation, either as part of a prenatal vitamin or as a special supplement.

Folic acid is also needed to produce the extra maternal and fetal blood cells needed during pregnancy. It has also been shown that, in certain populations, folic acid supplementation can prevent neural tube defects. Because of this, the Food and Drug Administration has approved adding folic acid to foods and making folic acid supplements available over-the-counter. Since the neural tube is formed so early in pregnancy, supplementation is recommended during periods of time when women are trying to conceive. Prenatal vitamins contain the recommended amount of folic acid and other vitamins and minerals.

Calcium is needed for the development of the baby's strong bones and teeth. The baby will take its calcium directly from the mother's own body, thus putting the mother at risk for osteoporosis later in life if she does not increase her calcium intake during pregnancy. Women who drink six or more glasses of milk daily will get the extra calcium they need. Women who cannot drink milk should choose other foods high in calcium, such as dark green, leafy vegetables, canned sardines, or calcium-fortified orange juice. Calcium supplementation may also be recommended.

Many women are lactose intolerant—they lack the enzyme lactase, which enables the body to digest the milk sugar lactose. These women experience gas and stomach pains when they eat dairy products, such as milk. Pregnant women who are lactose intolerant need to make sure they get enough calcium and protein from other sources. Some lactose-intolerant women find that they can eat cultured dairy products, such as cheese and yogurt, without having discomfort.

Vegetarians who eat milk and eggs should have no problem meeting their dietary needs during pregnancy. Vegans—who eat no animal products—must plan a little more carefully. Animal products are the most common source of vitamin B_{12}. Vegans should take supplements of this vitamin and be sure they get enough calcium, protein, and iron from other food sources.

Women who have PKU lack an enzyme needed to break down some amino acids—the building blocks of food. If they become pregnant, their fetuses are at risk for birth defects. If you have PKU, your doctor may have you follow a special diet, like the one you followed when you were younger. A diet low in the amino acid you cannot digest can help prevent the problems of PKU. If you follow this same diet before you become pregnant and throughout your pregnancy, you can reduce the risk of problems with the fetus.

Eating disorders are serious at any time in a woman's life, but they require particular attention during pregnancy. A pregnant woman who has struggled with her body image may find her increasing weight and growing waistline hard to bear, even though they are signs of a healthy pregnancy. Although many practitioners forget to ask about it in the initial interview, women with eating disorders need special assistance even in early pregnancy. Even if practitioners do ask, some women are very uncomfortable discussing their anorexia or bulimia. If a woman cannot tell her doctor, she should tell someone, so she can get help dealing with the changes that will accompany the pregnancy.

Exercise

Women who are active can usually stay active right through the end of pregnancy. A regular program of exercise can help a woman feel better and have more energy during pregnancy. Most sports and exercises are safe during pregnancy, but a woman should talk with her doctor if she has any questions. If a woman was relatively inactive at the start of pregnancy, a walking program or an exercise class designed especially for women who are pregnant will usually be beneficial. It is important to avoid over-heating, since sustained core temperatures of greater than 101°F may be associated with the development of fetal anomalies. If a woman experiences bleeding during pregnancy she should refrain from exercising until her physician says it is OK. Every pregnant woman needs to listen to her body—stopping if she feels pain, dizziness, discomfort, excessive fatigue, or irregular or rapid heartbeat. Any of these symptoms should be reported to the doctor.

A woman will tire more easily when she is pregnant and should tailor her workout accordingly. As she gains weight and her abdomen enlarges, her center of balance changes. As pregnancy advances, the pelvic bone becomes less stable, so falls occur more easily. Sports that require a fine sense of balance or sudden stops, such as gymnastics or bicycle riding, are not recommended. Activities that present a risk of falling or traveling at a high rate of speed, like snow or water skiing, should also be avoided. (See Chapter 9 for more information about exercising during pregnancy.)

Avoiding Hazardous Substances and Behaviors

What a woman avoids doing during pregnancy is just as important as what she does. She should avoid using alcohol, tobacco, and drugs, which threaten her own health and her baby's. Some prescription drugs and workplace hazards should also be avoided.

Alcohol. According to the Centers for Disease Control and Prevention, alcohol use during pregnancy has been identified as the leading preventable cause of birth defects. Alcohol crosses the placenta during pregnancy and can cause fetal alcohol syndrome (FAS) in the baby. Severely affected infants are mentally retarded and may have facial abnormalities. Less severely affected infants may have learning disabilities, especially in math and subjects that require abstract reasoning. It is not known how much alcohol—if any—is safe to drink during pregnancy. Women who drink more than two drinks each day and women who binge drink to the point of drunkenness seem to be at greatest risk for having children with FAS. The safest course is to give it up completely. A woman who had been drinking before she knew she was pregnant should talk with her doctor about how much risk she incurred during this interval.

Tobacco. It is strongly recommended that pregnant women who smoke quit. If they cannot quit, they should cut down as much as possible. Asking your partner to quit may help you quit too, and it will help to create a smoke-free environment for the baby after it is born. Miscarriage, premature birth, and low birth weight are more likely with pregnant women who smoke. School-age children who were born to women who smoked during pregnancy have higher incidence

wellness **tip**

Pregnant women who feel self-conscious taking a regular exercise class may want to look for special prenatal exercise classes, commonly offered at many hospitals, community centers, and YWCAs.

wellness **tip**

Tell your employer as soon as possible that you are pregnant. This will allow optimal planning to avoid hazards in the workplace and plan for covering your responsibilities during maternity leave.

of hyperactivity disorders and lower IQ scores. Children exposed to secondhand smoke in the home have higher rates of sudden infant death syndrome (SIDS), higher rates of upper respiratory infections, and more asthma.

Nicotine replacement patches and gums are now available without a prescription, but some are not recommended for use during pregnancy. A woman who wants to use these products in order to quit smoking should discuss it with her health care provider first. (Chapter 13 includes a detailed section on techniques for quitting smoking.)

Drugs. Street drugs pose a definite threat to the health and safety of a pregnant woman and her baby. For example, a woman who uses cocaine during pregnancy increases the chance that the placenta will tear away from her uterus too early (placental abruption), causing bleeding, reduced oxygen to the baby, and in the case of complete placental separation, rapid death of the infant. Babies born to cocaine-using mothers are often irritable and fussy. Babies born to heroin using mothers are not only irritable, they are also addicted to heroin and will experience withdrawal symptoms. If a doctor or nurse suspects that a pregnant woman is using drugs, she may ask for a urine drug screen. In some states, the doctor has the right to test the woman without her permission. A positive test may mean the baby is put in foster care after birth until the mother can prove she is drug-free.

Prescription Drugs and Medical Treatments. Some prescription medications, such as the acne treatment Accutane, can be harmful during pregnancy. A pregnant woman should tell her health care provider about any medications she uses—whether available without a prescription (over-the-counter) or prescribed by a doctor. If she seeks care from other health care professionals, she should also tell them that she is pregnant. Treatments can then be chosen that will be safe for both her and her baby.

Radiation can cause birth defects, but only at high exposures. Ordinary diagnostic or dental x-rays, especially with the abdomen shielded, do not place the infant at risk. On the other hand, doses of radiation used for certain other types of treatment, such as cancer, can be harmful to a fetus. If a pregnant woman develops cancer, she will need to work carefully with both her oncologist and her pregnancy care provider to weigh the risk of radiation to the baby against the risk of delaying her cancer treatment.

Occupational Hazards. Some substances in the workplace can be hazardous to pregnant women and their unborn babies. A pregnant woman who works with radiation or heavy metals should ask her safety manager or union representative about her routine level of exposure and discuss problems that could occur from higher accidental exposure. The radiation that comes from a computer screen is not harmful to a pregnant woman or her baby.

Domestic Violence. According to a recent study, as many as 23 percent of women seeking prenatal care are also experiencing physical or verbal abuse. Abuse often becomes more frequent during pregnancy, and it is not uncommon for the first episodes of abuse to occur during a pregnancy. Any woman who is being abused sexually, physically, or verbally needs to know that she is not the cause of the abuse, and she should not blame herself. She does, however, need to protect herself and her unborn baby. She needs to inform her doctor or midwife about the abuse. If she cannot talk to her provider, she must talk to someone she trusts. The national hot line number for victims of domestic violence is 800-799-SAFE(7233). (Chapter 14 provides specific information on domestic violence and recommended strategies for getting emergency and longer term assistance.)

Infections. The following infections can be especially harmful to a developing fetus if the mother becomes infected during vulnerable periods during the pregnancy:

- Sexually transmitted infections (syphilis, HIV, herpes, gonorrhea, chlamydia, human papillomavirus)
- Chickenpox (varicella)
- Fifth disease (parvovirus)
- Rubella (German measles)
- Mumps
- Cytomegalovirus
- Hepatitis
- Listeriosis
- Group B *Streptococcus*
- Lyme disease
- Toxoplasmosis
- Tuberculosis

If a woman is at risk for exposure to chickenpox, rubella, or mumps and has not developed natural immunity (by having the disease in her childhood), she should be vaccinated prior to attempting pregnancy. If she is already pregnant, she should avoid situations where she might be exposed to these infections and get immunized after delivery.

Some sexually transmitted diseases can affect the fetus during pregnancy (for example, syphilis), while others are acquired by the fetus during delivery (for example, chlamydia). It is very important for an infected woman to talk to her doctor about how she and her fetus might be affected.

Daily Living

Two questions commonly asked by pregnant women are: how will my pregnancy affect daily living, and what adjustments do I need to make to my daily routine? By making a few small changes, a pregnant woman can continue her normal routine while meeting the requirements for a healthy pregnancy.

Work. Sixty-five percent of pregnant women in the United States work outside the home in full- or part-time positions. Pregnancy need not interfere with a woman's work responsibilities if they pose no more risk to her than her average

Rights in the Workplace

Pregnant women need to know they have rights in the workplace. These rights are spelled out in three federal legislative acts:

- **The Pregnancy Discrimination Act** states that, in companies with 15 or more employees, women affected by pregnancy, childbirth, or related medical conditions must be treated the same as other applicants and employees on the basis of their ability or inability to work. In other words, if an employer makes special accommodations for employees with disabilities or those who can otherwise not perform their job, she must also do so for pregnant women. The Act also protects women from being fired, being refused a job, or being denied a promotion simply because they are pregnant.
- **The Occupational Safety and Health Act** sets forth specific guidelines for workplace safety, to protect workers from unreasonable harm. State and local laws also give employees the right to know what hazardous substances, if any, are used in their workplace.
- **The Family and Medical Leave Act** grants up to 12 weeks of unpaid leave a year for the birth, adoption, or foster care of a child; caring for a sick spouse or other family member; or caring for oneself if ill. Companies and organizations with fewer than 50 employees are not compelled to comply with this law.

daily activities. Most jobs can be continued throughout pregnancy with little risk to a woman's health or her baby.

Travel. Recreational and leisure activities are as important to a balanced life during pregnancy as they are at other times. All travel plans should be discussed with your health care provider. For travel within the United States, a pregnant woman is safe traveling before 22 weeks gestation, unless she is showing evidence of threatened miscarriage. Between the period of about 24 to 32 weeks gestation (and possibly longer), women should be certain an intensive care nursery is available near their destination, because babies born within these weeks of gestation will almost certainly require such a facility. After 35 weeks gestation, the baby will probably do well regardless of where it is born in the United States, though most airlines decline to carry pregnant passengers after 27 to 28 weeks gestation.

Sitting still for many hours is not recommended at any time during pregnancy, and the impact on your circulatory system becomes more pronounced as the abdomen enlarges. If traveling by car, frequent stops to walk around and stretch are advised.

Sex. Some pregnant women find that they have an increased sex drive, but morning sickness and sheer exhaustion make them feel unwell and worn out. It is recommended that a pregnant woman let her own comfort be her guide. Some pregnant women find that trying different positions for intercourse helps her partner avoid putting pressure on her growing abdomen. Women who feel uncomfortable, physically or psychologically, about intercourse can enjoy hugging and cuddling with their partner, as well as mutual masturbation or oral sex (referred to as noninsertive sex). During oral sex, however, it is important for a woman's partner to avoid blowing air into her vagina, which can be hazardous.

Feeling *Good*

There are many joys associated with planning a pregnancy, conceiving, and nurturing that pregnancy to term. For most women, however, this is a time with some unique physical challenges. Finding ways to feel good physically may take more than a little planning and determination.

Rest

Pregnant women tire easily. This is normal—and if a woman's partner does not understand, she can give him a 10-pound sack of sugar to carry around everywhere for a couple of days! Early in pregnancy, some women have interrupted sleep because of nausea and frequent urination. Pregnant women may have trouble sleeping in the last trimester also. It may be hard to find a comfortable position. Also, as the baby grows, it puts increased pressure on the bladder, so women find they have to get up several times a night to urinate. To make up for lost sleep at night, a pregnant woman may want to go to bed earlier and try to find times during the day to rest. Being well rested helps a woman feel better, of course, but it may also help ease or prevent morning sickness. Getting help with household tasks and paring down other responsibilities may also be a good idea.

Morning Sickness / Indigestion

Some women breeze through their pregnancies with no morning sickness at all. For others, it would be better called "morning, noon, and night sickness," with gastrointestinal symptoms that range from vague nausea to severe bouts of vomiting. Increased progesterone levels cause digestion to slow down, leading to nausea. Often, as the body adjusts, morning sickness stops after the first trimester, but a few women have persistent symptoms for longer periods. Women who experience morning sickness may find the following suggestions helpful:

- Keep something in the stomach at all times—an empty stomach seems to make nausea worse. Nibble on toast or light snacks throughout the day.
- If nausea is worse in the morning, eat something—such as a cracker—before you even get out of bed.
- Try to sip on room-temperature, sweet fluids if vomiting is a problem—it will help with the nausea and prevent dehydration.
- Find what types of food are tolerable and stick with them—bland starches, such as rice and bread, are usually good. You can concentrate on balanced nutrition as your symptoms subside.
- Avoid foods, cooking smells, and other strong odors that trigger your nausea.

After the morning sickness goes away, there is a relatively quiet period before the ongoing changes in a pregnant woman's body begin to make her more susceptible to indigestion or heartburn. As progesterone levels rise, the muscle that separates the esophagus from the stomach relaxes, and stomach acid may irritate the lower part of the esophagus. As the uterus enlarges, it pushes upward on the stomach and makes the problem worse. The following tips may help:

- Eat several small meals a day instead of a few large ones.
- Decrease fat content of the meals you eat (fat slows the stomach from emptying).
- Make note of foods that seem to cause stomach upset and avoid them.
- Avoid clothes tight around the waist.
- Avoid lying flat after eating—sit up or prop yourself up at about a 45-degree angle.
- When stomach upset occurs, it is generally safe to take over-the-counter antacids containing calcium. Before using other medicines designed to ease stomach symptoms, talk with your health care provider.

Backache

Backache is the most common physical complaint during pregnancy. Not only is the pregnant woman carrying additional weight, that weight is in the front. To compensate for her changing center of gravity, she has to throw her shoulders back, which puts even more strain on the lower back. The following suggestions may help prevent and relieve backache:

- Wear low-heeled, but not flat, shoes.
- Be sure that beds and chairs provide good support for the back.
- When sitting at a desk, rest your feet on a couple of telephone books.
- When standing for long periods, try to prop one foot on a small box and change positions frequently.

wellness
warning

If you vomit repeatedly and cannot keep anything down, call your doctor or midwife. You may need special care in a hospital.

wellness **tip**

During the last trimester, some pregnant women find it more comfortable to sleep on one side with a pillow under the abdomen and another between the knees. Some pillow manufacturers have even created a body-length pillow to facilitate finding a comfortable position in which to rest.

- Most maternity stores sell a supportive belt to be worn under the abdomen. (Unlike buying maternity wear that is larger so you can "grow into it," buy a belt that fits well now—it is elastic and will stretch over time anyway.)
- If you have to lift something, use your leg muscles rather than bending from the waist.
- A massage or warm compresses can relieve aching pain.

Constipation / Hemorrhoids

Constipation and hemorrhoids are common nuisances of pregnancy. Constipation may be caused by pregnancy hormones slowing the passage of food through the stomach and intestines, leaving more time for water to be drawn out of stools and making them hard. Hard stools are more difficult to pass. The growing fetus also makes having bowel movements more difficult.

Hemorrhoids are swollen veins in the rectum. Just like swollen veins in the legs and feet, these veins in the rectum get bigger as the fetus grows. They become symptomatic if you sit for a long time or when you strain a lot to pass hard stool. The most common symptoms are pain and itching. To limit both constipation and hemorrhoids, try the following suggestions:

- Drink plenty of fluids.
- Eat plenty of fiber-rich foods, including fruits and vegetables.
- Consider using a stool softener to decrease the straining and help pass bowel movements.
- Ice packs will help relieve both itching and pain. Hot soaks may also help.
- Consult a health care provider before using any products for relief of hemorrhoids.

Swelling

Some swelling, called edema, occurs in every pregnancy. This swelling affects the legs, ankles, and feet. It is worse at the end of the day and gets better when you prop up your feet or lie down. Some swelling of the hands may occur at night and gets better when you wake up and start moving around again. Sometimes swelling that does not get better with rest may signal the onset of pregnancy-associated complications, so a blood pressure check is appropriate to rule this out—especially if the face is swollen and other symptoms, such as headaches, are present.

Swollen veins are called varicose veins. They are common in pregnancy and can get quite large. They are genetically determined, so some women will not get them at all. Sitting with your feet propped up and wearing support stockings will help prevent and minimize the discomfort from these veins.

Mood Swings

A woman's changing hormone levels during pregnancy, combined with a constantly changing set of feelings—from joy and elation to anxiety and fear—about labor and delivery or the new baby, can cause mood swings throughout pregnancy. It is natural to feel happy and excited about pregnancy and to look forward to the birth of a baby with joy, but it is just as natural to feel miserable, confused, overwhelmed, or unhappy at times. The following suggestions can help a pregnant woman manage mood swings and feel in control of her emotions:

- Be sure to get enough rest, balanced with moderate exercise.
- Avoid too much sugar, chocolate, and caffeine.
- Talk about your feelings with a partner, close friend, or family member. They can provide support if you explain how you are feeling.
- Learn as much as possible about pregnancy, labor and delivery, and life with a new baby. Staying well-informed can help you feel more in control.

Getting Ready

Women who are pregnant for the first time can easily feel overwhelmed by all there is to learn and do as they get ready for a new baby. Friends and family members offer well-meaning advice, but it can sometimes be confusing and contradictory. Health care providers offer new information at every prenatal visit but cannot supply all the information pregnant women need.

Learn What to Expect

Childbirth preparation classes are offered by hospitals and childbirth educators. Varying from one weekend to six weeks in length, they describe all the details of labor and delivery, including how to tell when labor starts, what happens during labor, how contractions feel, what happens during delivery, and how it may feel to hold your infant for the first time. They cover pain relief options, including different types of anesthesia, as well as general instruction in nonmedical means of relieving labor pain, such as breathing exercises, focusing on objects, and massage. They usually talk about cesarean birth and other common complications. Most include information about breastfeeding and newborn infant care, such as bathing and diapering.

Most women who attend these classes also bring their partner or someone who has agreed to be their "labor coach." The classes explain what a coach can do to help the woman during labor, such as applying pressure to her lower back to ease contraction pain or helping her count or focus on her breathing to help her through contractions. A woman should bring her coach with her to all classes. If a woman and her coach plan a "natural" birth, they should take special classes devoted just to labor and delivery techniques.

Classes are also offered in both general baby care and first aid/CPR (cardiopulmonary resuscitation) for infants. Check with local hospitals and chapters of the American Red Cross. Baby care classes help new parents learn what to expect about life with a newborn: from sleeping and feeding, to elimination patterns (such as how many wet diapers a day is normal), strategies for calming a crying baby, and bathing and dressing needs. First-aid classes describe what to do when baby is hurt or injured. Classes in CPR describe what to do with an infant or young child who is choking or who has stopped breathing.

What to Buy—or Borrow—for Baby

One of the exciting parts about pregnancy for many women is setting up the baby's room or an area in her own room for the new baby. It is a good idea to make a list of needed items—clothes, a crib, infant bathtub, and so on—so that nothing will be forgotten. Remember, some items are essential and others only

wellness
warning

Intercourse is absolutely prohibited for women with active vaginal bleeding or leaking amniotic fluid. Women who have premature shortening or dilatation of the cervix may be advised to avoid intercourse. Women who have experienced a previous preterm birth or who are at risk for preterm labor should talk with their doctor about sexual activity during this pregnancy.

wellness **tip**

A popular baby shower idea is to have guests bring a frozen dish or a "promissory note" for a hot meal, in addition to, or instead of, a gift. Mothers-to-be go home with several meals all set to go.

recommended or helpful—or just for fun. With so many products on the market, it is easy to feel overwhelmed, especially for women on a budget.

Baby products are sold in discount stores, baby specialty stores and boutiques, baby "superstores," and general department stores. Comparison shopping is worthwhile, as prices can vary tremendously for the same type of item. With certain items, such as furniture, consider buying a product not especially designed for a baby. Small dressers sold by general furniture stores or discounters may be less expensive than those sold in baby specialty stores. Consider painting or refinishing an old, unused dresser or buying a new shade for an old lamp.

To save money, many new parents buy used baby items, either from consignment stores or at garage and yard sales. Look for items that are clean and in good shape. When purchasing used items, be sure they are safe. For safety reasons, it is recommended that items such as car seats and cribs, which are used constantly, be purchased new. If cribs are too old, they may not meet safety standards. Cribs should have less than 2 3/8 inches of space between slats, no cutouts in the headboard or footboard that could trap the baby's head, no knobs on the corners, and no more than two finger-widths of space between the crib and the mattress.

Some new parents are able to borrow baby clothing and other items, such as baby monitors, receiving blankets, or highchairs, from friends or family members with children. Borrowing can save parents a significant amount of money. Infants grow quickly—so baby items are usually in good condition, as they may only have been worn or used for a short period of time.

Planning Before the Baby Is Born

Preparing for the new baby encompasses many areas in addition to preparing for labor and delivery. The pregnancy months are a good time to accomplish many of these tasks.

Babyproofing. Even though it will be several months before the baby can grasp objects or crawl, a significant amount of babyproofing can take place during the pregnancy months. Store glass and breakable items in boxes or place them on high shelves or the mantelpiece. Purchase outlet plugs and drawer and cabinet latches. Crawl around your home on your hands and knees, looking for any small objects, such as safety pins or buttons, loose wires, protruding nails from furniture or tables, and so on. Set your water heater thermostat to below 120°F to prevent accidental scalding. Store throw pillows away from where the baby will sleep and play—they are a suffocation hazard. If anyone in your home smokes, begin training them to go outside to smoke.

Meals for the First Six Weeks. The first six weeks after the baby comes home are physically draining. Lost sleep, getting used to the baby, and caring for the baby 24 hours a day is exhausting. Many new parents find it practically impossible to eat well. It is a good idea to stock up on easy to fix meals or prepare casseroles, breads, and vegetable dishes that can be stored in the freezer.

Financial Planning. With a new baby come many extra expenses, and household income may be reduced during the mother's maternity leave or if she decides to

Baby's Checklist

When a new baby is on the way, there are many items you will need to buy or borrow. For others, you can put out the word that they would make welcome gifts. Some items will be needed at the onset—others will be needed over time. Here are some items to consider getting:

Nursery Items

- ☐ Crib—be aware that older models may not meet new safety standards
- ☐ Waterproof crib mattress
- ☐ Crib sheets and bumpers
- ☐ Receiving blankets or other small blankets
- ☐ Diaper changing table or changing top to fit on a dresser
- ☐ Bureau or storage unit for baby's clothes
- ☐ Wastebasket with lid or diaper pail for dirty diapers
- ☐ Baby monitor

Baby Clothes

- ☐ Diapers
- ☐ One-piece undershirts that snap between the legs
- ☐ One-piece footed sleepers (blanket sleepers for cold weather) or drawstring gowns (look for those with an elasticized bottom, not an actual drawstring)
- ☐ Hats
- ☐ Booties or socks
- ☐ One-piece or two-piece play outfits
- ☐ Sweaters and coats or snowsuits for fall/winter babies

Mealtime Equipment

- ☐ Nursing pads and bra for breastfeeding (breast pump, if expressing breast milk)
- ☐ Formula, if bottle-feeding
- ☐ Bottles, nipples, and bottle brushes, if bottle-feeding or expressing breast milk
- ☐ Bibs
- ☐ Unbreakable infant spoons and dishes

Bath Equipment

- ☐ Infant tub
- ☐ Soft washcloths and hooded towels
- ☐ Baby cleansing gel or soap
- ☐ Baby shampoo

Toiletries

- ☐ Cream for diaper rash
- ☐ Diaper wipes
- ☐ Baby comb and brush
- ☐ Small scissors with rounded tips or nail clippers
- ☐ Pain relief drops (acetaminophen, not aspirin) and medicine dropper
- ☐ Nasal aspirator (looks like a small rubber bulb) to remove excess mucus

Safety Items

- ☐ Car seat
- ☐ Outlet safety plugs and drawer latches
- ☐ Baby gate(s)
- ☐ Cushioned edge protectors for low tables and hearths (for when baby is older)

stay home permanently. It is recommended that a pregnant woman project new expenses, determine how much money she can save prior to the birth, and then construct a budget for when the baby is born.

Breastfeeding. Breastfeeding is a learned technique—for both mother and baby. If a woman chooses to breastfeed her baby, there is much she can do to prepare. She may take a breastfeeding class given by a lactation consultant (most hospitals today have in-house lactation consultants) or an organization that promotes breastfeeding (like La Leche League). Your doctor, midwife, or local telephone book can tell you where to find help in your area. There are books and videotapes in libraries and bookstores about breastfeeding that can be helpful. Family or friends who have had successful breastfeeding experiences are also very helpful. If the mother-to-be plans

Cloth or Disposable Diapers

Cloth or Disposable Diapers

Some people think cloth diapers are better for the environment and that disposable diapers are filling up the nation's landfills. In fact, the energy expended to heat the water to an appropriate temperature and the chemical detergents used to clean and disinfect cloth diapers effectively are also harmful to the environment.

Contrary to popular belief, disposable diapers are not the number one item clogging landfills—newspapers are. You may wish to read up on the subject of cloth versus disposable diapers in order to make your own well-informed decision.

to express (pump) breast milk so the father or other caregivers can feed the baby, electric breast pumps are widely available for rental or purchase.

Diaper Service. If a woman chooses to use cloth diapers, she can investigate various diaper services. These are usually listed in the Yellow Pages of a local telephone book. There is a wide variation in services and prices, so it is best to interview two or three services before making a decision.

Labor *and* Delivery

More and more women are taking an active role in planning their baby's birth. An important tool is the birth plan, in which a woman summarizes her preferences about what she wants—and does not want—for the birth of her baby. With the knowledge a woman gains from her health care provider and the childbirth education classes she attends, she will know what to expect during the different stages of labor and delivery and how she may be able to manage pain and increase her own comfort.

The Birth Plan

The birth plan is a written document in which a woman lists her wishes for labor and delivery. Many obstetricians and midwives offer a birth plan form that can be tailored by each mother-to-be. In order to develop a birth plan, it is recommended that the woman discuss her thoughts with her partner or labor coach and her doctor or midwife. (See Figure 18.5 for an example of a completed birth plan.)

One copy of the birth plan is kept by the woman, one given to the doctor or midwife, and one taken to the hospital to be entered into the woman's medical record. When you review your birth plan with your doctor and delivery nurse, don't be surprised that many of the personal touches you have included in your plan have become common practice in good birthing centers. Don't hesitate to ask about items that concern you.

A birth plan can be whatever a woman wants it to be. Here are some things a woman may choose to discuss in her birth plan:

- **Her labor partner(s).** Who they will be? What should they do during labor and delivery (help the woman count during breathing, cut the cord, and so on)? Should they be present in the operating room (if the hospital allows) in the event of a cesarean?
- **Pain relief.** What type does she think that she wants, under what circumstances, and when?
- **Labor positions.** Does she want to be free to move around during early labor? What type of position does she want to use for delivery?
- **Medical procedures.** Does her delivery center have policies about intravenous (IV) access being placed on arrival or can she opt to have it only when needed? Does she object to having her pubic area shaved and having an enema? What are her preferences about induction or augmentation of labor (bringing on or speeding up labor with medicine)? Does she want to avoid an episiotomy (cutting of the skin and muscles between the vagina and rectum to ease the baby out)? How does her provider deal with patient preferences with regard to

FIGURE 18.5 Sample Birth Plan

After discussing your preferences with your partner and
doctor, use this sample to develop your own birth plan.

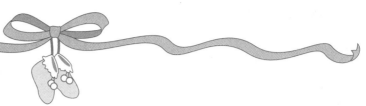

LABOR AND BIRTH PLAN

Name: _Margaret Wright_

Date: _4/28/98_

Support person to be present at birth: _Arthur Wright (husband)_

Additional support person to be present at birth: _Karen Worth (sister)_

My feelings about:

 Fetal monitoring: _Only if medically necessary (if baby is in fetal distress)._

 Activity in labor: _I would like to be able to move around as much as possible—walk, hospital tub, shower, etc._

 Medications: _I would like to try all methods of natural pain relief—massage, water (tub, shower), breathing—_
before drugs. I would prefer something like Demerol before an epidural. While I have never given birth, I consider
myself to have a high pain threshold.

 Episiotomy: _I am interested in trying all methods to prevent the need for an episiotomy, e.g. squatting/using_
gravity during pushing, massage with oil, etc. If medically necessary, I'll have an episiotomy.

 Delivery position: _No particular feelings._

 Initial bonding: _I would like the baby placed on my chest as soon as possible after birth and would like to_
try to breastfeed.

I would like doctor/baby's father/other [name] to cut the umbilical cord (circle one)

I do/do not mind if a student nurse observes the birth (circle one)

Things that help me relax: _classical music, holding hands, deep breathing, imagery (thinking about a calm, quiet place),_
people talking in a calm, focused manner.

Things that make me feel tense: _Being ignored or not taken seriously by medical staff, not having my questions answered,_
being kept in the dark.

My expectations of:

 Support person: _That Arthur and Karen will help me focus and breathe in order to manage pain, that they will_
stay with me the entire time, that they will be my "spokespeople" for getting my needs met and my thoughts
communicated in the hospital if I am having trouble doing so.

 Doctor or midwife: _That she will coach me with suggestions for different positions during contractions, that_
she will explain what's going on at each stage, that she will help me with breathing.

 Labor and birth: _I have some fear of the unknown but I know I am strong and am looking forward to it all being_
over with. I hope I can handle the pain. I am extremely excited about delivery and seeing my baby for the first
time—I know it will be exhilarating. I think about it all the time.

I plan to breastfeed/bottlefeed (circle one)

A male baby will/will not be circumcised (circle one)

 If circumcised: by MD/religious ceremony (circle one)

wellness
warning

Call your health care
provider right away if any
of the following arise:

- **Your water breaks (the
  membrane surrounding
  the fetus ruptures,
  spilling the amniotic
  fluid)**
- **You have bright red
  vaginal bleeding**
- **You have constant severe
  pain with no relief
  between contractions**

forceps delivery or vacuum extraction (using a device like a pair of spoons or a suction cup to ease the baby's head out of the vagina)? What about cesarean delivery?

- **Care of baby after birth.** Does she want the baby to be placed on her chest immediately after delivery? Does she want the baby in her room all the time (called rooming in) or does she want to put the baby in the hospital nursery and have the baby brought to her to nurse?
- **Pictures/videotaping.** Does she want a picture or videotape of the birth? Does her delivery center have policies about photography? If she plans to have the birth videotaped, she needs to test the camera equipment at home ahead of time (including the battery) and find someone other than her partner or labor coach to be the camera person (the partner or labor coach needs to focus on the mother). Remember, the point is to make a baby, not a movie. Also remember that these videos can contain some very private poses, so planning what she does and does not want photographed is important. A safe rule is not to videotape anything you would not show to your father-in-law without blushing.

Preparing for Labor

As the due date draws near, it is important that a pregnant woman be sure all her questions are answered and that she knows how to contact her doctor or midwife at the onset of labor. It is best to keep telephone numbers, instructions, and directions to the hospital or birthing center posted in a handy place. Following are the early signs of labor:

- Contractions at regular intervals that come closer together and increase in strength
- Contractions that continue even with movement, such as walking around
- Contractions in the back, coming around to the front

Contractions known as false labor are common. Such contractions may come and go, cease with movement, or may be felt primarily in the abdomen.

Once in labor, it may be some time before the woman needs to go to the hospital. Women are directed to try to rest and prepare for the big event. It is best to avoid eating anything heavy after the onset of labor because the stomach empties much more slowly and vomiting may make the labor experience unpleasant. It can also be a health risk if something other than regional anesthesia is needed. Many centers allow clear liquids and hard candy, so check with your doctor or midwife about what they feel is best for you.

Pain Relief

Most women experience pain during labor and delivery, but that experience is different for each woman. Every woman also differs in her ability to manage the pain she experiences; and each woman's ability to manage her pain may change in the course of labor and delivery. What is right for one woman may not necessarily be the best choice for another. A woman has many options for pain relief. Childbirth education classes describe medical and nonmedical options. Some women find that they can cope with the pain of labor with just nonmedical methods. For other women, medications are a welcome relief.

Packing Your Labor Bag

What you pack to bring to the hospital or delivery site will depend in part on how long you plan to stay. Stays at birthing centers are brief—rarely overnight—so fewer clothes are needed. You can use this checklist when deciding what to pack:

- ☐ Clothes for your stay (washable nightgowns or big T-shirts if you will not be wearing hospital gowns)
- ☐ Clothes for your trip home (a comfortable maternity outfit)
- ☐ Toiletries (hairbrush or comb, toothpaste and toothbrush, deodorant, shampoo, any contact lens solutions you need, makeup if you choose to wear it)
- ☐ Comfort aids for labor
  - ☐ Focal point item
  - ☐ Socks
  - ☐ Extra pillows (some women feel more comfortable with pillows from home)
  - ☐ Massage tools
  - ☐ Lip balm
  - ☐ Drinks/light snack for partner/coach—and for you if your site and provider allow it
  - ☐ Tapes, tape player, reading material, cards, or games
- ☐ Clothes for the baby to wear home
- ☐ Personal telephone book and change for making telephone calls
- ☐ Separate list of people to call after the baby is born; helpful to record telephone numbers on this list, since others will often make these calls for you.

Nonmedical methods include the following:

- Use of relaxation and breathing exercises
- Concentration on a focal point (a photograph, knickknack, or other small object)
- Massage
- Distractions, such as music, TV, games

A variety of pain relief medications can be used to alter the pain experience. There are analgesics (which lessen the pain) and anesthesia (which blocks all sensations). Analgesic medicines diminish the pain but do not take it away completely, especially at the peak of contractions and near delivery. Those agents can also cause drowsiness and difficulty concentrating. These agents are usually not given near delivery because they can sedate the baby after it is born.

Anesthesia may be local, regional, or general. Local anesthesia numbs just the area where it is injected. It is good for doing an episiotomy or repairing a laceration.

Regional anesthesia numbs a wider area and can be used in several different ways:

- **Pudendal block**—an injection that blocks pain between the vagina and the rectum. It is good for relieving the pain of delivery and is given just before delivery. It is a good choice when obstetrical forceps or a vacuum device is needed. It is also a good choice when an episiotomy is needed, but it does not relieve contractions felt in the uterus. It has limited side effects.

- **Epidural block**—an injection made through a tiny teflon catheter inserted in the small of the back that relieves pain and causes numbness from the waist down. It is a powerful pain relief method used by many women. It can relieve the pain of contractions as well as pain during labor—whether it is a vaginal delivery or cesarean section. A woman who has an epidural has less control of her "voluntary" muscle activity, so she will no longer be able to walk around during labor or may not be able to push as effectively. This may increase the need for use of obstetrical forceps or vacuum extraction, and may lengthen the delivery stage of labor. When it is given before the woman's labor has progressed far enough, it may slow the labor process. A common side effect after epidural placement or re-injection is a temporary drop in the mother's blood pressure. Sometimes oxygen is given to the mother during this time in an effort to prevent slowing of the baby's heart rate. In very few instances, women complain that they are having trouble breathing, and this is because they can no longer feel the abdominal muscles that assist with respiration.
- **Spinal block**—an injection also made in the small of the back, which lasts an hour or two, since a catheter cannot be left in place to inject more medicine. It is used for delivery, especially when forceps are needed. Side effects are like those of the epidural, though spinal block is more likely to cause headaches.

In deciding on pain relief, a woman should consider the following:

- Her pain tolerance and other supports available to her
- Where she plans to deliver (a full range of anesthesia services are more likely to be available in a hospital than a birthing center)
- Side effects of medications
- Personal health and injury history
- Previous labor and delivery experiences

What Happens in Labor

Labor and delivery are divided into three stages: the first, second, and third stage. In each stage, there are things you can do to help labor along and to feel better.

First Stage. The first stage is also divided into three parts: early labor, active labor, and transition. It is the longest stage and lasts from the time contractions begin to the time the cervix is completely open.

Early Labor. Early labor lasts from the time labor begins until the time the cervix is about halfway dilated (five centimeters). During this time contractions start off mild and irregular, then get progressively stronger and more regular. You may pass some bloody or pink mucus, which is the mucus plug that collected in the closed cervix. During early labor, if all is going well, you are likely be more comfortable at home. You can do the following things to keep from going to the hospital or birthing site too early:

- Rest between contractions.
- Take walks with your partner or coach.
- Take a warm bath or shower (do not take a bath if your water has broken and contractions have not yet begun).
- Use breathing and relaxing exercises.
- Keep your mouth moist and drink clear fluids (if permitted).
- Call your health care provider and let her know you have begun labor. Your provider may ask you questions to determine when you should go to the hospital or birthing center.

Active Labor. In active labor, contractions become stronger, more regular, and closer together. Active labor lasts from five to eight centimeters of dilation. You may have a gush or trickle of fluid from your vagina (when your water breaks), or you may pass your mucus plug. During this time, try the following:

- Use breathing and relaxing exercises.
- Walk with your coach if it is safe.
- Have your coach massage your back.
- Urinate often (an empty bladder makes room for the baby's head to move down).
- Lie on your side if you are in bed (this position gives the baby the most oxygen).
- Ask for pain relief if you want it.

Transition. Transition is the hardest part of labor. Contractions are the strongest, and they seem to come on top of each other, giving you no time to rest in between. It lasts from eight centimeters of dilation until ten, when the cervix is completely open. During this time, try the following:

- Take the contractions one at a time.
- Stay focused—do not let the contraction get ahead of you.
- Use breathing exercises.
- Change positions often.
- Work with your coach, letting him or her know what would feel good (ice chips, a cool cloth, a massage).
- Tell your coach, doctor, or nurse if you feel like pushing (you should not push until the cervix is completely open).

Second Stage. In the second stage, a combination of contractions and pushing moves the baby out toward birth. This stage ends when the baby is born. It can last only a few minutes or be an hour or two of hard work. Your contractions will be spaced further apart. If you need an episiotomy, it will be done during this stage. Try the following now:

- Find a comfortable position.
- Push with contractions.
- Ask for a mirror if you want to see the baby's head.
- Rest between contractions.

- Focus your efforts as your care provider(s) instruct.
- Stay calm.

Third Stage. The third stage, when the placenta is pushed out, is the shortest. It usually lasts only 15 minutes or so. Now you can try the following:

- Breastfeed your baby if you wish.
- Push when asked.

Immediately After Birth

Right after she gives birth, a new mother is carefully checked by her health care provider to be sure that everything is OK. Her blood pressure, temperature, and other vital signs are checked from time to time until she is discharged from the hospital or birthing center. If she had an episiotomy or cesarean section, her incision and stitching are also checked.

Rooming In. As indicated in the birth plan section, some new mothers may wish to keep the baby in the room with them. Rooming in provides many benefits. It gives mom and baby extended time to bond, and it makes feeding the baby easier. Mom will be able to feed the baby on demand (whenever the baby wants to feed) rather than on a schedule or when the nurse brings the baby. Rooming in may be the only choice at birthing centers, as many do not have an infant nursery. Even there, though, a new mother can have breaks from the baby when she needs them to rest.

Infant Care Education. Surrounded by health care providers, a new mother has several opportunities to gain valuable advice and information about infant care. Her doctor or midwife can give her advice. The nursing staff at the site where she delivers is trained to teach new mothers about diapering, dressing, feeding, and bathing the baby, as well as offering advice on other topics, such as burping, gas pains, and warning signs of illness. Hospitals may offer classes or videos that teach infant care skills.

Length of Stay. Stays after delivery are far shorter today then they used to be. In the past few years, health insurance plans have attempted to make stays even shorter. Recently, many state legislatures throughout the country have limited the insurance industry's intrusion into medical decision making. In those states, a new mother must be allowed to stay in the hospital for two days after a normal vaginal birth and four days after a cesarean if she needs the services provided there. If she elects early discharge, it is important that the baby be taken to the pediatrician for follow-up sooner than the standard two-week checkup.

Congratulations—
It's a **Baby**

Once a woman has delivered her first baby, her life will never again be the same. Some changes will be wonderful, and others will be more challenging, but life will definitely be different. There will be some sacrifices, such as limited sleep, that need to be made for the baby early on, but usually within a few months, the biggest adjustments ease into a new, more comfortable routine.

Changes are often easier to handle if anticipated. Knowing what to expect—and reading up on as many tips, strategies, and suggestions as possible for dealing with the unexpected—will help a woman not only survive the first several weeks after delivery, but also enjoy getting to know her new baby.

Baby Boot Camp

Caring for a new baby is a lot of work, and it is 'round-the-clock work. The first six weeks after a baby is born can be thought of as "baby boot camp"—with baby as the drill sergeant. The constant feeding, diapering, dressing, undressing, bathing, and trying to calm fits of crying—on top of a lack of sleep—can be physically draining and emotionally overwhelming. A new mother *will* survive, but understanding what to expect will make things a lot easier. Most new moms feel a little overwhelmed by the responsibilities of a new baby. And, there is no way to prepare in advance for the sleep deprivation and endless demands on her energy. Having a supportive partner, extended family member, or other help is especially needed during the first one or two weeks.

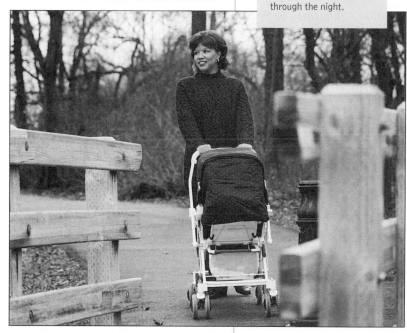

When caring for your newborn, it is important for your physical and emotional wellness to get out of the house with your baby as often as possible. Exposure to daylight will also help your baby learn to sleep through the night.

Feeding. Newborn babies sleep off and on around the clock and wake when they need to be fed. Their stomachs are too small to hold much liquid, so they get hungry and wake up. In the early days, a new mother can expect to feed a baby every two to three hours. Keep in mind that the time between feedings is from the start of one feeding to the start of another. So, if the baby is feeding every two hours and a feeding takes 45 minutes, there is only really only 1 hour and 15 minutes of "rest."

Experts agree that mother's milk is the best food for babies. Breast milk is nutritionally complete, always available, always the right temperature—and free. In addition, it provides the mother's antibodies, which can protect the baby from infection and build up the baby's own immune system.

Some women cannot breastfeed. They may try it, but for a variety of reasons it just does not work. Women with illnesses or who take medication should check with their doctors about whether breastfeeding is safe for them, since some viruses and most drugs will be passed on to the baby in breast milk.

Some women choose not to breastfeed—again for a variety of reasons. Formula will provide the baby with all the needed nutrients, and it can be used by any mother, regardless of her health or medication use. It gives the baby's father, other family members, and caregivers a way to share special closeness with the baby, too (although if a woman expresses breast milk, others can enjoy feeding the baby as

Feeding and Bonding

Because a new mother spends so much time feeding her baby, she may choose to also listen to the radio or watch TV during that time. While these activities are fine, it is important that she also use this time to bond with her baby.

It is unsafe to prop the bottle up while it is in the baby's mouth and leave the baby alone. It is also unhealthy for newly emerging teeth if the baby falls asleep with the nipple in her mouth. Leaving the baby alone with a bottle also means missed opportunities to cuddle and talk or sing to her.

well). Formula frees the mother from having to be baby's sole provider, if this an issue with her. Some mothers may like the fact that because formula is harder to digest than breast milk, babies may go longer between feedings on formula.

Bottle feeding has some disadvantages. In addition to not providing antibodies, it is more expensive (bottles, nipples, formula, cleaning brushes, and so on). It can also be inconvenient. Formula has to be prepared in batches unless a ready-to-serve type is purchased, which increases the cost even more. Formula from liquid concentrate or powder has to be refrigerated and only keeps up to 48 hours. Bottles must be carefully cleaned—and sterilized—for a newborn. There may also be more food allergy and colic in formula-fed infants.

Why Babies Cry. Crying is the only way babies can communicate with the outside world. Crying does not always mean the baby is hungry—she may be tired, wet, lonely, or too hot. New moms often can tell which unmet need is being communicated by each type of "cry." Crying is healthy, normal, and does not hurt the baby. Entire books have been written on the subject of how to calm a crying baby. Following are some of the more common approaches:

- Start with a diaper check and change if wet or soiled.
- Check for loose tags or too-tight clothes that could irritate the baby.
- Try to determine if the baby is too hot (take off some clothes) or too chilly (put on another layer).
- Offer a bottle or the breast if it has been an hour or so since the baby ate.
- Hold the baby in different positions and walk around or provide a change of scenery.
- Try amusements, like a baby swing.

A woman and her baby will both feel frustrated when the cause of crying is hard to determine. It takes time for each to learn to read the other's cues, but this, too, will happen with time. Most experts agree that routinely letting a baby "cry it out" unattended does not help babies and in fact can harm the mother–baby bond. Sometimes, though, babies cry just because it is something they can do. It will not hurt a baby to be left in a safe place, like the crib, on occasion for five or ten minutes while mom goes somewhere quiet and recoups her strength or uses the restroom.

Postpartum Blues

With so many new responsibilities as well as changing hormone levels after birth, it is completely normal for a new mother to feel tired and blue at times. These "baby blues" commonly occur at about the third or fourth day postpartum. They generally last a short time and go away by themselves. While experiencing the blues, a new mother needs to get enough rest and ask her partner, family, and friends for help and extra support.

Sometimes the baby blues do not get better. A condition called postpartum depression (PPD) is the most common emotional disorder that can occur anywhere from two weeks to one year after delivery. PPD is characterized by sadness, tearfulness, marked irritability and mood swings, fatigue, sleeplessness (not related to the baby), and in some cases, confusion and forgetfulness. Its symp-

Helping Baby Sleep Through the Night

The following guidelines can help your baby learn to tell night from day and help her sleep through the night. Remember, it is easier to prevent sleep problems before six months of age than it is to treat them later.

Newborns

- Place your baby in the crib when she is drowsy but awake. This is the most important step of all. Your baby's last waking memory should be of the crib, not of you or of being fed. She must learn to put herself to sleep without you. The baby may not go to sleep right away—it may take up to 20 minutes or so. If she is crying, rock her and cuddle her. But when she settles down, try to place her in the crib before she falls asleep.
- Hold your baby for all crying during the first three months. Always respond to a crying baby. Babies cannot be spoiled during the first three or four months of life.
- Carry your baby for at least three hours a day when she is not crying. This will reduce fussy crying.
- Do not let your baby sleep for more than three consecutive hours during the day. In this way, the time when your infant sleeps the longest will occur during the night.
- Keep daytime feeding intervals to at least two hours for newborns. Do not let her get into the bad habit of eating every time you hold her. That is called grazing.
- Make middle-of-the-night feedings brief and boring. Do not turn on the lights, talk to her, or rock her. Feed her quickly and quietly. This approach will lead to longer periods of sleep at night.
- Do not awaken your infant to change diapers during the night. The exceptions to this rule are soiled diapers or times when you are treating a bad diaper rash.
- Do not let your baby sleep in your bed. Once your baby is used to sleeping with you, a move to her own crib will be extremely difficult.
- Give the last feeding at your bedtime (10 or 11 PM).

Two-Month-Old Babies

- Move your baby's crib to a separate room from yours. If this is not possible, at least put up a screen or cover the crib railing with a blanket so that your baby cannot see your bed.
- Try to delay middle-of-the-night feedings. By now, your baby should be down to one feeding during the night.

- Never awaken your baby at night for a feeding except at your bedtime.

Four-Month-Old Babies

- Try to discontinue the 2 AM feeding before it becomes a habit. If you do not eliminate the night feeding at this time, it will become more difficult to stop as your child gets older. If your child cries during the night, comfort her with a back rub and some soothing words instead of with a feeding.
- Do not allow your baby to hold her bottle when not feeding or take it to bed with her. Babies should think that the bottle belongs to the parents.
- Make any middle-of-the-night contacts brief and boring. All children have four or five partial awakenings each night. They need to learn how to go back to sleep on their own. If your baby cries for more than five minutes, visit her but do not turn on the light, play with her, or take her out of her crib. Stay for less than one minute. If the crying continues, you can check your baby every 15 to 20 minutes, but do not take her out of the crib or stay in the room until she goes to sleep. (Exceptions: You feel your baby is sick or afraid.)

Six-Month-Old Babies

- Provide a stuffed animal, doll, or blanket for your child to hold in her crib. At this age, children start to become anxious about separation from their parents. A soft, friendly toy can comfort your child when she wakes during the night.
- Leave the door to your child's room open. Children often become frightened when they are in a closed space and are not sure that their parents are nearby.
- During the day, respond to separation fears by holding and reassuring your child. This will lessen nighttime fears.
- Make visits for middle-of-the-night fears prompt and reassuring. For mild nighttime fears, check on your child promptly, but keep the interaction as brief as possible. If your child panics when you leave, stay in her room until she is calm. Do not hold her. Provide whatever she needs for comfort without turning on the lights or talking too much. At most, sit next to the crib with your hand on her. This will calm even a severely upset infant.

Source: Adapted from *Your Child's Health*, B.D. Schmitt, MD, Bantam Books, 1991.

toms are similar to those of other depressions (see Chapter 12 for more information on depression). In addition to the mother's own psychological and physical discomfort, these symptoms can also cause marital difficulty and interrupt the baby's emotional development. Having postpartum depression is not a reflection of your parenting skills. Moms with PPD are not "bad" mothers. Postpartum depression is a serious medical condition, but it is treatable. Symptoms should not be ignored.

Women who are depressed for more than two weeks, cannot perform their usual activities, no longer take pleasure in the activities and interests they previously enjoyed, have trouble eating or sleeping, or worry that they might hurt themselves or their baby should call their doctor or midwife right away for help. Treatment for PPD includes a thorough assessment of the individual's situation and needs, education, therapy, and medications, as indicated. Support groups, such as the national DAD groups (Depression after Delivery) also exist for women with PPD. The recovery rate is excellent once the disorder is properly diagnosed.

Postpartum psychosis (PPP), which only occurs in one or two out of every 1,000 postpartum women, is the most serious postpartum disorder. It is caused by biological, hormonal, and genetic factors. Women with PPP may lose touch with reality, become paranoid, hear or see things that are not really there and experience irrational fears or beliefs. Short-term hospitalization and carefully-monitored medication are usually necessary.

Childcare

Another important decision for a woman to consider is who will care for her baby. Many women today work, either because they enjoy their career or because they need the money or both. While some women decide to stay at home after the birth of their child, others go back to work within weeks or months after birth. Options for childcare include you, your partner, a nanny, family day care, or a day care center.

There are many ways to find a good day care provider. Providers can be found through the following:

- Word of mouth
- Employer-sponsored day care
- Church, temple, YWCA, or other local groups
- Nonprofit referral services
- Advertisements on a bulletin board or in the newspaper
- Government clearinghouses

Look at these qualifications in a day care provider:
- Licensing
- Number of children cared for
- Special training (in childcare, CPR/first aid)
- Views similar to your own on issues, such as discipline, TV, and toilet training
- Clean and nonsmoking environment

Take a site visit to help make your decision. Make sure that safety precautions are taken, see how the children spend their time, and check the overall appearance of the site and whether the children appear happy.

Women also need to consider financial factors when choosing day care. Nannies and day care centers are generally the most expensive, while care by family, friends, or family day care providers is less costly. It is also important to consider tax issues. Women who use a day care center or a family day care provider who declares the income to the Internal Revenue Service (IRS) can obtain a tax break on federal income taxes. Women who pay for in-home care, however, will likely have to pay taxes on their employees' earnings.

Some women decide not to return to work. For them, the rewards of raising their child outweigh any financial sacrifices they may have to make. However, even women who stay at home may need childcare, for example, in order to run errands or take care of other interests and commitments. It is becoming increasingly common for fathers to be the ones who stay at home with the children. In fact, there are approximately 2 million stay-at-home dads in the United States.

Another Baby?

Unless a woman's health care provider has given her special reason to postpone resuming sex, she can resume sexual activity approximately six weeks after delivery. If she is

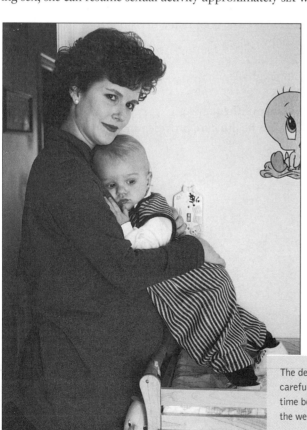

The decision to have another baby should be made carefully. A mother needs to take adequate recovery time between pregnancies, both for her own health and the well-being of the children.

breastfeeding, it may be a while before a woman's period returns, which has led to the myth that it is impossible to become pregnant during this time. Breastfeeding does limit the potential for pregnancy because it is common for a woman not to ovulate during the first six months after delivery if she is offering the baby no other kind of nourishment besides breast milk. However, it would be unwise to depend on breastfeeding as a form of birth control, since ovulation occurs before the onset of the period, and there is no reliable way to know when ovulation will resume.

If a woman wishes to avoid pregnancy, she needs to explore a reliable method of birth control. If she used a diaphragm before deciding to become pregnant and wants to do so again, she will need to be refitted. When making a decision about the best method of birth control for her, a woman can discuss the options with her doctor or midwife.

When a woman does decide to try to get pregnant again, adequate spacing between children is recommended for both her benefit and her children's. Having children places extreme demands on a woman's body, and it takes a while for her body to replenish its store of nutrients and physically heal from the birth. How far apart a couple chooses to space their children is a personal decision, but it is important to consider such factors as the health and well-being of the mother, how well-adjusted the couple is to their firstborn, finances, whether the couple had difficulty getting pregnant the first time around, and many other factors.

What *You* Can Do

Women who are pregnant or thinking about starting a family can educate themselves and their partners about what to expect. The better informed a woman is about her pregnancy, the better able she is to make decisions in the best interest of her health and that of her baby:

- Begin prenatal care early in pregnancy.
- Lead a healthy lifestyle.
- Plan ahead for the new member of the family.
- Plan your care and include your health care provider and partner in decision making.

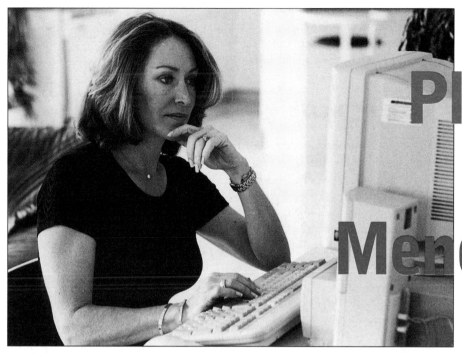

Chapter 19

Planning *for* Menopause

A mong women's issues, menopause is the health issue that is most charged with myths and misperceptions. If menopause represents a transition from one life stage to another, is it a natural state or a medical condition?

Studies show that while women consider menopause to be a biological event, like pregnancy, most do not anticipate negative effects on their physical or mental health. In fact, most women have either positive or neutral feelings about menopause. The negative feelings surrounding menopause are probably reflective of our youth-oriented culture in which anything connected with aging usually has negative associations. It is interesting to note that in cultures where women gain respect and authority as they transition out of the childbearing years, this time is happily anticipated, and women experience fewer negative menopausal symptoms.

Developing your own positive attitude about this transitional time requires some basic understanding of the biological events that are taking place. What are hormones? What role do they play in menopause? What are the typical symptoms of menopause? Why are postmenopausal women at increased risks for developing certain diseases? How could a healthy lifestyle have a positive impact on the menopausal experience itself and on the years that follow?

Hormones: *The* Body's Messengers

Hormones are chemical substances that are released into the blood stream to deliver "messages" to other organs. These messages are instructions, which tell the "target" cells to take certain actions.

wellness **tip**

If you have abnormal bleeding, talk with your doctor about performing an endometrial biopsy. This simple office test can often determine if you have endometrial hyperplasia—an excessive growth of cells in the lining of the uterus (endometrium). Left untreated, this condition can lead to endometrial cancer.

From the onset of puberty through menopause a woman's reproductive hormone levels rise and fall monthly as they orchestrate the complex chain of events that allow her to bear children. As a woman approaches menopause this careful orchestration begins to falter and there is a gradual reduction in her hormone levels. This period is known as perimenopause.

Perimenopause

Declining hormone levels account for the physical symptoms associated with the perimenopausal time. In fact, most events usually attributed to menopause are really the events of the perimenopausal period. For most women this transition lasts approximately four years and occurs between the ages of 45 and 55. In other countries this time is called the "climacteric," which translates to "rungs of a ladder." (Menopause itself is actually a medical term that means it has been at least a year since a woman's last menstrual period.)

What Happens During Perimenopause?

As women age, their ovaries become less able to produce the hormones estrogen and progesterone, altering the menstrual cycle. This process occurs slowly, so many women are not aware of it until their menstrual cycle begins to change. Their menstrual cycle may become longer or shorter. Their menstrual flow may become heavier or lighter. Some women may not ovulate with each cycle and their fertility is markedly reduced. Your doctor will want to know if you have any of the following symptoms:

- Change in your monthly cycle
- Heavy bleeding
- Longer period of bleeding
- Bleeding more frequently than every three weeks
- Bleeding during intercourse

During this time, some women begin to experience the classic physical symptoms associated with menopause, like hot flashes, weight gain, sleep problems, vaginal dryness, and lack of lubrication during intercourse. Some experience occasional emotional symptoms, like mood swings, irritability, memory lapses, or depressed mood. All of these symptoms may be related to fluctuating or declining estrogen levels. Just knowing that these symptoms have a physical cause can help some women cope more easily.

There are other changes taking place during perimenopause that do not cause any symptoms but which may significantly affect the quality of a woman's life. Even though estrogen's primary role is related to reproduction, it also protects bones and lowers the cholesterol that forms fatty deposits that cause hardening of the arteries. When estrogen levels drop, bones lose this protection and can become less dense, leading to a condition called osteoporosis, or "brittle bone disease." This process is a natural part of aging, but it speeds up as estrogen levels fall. Likewise, the risk of cardiovascular disease increases as estrogen levels drop. (Heart disease and osteoporosis are discussed in more detail later in this chapter, and in Chapters 20 and 25.)

Preparing for Perimenopause

There are several steps, such as focusing on and maintaining a healthy lifestyle, that you can take to prepare your body and mind for perimenopause. These include making changes in your diet, choosing and sticking to a regular exercise program, avoiding harmful substances, and getting routine health care.

Diet. A well-balanced diet is essential for good health during every stage of your life, including your adult years. Making the right food choices prior to and during perimenopause can help keep you at a healthy weight and reduce your risk of developing osteoporosis, heart disease, and diabetes. Consult the Food Guide Pyramid (see Chapter 8) to determine how many servings of each food group you need to get the nutrients your body requires.

Adult women, however, may not receive all the nutrients they need for good health simply by eating the quantities of food specified by the Food Guide Pyramid. Following are some of the more common nutrients that women must be certain to take as they near midlife:

- **Calcium.** You can reduce your risk of developing osteoporosis by taking at least 1,000 milligrams of calcium each day. If you do not get enough calcium from foods, or if you are lactose intolerant, you can take supplements that contain calcium.
- **Vitamin D.** This vitamin is important for menopausal and perimenopausal women because it helps the body absorb calcium. You can get adequate amounts of vitamin D from multivitamins (which usually contain a full daily dose of vitamin D), vitamin-D fortified milk, and spending a portion of each day outdoors (when exposed to sunlight the body manufactures vitamin D).
- **Iron.** During the perimenopausal years, women can lose up to 20 milligrams of iron each month (while they are still menstruating). You should have 15 milligrams of iron a day before menopause and 10 milligrams a day after. See your doctor about supplements if you are not getting enough iron from food.

See Chapter 8 for an in-depth discussion of nutrition.

Exercise. Moderate exercise will help you maintain a healthy heart, strong bones, and an ideal weight. It will also help you gain strength and energy, reduce stress, and even decrease some of the symptoms of menopause, such as hot flashes and sleep deprivation.

Thirty minutes of moderate exercise a day is generally recommended in order to stay healthy. Although many women complain about not having enough time to exercise, you do not have to go to the gym in order to get a good workout. Everyday activities, such as walking, gardening, and playing with your children, constitute moderate exercise, and they are an excellent alternative if time or expense prevents you from exercising in a health club or gym. (See Chapter 9 for more information on exercise.)

wellness **tip**

Try to get the majority of your calcium from food sources. Take a tip from Finnish women, who consume large amounts of dietary calcium—their fracture rates are among the lowest in the world. If you need to use calcium supplements, make sure to take them with food. If you are lactose intolerant, try calcium-enriched orange juice, which provides as much calcium per glass as milk.

wellness **tip**

The average woman enters menopause close to the age at which her mother did. If your mother had an early or late menopause, you may follow a similar pattern.

Avoiding Harmful Substances. Certain substances, such as alcohol and tobacco, are harmful to women throughout the life cycle. Alcohol use can interfere with a woman's bone growth and calcium absorption, increasing her risk of osteoporosis. Women who drink heavily are more likely to have high blood pressure, develop cirrhosis of the liver, and reach menopause earlier. Smoking cigarettes promotes bone loss, along with its many other negative effects on health. (See Chapter 13 for a discussion of the many health risks associated with smoking.) Sensible drinking (one to two drinks per day) and not smoking are healthy habits anytime, but gain importance as you approach menopause.

Routine Health Care. As women age they are more prone to illnesses that would benefit from early detection and treatment. Routine checkups can help detect these conditions. (See Chapter 6 for more information about routine checkups during your forties and fifties.)

Menopause

The average age of menopause in the United States is 51 years. Since the average life expectancy of women is approximately 85 years, the average woman will spend nearly 40 percent of her life in the postmenopausal period. By the year 2000 over 50 million American women, more than one-third of the entire United States population of women, will be at or beyond the age of menopause.

The term menopause, as stated earlier, literally means the last menstrual period. The diagnosis for menopause is made in hindsight, since most women do not realize at the time that they are having their last episode of menstrual bleeding and that no further menstrual periods will follow. Over time, the ovaries produce lower amounts of hormones, most specifically estrogen but also progesterone and testosterone. This decrease in hormone levels brings a predictable set of changes associated with menopause.

When menopause occurs naturally in a woman around age 50, the changes are gradual. Menopause can also occur suddenly, however, after any type of surgery that results in removal of the ovaries. If a woman has just one ovary removed she will continue to produce adequate amounts of hormones and should experience menopause at the usual time. If both ovaries are removed before natural menopause, however, her hormone levels drop suddenly and she will experience a dramatic onset of menopausal symptoms unless replacement hormones are provided.

Body Changes During Menopause

Symptoms vary tremendously from one woman to another. Some women have difficulties coping with menopause—and this is completely normal—whereas others barely notice the changes taking place.

As hormone levels drop the first thing most women notice is a change in menstrual cycles. The body stops producing enough estrogen to thicken the lining of the endometrium, and periods stop. The reduced estrogen results in many of the physical and mental symptoms of menopause, although it may be difficult to distinguish some of these changes from what we consider "normal aging."

Hot Flashes. Most women experience hot flashes (sometimes called "hot flushes" or "night sweats") during menopause. The most common symptom of hot flashes is a sudden wave of heat—often focused in the face, neck, and chest—rushing through the body. The affected areas usually redden during the feeling of heat, but the flush fades as the body restores itself to normal temperature. Sweating sometimes occurs during the drop in body temperature and may be followed by chills.

While the exact cause of hot flashes is unknown, experts believe that decreasing estrogen levels cause the hypothalamus, the gland that controls body temperature, to malfunction in a minor way. This "malfunction" causes the hypothalamus to act as though your body is too warm and it attempts to cool you off. It sends a message to the blood vessels to dilate, allowing heat to escape from the body. These dilated blood vessels account for the reddening of the face, neck, and other areas. Some women sweat during a hot flash, since sweating is the primary means by which the body cools itself.

Hot flashes may come on suddenly at any time of the day or night. Some women may become anxious during hot flashes because of the increase in heart rate. This should not be a cause for concern, however, since hot flashes are not harmful to women's health. They are more of a nuisance, sometimes interfering with concentration and with sleep.

wellness **tip**

Be alert to what can trigger hot flashes. Here are just a few: spicy foods, alcohol, hot drinks, caffeine, hot weather, overly heated rooms, eating too quickly, and stress. Make any necessary adjustments, such as turning down the thermostat and dressing in layers (so you can easily take off layers if you have a hot flash). Keep your bedroom as cool as possible.

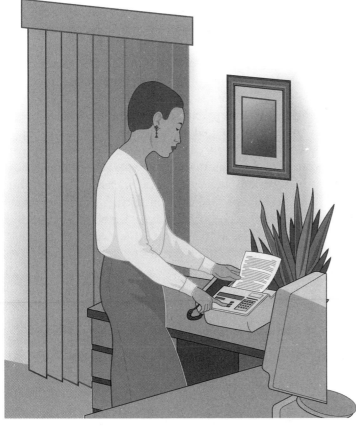

FIGURE 19.1 **The Effects of Menopause**
Each woman has different physical and psychological symptoms during menopause, and some experience none at all. Here are some of the more common symptoms that women experience during menopause.

- Hot flashes and sweating

- Fatigue

- Insomnia

- Vaginal dryness

- Increased risk of having urinary tract infections and developing incontinence

- Sleep disturbances, which can cause mood changes, irritability, or poor concentration

- Increased risk of osteoporosis

- Increased risk of heart disease

wellness **tip**

If you are having trouble sleeping, avoid drinking alcoholic beverages for several hours before bedtime. Alcohol can affect your pattern of sleep and, as its effects wear off, it may actually cause you to wake up during the night. (See Chapter 10 for more helpful hints on sleeping well.)

To help ease or reduce the incidence of hot flashes, consider the following:

- **Exercise.** Studies show that moderate exercise (a total of three to four hours a week) reduces the severity and frequency of hot flashes.
- **Relaxation.** If you find that stress is a trigger for hot flashes, deep breathing and other relaxation techniques may help.
- **Food choices.** Avoid sweets and eat every four to five hours to keep your blood sugar level more even. Increase your intake of foods containing vitamin E (sunflower seeds, almonds, crab, sweet potatoes, fish, wheat germ, and whole wheat bread). Watch your intake of hot foods, spicy foods, alcohol and caffeine, which can trigger hot flashes.
- **Clothing and sheets.** Wear clothing and purchase sheets made of breathable fabrics, such as 100% cotton.

Fatigue and Insomnia. Fatigue and sleep disturbances are a common part of the perimenopausal period. Perimenopausal and postmenopausal women may be chronically deprived of REM sleep (the most restful phase of the sleep cycle) due to conditions, such as night sweats (hot flashes that occur during sleep). This lack of sleep can begin to affect memory and concentration, and sometimes can result in irritability. In fact, many of the mood changes associated with menopause are only indirectly related to falling estrogen levels. Sleep deprivation and fatigue are the primary reason for mood changes during menopause.

Vaginal Dryness. The vaginal lining is very estrogen dependent, so as estrogen levels begin to decrease, the vagina begins to change. The vaginal tissues become thinner, lose their elasticity (their ability to stretch), and may feel dry. Vaginal tissues are also less supple, and they are unable to support the bladder and urethra as well as they did when estrogen levels were higher. In addition, the vaginal tissues are more prone to injury from trauma or infection. They also provide less lubrication, sometimes making it difficult to have intercourse. A water-based lubricant can be helpful in supplementing natural lubrication for intercourse. Petroleum-based products should not be used in the vagina, because they cause irritation. Petroleum-based products can also damage latex condoms.

Vaginal changes are often the first sign that the body has begun the gradual changes of the perimenopausal period. Women often experience decreased lubrication for intercourse long before hot flashes or menstrual changes become noticeable. As the vaginal aging process continues some women feel a sense of "discomfort" that is related to dryness in the vagina. A new class of "bioadhesive" lubricants has been developed to help relieve this uncomfortable dry feeling. It is also helpful to avoid alcohol, caffeine, diuretics, and antihistamines, all of which have drying effects on the mucus membranes throughout the body.

Sexuality. Nowhere does the combination of menopause and natural aging cause more difficulty than in the area of sexuality. During this time, both women and men may experience changes in their level of sexual desire, changes in arousal, and difficulty with orgasm. Premenopausal sexual activity and enjoyment are the primary factors in determining sexual function in the postmenopausal period. But there are also hormone-related physical changes and changes in reproductive anatomy that can affect a woman's sexuality during this time. Other factors, such as sexual or health problems (either the woman's or her partner's), medications, and the availability of a partner may also affect the sexual expression of perimenopausal and menopausal women.

Disorders of desire are often related to psychological factors. Menopause is a time when some women feel that they are less attractive because of their age. There may also be difficult life situations—such as loss of a parent, loss of a partner, or serious illness of a loved one—that can have a profound impact on sexual desire. The chronic fatigue often associated with the perimenopausal period may also decrease a woman's interest in sex.

Arousal disorders are more likely to be caused by physical factors. As estrogen levels fall, the vagina produces less lubrication during intercourse. This lack of lubrication can affect a woman's sense of arousal, and it may cause enough pain to inhibit sexual desire and orgasm.

Other women actually experience increased levels of desire and orgasm during this time. On a psychological level, some women say that their sexual desire increased because the possibility of unplanned pregnancy is no longer an issue. Others note that their careers are stable and their children are grown, so they have more time and energy to devote to their partner and their sexuality. On a physical level, the ovaries continue to produce a small amount of testosterone, even after they have lost the ability to produce estrogen and progesterone. Since testosterone is the hormone that provides one's sex drive, some women report increased sexual desire during this time. This phenomenon is not seen in women who have surgical menopause, and have had their ovaries removed.

Urinary Tract. Approximately one in six women over the age of 45 develop urinary tract problems. Perhaps the most common urinary tract problems during peri- and postmenopause are urinary tract infections and urinary incontinence.

Urinary Tract Infections. Symptoms of urinary tract infections may include burning or pain during urination, urine leakage, feeling like you need to go to the bathroom very often (even when your bladder is empty), and blood in the urine. It is very important to see a doctor if you have any of the above symptoms, since an untreated urinary tract infection can spread to the kidneys, causing permanent damage. The following tips can help reduce incidence of these infections:

- Urinate as soon as you feel the urge and after sex.
- After urinating, stand for ten seconds, then sit and empty your bladder again.
- Wear cotton underwear or underwear with a cotton crotch panel.
- Drink plenty of water every day.
- Drink cranberry juice often.

Incontinence. While it is commonly diagnosed in women of all ages, incontinence, leaking urine when you cough or sneeze or loss of bladder control, is also seen in menopausal women to varying degrees. New onset or worsened incontinence in menopausal women is usually caused by weight gain and the progressive weakening of the muscles that control urination. Pelvic muscle exercises, known as Kegels, performed daily can strengthen these muscles, thus improving

wellness **tip**

Women who do not smoke can sometimes use oral contraceptives into their forties and fifties. This can lower their risk of ovarian cancer and endometrial cancer. The protection lasts even after you stop taking the pill.

Kegel Exercises

Exercises used to strengthen the muscles that surround the openings of the urethra, vagina, and rectum are called Kegel exercises. It is important to use the right muscles and to learn how to do the exercises properly. At first, a doctor or nurse will show you how to do Kegel exercises. You will be asked to squeeze your vaginal muscles around her finger during a pelvic examination to check whether you are using the proper muscles. When you begin the exercise program at home, place a hand on your abdomen to make sure you don't squeeze the muscles of your abdominal wall. Do not squeeze your thighs or buttocks. Squeeze your pelvic muscles for 10 seconds, 10 to 20 times in a row, 2 to 3 times a day. After performing Kegel exercises regularly for at least six weeks, your ability to hold urine should improve.

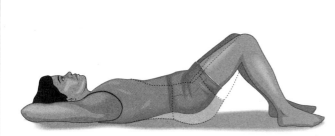

STEP 1 Lie on the floor with your knees bent. By tightening your pelvic muscles, raise your pelvis slightly off the floor. (The muscular contraction should feel the same as when you try to start and stop the flow of urine.) Do not contract your abdominal, thigh, or buttocks muscles. Hold for a count of ten.

STEP 2 Relax the muscle completely for a count of ten. Do ten repetitions of the exercise. Try to perform the exercise three times each day.

FIGURE 19.2

Kegel Exercise

The Kegel exercise strengthens the pelvic muscles and can help improve bladder control. Once you have learned the Kegel technique, you can do this exercise virtually anywhere, while sitting or standing, even on the telephone or in the car.

bladder control (see Figure 19.2). Also, hormone replacement therapy may help some women overcome this condition. Incontinence is a medical condition that can be treated and should be discussed with your doctor.

Mental Outlook. While depression, irritability, and lack of confidence are still considered "symptoms" of menopause, doctors remain uncertain as to whether these "symptoms" that accompany menopause are caused by physical and hormonal changes or are simply coincidental. In fact, studies show that prior depression is the most common attribute among women who experience depression around the time of menopause. In other words, most women who experience depression during menopause have also experienced depression at earlier points in their lives. On the other hand, it has been shown that women who have a long perimenopausal stage (more than 27 months) are more likely to have depressive symptoms than those who do not. So are changes in mood a result of hormones or circumstance?

While there is no definitive answer to the question, theories abound. Following are four theories that attempt to explain the association between depression and menopause:

- **Biochemical theory.** This theory states that the decreasing levels of estrogen during perimenopause cause biochemical changes in the brain, resulting in depression.
- **Symptom theory.** This theory states that the physical changes caused by decreasing estrogen levels lead to depression. For example, women often experience depression due to menstrual problems during menopause.
- **Psychoanalytic theory.** This theory views menopause as an important event in a middle-aged woman's life that threatens her self-concept. Feelings of anxiety

result in lack of confidence and depression. The social expectations surrounding aging can increase the anxiety.

- **Social circumstances theory.** This theory states that menopause does not necessarily *cause* depression but just happens to coincide with circumstances and life events that cause depression.

Osteoporosis. A woman may not be aware of changes taking place in her bones, but as she ages, more bone is broken down than is replaced by new bone. As estrogen levels drop, the process accelerates. Bones lose their density and become weak and brittle. Weakening vertebrae, in the backbone, are usually the first to fracture and can cause what is known as "dowager's hump." Women are also at risk of hip fractures, with markedly increased rates after age 75. Osteoporosis can have a serious impact on a woman's mobility, independence, and health. (A detailed discussion of osteoporosis and recommendations for reducing the risk of this condition appear in Chapter 25.)

Heart Disease. Menopause affects the heart in at least two major ways. Until the onset of menopause, estrogen naturally protects the heart and blood vessels. It has a positive effect on a woman's total cholesterol, lowering LDL (low-density lipoprotein, the "bad" form of cholesterol) and increasing HDL (high-density lipoprotein, the "good" form of cholesterol). A woman's risk of heart attack increases as estrogen levels drop as she approaches and goes beyond menopause. By age 65 a woman's risk approaches that of a man's, unless she uses estrogen therapy. One of the authors of the Nurses Health Study, a long-term study of 122,000 nurses, estimates that 90 percent of heart disease cases could be eliminated if people changed their lifestyle. (See Chapter 20 for a full discussion of heart disease and suggestions for lifestyle adjustments that can lower your risk.)

Estrogen's other major effect is to keep blood vessels more supple. Estrogen maintains a blood vessel's ability to dilate in response to stress, rather than go into spasm. This is crucial to reduce angina, heart attacks, and blood clots within the arteries of the heart. Thus, as a woman reaches menopause, her risk of these conditions increases.

Hormone Therapy

A woman can take hormones to help ease the symptoms of menopause as well as prevent other health problems down the road. Hormone therapy presents both benefits and risks, and the topic is continually being studied. Hormone therapy has traditionally been prescribed for about three to five years to offset the symptoms of hot flashes and insomnia. What is at the heart of the controversy is the issue of long-term hormone therapy, and which hormones to use.

Those health professionals who espouse the benefits of long-term hormone therapy (even starting therapy prior to menopause) claim that it lowers the risk of osteoporosis, heart disease, and Alzheimer's disease, and helps women maintain their health longer. Those who object cite studies that show that long-term therapy increases a woman's risk of breast cancer, blood clots, gallbladder disease, and uterine cancer. They maintain that women have long lived well into old age, despite the reduced levels of estrogen that occur after menopause. The Nurses Health Study found that women between the ages of 60 and 64 who took hor-

The French Connection

Can Americans learn something about lowering their risk of heart disease from the French? While the French diet is full of fat and most French smoke, they suffer 40 percent fewer heart attacks than Americans.

Researchers believe a moderate intake of alcoholic beverages (one to two per day), especially red wine, which contains phenolic compounds that limit the oxidation of low-density lipoprotein (LDL), may play a role. (Recent studies suggest that grape juice also has this benefit.) Others say the French also eat more fresh fruits and vegetables, eat (and live) at a more relaxed pace, and use more olive oil than Americans.

mones for at least five years increased their risk of getting breast cancer by 71 percent and increased their risk of dying of breast cancer by 45 percent. However, more recent studies show a 16 percent lower risk of dying of breast cancer in women who have postmenopausal hormone replacement. Some researchers feel, however, that short-term studies do not adequately demonstrate the risks of breast cancer, because breast cancer may grow in the body for 16 to 20 years before it is detected. Short-term studies cannot differentiate between breast cancer occurring earlier with hormone therapy from breast cancer occurring when it would not have otherwise occurred.

The risks and benefits of hormone therapy are subject to ongoing scientific evaluation through two major research initiatives. One is the Postmenopausal Estrogen/Progestin Interventions (PEPI) Trial launched in 1991 by the National Institutes of Health (NIH). This three-year study supported results of numerous other medical trials that concluded that hormone therapy produces significant changes in cholesterol, thus reducing a woman's risk for cardiovascular disease. The PEPI Trial included nearly 900 women who were followed to evaluate the impact of therapy on the risk of heart disease. The results of this study indicated that all of the regimens followed produced higher HDL levels and decreases in LDL and fibrinogen (a substance in the blood that promotes blood clotting), further protecting against heart disease. None of the hormone regimens studied had a negative impact on blood pressure.

Despite the findings of the PEPI Trial, the three-year period was not considered adequate to draw a conclusion that hormone therapy actually reduces the incidence of heart disease. This question may be answered by another study that is currently under way. The Women's Health Initiative is a large clinical trial, orchestrated by the NIH, following postmenopausal women for nine years to measure the effects of hormones on the rate of heart attack and other medical conditions, such as breast cancer.

In order to make your own informed choices about long-term hormone therapy, familiarize yourself with the risks and benefits and the various types of regimens available. Read articles on short- and long-term therapy from a variety of professional and lay sources, in order to get a balanced view. Discuss your concerns and questions with your doctor, in the context of your own health needs, so you can make the decision that is right for you.

Regimens for Hormone Therapy. In the 1960s women in the United States were encouraged to take estrogen replacement therapy to combat heart disease, fractures, and vaginal dryness, as well as other symptoms of menopause. Although the beneficial effects of estrogen were confirmed, it soon become apparent that postmenopausal women who used estrogen had an increased risk for cancer of the endometrium, especially in the high doses taken then. In response, progestin, a synthetic form of the hormone progesterone, was added to the estrogen regimen in women who had not had hysterectomies (removal of the uterus), allowing the uterus to shed the endometrial buildup, protecting them from the development of endometrial cancer. This estrogen-plus-progesterone combination is the form of hormone replacement therapy (HRT) typically prescribed today. The doses of estrogen are much lower and can be combined with either synthetic or natural forms of progesterone. Estrogen and progesterone can be given sequentially or in combination. Each woman's tolerance is different, and the dosages and method of administration need to be adjusted to find the right combination. (In some cases, testosterone is given to women with a significantly lowered sex drive.)

Estrogen. There are both synthetic (chemically manufactured) and natural forms of estrogen. Natural forms and synthetic forms are used for hormone therapy, whereas only synthetic estrogens are used for oral contraceptives. Estrogen can be given in the form of a pill, skin patch, or vaginal cream. It is recommended that women who use estrogen vaginal creams also take progestin to reduce their risk of endometrial cancer. The vaginal creams relieve vaginal dryness but may not protect against heart disease or osteoporosis at the same rate that other forms of estrogen therapy do. Most women take estrogen therapy in pill form.

Estrogen is produced naturally by the body in three forms:

1. **Estradiol**—a potent hormone produced by the ovaries.
2. **Estrone**—a hormone converted from estradiol and also found in body fat.
3. **Estriol**—a hormone converted from estrone and produced by the placenta during pregnancy.

After menopause, the production of estradiol by the ovaries decreases, and estrone becomes the main form of estrogen. Both estradiol and estrone are potent forms of estrogen, and their reduced levels during and after menopause can be supplemented by either synthetic or natural sources of estrogen.

The most commonly prescribed oral estrogen for postmenopausal women is Premarin, derived from a natural source. The estrogen and other hormone substances in Premarin are obtained from the urine of pregnant mares. This form is called conjugated equine (meaning from a horse) estrogen. It is taken in pill form, and as it goes through the digestive system, it is converted by the liver into estrone and estradiol. This process also helps lower LDL cholesterol and raise HDL cholesterol levels (helping to protect against heart disease). Other natural sources of estrogen include phytoestrogens, which are found in plant products, such as legumes and soy bean curd. Phytoestrogens contain high levels of estrogen.

Skin estrogens are made in laboratories and can contain any combination of estrogen and other hormone substances. The skin patch form of therapy uses a patch that adheres to the skin and releases a steady flow of estradiol. A new patch is applied once or twice a week, usually to the woman's abdomen. Estrogen administered in this manner goes directly into the bloodstream. Because it does not go through the digestive system like pills do, the patch is a good choice for postmenopausal women with liver or gallbladder disease. The patch does not improve HDL levels but does reduce LDL levels as much as the pill form, and improves blood vessel tone to protect against heart disease. It also protects against bone disease and some of the physical symptoms of menopause.

Progesterone. Progesterone is the hormone produced by the ovaries during the second half of the menstrual cycle. Progesterone controls the buildup of the endometrium that can occur when estrogen is taken alone. Progesterone, like estrogen, comes in synthetic and natural forms. The synthetic form of progesterone is called progestin. Progestins are given as pills. They act similarly to

wellness
warning

About one-third of women over 50 who are prescribed hormone therapy never fill their prescriptions, and it is estimated that up to half of those who start therapy stop by the end of one year. The reasons are fear of cancer and uncomfortable side effects, both of which can be discussed and controlled.

progesterone, which causes the lining of the endometrium to shed during the menstrual period.

Natural progesterone, also known as micronized progesterone, may be a good alternative for those who have side effects from synthetic progestins. Natural progesterone has been shown in the PEPI Trial to be as effective as synthetic versions in protecting women from endometrial cancer and more effective than progestins in elevating HDL levels, and thus protecting against heart disease. Researchers have found that natural progesterone more closely matches the molecular structure of the progesterone found in females than synthetic versions. Natural progesterone can be obtained from soy products, such as tofu, soybeans, soy milk, soy flour, soy cheese, and yams. It can be supplied as oil-based capsules, tablets, suppositories, or cream. Proponents of natural progesterone also claim that its use is not associated with common side effects linked to progestins, such as mood swings, fluid retention, and headaches.

Preliminary findings regarding postmenopausal use of natural progesterone are promising; however, the drug is relatively new to the scientific community and there is a lack of good data to support its use. Further supporting information is unlikely to be forthcoming because, as a natural substance, natural progesterone cannot be patented, nor does it require approval of the Food and Drug Administration. As a result, pharmaceutical companies have no incentive to study and market the drug. Without scientific backing, physicians are hesitant to prescribe the drug. It can be obtained in some health food stores and through mail order pharmacies that prepare the product, such as the Women's International Pharmacy (800-279-5708). Cream-form brands include Pro-Gest, Progenol, Ostaderm, and Progesterone.

Testosterone. The ovaries also produce testosterone, a hormone that occurs in much higher levels in men. After menopause, testosterone production decreases, although the ovaries continue to produce small amounts. Its role is not well understood, but it is thought that testosterone is responsible for a woman's libido or sex drive. Postmenopausal women who experience a significantly lowered sex drive may consider testosterone therapy, which can enhance the libido and improve a woman's sense of well-being. Testosterone therapy can be administered by injection or orally, in combination with estrogen. Long-term effects are not known. There are concerns that giving testosterone counteracts some of the benefits of estrogen in preventing heart disease, although this effect has not been proved.

Administration of Hormone Therapy. Although some doctors initiate low-dose HRT during perimenopause to reduce symptoms and smooth the transition to full HRT, traditionally doctors do not initiate hormone therapy until they are sure a woman has had her last menstrual period. They usually wait until a woman has not had a menstrual period for a year or they test the levels of follicle-stimulating hormone. Follicle-stimulating hormone is produced by the pituitary gland to stimulate an egg to mature and be released at ovulation. After menopause, there are no more eggs to release. Follicle-stimulating hormone levels increase sharply as a way of signaling the ovaries to respond. An elevated follicle-stimulating hormone level, measured in a blood test, confirms menopause.

Hormone therapy can be given continuously, on a daily basis, in cycles, or in a combination. Some of the commonly used hormone replacement therapies are described below:

- **Cyclic or cycled therapy.** Estrogen is given daily during 25-day cycles and progestin is given for the last 10 to 15 days of that cycle (days 10 or 15 to day 25, depending on the doctor's directions). Both hormones are stopped after 25 days and are not taken for three to six days. With cyclic therapy, some bleeding occurs after the hormones are stopped. Cyclic therapy may be adjusted to use progestins every two or three months rather than monthly if a woman is closely monitored for endometrium buildup.
- **Continuous-combined therapy.** Estrogen and progestin are taken daily. Bleeding may occur irregularly for the first few months but eventually will stop. Most women do not have any bleeding after one year.
- **Transdermal patch.** Estrogen can be delivered in a time-released fashion through a patch on the skin. If a woman still has her uterus, she will need to use progestins in a cyclic or continuous therapy.

Estrogen may be given by itself to some women, such as those who have had their uterus removed and thus are not at risk of endometrial cancer. Most women who have a uterus take a combination of estrogen and progestin. Women who experience side effects from progestin may opt for natural progesterone or elect estrogen-only therapy with regular endometrial sampling to rule out endometrial hyperplasia. Dosages and routes of administration can be adjusted to reduce side effects.

Benefits. Hormone therapy can relieve the symptoms of menopause as well as lower some long-term risks. The effects are still being studied, but there is evidence to support certain benefits:

- **Alleviates menopausal symptoms.** Hormone therapy controls hot flashes and relieves insomnia. It can also relieve irritability, memory loss, and anxiety.
- **Aids sexual function.** Estrogen helps lubricate the vagina, keeping it moist and easing intercourse. The addition of testosterone can improve a woman's sex drive as well as have a positive effect on her mood and overall sense of well-being.
- **Improves urinary function.** By softening the tissues around the urethra and keeping the pelvic muscles firm, estrogen reduces urinary incontinence and bladder infections.
- **Reduces risk for cardiovascular disease.** Estrogen elevates HDL levels, lowers LDL levels, and decreases levels of fibrinogen. Estrogen reduces the development of plaque, normalizes blood vessel function, and helps prevent angina (chest pain) and heart attacks from blocked arteries.
- **Prevents osteoporosis.** Estrogen slows the process of bone loss and increases bone formation, thus helping prevent osteoporosis. It reduces the loss of calcium from the body and helps bones absorb calcium, which improves strength.
- **Additional benefits.** Estrogen can have a positive effect on mood and can prevent short-term memory loss. It can also help protect against Alzheimer's

wellness **tip**

It is recommended that women who choose hormone therapy have annual breast and pelvic examinations, as well as screening mammograms at regularly scheduled intervals.

Contraindications for Hormone Therapy

Following are absolute and relative contraindications for hormone therapy.

Absolute Contraindications. Women with the following conditions should not take hormone therapy:

- Unexplained vaginal bleeding
- Acute liver disease
- Breast cancer
- Active thrombophlebitis or thromboembolic disorders
- Endometrial cancer

Relative Contraindications. Women with the following conditions may have a slightly increased risk of problems with hormone therapy and should consider the risk in light of the benefits:

- Chronic liver dysfunction
- Seizure disorders
- Uncontrolled hypertension
- Elevated triglycerides
- Migraine headaches
- Thrombophlebitis
- Endometriosis
- Gallbladder disease

disease. This disease, which causes early senility, is more common among women than men. There is also some evidence that estrogen protects against cancer of the colon.

Risks. Hormone therapy is not for everyone. It can be especially risky for women who have had certain types of cancer that are aggravated by estrogen, such as cancer of the breast or endometrium. In some cases, however, the benefits outweigh the risks. A woman should be absolutely sure she understands the risks of hormone therapy and should consider them in relation to the benefits. For instance, a woman who has a history of breast cancer in her family may also have factors in her history that increase her risk of heart disease. Your doctor can help you work through these issues and make informed choices.

Endometrial Cancer. The use of estrogen alone increases the risk of cancer of the endometrium. Adding progesterone counteracts this risk.

Breast Cancer. Some studies have shown that the risk of breast cancer increases in women who take estrogen. Other studies have not supported these findings, however. If there is an increased risk, it seems to be very small. It is not clear whether the breast cancer occurs in women earlier on HRT or in women who would not ever have developed breast cancer.

Thromboembolism. A blood clot can form in one part of the body and move through the blood vessels to lodge elsewhere and block the blood supply. Estrogen increases production of substances that promote blood clotting. Although this characteristic may increase the risk of thromboembolism in women using oral contraceptives, the lower doses of estrogen used in hormone therapy have not been linked with an increased risk of thromboembolism. The risk could be higher in women who smoke, however, or during the first month of hormone use if the woman has been postmenopausal for some time.

Weight Gain. Some women are concerned that hormone therapy causes weight gain. There is no evidence this is true. Menopause in general is associated with a slight weight gain. In one study, women treated with estrogen had a lower weight gain than untreated women.

Side Effects. Side effects of hormone therapy include bleeding caused by progestins. Just as progesterone triggers bleeding in the second half of the menstrual cycle before menopause, it can cause bleeding after menopause. In some cases this side effect does not continue for an extended time. Other side effects include fluid retention and breast soreness and symptoms similar to premenstral syndrome (PMS).

Natural Alternatives to Hormone Therapy

For women who are unable to tolerate hormone therapy, natural alternatives are available:

- **Preventing bone loss.** Therapies that are effective in preventing bone loss include sodium fluoride, calcium carbonate, alendronate, and intranasal salmon calcitonin.
- **Controlling hot flashes.** Alternatives to control hot flashes include clonidine (a blood pressure medication), which can be given in a patch, and natural progesterone cream.

When Extra Pounds Creep Up

Women tend to gain weight as they age, placing them at increased risk for heart disease. Extra weight poses health problems, such as joint or back pain or shortness of breath, and also keeps women from looking and feeling their best. To curb weight gain that occurs with age, it is recommended that women limit high-fat and calorie-rich foods, eat a variety of low-fat, high-fiber, and nutrient-dense foods, and balance calorie intake with physical activity. Regular exercise also builds muscle mass and raises your metabolic rate; in turn, these two benefits raise the number of calories burned during everyday activities.

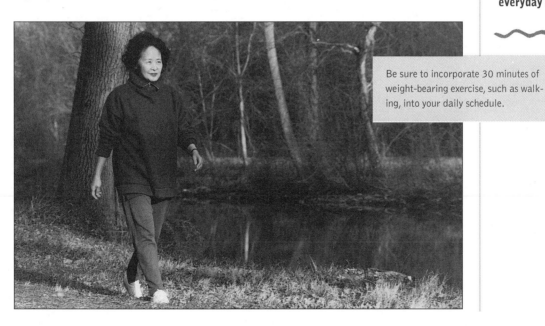

Be sure to incorporate 30 minutes of weight-bearing exercise, such as walking, into your daily schedule.

wellness **tip**

Contact the Social Security Administration to find out when you will become eligible for social security benefits and how much you and, if applicable, your spouse will receive.

- **Vaginal dryness.** For women who cannot take estrogen, vaginal dryness may be relieved with the use of a water-based lubricant gel or vitamin E oil.

A **Healthy Lifestyle** *to* **Manage** Menopause

As with all of a woman's life stages, a healthy lifestyle plays a significant role in helping a woman positively handle the myriad changes that menopause brings. Following are some suggestions to promote your health, whether or not you take hormone therapy:

- **Diet.** Eat a balanced diet low in fat, especially saturated fat (such as animal fats, which harden at room temperature). Make sure you get adequate amounts of calcium from calcium-rich foods, not just supplements.
- **Exercise.** Weight-bearing and impact exercises can build strong bones. Try to do some form of weight-bearing exercise, such as jogging or walking with weights, for 30 minutes daily.
- **Alcohol.** Drinking moderate amounts of alcohol can increase estrogen levels and has been linked to an increased risk of breast cancer. If you drink, moderation is advised.

Daily Calcium Requirements and Calcium-Rich Foods

The 1994 National Institutes of Health Consensus Development Conference on Optimal Calcium Intake recommends more calcium for women than the original Recommended Dietary Allowance (RDA) requirements:

- 1,000 mg/day for premenopausal women aged 25 to 49
- 1,000 mg/day for postmenopausal women aged 50 to 64 who are taking estrogen
- 1,500 mg/day for postmenopausal women aged 50 to 64 who are not taking estrogen
- 1,500 mg/day for all women aged 65 and over

The average American women only gets half this much from her diet, with or without supplements. For best absorption and safety, calcium should be from calcium-rich food. However, if supplements are used, take them with food.

Calcium-rich foods :

- Milk (skim or 1% low-fat)
- Calcium-enriched orange juice
- Nonfat plain yogurt
- Low-fat cottage cheese
- Cheddar cheese
- Grated Parmesan cheese
- Gruyere cheese
- Canned pink salmon with bones
- Canned sardines with bones
- Mackerel
- Dried figs
- Cooked rhubarb with sugar added
- Blackstrap molasses
- Broccoli
- Collard greens
- Kale
- Bok choy
- Mustard greens
- Turnip greens
- Soybeans
- Baked beans
- Tofu
- Cheese pizza

Remember, consuming vitamin D with your calcium helps your body absorb calcium.

- **Routine health care.** Have an annual physical examination, including breast and pelvic examinations, a Pap test, mammogram, complete cholesterol analysis, and measurement of blood pressure. Make sure you ask your doctor to explain the results, in language you can understand. It is also recommended that you perform a monthly breast self-examination and seek medical evaluation if you notice any changes.

The Postmenopausal *Years*

Given current life expectancy rates, over a third of a woman's life is spent in the postreproductive years. It is estimated that 50 percent of women who reach age 50 will live to age 90. Many women see the postreproductive years as a time of liberation, when they are free to focus on their careers, relationships, and interests. Although there are demands at this stage of life, just as there are at other stages, there also are opportunities. Many women are able to retire from their full-time job, whether it be a career or that of a homemaker, and branch off into new areas, such as pursuing personal interests or volunteer work. Women also may find new ways of relating to their partners or expanding their circle of friends. Regardless of individual circumstances, menopause can be considered the beginning of a new and rewarding life cycle.

Retirement. A key element of the American dream is to retire to a life of leisure, comfort, and financial security. Unfortunately, reality paints a darker picture. Around the middle of the twentieth century, when age 65 was a typical retirement age, most people lived only 10 or 12 years after they stopped working. Today, with longer life expectancy and earlier retirement ages, many people now may live the last quarter of their lives after they leave their jobs. Many retire early to embark on new careers or part-time work.

The Health and Retirement Survey is a long-term study underway at the University of Michigan to provide insight into work, retirement, and midlife family roles in the 1990s for individuals between the ages of 51 and 61. Initial findings show that people in this age group not only want to continue working but also are actively engaged in family roles and responsibilities. About 70 percent of married couples in midlife are part of four-generation families, and they provide substantial assistance, personal and financial, to both their adult children and their parents. About two-thirds of respondents have living parents or parents-in-law. About one-third of older parents are frail, need personal care, or require supervision. In response to these trends, new patterns of living and caregiving are emerging, and health care costs and quality of life are becoming ever more critical issues.

Although many older women are able to retire with enough money to meet their basic needs and enjoy some leisure activities, some face poverty for the first time in old age. Retirement savings often must be used for expensive medical treatment or to supplement fixed incomes, and many older women outlive their assets. It is never too early to plan for retirement.

Women on average earn lower salaries than men, which limits retirement benefits. Benefits, including pensions and Social Security payments, are calculated

---

Financial Planning

Keep a record of the following information, and note the location of papers and property, to aid in financial planning:

- **Sources of income**
- **Assets and deeds**
- **Will**
- **Social Security information**
- **Investments**
- **Insurance policies**
- **Bank accounts**
- **Income tax returns**
- **Liabilities (debts)**

on average lifetime earnings, so time spent at home rearing children reduces both pensions and Social Security income in later life. Women are also more likely to work part-time and to work for employers who do not offer pension benefits. Although Social Security is intended to supplement other forms of retirement income, for the majority of women over age 65 it is their only source of support.

Many older women do not receive the benefits they are eligible for, either because they do not know about them or because they do not know how to get them or because they do not want to seek assistance. Those for whom English is a second language may not understand how to get payment. Only half of older persons who are eligible for Social Security income actually receive benefits.

Retirement, just like other aspects of a person's life, is best when it is planned for. The ability of government programs to support the increasing number of individuals approaching retirement is questionable. It is a good idea to consult a financial adviser well before retirement and to develop a long-term plan that will cover all contingencies. It may be worthwhile to consider additional insurance coverage to protect against long-term disability.

Caregiving. It is not unusual for a woman in her sixties to be the primary caregiver for a parent, an aging spouse, a friend, or even grandchildren. About 2.2 million people in the United States have daily personal care responsibilities for an older person, and the majority of these caregivers—72 percent—are women. When the person being cared for has a disability, the emotional and physical burdens on the caregiver can be overwhelming. Caregivers often suffer mental or stress disorders, family strains, career disruption, and financial hardships. One of the key factors in dealing with these problems is support from relatives and friends. People who have a strong personal support network are better able to cope with the stress of caring for an elderly parent or a family member with a disability, such as Alzheimer's disease.

Caregiving responsibilities usually include helping with meals, shopping, and other daily activities. Caregivers of older persons who are still living in their own homes usually help them with daily functions, such as eating, bathing, dressing, and using the bathroom.

Caregiving Resources. Although being a caregiver can be stressful, it is not always a burden. If you are a caregiver of an elderly parent, there are many resources available to you:

- **Workshops and seminars** on caring for elderly parents (check with your local community or adult education center, YWCA, or community college)
- **Eldercare consultants,** who will help you develop specific strategies for your particular situation
- **Community-based programs,** such as Meals on Wheels, which delivers hot meals to people who are homebound
- **Home health aides,** who provide care for a portion of each day in an elderly person's home

Caring for an elderly parent is demanding. It is vital that you also take time to take care of yourself. If you are not in good mental and physical health, care-

Caregivers' Checklist

People providing care to another may find the following points helpful:

- Reassure the person being cared for by expressing support and showing that you can be depended upon to help solve problems.
- Become informed about areas relating to the person's situation. This may include familiarity with legal matters (will and property ownership), financial arrangements, health care resources, support services, housing and recreation resources, and knowledge about aging processes.
- Obtain a professional assessment of the older person's problems. Seek out health professionals trained in caring for older persons by calling your local medical society, hospital, or medical school. A lawyer or a financial adviser may also be of assistance.
- Help the person retain control of her affairs as much as possible. Limits often have to be placed on autonomy due to illness, finances, or for other reasons, but the older person's participation in making decisions is still almost always possible.
- Share caregiving responsibilities with family, friends, professionals, and paid helpers. Do not try to do everything alone.
- Brainstorm with family and friends about ways to help an older family member remain active.
- When making a change, start with the smallest step possible. This will help you avoid becoming overwhelmed if many difficult decisions have to be made; they may not all have to be made at one time.
- Seek professional counseling if a situation or relationship with an older person becomes too demanding.
- Take time off for yourself. You also need recreation and time to pursue personal interests. Be honest with the older person about the limitations on your time and energy.

Source: Adapted from *Who? What? Where? Resources for Women's Health and Aging.* National Institute on Aging, 1992.

giving will be more stressful. Eat right. Exercise. Get plenty of rest. And most importantly, set limits. You will never be able to do as much for your parents as they did for you. Adjust your expectations accordingly. Do your best, but do not try to be superwoman.

Caring for the "Oldest Old." One aspect of elderly care involves what is called the "oldest old," those who are 85 and older. As the oldest old grow in numbers, more and more people of retirement age will find themselves caring for older relatives. Between 1960 and 1990, this group grew at the amazing rate of 232 percent. As the numbers continue to increase, the 85 and over age group could make up almost a fourth of the older population. According to the U.S. Bureau of the Census, women in this age group, most of them widows, outnumber men by two to one. Women are more likely to be poor and more likely to be institutionalized than are men. The rapid increase in this age group can have a major economic and social impact. Many will need nursing homes and other forms of long-term

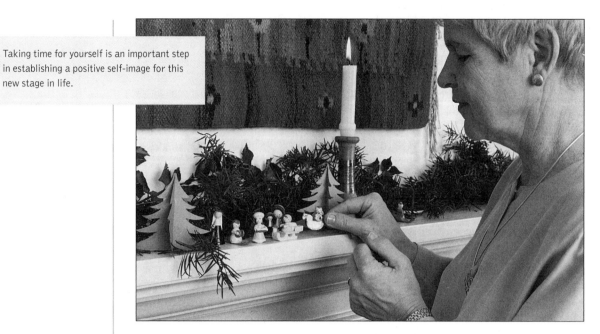

Taking time for yourself is an important step in establishing a positive self-image for this new stage in life.

care, and most will need some form of help in activities of daily living. Many of these services are not covered by Medicare. (For further information on health coverage, see Chapter 3.)

Cultural Differences in Caregiving. There are cultural differences among ethnic groups in their approach to caregiving. In one study, African American women were more likely to rely on family members and friends for help with housekeeping tasks after leaving the hospital, while white women were more likely to do the housekeeping themselves. Certain minority groups tend to have and rely on social networks for support. These groups may perceive caretaking to be less of a burden. Social networks and caregiving approaches will assume greater importance as the need for such services increases in the next century.

Changing Self-Image. Many women go through a change in their appearance after menopause. There is a tendency to gain weight, and the weight accumulates around the waist. Hair and skin also become drier. Breasts lose their fatty tissue and may thin out or sag. These changes can negatively effect a woman's self-esteem, especially in today's youth-conscious society. Women in other cultures have fewer problems with menopause than those in the United States. It has been theorized that this ability to handle the changes of menopause so well is related both to diet and a more accepting attitude toward aging itself.

The thin, youth-oriented ideal with which women are faced is unrealistic and even unhealthy for most women, particularly if they are menopausal. It is far preferable to maintain a healthy weight and to gain reassurance from a healthy lifestyle than to strive for an unrealistic body image and suffer the physical consequences. Good health fosters self-esteem and independence.

Health professionals today generally agree that the mind and body are integrally linked. A healthy body is the first step toward a healthy mind, and vice versa. Being aware of stressors, and taking steps to alleviate them, can help promote a healthy mind-body connection. This positive outlook is especially helpful for postmenopausal women who may be "putting themselves first" for the first time in many years, after raising a family. Taking personal time for themselves may be an important step in establishing a positive self-image for this new stage.

Relationships. Many postmenopausal women struggle with new facets of their relationship with their partners. There may be changes in their sexuality based on changing levels of sexual drive as well as other conditions that may exist. Overall, women are less affected than men by changes in their sexuality. As they age, men are more prone to impotence, the inability to get or keep an erection. It may take longer to get an erection, and the erection may not be as firm or last as long as in earlier years. Impotence may be further worsened by health problems, such as heart disease, hypertension, and diabetes. Although illness or disability can affect sexuality, even the most serious conditions should not prevent a satisfying sex life. (For further information on sexual function, see Chapter 16.)

Sexuality is only one aspect of a relationship, however. Older couples may have the added concerns of aging, retirement and other lifestyle changes, and illness. For retired couples who have been accustomed to both or one partner's going to work every day for many years, being constantly in each other's company may be a source of stress. These problems, as well as illness—such as cancer, stroke, or senility—can cause psychological difficulties. It may be helpful to talk to a counselor to sort through these feelings.

Many postmenopausal women are widows. Half of all women over age 65 live as widows. Becoming a widow, and facing the end of a relationship that often has lasted most of a lifetime, can cause profound grief. The period of most intense grief can last from a few months to a year or more. It is normal for women to feel despair or depression, irritability, or even anger. Loneliness is also common. Women may need help with social and psychological problems and with finding social activities and friends.

What *You* Can Do

As women approach menopause, they confront choices that will affect a major portion of their lives still before them. Self-education and increased awareness can equip women to handle challenges, make informed decisions, and take an active role in ensuring a smooth transition from one life cycle to the next:

- Follow a healthy lifestyle tailored to your particular needs.
- Maintain a healthy diet, making sure to include adequate amounts of vitamin D, vitamin E, calcium, and iron.
- Learn about the powerful effects of hormones and their role in normal physiological function.
- Follow your menstrual cycle and be alert to symptoms and changes.
- Monitor signs of impending menopause and talk with your doctor about approaches to menopause so you feel comfortable and in control.

Maintaining the Balance of Wellness:
Systems and Diseases

The intricate systems in the human body that keep us alive and thriving operate in a balance that needs lifelong care. A normal, healthy body is naturally designed to maintain its own balance, but external influences, such as lifestyle choices and environmental factors, as well as genetic risk factors, can threaten that balance.

Part IV of this book will help you learn important facts about what makes the major body systems vulnerable to disease and what preventive steps you can take to improve your chances for enjoying good overall health and a high quality of life. You will learn about lowering your risk of cardiovascular disease and can-

cer, preventing and fighting infections, keeping your metabolic system healthy, keeping your senses sharp, and maintaining a strong musculoskeletal system.

Sometimes focusing on the causes of disease can lead to anxiety and fear. The discussions in Part IV are designed to reassure you that disease can often be prevented and risk can very often be lowered. These chapters encourage you to learn as much as you can about the body systems or diseases that you are particularly concerned about and to make any necessary changes to help prevent serious illness.

Chapter 20

Lowering *Your* Risk for Cardiovascular Disease

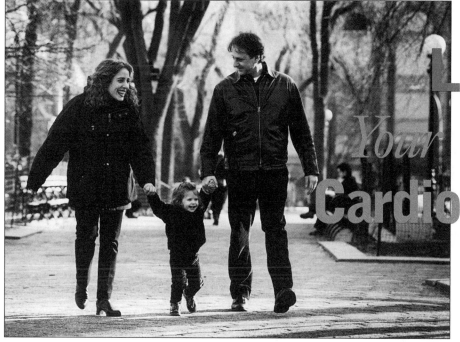

A major focus of a wellness program is improving the health of your heart. This vital organ, literally the life center of the body, must be exercised and cared for with the same attention as your muscles, skin, and bones. It is important to familiarize yourself with the early warning signs of heart disease, methods of early detection, and ways to lead a healthy lifestyle in order to minimize your risk of heart disease, especially if it runs in your family. Consider these sobering statistics about heart disease and women:

- Cardiovascular disease, affecting the heart and circulatory system, is the leading cause of death in women.
- One out of every ten women aged 45 to 65 and one out of every three women over age 65 has some form of major heart or blood vessel disease.
- Over one-half million U. S. women die of cardiovascular disease each year. That's more than twice the number of women who die from all types of cancer combined each year.
- Coronary artery disease is the leading killer in the United States, accounting for approximately 480,000 deaths in women each year.
- In women aged 35 to 74, the death rate from heart disease for African American women is about 1.5 times that of white women and two times that of women of other races. Heart disease is the number one cause of death in African American women over 35 years of age.
- Women are more likely than men to die of their first heart attack and to have a subsequent heart attack.
- Heart attacks are unrecognized more often in women than in men, and treatment is often delayed.

Despite these facts, many women fear cancer and wrongly think of heart disease as affecting mostly men. Nothing could be further from the truth. Whether you are 15 or 65, there are measures you can take right now to improve the health of your heart.

Women usually develop heart disease about 10 to 20 years later than men. A woman's risk of heart disease increases dramatically after menopause, when the heart-protecting properties of estrogen are gone. By age 65, a woman's risk is virtually the same as that of a man's.

Until recently, little research has been done on heart disease in women. Most of the information has come from studies done on men. Reasons cited for why women are not studied include the possibility of pregnancy and risk to the fetus, the influence of changing hormone levels, the absence of heart disease in young women, and the confusion caused by the existence of other illnesses in older women, who are more likely to have heart disease. However, new research projects currently under way are designed to turn those tables. The Nurses Health Study, begun at Harvard University in 1976, is an ongoing study that has revealed much new information about heart disease in women. Another major study, the Women's Health Initiative, is being conducted by the National Institutes of Health to evaluate health problems of older women, including heart disease.

As new information emerges, it becomes clear that women need to be aware of their risks and what they can do to lower them. The key to a healthy heart is preventing or delaying the onset of disease. Fortunately, many of the factors that pose a risk of heart disease can be modified by changes in lifestyle. A lifestyle that contributes to a healthy heart also is good for general health and well being.

The **Cardiovascular** System: **A Primer**

In simplest terms, the cardiovascular system is the network that circulates blood through the body, delivering oxygen to organs and tissues and removing waste products. The main player is the heart, which serves as the central pumping station. It is supported by a system of blood vessels—arteries and veins, connected to smaller arterioles and venules, and finally to tiny capillaries.

The heart is a muscle made up of four chambers: The right and left atria and the right and left ventricles. The heart contracts and expands to move blood through the chambers and to the rest of your body. A system of valves, which open and close, regulates the flow and ensures

FIGURE 20.1

The Heart

The heart is the central pumping station of the body. It pumps oxygen-rich blood from the lungs through the body and forces waste-laden blood back from the body to the lungs, where waste is removed and the blood is renewed with oxygen.

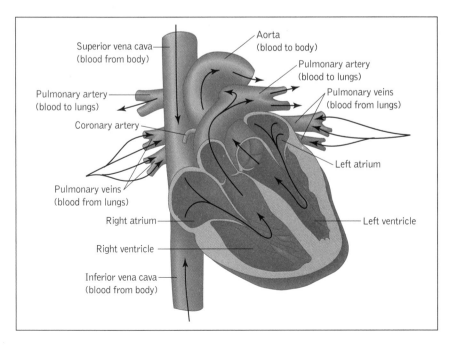

- Superior vena cava (blood from body)
- Aorta (blood to body)
- Pulmonary artery (blood to lungs)
- Pulmonary veins (blood from lungs)
- Pulmonary artery (blood to lungs)
- Coronary artery
- Left atrium
- Pulmonary veins (blood from lungs)
- Right atrium
- Left ventricle
- Right ventricle
- Inferior vena cava (blood from body)

that the blood moves in only one direction. A series of electrical impulses causes the chambers of the heart to contract and move blood. These impulses signal the heart to beat in the sequence required for proper function.

A complex sequence of events continuously renews and enriches the blood, enabling it to provide the body with life-giving oxygen and nutrients and remove the by-products of expending energy. Arteries carry oxygen-rich blood to all parts of the body, including the heart, which is supplied by the coronary arteries. As blood circulates, oxygen fuels the body's functions, and carbon dioxide, a waste product, enters the bloodstream. The oxygen-depleted blood is returned to the heart via the veins.

Blood enters the heart through the right atrium. The heart relaxes, allowing the blood to flow into the right ventricle. Once filled, the right ventricle contracts, sending the blood to the lungs through the pulmonary artery. In the lungs, the blood receives a fresh supply of oxygen, and carbon dioxide is expelled. The oxygen-rich blood is returned to the heart and enters the left atrium. From there it flows into the left ventricle, where it is pumped to the rest of the body.

Each heartbeat pumps blood through the system. By expanding and contracting, the heart exerts a powerful force. Blood pressure is the force created by the heart as it pushes blood into the arteries and through the circulatory system. Blood flows through the arteries into smaller branches, the arterioles. The walls of the arterioles can expand or contract. When they expand, blood flow increases and resistance to blood flow is reduced. Likewise, when they contract, blood flow decreases and resistance increases.

The beat of the heart follows a specific pattern or rhythm, but the rate can be influenced by a number of factors—including emotional reactions, chemicals, and hormones—that allow the heart to respond to new demands. Other factors that can affect the heart include a problem with its structure or function, such as a defect in a valve or an irregularity in the heartbeat, or a disease process taking place, often silently, over time.

Types of
Cardiovascular *Disease*

Some forms of cardiovascular disease are congenital—that is, they appear at birth—whereas others are acquired. Often heart disease may be building for a long time without any warnings. Some forms of heart disease have related causes and stem from a process called atherosclerosis.

Atherosclerosis

With age, the walls of arteries thicken and harden. A form of this thickening is atherosclerosis. In the lining of the arteries, deposits of fatty substances build up to form what is called plaque. As the openings of the arteries narrow, the heart needs to work harder to push blood through them. Plaque or blood clots where plaque occurs can block the flow of blood to the organs served by the blood vessels, such as the heart and brain, resulting in a heart attack or stroke.

Atherosclerosis is a slow, progressive condition that may begin as early as childhood. It is thought to occur as a result of damage to the wall of the artery. Damage

---

The Components of Blood

Each person has about ten pints of blood that are recirculated once every minute at rest and even more often with exercise. About half of your blood is made up of blood cells, while the rest is a fluid called plasma. There are three types of blood cells:

- **Red cells carry and promote the exchange of oxygen and carbon dioxide.**
- **White cells fight disease.**
- **Platelets, or thrombocytes, are responsible for blood clotting.**

can come from high blood pressure, high levels of cholesterol and fats, smoking, infection, or other forms of irritation—all of which worsen the condition.

Coronary Heart Disease

Also called coronary artery disease, coronary heart disease is one of the most common forms of cardiovascular disease. It occurs when one of the arteries supplying blood to the heart is blocked. Narrowing of the arteries by atherosclerosis or a blood clot blocking a key artery can lead to symptoms of coronary artery disease. Sometimes symptoms occur when the coronary artery goes into spasm, temporarily cutting off the blood supply. If the blood supply remains totally blocked, a heart attack will occur. Lack of oxygen causes injury to the part of the heart muscle being served by the artery, and the heart can be damaged permanently.

If the blood supply is temporarily reduced, angina (chest pain) can occur. Angina is a symptom that the heart is not getting enough blood or oxygen to support the demands being placed on it. Although the blood supply may be sufficient for normal activities, it cannot support additional demands, such as from exercise or emotional excitement. Angina is often a warning sign of a more serious heart condition that could lead to a heart attack.

Stroke

Just as a blockage of an artery leading to the heart can cause a heart attack, blockage of an artery leading to the brain can cause a stroke. A stroke can occur as a result of atherosclerosis narrowing the arteries or a blood clot lodged in an artery. It can also result from bleeding when a blood vessel ruptures. When part of the brain is deprived of oxygen, it dies, losing its function as well as the function of the part of the body it controls.

Often a stroke may be preceded by a transient ischemic attack (TIA), the temporary interference with blood supply to the brain, also called a mini-stroke.

FIGURE 20.2
The Warning Signs of Heart Disease
If you experience any combination of these symptoms, see your doctor immediately.

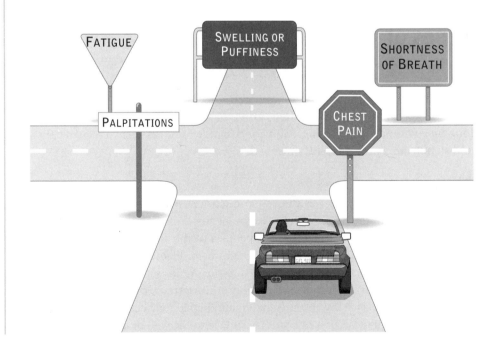

Over one-third of people who have had one or two TIAs will later have a stroke. When they will have the stroke is less clear—it could be days, weeks, months, or even years before a major stroke. The important warnings of a stroke, however, should be heeded.

During a TIA, the blood supply of the brain is temporarily blocked, either by a clot or blood vessel spasm. The symptoms are similar to those of a stroke and usually last a few minutes. By definition, a TIA lasts less than 24 hours. After the attack, symptoms go away and the person returns to normal.

A person experiencing a possible TIA must receive prompt medical attention to determine the cause or find any other condition that could be present. Early care could help prevent serious problems associated with a stroke.

Thrombosis

The formation or presence of a blood clot inside a blood vessel or cavity of the heart is called thrombosis. A thrombus is the clot that is formed; the plural of thrombus is thrombi. As mentioned previously, clots can form in the arteries that lead to the heart and brain resulting in heart attack and stroke, respectively. Clots can also form in one place and be carried through the blood system, lodging in another vessel. This is called a thromboembolism.

At one time it was thought that women who took oral contraceptives were at a higher risk of thromboembolism. This risk was related to the higher dosages of estrogen found in early forms of oral contraceptives. With the lower doses used today, this risk is no longer a significant threat. The risk of thromboembolism remains, however, for women on the pill who smoke, especially women over age 35. These women need to choose another form of birth control. Since smoking alone is a risk factor for heart disease and stroke, it is strongly recommended that women who smoke quit.

Congenital Defects

A heart problem that appears at birth is called a congenital heart defect. For example, the mother's exposure to a virus, such as rubella (also called German measles), during pregnancy may cause the fetus' heart or blood vessels near the heart to not form properly before birth. Such a defect can also occur as one aspect of a genetic disease that affects multiple parts of the body. Finally, congenital heart defects can occur if the mother drinks large amounts of alcohol or takes drugs, such as cocaine, while she is pregnant.

Congenital heart defects can be minor and not apparent right away, gradually worsening with time, or they can be life-threatening from birth. They can affect the heart itself, the valves and walls that separate the chambers, or the vessels leading to and from the heart. In most cases, defects either obstruct blood flow or cause blood to flow in an abnormal pattern. Some defects are openings in the heart that interfere with circulation. Others are obstructions or narrowings, called stenosis, that can occur in heart valves, arteries, or veins and block blood flow.

The severity of the defect often determines the severity of the symptoms and how soon after birth the symptoms first appear. Symptoms vary and often are the result of a lack of oxygen. They can include shortness of breath, dizziness, and turning blue. If a defect is recognized right away, as in a newborn baby, it may be possible to treat the defect before any serious damage occurs. Usually treatment

---

Symptoms of a Stroke or Transient Ischemic Attack

A stroke is a permanent loss of body function. A transient ischemic attack (TIA) is a temporary (less than 24 hour) loss of function. Both a stroke and a TIA may affect the body in a similar way:

- **Weakness and clumsiness in an arm, a leg, or a side of the face or body**
- **Loss of feeling in an arm, a leg, or the side of the face**
- **Dimness or loss of vision, especially in one eye**
- **Loss of speech or difficulty speaking or understanding speech**
- **Dizziness, double vision, or staggering**
- **Confusion or inability to think clearly**

If symptoms of a stroke or TIA occur, prompt medical attention should be sought. Thrombolysis or other treatment may stop the stroke or reduce damage but are only used at the onset of symptoms. Medication or treatment can be given to prevent recurrent strokes or TIAs.

involves surgery to either close an opening that should not be there or open an obstruction. New techniques may allow defects to be repaired without major operations. In some cases life-long medical care may be required.

Structural Heart Disease

Sometimes the heart has a structural defect that keeps it from working efficiently. The demands on the heart may be too great, or the mechanics of the heart itself are somehow not working right. All the parts must work in sequence for proper function, so a problem in the structure of the heart can be serious. Some structural problems include defects in the valves, congestive heart failure, and pericardial disease. These are usually diagnosed by examination and the use of echocardiography.

Valves. Heart murmurs can occur because of a defect in a valve that separates the chambers of the heart. The valve may not close completely, allowing blood to flow backward through the valve. The valve also may not open completely, preventing blood from moving from one chamber to another. A diastolic murmur occurs between beats, when the heart is relaxed. A systolic murmur occurs during a contraction, when the heart beats. Murmurs are graded according to loudness on a scale of 1 to 6, with 1 being the softest.

A problem in a valve can be minor, without symptoms, or major, requiring surgery to repair or replace the defective valve with a new one. New technologies may allow the valve to be repaired without major open-chest surgery. Problems in

Varicose Veins

Veins in the legs have thin walls and valves, which keep blood flowing in one direction. Sometimes the valves in the legs break under the pressure, and blood flows backward and collects in pools that bulge outward. These cause swollen blood vessels, which become varicose veins.

Women are four times more likely than men to have varicose veins. Their hormones weaken the vein walls, and the changes that accompany pregnancy can promote varicose veins.

Varicose veins are rarely dangerous, but they are unsightly and can be uncomfortable. Treatment is available to close the vein and reroute the blood supply. Following are some tips for preventing varicose veins:

- Stay active—avoid standing or sitting for long periods and exercise the calf muscles as much as possible.
- Raise your legs higher than your hip level or over your head to aid blood flow out of the veins.
- Avoid becoming overweight.
- Avoid lifting heavy objects and straining.
- Don't smoke.
- Avoid tight shoes or clothing that restricts blood flow.
- Some medications can strengthen the walls of blood vessels and reduce the incidence of varicose veins. Check with your doctor to see if these may help you.

valves can be congenital, or they can result from damage from conditions, such as pregnancy, fever, thyroid problems, medication, or anemia. Any valve can be damaged; however, mitral valve prolapse and aortic stenosis are the two that are of special concern in women.

Mitral Valve Prolapse. Mitral valve prolapse (MVP) affects the valve that separates the left atrium and left ventricle of the heart. The flaps of the valve become enlarged, thickened, or elongated and do not close smoothly when the heart beats, collapsing back into the left atrium. A variable amount of blood flows backward through the valve, causing the murmur, called mitral regurgitation.

In many cases MVP does not cause symptoms. In other cases, it causes stabbing chest pain or skipped heartbeats. Women with this condition may be at risk for bacterial endocarditis, and need to take antibiotics before having surgical or dental procedures that may introduce bacteria into the bloodstream. In the past, MVP was often diagnosed in patients who had a slight murmur and symptoms of skipped beats. Criteria for the medical diagnosis of MVP have changed in the past few years, however, so many people who once believed that they needed antibiotics are now being told they do not. In most situations, MVP is a minor concern, but it should be followed to make sure that rare but significant problems are identified and treated.

Aortic Stenosis. Aortic stenosis may be caused by a congenital defect or develop because of damage from other causes, such as rheumatic fever. The valve connecting the left ventricle to the aorta (the blood vessel that carries blood to the rest of the body) is narrowed, obstructing the flow of blood out of the heart. The valve can become calcified, further limiting blood flow. This can lead to angina, dizziness, sudden low blood pressure, and arrhythmias in advanced stages. Treatment requires surgery to replace or repair the valve.

Congestive Heart Failure. If the heart muscle is damaged or overworked, it can fail to perform. The damage can come from a heart attack, atherosclerosis, high blood pressure, a virus, or a congenital or acquired defect. The damaged heart lacks strength and enlarges as it tries to continue to function. As the damage progresses, the heart is less efficient as a pump and the whole circulation process becomes less effective. Blood backs up into the lungs, causing fluid to collect and making it difficult to breathe. In more severe cases, blood backs up in the right side of the heart. This affects the veins, causing congestion or swelling in the tissues of the ankles and legs as the body struggles to return blood to the heart.

Most causes of congestive heart failure can be treated with medications, surgery, or transplantation in severe cases.

Pericardial Disease. The heart and base of the major blood vessels are surrounded by a fibrous sac called the pericardium. The pericardium can become inflamed, resulting in pericarditis. This inflammation is associated with fluid production and can be caused by infection, injury, connective tissue disease (such as rheumatoid arthritis or lupus erythematosus), cancer, exposure to drugs or radiation, or a buildup of toxic substances in the body. The fluid causes the pericardial sac to rub against the heart, causing pain or rhythm disturbances. Often pericarditis

wellness
warning

Some infections can affect the heart, especially viruses accompanied by a high fever. If you have had such an illness and experience chest pain or shortness of breath during it or afterward, see a doctor.

affects young people with seemingly no cause, but it occurs days or weeks after a viral infection. Pericarditis can come on quickly, or it can slowly progress and become chronic, often with no symptoms. In most cases, if it is found early, the condition can be treated with success.

Regardless of the cause, most women feel pain at the onset of pericarditis. The pain may be either sharp or dull and pressing. The pain may worsen with deep breathing and lying flat and lessen with sitting up and leaning forward. Fever may be present. One sign that is usually present is what is called a friction rub. This scratchy or grating sound at certain times in the heartbeat is caused by the sac rubbing against the heart and can be heard by the doctor with a stethoscope.

Pericarditis usually heals on its own when the cause is corrected. Treatment involves use of nonsteroidal anti-inflammatory drugs, such as aspirin, as well as treatment of any underlying cause. In some cases, pericarditis will recur, requiring treatment with corticosteroids.

Pericarditis can become chronic in some people and pose more serious problems in the form of pericardial compression. (The medical term for this type of compression is tamponade.) Treatment of pericardial compression is removal of a portion of the pericardium and the fluid causing the pressure.

Arrhythmia

An abnormality in the pattern of the heartbeat is called an arrhythmia. It can interrupt the heart's natural rhythm and cause it to beat too fast, too slow, or irregularly.

In the heart, certain fibers function as the heart's natural "pacemaker," triggering the sequence of signals that cause the heart to beat. When this sequence is interrupted, or when the natural pacemaker of the heart develops an abnormality or is taken over by another part of the heart, arrhythmias occur. Various forms of arrhythmias are skipped or ectopic beats, bradycardia, tachycardia, and fibrillation. These are usually identified on an electrocardiogram, a Holter monitor test, or more sophisticated diagnostic tests.

Skipped or Ectopic Beats. Skipped or ectopic beats may start in the atria or ventricles. Often, they occur during times of stress and may be single or multiple beats, like a jump or brief flutter. Ectopic or skipped beats are sometimes controlled with medication, but usually they are managed by limiting stress or stimuli, such as caffeine.

Bradycardia. Bradycardia means the heartbeat is too slow, resulting in dizziness, fatigue, and a feeling of faintness. These symptoms occur because the body is not getting enough oxygen. The condition can be corrected by treating the cause of the slow heart rate (such as thyroid disease) or by replacing the heart's natural pacemaker with a mechanical one, which is usually implanted under the skin. This device transmits a signal that triggers the heart to beat at a more normal speed.

Tachycardia. Tachycardia is when the heart beats too fast, usually in a regular pattern. It can produce feelings of heart palpitations, rapid heart fluttering, dizziness, or feeling faint. If the heart beats too rapidly, it does not have time to fill with blood, so its ability to circulate blood is inadequate. Tachycardia most commonly starts in the upper heart chamber and may be treated with medications or newer procedures, such as radio frequency ablation, that can repair the heart and prevent recurrence. If tachycardia starts in the ventricles, it is life-threatening and requires immediate medical attention.

Fibrillation. In some cases, either the upper (atria) or the lower (ventricles) chambers may quiver instead of contracting and pumping. This is called fibrillation—either atrial or ventricular, depending on the location. Atrial fibrillation usually occurs at a rate that still allows the heart to fill with blood, so it is usually not life-threatening. However, it can result in blood clots, because not all the blood moves from the atrium to the ventricle. The remaining blood has a tendency to pool and form clots, which can become dangerous if they break loose and lodge in other parts of the body. Ventricular fibrillation is a life-threatening emergency.

Normal heart patterns often can be reinstated with medications or an electrical shock, using a device called a defibrillator. It is important that care be provided immediately.

Risk *Factors* of **Cardiovascular** *Disease*

It is well-known that certain factors, such as hypertension, diabetes, and smoking, as well as heredity, increase a woman's risk of cardiovascular disease. By being aware of factors that increase the risk of heart disease, you can take steps to protect yourself.

Identifying Personal Risks

A woman's risk of heart disease is based on her history, both family history and personal history. Heart disease in a close relative at an early age (before age 50) could be a sign that the disease may occur in other relatives.

The presence of a risk factor does not mean you will get heart disease, but it does increase the odds, especially if more than one factor applies. Some of these factors can be modified, whereas others are beyond a person's control. Familiarizing yourself with risk factors provides guidance in assessing personal risk and developing a plan to combat cardiovascular disease. Following is a profile of factors that increase the risk of heart disease:

- **Heredity.** Having a parent, grandparent, brother, or sister who had heart disease or a heart attack before age 50 is a factor.
- **Race.** African American women develop heart disease more often than white women, and they die from it more often. Heart disease is the number one cause of death in African American women over age 35.
- **Gender.** Men are more likely to have heart disease at a younger age than women.

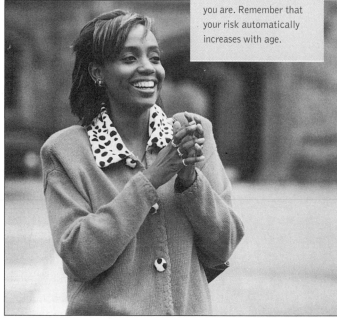

Your risk for heart disease is based on personal and family medical histories (which will indicate, for example, whether you are hypertensive or if you have a family member with heart disease) and certain lifestyle factors, such as whether you smoke and how active you are. Remember that your risk automatically increases with age.

Symptoms of Angina and Heart Attacks

Angina—a temporary lack of blood flow to the heart muscle—may be felt as a heavy pressure radiating to the neck, arms, or jaw and lasting minutes. It is usually brought on by exercise and relieved by rest. But in some older women, and especially in those with diabetes or high blood pressure, the chest discomfort may not be felt. Instead, they may often experience breathlessness, stomach distress, fatigue, or a feeling of weakness or being "sick." Women who are not active physically may feel these symptoms after meals or at times of emotional stress.

Symptoms of a heart attack often include chest pressure that lasts 20 minutes or more and does not abate with rest or change of position. The discomfort may be mild or severe and sometimes radiates into the jaw, abdomen, back, shoulders, or down the left arm. Other symptoms include nausea, sweating, shortness of breath, or what is described as a sense of impending doom.

Often, women who are having a heart attack, like some women with angina, may not feel chest pain or discomfort but have indigestion and trouble breathing. Some women experience any of a variety of symptoms, including a sensation of inhaling cold air or a feeling of weakness and sluggishness. They also may feel a hot stabbing pain, pressure, or sick feeling starting between their breasts, and running into their back or stomach, or into their armpits.

In the event of a heart attack or suspected heart attack, obtain care immediately. Contact emergency cardiac care services. Cardiopulmonary resuscitation (CPR) can be administered if the victim has lost consciousness. Thrombolysis, or clot busters, can be given to help reopen vessels. The sooner treatment can be given the less damage there may be to the heart and the better the outcome. Heart attacks can lead to severe disability or death.

- **Age.** Women develop heart disease at a later age than men, but by age 65, a woman's risk is about equal to that of a 65-year-old man.
- **Diabetes mellitus.** Approximately 80 percent of women with diabetes suffer from heart disease at some point in their lives, and they have an equal risk for heart disease as men the same age without diabetes.
- **Hypertension.** High blood pressure increases the risk of heart attack and stroke.
- **Abnormal lipid levels.** Increased levels of triglycerides and low-density lipoproteins (LDL)—"bad" cholesterol—and low levels of high-density lipoproteins (HDL)—"good" cholesterol—contribute to atherosclerosis, coronary heart disease, and stroke.
- **Obesity.** Being overweight increases the risk of heart disease and can lead to other illnesses, such as hypertension and diabetes, that contribute to heart disease. Obesity concentrated in the waist area poses the greatest risk.
- **Smoking.** Cigarette smoking increases the risk of heart disease and stroke as well as hypertension and numerous other disorders that can lead to heart disease.
- **Inactivity.** Leading a sedentary lifestyle (lack of activity) often contributes to obesity, having hypertension, and abnormal lipid levels.
- **Stress.** Unresolved stress, especially in areas you have little control over, can increase other cardiac risk factors and lead to heart disease.
- **Blood vessel irritants.** Certain chemicals in the bloodstream, such as nicotine, can damage the blood vessel lining and lead to the development of plaque or heart attack.
- **Hormone status.** After menopause (surgical or natural), a woman's risk of heart disease increases 40-fold.

In combination, many of these risk factors in one person can be deadly. The good news is that much of the risk can be lessened by changes in lifestyle, diet, and exercise.

Hypertension

High blood pressure, or hypertension, can be considered a disease in and of itself. Although it often has no symptoms and is rarely the direct cause of death, it is a major risk factor for coronary heart disease, stroke, congestive heart failure, and kidney failure. For this reason hypertension has been termed "the silent killer." When symptoms occur they can include dizziness, headaches, fatigue, shortness of breath, insomnia, or anxiety.

In the United States, an estimated 25 percent of white women and 30 percent of African American women have high blood pressure. Although in some cases high blood pressure can be caused by another medical condition, in most cases the cause is not known. Obesity, kidney problems, overuse of salt in people who are sensitive to salt, smoking, heavy consumption of alcohol, diabetes, use of certain medications, and lack of exercise can contribute to high blood pressure. Blood pressure increases with age. In young adulthood and early middle age, high blood pressure occurs more often in men than in women; thereafter, the reverse is true. By age 65, more than half of American women will have high blood pressure. High blood pressure appears to run in families and is more likely to occur and to be more severe in African Americans, who also tend to have diets higher in salt.

Hypertension occurs when arterial blood vessels constrict or narrow, creating resistance against blood flow, much like water in a hose that is being squeezed. The heart must work harder to pump blood throughout the body, which places stress on the heart. The presence of atherosclerosis can worsen the condition, further narrowing the blood vessels. It is thought that hypertension also injures the lining of the blood vessels, causing plaque to develop.

Blood pressure is expressed as diastolic and systolic pressure. It is often referred to as one number over another, for instance, 130 over 85, or 130/85. The first, or top, number is the systolic pressure, the force of blood against the blood vessel walls when the heart muscle contracts. The second, or bottom, number is

wellness
warning

Many negative effects of hypertension can be prevented if the patient's blood pressure is brought under control and kept at normal levels. For this reason, have your blood pressure checked regularly and, if it is high, seek medical attention, along with the recommended lifestyle changes. If you are at risk for high blood pressure, the lifestyle changes made now, before you develop high blood pressure, may slow or prevent its development.

Measuring Blood Pressure

The following techniques are recommended to obtain an accurate blood pressure reading:

- Do not smoke or drink caffeine (including sodas) within 30 minutes before the measurement.
- You should be relaxed, having rested for at least five minutes before having your measurement taken. You should not speak or chew gum during measurement.
- Sit with your legs uncrossed and your bare arm supported and at heart level.
- Have two or more readings taken at two-minute intervals. The results of the readings should then be averaged. The doctor may also check your blood pressure in other positions, such as standing, especially if you are on blood pressure medication.
- If the first two readings differ by more than five mm Hg, additional readings should be obtained.

You can measure your blood pressure at home using inexpensive devices. These readings may be more accurate than those in a health care setting, because you are less likely to be stressed. It is important to understand fully how to use and calibrate the device and to follow instructions carefully.

wellness **tip**

It is natural to be anxious in a hospital or doctor's office. This can cause your blood pressure to increase, a reaction called "white coat syndrome." Blood pressure may return to normal once you are home in comfortable surroundings. Try to remain seated for a few minutes with legs uncrossed, not chewing gum or speaking when your blood pressure is taken.

TABLE 20.1

Classification of Blood Pressure for Adults Aged 18 Years and Older

CATEGORY *	SYSTOLIC	DIASTOLIC
NORMAL	Less than 130 mm Hg	Less than 85 mm Hg
HIGH NORMAL	130–139 mm Hg	85–89 mm Hg
HYPERTENSION		
Stage 1 Mild	140–159 mm Hg	90–99 mm Hg
Stage 2 Moderate	160–179 mm Hg	100–109 mm Hg
Stage 3 Severe	180–209 mm Hg	110–119 mm Hg
Stage 4 Very Severe	210 mm Hg or higher	120 mm Hg or higher

* The category of blood pressure of an individual is determined by the greatest level obtained, from either systolic or diastolic measurements.

Source: Joint National Committee on Detection, Evaluation, and Treatment of High Blood Pressure. Archives of Internal Medicine 153:154, 1993.

the diastolic pressure, the force of blood against the blood vessel walls when the heart relaxes. The numbers are the units of measurement in millimeters of mercury (mm Hg). The device used to measure blood pressure is called a sphygmomanometer, which displays the blood pressure with a column of mercury. It can also be measured with electronic devices.

Elevations in either the systolic or diastolic pressure, or both, are unhealthy and pose a health risk. Blood pressure is classified as normal, high normal, or stages 1 to 4 of hypertension (Table 20.1). In the general population, risks are lowest for adults with an average systolic blood pressure less than 120 mm Hg and an average diastolic pressure less than 80 mm Hg (120/80).

Blood pressure readings obtained in a hospital or doctor's office may not reflect a woman's true levels. Some people have what is referred to as "white coat syndrome," anxiety about being in the presence of a medical professional; this syndrome can cause blood pressure to be unnaturally high. Repeated blood pressure measurements determine whether high levels persist and require attention. High blood pressure readings should be confirmed on at least two subsequent visits during one to two weeks.

Blood pressure can be lowered by a combination of lifestyle changes and, if needed, medication. Borderline high blood pressure can often be controlled by losing weight, limiting intake of salt and caffeine, drinking less alcohol, and stopping smoking. A diet low in salt and high in fruits, vegetables, and low-fat dairy products has been shown to be effective in lowering blood pressure. Exercise also can help lower blood pressure and relieve stress, another risk factor. More severe hypertension usually requires medication in addition to these lifestyle changes.

Diabetes

Diabetes is a disease in which the body is unable to use glucose, a form of sugar from which the body derives energy. Glucose is produced from foods and, with the help of a hormone called insulin, converted into energy. When there is not enough insulin, or when the body resists the effects of insulin, levels of glucose in the blood increase, resulting in what is called "high blood sugar," or diabetes. Diabetes is sometimes referred to as glucose intolerance or insulin resistance, both of which contribute to heart disease.

People with diabetes are more likely to have heart disease and to have it at an earlier age. This is especially true for women with diabetes, who are two to five times more likely to have a cardiovascular disease than women the same age without diabetes. Even borderline diabetes poses a significant risk. Women with diabetes get cardiovascular disease at the same rate as nondiabetic men the same age. Approximately 80 percent of adults with diabetes die from cardiovascular disease, and women with diabetes die at a younger age than men with diabetes. High blood pressure, high cholesterol, and obesity—conditions that often accompany diabetes—add to the risk.

Diabetes accelerates atherosclerosis, increasing the possibility that a blood vessel can become narrowed and restrict blood flow. This can occur in the blood supply to the legs, reducing circulation and causing pain and cramping with activity. Even smaller arteries can be damaged by diabetes and affect vision, kidney function, and healing ability.

Control of diabetes does not necessarily lower the risk of heart disease. However, stopping smoking, keeping blood pressure and cholesterol levels down, exercise, weight control, and a healthy diet can have a positive effect on diabetes as well as on cardiovascular disease. (For more information about diabetes, see Chapter 23.)

Cholesterol

Cholesterol is a fatlike substance in the cells of the body and the blood. The main ingredient of cholesterol is saturated fat. The liver naturally makes about 1,000 milligrams a day of cholesterol from saturated fat. Another 400 to 500 milligrams or more come from foods that contain cholesterol. It is found in fish, meat, eggs, certain plants, and dairy products. Although cholesterol is needed for certain bodily functions, too much of it can lead to atherosclerosis and coronary heart disease.

Lipoproteins transport cholesterol and fat through the bloodstream to and from the various parts of the body. Lipoproteins are made up of protein, cholesterol, and triglycerides, a form of fat produced by the liver that helps store fat in body tissues. HDL contain high levels of protein and low levels of cholesterol, and LDL contain low levels of protein and high levels of cholesterol. Both forms contain small amounts of triglycerides.

Most of the cholesterol in the body—60 to 80 percent—is carried by LDL. Cholesterol is carried from the liver and into the blood, where it circulates through the body and is used by the body. Excess LDL is converted by reacting with free oxygen radicals in the bloodstream, so it can build up inside the walls of arteries. This residue buildup is referred to as plaque, the hallmark of atherosclerosis. Therefore, high LDL levels are a risk factor in coronary heart disease and stroke.

HDL can remove LDL from plaque in blood vessel walls, carrying it back to the liver to be excreted. The higher the HDL level, the lower the risk for heart disease.

Controlling Cholesterol Intake. In order to control your cholesterol intake from foods, you need to know about the two major types of dietary fats: saturated fat and unsaturated fat. Saturated fat, such as that found in red meat, is a key contributor to high blood cholesterol levels. Unsaturated fats, such as canola oil, can be polyunsaturated or monounsaturated. On food labels, saturated and unsaturated fats together make up the total fat content of the food product.

A diet high in saturated fat will cause the liver to produce too high levels of cholesterol, causing excess levels of cholesterol to circulate in the blood and build up in the arteries. When the diet is low in saturated fats, the liver produces lower levels of cholesterol and less is available to circulate in the blood and build up in the arteries.

Measuring Cholesterol. Before techniques to measure LDL and HDL levels were available, total cholesterol—approximately equal to LDL + HDL—was all that could be measured. In fact, many older statistics and recommendations are based on the total level. Currently, experts agree that a total cholesterol level of greater than 260 places a person at twice the risk of heart attack as someone with a total cholesterol level of less than 200. However, in women, the link between high cholesterol and heart attack is not as strong as in men.

A healthy body has low levels of LDL and high levels of HDL. (Triglycerides, harmful fats in the blood, may also play a role in heart disease, depending on how the levels relate to HDL and LDL. Triglycerides are discussed later in this section.) For every one percent increase in total cholesterol levels, the risk of heart attack increases two to three percent. These figures are based on the risk in middle-aged men, however. It is not known what total cholesterol level is healthiest for women, mainly because the total cholesterol level in women is often made up of more HDL, the "good" cholesterol.

Role of Stress

Stress has often been linked to many medical problems, including hypertension and heart disease. Although there is no denying that too much stress can have a harmful influence, stress can also be a positive force. It can motivate us and stimulate creativity, provided stress is harnessed and directed. When it becomes a source of frustration, however, stress can undermine your health.

The brain and the central nervous system respond to feelings of distress by producing the chemical adrenaline. This surge of adrenaline creates the "fight or flight" response that is the body's way of defending itself. Oxygen needs, respiration, heart rate, blood pressure, and cholesterol levels increase. Sustained levels of stress result in sustained levels of these responses, which can promote atherosclerosis.

Individuals with certain personality types labeled as type A (aggressive, achievement-oriented) were once considered susceptible to heart disease. This is no longer thought to be completely true. Rather, the risk may arise with ongoing feelings of hostility, frustration, urgency, or cynicism. Such feelings often occur in individuals exposed to prolonged stress that they cannot control or do not handle well. Also, those under stress are more likely to turn to behaviors that contribute to high blood pressure or heart disease, such as alcohol and tobacco use and poor eating habits.

Levels of HDL are especially important to women because they are a better predictor of heart disease in women than LDL levels. Higher HDL levels offer women protection against heart disease, a benefit that may be linked to the presence of the female hormone, estrogen.

Women need to have both types of cholesterol and triglyceride levels measured in order to assess their cardiac risk. This measurement is called a lipid profile, in which individual levels and their ratios to total cholesterol are assessed. A lipid profile is much more accurate than measuring just total cholesterol in predicting risk.

Cholesterol is measured in milligrams per deciliter (mg/dL) of blood. Ideally, HDL levels should be about 55 mg/dL; less than 45 in women (35 in men) is considered low, and over 70 in women (60 in men) is high. For every increase in HDL of 10 mg/dL, there appears to be a 50 percent decrease in heart disease risk. The ratio of HDL to total cholesterol can be a useful guide to the risk of heart disease. Following are sample ratios (total cholesterol divided by HDL):

	Ratio	Example
Good	Less than 3.5	Total cholesterol of 160; HDL of 70
Moderate risk	3.5–6.9	Total cholesterol of 220; HDL of 44
High risk	7.0 or greater	Total cholesterol of 260; HDL of 35

The National Cholesterol Education Program (NCEP) recommends that women over age 20 have their cholesterol level checked once every five years. If either LDL or total cholesterol levels are too high, further testing, counseling about diet, or medication may be required. Some physicians recommend more frequent checks, especially if a woman has other risk factors for heart or blood vessel disease, has experienced a change in weight or activity level, or if she has been ill (with thyroid disease or after any significant illness).

The NCEP recommends a two-step diet for those with high or borderline total cholesterol or LDL levels. Step one is followed for three months, after which cholesterol is remeasured. If levels remain high, step two is implemented. If total levels remain elevated (higher than 190 mg/dL on a diet or 160 mg/dL on a diet in the presence of two other risk factors), medication needs to be given. It is recommended that women with diagnosed heart disease attempt to lower their LDL cholesterol levels to less than 100 mg/dL through diet or medication or both. Talk to your doctor if you have specific concerns about your lipid level.

Triglycerides. Although the exact role of triglycerides in heart disease is unknown, it is generally thought that high levels increase risk for heart disease, possibly by forcing more LDL into plaque. Many people with low HDL and elevated LDL levels also have high triglyceride levels. Triglyceride levels should be measured, even if total cholesterol

wellness **tip**

Do not rely on cholesterol tests in shopping malls— the results may not be very accurate. It is recommended that you use a certified laboratory, preferably after you have been fasting for 12 to 14 hours. If results are high, confirm them by having the test repeated. Nonfasting tests may cause a high triglycerides reading and possibly affect the high-density lipoprotein (HDL) level as well.

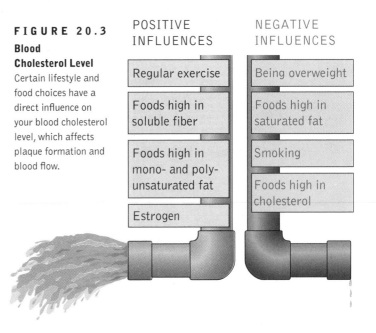

FIGURE 20.3
Blood Cholesterol Level
Certain lifestyle and food choices have a direct influence on your blood cholesterol level, which affects plaque formation and blood flow.

POSITIVE INFLUENCES

Regular exercise

Foods high in soluble fiber

Foods high in mono- and poly-unsaturated fat

Estrogen

NEGATIVE INFLUENCES

Being overweight

Foods high in saturated fat

Smoking

Foods high in cholesterol

National Cholesterol Education Program Recommendations for Lowering Cholesterol

Step One

- Keep total fat intake to less than 30 percent of total calories.
- Keep saturated fat intake to less than 10 percent of total calories.
- Increase polyunsaturated fat to 10 percent of total calories.
- Make monounsaturated fat 10 to 15 percent of total calories.
- Make carbohydrates 50 to 60 percent of total calories.
- Make protein 10 to 20 percent of total calories.
- Reduce cholesterol intake to less than 300 milligrams/day.
- Adjust total calories to achieve and maintain desirable weight.

Step Two

- Reduce saturated fat intake to less than 7 percent of total calories.
- Reduce cholesterol intake to less than 200 milligrams/day.

Source: National Cholesterol Education Program Expert Panel on Detection, Evaluation, and Treatment of High Blood Cholesterol in Adults, 1993.

values are normal. For an accurate triglyceride reading, you must fast for 12 to 14 hours before the test. Following is the NCEP classification of triglyceride levels:

Desirable	Less than 200 mg/dL
Borderline	200–239 mg/dL
High	Greater than 240 mg/dL

Levels higher than 200 are cause for concern to women. Levels higher than 240 require immediate attention including dietary changes to bring the changes down.

Triglyceride levels increase after eating fatty foods. Eating less sugar, losing weight, avoiding alcohol, and exercising can help lower levels.

Estrogen and Cholesterol. The female hormone, estrogen, promotes high levels of HDL, which protect women against atherosclerosis and heart attacks. It also lowers LDL cholesterol. When estrogen production drops after menopause, the ratio of LDL to HDL rises, and a woman's risk of heart disease increases. Postmenopausal hormone therapy has been shown to reduce this risk.

The Postmenopausal/Estrogen Progestin Interventions (PEPI) Trial—a 1991 National Institutes of Health study of 900 women to evaluate the impact of hormone therapy on the risk of heart disease—looked at the effect of estrogen and the addition of various forms of progesterone in lipids. Estrogen alone had the most beneficial effect but was associated with an unacceptable buildup in the endometrial lining. This endometrial buildup was completely prevented by the addition of natural or artificial progesterone (progestin). Estrogen and natural progesterone had the next most favorable benefit on lipids, followed by the estrogen and progestin combination.

Early Symptoms

As stated earlier, symptoms of a heart attack or stroke may differ in women and men. Women need to be alert to symptoms, such as shortness of breath, fatigue, weakness, abdominal or throat discomfort, and tightness or heaviness in the chest or arms. These symptoms are especially important in women with the presence of cardiac risk factors. Any evidence of heart disease must be checked immediately by a doctor.

Women are more likely to suffer silent or unrecognized heart attacks than men. They are less likely than men to get prompt treatment, which would prevent damage to the heart, when they are having a heart attack. Women more often die during their first heart attack than men do. After they have had a heart attack, women are less likely than men to have cardiac rehabilitation. Bypass surgery has a higher death rate and is often less successful in women than in men. Some say this is because women have smaller arteries and thus are not as easily treated; others feel it is because women are more ill than men when they finally receive treatment.

You can, however, help protect yourself from the consequences of heart disease:

- Know your risk factors and do what you can to reduce them.
- Be alert to early warning signs and symptoms.
- Seek care at the first sign of a problem.
- Make sure that your health concerns receive proper attention.

Once it occurs, heart disease does not go away. Early and appropriate treatment, however, can make a difference in preventing heart damage and improving your quality of life.

Check **It Out**

Routine checkups can help detect health problems early, before you may be aware of them. They also give you an opportunity to discuss questions or concerns with your doctor. If problems are found, further tests may be needed. If you have symptoms or risk factors for heart disease, your doctor is likely to order tests to further evaluate the situation. If your doctor does not order additional tests or you feel she is not giving your concerns adequate attention, speak to her about your concerns and get a second opinion if needed. Because heart disease is often overlooked or undertreated in women, you may need to be assertive in order to get the attention you require.

Routine Checkups

Many women have a routine checkup annually. Some may need an examination more often, whereas others can go longer between examinations. The frequency depends on whether health problems exist. It is a good idea to have a routine examination periodically, however, so your doctor can follow your health and detect any changes. (Part II of this book gives complete information on routine checkups.)

During a routine examination, the doctor or nurse will check your blood pressure and examine your heart, lungs, and other body parts. Your lipid level may also be checked, along with your blood sugar and other appropriate tests. During this examination, your doctor can discuss with you changes in your lifestyle that may decrease your risk of heart disease. Following are the most effective steps:

- Stop smoking.
- Change your diet to increase fiber and limit fat, saturated fat, and cholesterol.
- Maintain a proper weight.
- Moderate alcohol intake.
- Increase the amount of exercise with moderate daily activity.
- Discuss hormone therapy if you are postmenopausal.

If you have any concerns about your health, discuss them with your doctor. Together you can work out a plan for a healthy heart. Your doctor will suggest further tests depending on your age or any risk factors.

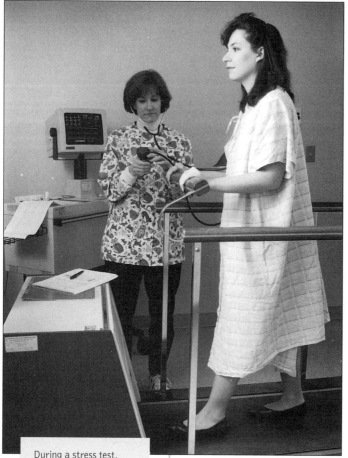

During a stress test, blood pressure and heartbeat are monitored to determine whether the heart is getting an adequate supply of blood.

Special Assessments

Special tests are available to view the heart's function and assess its rhythms. Some of these tests are new and very sophisticated. Some monitor the signals of the heart as it beats, and others create images of the heart and its function. All help evaluate the heart for possible problems. Most were standardized using men as patients, so it is important that your doctor pay attention to differences in results based on gender to ensure that her interpretation of test results is accurate for her female patients.

Electrocardiography. The electrical impulses that trigger the beating of the heart can be read and recorded with electrocardiography (ECG). Electrical sensors are placed on the skin at various points on the body. The electrical signals produced by the heart are picked up by the sensors and recorded on an electrocardiogram. Depending on the pattern of the signals, they may show an irregularity in the heartbeat, a lack of blood flow to the heart, or damage to the heart or its electrical system from a heart attack or other condition. The ECG may be done in a resting state or while the person is exercising.

Holter Monitor. How the stresses of daily living affect heart rhythm can be assessed with a Holter monitor, a miniature ECG with a tiny recording device. This device is connected to a person for a 24-hour period to assess how well her heart responds to normal day-to-day activities. The Holter monitor is usually used when tachycardia, bradycardia, and ectopic or irregular beats are present or suspected and can assist your doctor in treating them.

Stress Test. An exercise stress test can assess the heart's ability to meet demands. The test is designed to stress the heart to see how well it can perform. The harder the body works, the more oxygen and blood it needs to fuel the extra effort. The test can show if the heart is getting an adequate blood supply. This test also may be performed to determine the level and type of activity that would be appropriate for a woman beginning an exercise program.

During a stress test, one's heart rate, breathing, blood pressure, and heart rhythm are monitored. The test is usually done with a continuous ECG while the woman being tested walks on a treadmill or pedals a stationary bicycle. The speed and difficulty are gradually increased to monitor how her heart responds and to measure her endurance. Her oxygen level can be checked by a monitor attached to her finger when she exercises. After the test, the blood pressure and heartbeat are monitored for several more minutes. The test can be stopped at any time if discomfort occurs, and it is considered safe when done with medical supervision. Stress testing is moderately reliable in diagnosing coronary artery disease in men but much less reliable in women. Often, ECG abnormalities occur in women that are not caused by blood vessel narrowing. Imaging of the heart with echocardiography or nuclear perfusion imaging is more accurate, especially in women. These two tests are discussed below.

Echocardiography. Sound waves can be used to assess the size, shape, and motion of the heart structures by directing them into the heart and recording what bounces back with a special device. The recorded sounds are then converted into an image that can show the structure and function of the heart.

Echocardiography during exercise can show heart motion and its response to stress. This test helps clarify if coronary artery disease is present. It is very useful, especially in women, where the ECG stress test is much less reliable.

Sound waves can also be used to assess movement without creating a picture. Audible signals can help analyze the flow of blood through veins, arteries, and the heart. They can be used to see if there is an obstruction in a vein or artery or if there is a valve problem.

Nuclear Perfusion Imaging. In nuclear perfusion imaging, a small amount of radioactive material, called a tracer, is injected into the vein during stress testing. This tracer attaches to blood cells and flows with them to the heart. Using a nuclear scanner, the doctor can take "pictures" of this blood flow while the patient is at rest and while she is exercising. The doctor then compares the rest pictures with the exercise pictures. A lack of blood flow during exercise means that the patient may have a narrowed blood vessel serving part of the heart— coronary artery disease. Certain new tracers, such as technetium 99-m sestamibi, give better results in women than older tracers, such as thallium, especially when used with a newer technique that shows heart motion, called gated SPECT.

Angiography. Also known as arteriography or cardiac catheterization, angiography is used to show the negative image or outline of blood flow through the arteries. It can detect areas of narrowing or blockage in the arteries. A thin, flexible, hollow tube (or catheter) is threaded through an artery of an arm or leg and moved into the heart. A dye that shows up on x-ray is then injected, and the heart and blood vessels are filmed as the heart pumps it through the coronary arteries. The picture is called an angiogram or arteriogram. This technique is the "standard" against which all other tests for evaluating the blood flow to the heart and its blood vessels are compared.

Keeping *Your*
Heart Healthy

There are many ways you can protect your heart and maintain your health. Through proper diet, regular exercise, stopping smoking, avoiding harmful substances and excessive amounts of alcohol, and maintaining normal blood pressure and lipid levels, you can do your part to combat heart disease. At the same time, you can also help prevent other disorders that are often linked to the risk factors for heart disease.

wellness **tip**

The so-called "Mediterranean diet," rich in fruit, vegetables, bread, wine, fish, and canola or olive oil, may help reduce the risk of heart problems, including angina, stroke, heart failure, and blood clots.

Choosing a Healthy Diet

A diet that is beneficial against heart disease also helps prevent other diseases, such as cancer and diabetes. In general, a healthy diet involves eating a variety of foods that are low in fat, saturated fat, and cholesterol, and high in fiber and limiting the intake of calories to maintain a healthy weight.

Dietary Guidelines. The American Heart Association has issued dietary guidelines for the prevention of heart and blood vessel disease. Following is a summary:

- **Eat a variety of foods.** Choose foods from all food groups, including fruits and vegetables; nonfat and low-fat dairy products; whole-grain breads, cereals, pasta, starchy vegetables, and beans; and lean meat, skinless poultry, and fish.
- **Balance food intake with physical activity.** This will help you maintain a healthy weight. Excess weight increases cholesterol and high blood pressure as well as promoting heart disease, diabetes, stroke, and certain cancers. Experts recommend 20 to 30 minutes a day of moderate exercise.
- **Eat foods low in fat, saturated fat, and cholesterol.** No more than 30 percent of total calories should come from fat. Saturated fat should be limited to 8 to 10 percent of total calories, with the remainder coming from polyunsaturated (up to 10 percent) and monounsaturated (up to 15 percent) fats. Less than 300 mg/dL of cholesterol should be consumed in a day. These amounts can be found on food labels. Switch from butter to soft margarine products, which are lower in saturated fats and trans fatty acids and are cholesterol free.
- **Eat lots of fruits, vegetables, and whole-grain products.** Between 55 and 60 percent of total calories should come from these sources, which are low in fat and high in vitamins, minerals, fiber, and complex carbohydrates.
- **Use sugar and salt in moderation.** Diets high in sugar are usually high in calories and low in complex carbohydrates, fiber, and essential vitamins and minerals. Salt promotes high blood pressure in salt-sensitive individuals and should be limited to six grams per day.
- **Drink alcohol in moderation.** Those who drink alcohol should limit their intake to two drinks or less per day. Those who do not use alcohol should not start.

Calcium may help lower blood pressure in addition to preventing bone loss in women. A low-fat diet may prevent women from getting enough calcium, so

The Difference Among Oils

Coconut oil, palm kernel oil, and palm oil are high in saturated fats and are often used in processed foods. Read food labels carefully. Corn oil, peanut oil, and canola oil are unsaturated fat, and olive oil is monounsaturated, and thus healthier. Oil is fat, however, so avoid eating fried foods and watch the calories. Olestra, an oil that is not absorbed by the body, is now available in certain products, such as potato chips. While the use of Olestra in large quantities has side effects, such as diarrhea or loss of fat-soluble vitamins, it is an acceptable alternative for people who should restrict their fat intake, if used in moderation.

you may need to take a supplement to reach the recommended levels of 1,000 milligrams per day for menstruating women and 1,500 milligrams per day for postmenopausal women. Make sure the amount of calcium measured is elemental calcium. Calcium carbonate should be taken with food, while other forms of calcium should be taken on an empty stomach. Magnesium also may protect against heart disease and is often given with calcium. Drugs used to treat certain heart diseases and prevent sodium and water retention can also deplete potassium. This element is essential for the body's growth and maintenance. Women need to be sure they are consuming adequate amounts, especially if they are taking medication. (See Chapter 8 for more information on eating for wellness.)

Special Diets. A vegetarian diet high in complex carbohydrates and low in sugar and saturated fats can be very healthy for the heart. However, women who follow vegetarian diets need to be sure to include foods that provide the essential nutrients found in meat and fish, particularly protein and vitamin B_{12}. If a woman eats a variety of foods to provide a nutritious diet, a vegetarian diet high in fiber and low in fat should be healthy for her heart.

"Yo-yo" dieting, in which a lot of weight, such as ten or more pounds, is lost and gained over and over, is unhealthy and linked to heart disease. Such diets can double the risk of getting heart disease and dying from it. It is not known how these diets affect heart disease but, as with many aspects of health, moderate and regular habits are often the best.

Asian women, who typically eat low-fat diets, have a low incidence of heart disease as well as a low risk of certain cancers that often occur in women who consume high-fat diets. It is thought that protection may come from phytoestrogens in the Asian diet. These substances are natural estrogens from plants that are found in many foods, such as oilseeds, bran, whole cereals, vegetables, soybeans, chickpeas, and fruits. Phytoestrogens act biologically like natural estrogens, which also protect women from heart disease. The role of phytoestrogens is still being studied, but they do seem to have a beneficial effect on the prevention of heart disease as well as the symptoms of menopause.

Weight Control. It has been estimated that 70 percent of women with coronary heart disease are overweight. Being 10 percent over the ideal weight increases the risk of heart attack by 30 percent. Weight loss reduces cholesterol and blood pressure levels, thus reducing the risk of heart disease.

By following general guidelines for good heart health, women can also reduce weight and look and feel better. Reducing saturated fat also helps reduce the number of calories and aids in weight control because most saturated fats are high in calories. Regular exercise—another factor that reduces the risk of heart disease—also promotes weight loss.

The total overall weight is an important factor, but women also need to watch how their weight is distributed. A waist-to-hip ratio of greater than 0.8:1 (that is, your waist is larger than your hips) has become an important signal of heart disease. Why having body fat centered around the middle increases the risk of heart disease is not known, though losing weight in this area reduces your risk.

wellness **tip**

Omega-3 fatty acids are found in certain kinds of fish. Some researchers believe they may help prevent heart disease, but the benefit is not certain. What is known is that most fish is lower in cholesterol and fat than red meat and thus healthier. The current recommendation is to eat fish or seafood at least once a week to reduce cardiac risk.

Calculating Your Waist-to-Hip Ratio

You can determine one of your risks of heart disease by calculating your waist-to-hip ratio.

A good result is less than 0.8:1 in women (1:1 in men). For example, a woman whose hips are 36 inches should have a waist of 28.8 inches or less. (A man with 34-inch hips should have a waist of 34 inches or less.) Risk increases with a higher ratio. Lowering your waist measurement by diet and/or exercise will lower your waist-to-hip ratio and has been shown to reduce your risk of developing coronary artery disease. Many physicians do not actually calculate the waist-to-hip ratio when the ratio is obvious. If the ratio is not clear, it should be measured in order to identify the risk and serve as a baseline for improvement.

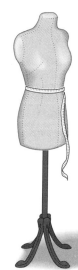

STEP 1 Measure your waist at the navel.

STEP 2 Measure your hips at the widest point.

STEP 3 Divide the waist measurement by the hip measurement.

EXAMPLE   Waist   30 inches
                     Hips   38 inches
                     30 ÷ 38 = 0.79
                     Round to nearest tenth.
                     Ratio   0.8:1

FIGURE 20.4

Calculating Your Waist-to-Hip Ratio

Follow these three steps to determine your waist-to-hip ratio.

Exercise

Exercise improves many of the factors associated with the risk of heart disease. Exercise lowers blood pressure, reduces LDL cholesterol and triglycerides in the blood, raises HDL cholesterol, helps control weight and burn calories, strengthens the heart and lungs, and promotes the body's ability to use oxygen. It also reduces stress levels and can help prevent diabetes and certain cancers. Exercise helps keep blood flowing, which lowers the risk of clots, and reduces resistance to insulin, a factor in both heart disease and diabetes. Despite such a strong argument for the benefits of exercise, only 50 percent of those who begin an exercise program continue it beyond six months. The benefits of exercise last only as long as the person is exercising.

Aerobic Exercise. Exercise that increases the heart rate to a certain sustained level for 15 to 20 minutes a day can strengthen the heart and increase the body's ability to work more efficiently. In order to be effective, the target heart rate must be reached (see Chapter 9 for more information on target heart rate and exercise). Exercise is considered "aerobic" when it draws energy from oxygen in the body. Such exercise builds a stronger cardiovascular system and allows a person to work harder while expending less effort. It makes the heart more efficient in delivering blood to the muscles and the muscles more efficient in using oxygen. Exercise can improve the performance of healthy people as well as those who have heart disease.

Exercise Guidelines. To offer cardiovascular conditioning, exercise must be aerobic, increasing and sustaining the heart rate. Exercise also can be done for strength, building muscles and their supporting structures and bones. Such exercise also promotes flexibility, allowing women to remain active and agile. An ideal exercise program includes stretching, aerobic exercise, and strength-building exercise.

Special Precautions. Women with a heart condition or other health problems can still exercise. Women who have two or more risk factors for heart disease or who are over age 40 and have not been exercising should consult a physician before beginning an exercise program. Women with cardiovascular disease can exercise at a moderate level under a doctor's supervision. Before beginning a program, the doctor may recommend an exercise stress test to assess possible risks and see what level of activity can be safely tolerated. The test may be repeated annually or as needed, depending on the individual situation.

Exercise training can be useful in the treatment of coronary artery disease and helps keep it from progressing. The type and level of activity depend on the nature and extent of the disease. Precautions should be taken to avoid injury, however. A health professional can monitor the following signs and symptoms to help establish a safe and effective pace:

- **Symptoms.** Watch for chest discomfort, shortness of breath, faintness, or weakness with activity.
- **Heart rate.** Watch for sudden increases of more than 20 beats per minute over resting, or heartbeat irregularities.
- **Blood Pressure.** This should be under control at the start of the program and monitored during and after exercise.

Once tolerance to exercise has been established, women with heart problems are encouraged to be active. Walking is an ideal form of moderate exercise and is often well suited to those with or without a heart condition.

Smoking Cessation

Women who smoke are two to four times as likely as nonsmoking women to have a heart attack. The more a woman smokes, the more she is at risk. Even one to four cigarettes a day increases the risk, and low tar and low nicotine cigarettes are no less harmful. Smoking permanently damages the lining of the arteries, allowing plaque to build up and atherosclerosis to progress. It also increases blood pressure and causes blood vessels to spasm and narrow. Smoking can reduce the flow of oxygen to the heart and can mask symptoms of a heart attack, producing a silent attack that is not recognized and therefore may not receive proper treatment.

Many of the negative effects of smoking can be reversed—the sooner a woman quits the better. The benefits of quitting smoking begin right away, and the maximal benefits for reducing the risk of heart disease can be reached within two years. However, some vessel damage from smoking persists, so it is best never to start smoking.

There is no denying that it is difficult to quit smoking. Nicotine, the main harmful ingredient in tobacco, is physically and psychologically addictive, and withdrawal has negative physical effects. Fortunately, these effects are short lived, lasting on average about two weeks. Exercise and a change in eating habits can help relieve these negative effects as well as the weight gain that often accompanies quitting. A woman who is trying to quit can find support groups to help, and her physician can recommend aids, such as nicotine replacement patches and gum, or medications to ease the transition. Quitting smoking can be a major step in adopting a lifestyle that promotes a healthy heart. (For further information on smoking cessation, see Chapter 13.)

wellness
warning

Passive, or secondhand, smoke is a major health hazard, raising heart disease and cancer risk, and can make some people ill. Women, such as waitresses, whose workplaces allow smoking have been shown to have up to 2 to 4 times the risk of coronary artery disease.

Preventive Measures

There are other measures women can take to help prevent heart disease. Some of these suggestions are commonly known to help in both men and women, and others are unique to women, relating to prolonging their special hormonal protection.

Aspirin. While aspirin is known to be life-saving in patients having an acute heart attack, its use for prevention in women has been more controversial. Studies, performed mostly on men, have found that taking a low-dose aspirin tablet every day lowers the risk of heart attack. It has now been shown that low-dose aspirin has a similar benefit in women at increased risk for coronary artery disease. Aspirin is routinely used by male and more recently by female patients who have had heart attacks to help prevent a future attack. It may also benefit healthy people who have never had a heart attack. Aspirin also prevents the development of recurrent strokes or a stroke after a transient ischemic attack, sometimes called a TIA or mini-stroke. Before taking aspirin on a long-term basis, however, women should weigh their risks for heart disease against possible complications, including the tendency to bleed. Aspirin should not be taken by women who have liver or kidney disease, peptic ulcer, gastrointestinal bleeding or disease, any bleeding problems, or allergy to aspirin or aspirin-like medication. It is best to discuss long-term aspirin use and dosage with your doctor. Researchers are not certain whether aspirin's main benefit is its ability to thin the blood or its ability to reduce inflammation in blood vessels.

Alcohol. It has been shown that one to two glasses of red wine a day helps lower the risk of heart disease in men. One large study found that women who drank three to nine glasses of red wine per week had half as much coronary heart disease as those who did not drink. This does not mean that women who do not drink should begin to do so. It does mean that one drink a day does not do significant harm and may have some benefit. Studies show white wine and grape juice may have similar benefits.

Estrogen Therapy. The hormone estrogen keeps arteries elastic and healthy. It also keeps HDL cholesterol levels high and LDL cholesterol levels low, creating a favorable lipid profile. Estrogen helps lower blood pressure, reduces the blood's ability to clot and form plaque, and helps arteries relax when stressed, reducing spasms that can cause blockages. After menopause, this protection ceases and a woman's risk of heart disease approaches that of a man, unless she is on hormone replacement. (For more information on hormone therapy, see Chapter 19.)

Antibiotics. Women who have heart murmurs or disorders of the valves of the heart are more likely to get bacterial endocarditis. This is a bacterial infection of the heart valves or the lining of the heart. It is more likely to occur during certain dental or surgical procedures that could involve some bleeding. The bacteria could be introduced into the blood stream during such procedures and lead to infection. Women who have abnormal blood flow from congenital or acquired heart problems, those who have had their heart valves replaced, or those who have had endocarditis should take antibiotics before a procedure to prevent the infection. Be sure to tell your doctor or dentist if you have such a condition so medication can be given in advance. Also, if you have one of these conditions and have been taking antibiotics, you should recheck with your doctor as to whether this practice is still necessary and whether the antibiotic regimen should be changed.

Therapy for
Heart Disease

Some medications can be used to treat problems linked to heart disease, although the first line of therapy is usually a change in lifestyle. If weight loss, exercise, diet changes, hormone therapy, and smoking cessation are not effective, medications may help support these measures. They can reduce high blood pressure, lower LDL cholesterol and triglyceride levels, reduce inflammation, break up blood clots and lessen their ability to form, or replace the protective effects of estrogen. In some cases, procedures or surgery may be required. The procedures can be used for diagnosis, treatment, or both. Regardless of the form of therapy used, it is important to continue an exercise program and lifestyle geared to a healthy heart.

Medications

There are many types of medications used to combat high blood pressure, prevent or treat coronary artery disease, improve lipid levels, or try to stop a heart attack or stroke. These medications work in different ways, with varying degrees of effectiveness. Some work better in certain people than in others. A woman who has trouble with one type of medication or who experiences uncomfortable side effects can ask her doctor to recommend another medication.

Angiotensin-Converting Enzyme Inhibitors. Often the first course of drug therapy for lowering hypertension or heart failure, angiotensin-converting enzyme (ACE) inhibitors change the tone of the blood vessel walls and their ability to transport sodium. Mild side effects, such as coughing, are common; rash, loss of taste, fatigue, and headaches occur less often. A serious allergic reaction called angioedema occurs infrequently and is characterized by swelling in the face or throat. This condition requires immediate medical attention. Newer medications called angiotensin receptor blockers provide the same benefit but work through a different point in the system and may have fewer side effects. These medications should not be used during pregnancy.

Calcium Channel Blockers. By blocking calcium from entering special channels within muscle cells, calcium channel blockers reduce the force of contractions of muscle cells in blood vessels, preventing arteries from going into spasms. They cause coronary and other arteries to open, allowing better blood flow, lowering blood pressure. Calcium channel blockers are also used to treat coronary artery disease. These medications may cause constipation. They do not affect body or blood levels of calcium. Long-acting, or sustained-release calcium channel blockers, appear safe and effective, while the use of high-dose, short-activity (older) formulations should be avoided. This class of drugs is popular among women because of its

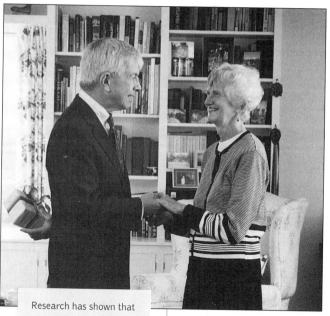

Research has shown that strong, long-term relationships, particularly those with a spouse or partner, can reduce your risk of developing heart disease.

low side effects; however, its association with other diseases is still being studied.

Diuretics. Long used for controlling blood pressure, diuretics in low doses cause dilation of blood vessels, which lowers blood pressure. When higher doses are used, water, along with sodium and potassium, is excreted. This action results in less volume of blood and fluids to be circulated, helpful in congestive heart failure and high blood pressure. Diuretics, however, can also deplete potassium and magnesium in the body and increase cholesterol levels. They are often used in combination with other medications.

Beta-Blockers. Used in the treatment of hypertension and coronary artery disease, beta-blockers block the effect of stimulants, such as adrenaline and stress, on your body. The heart rate slows and the heart muscle does not have to work as hard. Some forms of beta-blockers cause side effects, such as fatigue, cold hands and feet, depression, sleep disturbances, and decreased alertness. Newer products have fewer side effects. Although they can decrease the level of HDL, a cause for concern, beta-blockers are very powerful in reducing death rates from high blood pressure and coronary artery disease.

Alpha-Blockers. When alpha-blockers are used in the treatment of hypertension, blood vessels open and the lipid profile improves. Alpha-blockers decrease total and LDL cholesterol. Side effects include incontinence, weakness, fatigue, dizziness, and mild fluid retention. Nasal stuffiness also can occur.

Vasodilators. By relaxing the muscles of the walls of arteries, vasodilators can reduce blood pressure. Side effects include headaches, rapid heartbeat, and fluid retention.

Nitrates. Nitrates taken in the form of a pill held under the tongue, swallowed, or sprayed into the mouth, relieve angina and congestive heart failure by reducing the work of the heart and dilating arteries and veins. Nitrates are also available in patch or cream form. These medications may lose their effectiveness unless the body is given several hours each day to allow their effects to wear off.

Cholesterol-Lowering Drugs. Medications used to lower cholesterol include bile acid binding resins, nicotinic acid (niacin), and what are called the "statin" drugs—lovastatin, simvastatin, fluvastatin, pravastatin, and atorvastatin. By effectively lowering LDL cholesterol levels, and often raising HDL levels, these medications have been proven to prevent second heart attacks in women. Recent studies suggest they also reduce the risk of first heart attacks in women with elevated LDL. These medications should be used in combination with diet for lipid therapy. Nicotinic acid and the statins are metabolized in the liver and may cause liver enzyme abnormalities, and less commonly, muscle damage.

Thrombolytic Therapy. Medications, called thrombolytics or "clot busting" drugs are given at the first sign of a heart attack to break up a clot. Other drugs are given to prevent clotting or further clotting. Standard treatment is the drug aspirin, often combined with the blood thinning drug, heparin.

Medications called platelet inhibitors are now being used to reduce clotting by reducing platelets, the blood cells that clump together to form a clot. Aspirin is the best known of these drugs. Platelet inhibitors may also be used to prevent second heart attacks or strokes from occurring. It is important that the drug be given as soon as possible to limit damage to the heart or brain.

Antiarrhythmic Drugs. These medications are used to suppress abnormal heart-beats and help regulate the heart's rhythm. People taking antiarrhythmic drugs often need to have their dosage adjusted or blood level measured, and they may experience many side effects. These drugs are often reserved for more serious or life-threatening situations.

Cardiac Procedures and Devices

Heart disease may be treated with methods other than medication. These procedures, surgeries, and devices can be fairly routine and uncomplicated, such as inserting a pacemaker to regulate the heartbeat. They can also be major, such as complicated bypass surgery to reroute blood flow to the heart. Before any procedure or surgery is performed, it is important for a woman to be aware of the risks, benefits, alternatives, and possible outcomes so she can make an informed decision.

Pacemaker. When the heart's natural rhythm is disturbed for some reason, it may be necessary to correct the condition with a pacemaker. This small, battery-operated device takes over for the heart when the heart does not beat properly on its own, signaling it to contract and expand. It can be implanted under the skin as a permanent device or used outside the body on a temporary basis. Electrical signals are sent to the heart when needed, triggering it to beat. Pacemakers turn off automatically when they are not needed and start up again when the heart slows to a certain level.

Women who wear pacemakers must be aware that these devices can be affected by outside sources, such as very old microwave ovens (the new ones are safe), radio or radar transmitters, or electrical shavers. Also, some equipment used by doctors or dentists and airport security systems can affect pacemakers. It is a good idea to tell all health care providers if you have a heart condition or are using any devices, such as a pacemaker.

Defibrillator. Sometimes the heart loses its natural, regular rhythm and begins beating rapidly and irregularly. In severe cases, the heart may beat so rapidly it is unable to pump blood and merely quivers. An electronic device called a defibrillator can "jumpstart" the heart with an electric shock and restore the regular rhythm. A defibrillator can be placed externally on the chest, or it can be surgically implanted in women with recurrent problems. The use of this device helps reestablish the normal beating of the heart and is included routinely as part of emergency cardiac care services.

Cardiac Catheterization. Blocked blood vessels can be identified through cardiac catheterization, usually referred to as an angiogram. A long, hollow plastic tube called a catheter is inserted into a blood vessel through a tiny incision in the upper thigh or arm. After the catheter is moved through the blood vessel and into the heart, a dye is injected through it. This dye can be viewed with x-ray imaging, revealing the coronary arteries and any blockages. This is the standard test for determining blood vessel blockages.

Angioplasty. Narrowed or blocked coronary arteries can be widened with a procedure called angioplasty. The procedure may use balloons, lasers, or stents to open the arteries and keep them open. Angioplasty is often performed on those who have disease involving only one or two blocked arteries, where more involved surgery is not needed.

In balloon angioplasty, the cardiologist guides a catheter inside an artery to the point where it is clogged. Inside the catheter is a deflated balloon. Once it reaches the blocked area, the balloon is inflated, widening the opening. The balloon and catheter are then withdrawn.

In laser angioplasty, a high energy laser is placed inside the catheter. As the tip is guided to the blocked artery, the laser emits pulsating beams of light. The laser beam vaporizes the plaque inside the artery, breaking it down. Laser angioplasty is followed by balloon angioplasty.

A stent procedure may be used to help an artery opened by angioplasty to stay open. A stent is made of wire mesh that can be inserted into an artery to prop it open. The mesh tube is collapsed over a balloon that is guided by a catheter to the recently opened area. When the balloon inflates, the stent expands. It remains to support the opening after the balloon is withdrawn.

Angioplasty is not for everyone. It is best used for those who have significant blockage in limited areas. Complications are infrequent but can arise, such as a torn artery or a blood clot that can lead to a heart attack. Angioplasty, especially with laser or mechanical devices, is less effective in women than in men in clearing an obstruction, possibly because women's blood vessels are often smaller. Once the obstruction is cleared, however, the blood vessels are more likely to stay open in women than in men. Overall, the artery recloses in about 25 to 30 percent of those who have conventional angioplasty, a condition called restenosis. These individuals require a repeat procedure or more involved surgery.

Coronary Bypass Surgery. If one or more of the arteries supplying the heart become blocked they can be bypassed. Just as a highway bypass diverts traffic around a congested area, bypass surgery goes around the clogged arteries and creates new paths. A blood vessel used to make the new route (called a graft) is taken from another part of the body, usually a vein from the leg or an artery from inside the chest. The surgeon attaches one end of the graft to the aorta, the large artery leaving the heart, and the other end to the coronary artery beyond the area that is blocked. Blood flow is then restored through the new bypass.

Bypass surgery is major surgery, requiring opening the chest through the breast bone. The results are not permanent, and blockage can develop in the graft or in the joined areas within ten years of surgery. Women are twice as likely as men to die during or shortly after the procedure, possibly because they are older and more ill when they undergo it. For these reasons, women may consider other ways of treating heart disease before resorting to surgery, including lifestyle modifications and/or use of medications.

In selected cases, a new procedure called "keyhole" or minimally invasive bypass surgery can be used to bypass blockages in the coronary arteries without opening the breastbone. This procedure shows promise as a way to treat serious heart disease without a major procedure or a long hospitalization.

A **Positive** Outlook *for* **Women** *with* **Heart Disease**

Women who have a heart problem can benefit from long-term changes in their lifestyle that include a healthy, low-fat diet; regular, moderate exercise; reduction in stress; and in some cases, medication. Such lifestyle changes and medications can help control heart disease and even reverse some of the risk factors.

Cardiac rehabilitation involves a monitored program of exercise and lifestyle changes and is often recommended after a cardiac event. Although women are less likely to be referred for cardiac rehabilitation, those who participate in such programs do show significant improvement. However, women tend to have a higher dropout rate than men and should be encouraged to find and stay with a program they can follow.

Women with coronary heart disease are more likely to be depressed and anxious and less likely to resume sexual activity than men. It is natural to be distressed when faced with a chronic disease, but life does not end when heart disease develops. With a doctor's advice, women with a heart problem can enjoy activities of moderate intensity, including sex. Exercise stress testing is routinely done after heart attacks or cardiac procedures restoring blood flow and can help establish a safe level of activity that can be used as a general guide for daily living.

What *You* Can Do

The biggest threat to a woman's health is heart disease. Leading a healthy lifestyle will reduce your risk of heart disease as well as other life-threatening conditions. Following are the components of a lifestyle for a healthy heart:

- Eat a healthy diet high in complex carbohydrates and fiber and low in saturated fat and cholesterol. Make easy diet changes, such as switching from butter to soft margarine products or choosing low-fat frozen yogurt instead of ice cream.
- Engage in moderate exercise, such as walking, climbing stairs, or playing with young children, at least 20 to 30 minutes a day.
- Do not begin to smoke, or if you already smoke, get help in quitting.
- Achieve and maintain a reasonable weight for your body frame and height.
- Keep blood pressure and cholesterol levels down. Make sure you know your blood pressure and all your lipid values: LDL, triglyceride, and HDL.
- Get regular checkups, review and reduce your risk factors, know your family history, and discuss any signs of problems promptly with your doctor.

Reducing *Your* Risk *for* Cancer

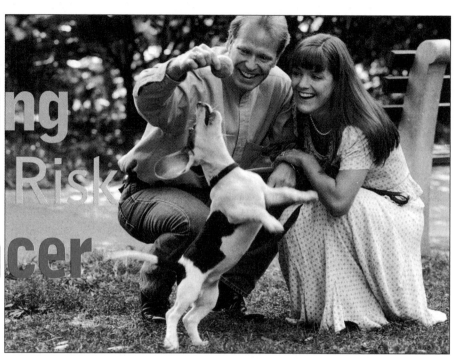

Many experts believe that a large number of cancer cases are preventable. This is welcome news in today's world, where cancer is undoubtedly the disease people fear most. It can be a devastating illness, claiming the lives of half a million Americans each year. There is no way, of course, to guarantee that you will never get cancer. No prevention strategy is foolproof. However, reducing your *risk* of developing cancer is something you *can* control—simply by how you live your life. Taking certain steps can make cancer less likely and can bolster your immune system to keep you healthy. In addition, getting regular checkups and screenings, and being aware of key symptoms, can help ensure that *should* cancer strike, it will be caught early, when it is most likely to be treated successfully.

On average, a person diagnosed with any cancer has about a 54 percent chance that the disease will be cured or controlled. And the outlook is far better with specific cancers, including breast, cervical, and uterine cancers. Cancer was a little-understood disease for centuries, but in recent years, researchers have made progress in unlocking its secrets. The cancer mortality rate for Americans of all ages fell nearly 3 percent between 1991 and 1995, a significant decrease and the first sustained decline since national records were initiated in the 1930s. This is in contrast to a 6.4 percent increase in cancer deaths between 1971 and 1990. For women, important signs of advances in the battle against cancer were a 6.3 percent drop in breast cancer deaths during the first half of the 1990s and a 9.7 percent drop in deaths from cervical and uterine cancers.

Cancer *Basics*

Cancer is a term applied to more than 150 diseases that can emerge anywhere on or in the body. All cancers have a key feature in common: uncontrolled cell growth.

Cells are the body's building blocks. Under a microscope, a normal body cell is round, oblong, or cubelike and has certain predictable features. All cells contain thousands of genes, which you inherit from your parents and pass on to your children. Genes, made up of DNA (deoxyribonucleic acid), determine all your physical, biochemical, and physiological traits. Genes also tell cells how to behave and when to divide. Cells replicate constantly, with old ones dying out as new ones are formed. Every so often, for reasons not well understood, a new cell is formed with an altered genetic code. This change, called a mutation, does not always lead to cancer, but it can increase a person's vulnerability.

Cancer experts (known as oncologists) believe that cancer arises not from one major event that turns a cell cancerous, but from multiple assaults. A vulnerable cell may be hit over and over by harmful substances, such as chemicals, viruses, and radiation, so that damage accumulates. Once a critical point is reached, the cancer "switch" turns on.

Recent research has focused on the role of so-called free radicals in the formation of cancer. Free radicals are molecules that have either a positive or negative chemical charge, unlike the majority of the molecules in the body that are balanced by positive and negative energies and are therefore neutral. Free radicals search for oppositely charged molecules to balance themselves, and they can damage healthy cells. If a free radical comes in contact with another radical, both are eliminated. If a free radical comes in contact with a nonradical, another free radical is produced. When your body is healthy and in balance, substances known as antioxidants prevent free radicals from getting out of control. (Antioxidants can be found in a variety of foods, especially fruits and vegetables.)

Cancer cells can be identified when examined under a microscope because they have abnormal DNA or chromosomes and may have irregular shapes and borders. How much they differ from normal cells can vary greatly, however. Some malignant cells are wildly atypical, while others still have many characteristics of healthy cells. Whereas normal cells grow and divide systematically, cancer cells multiply recklessly and start to infiltrate nearby healthy tissue. Unless they are stopped, these cancer cells will continue to spread, harming healthy organs and body systems.

Cancer *Prevention*

Sometimes it seems as if everything gives you cancer. When you hear reports about the increased risks of cancer from, for example, pollutants in the air and water, asbestos in old buildings, or secondhand smoke, preventing cancer may seem impossible.

Cancer actually stems from a complex interplay of genes and environmental factors. All cancer is genetic, in that it is triggered by altered genes, but only a small portion of cancer is inherited—passed from one generation to the next. In

TABLE 21.1

Incidence Rate of Specific Cancers per 100,000 Women, 1990–91

CANCER SITE	INCIDENCE
Breast	109.8
Lung	41.6
Colon and Rectum	39.5
Uterus	21.4
Ovary	15.0
Non-Hodgkin's Lymphoma	11.9
Melanoma	9.7
Cervix	8.6
Pancreas	7.8
Bladder	7.5
Leukemia	7.3
Thyroid	6.7
Mouth and Pharynx	6.1
Kidney	6.0
Brain and Nervous System	5.3
Stomach	4.9
Multiple Myeloma	3.4
Hodgkin's Disease	2.4
Esophagus	1.9
Liver	1.9
Larynx	1.6

Source: *Cancer Rates and Risks*, 1996. National Cancer Institute, Division of Cancer Prevention and Control. 1996.

fact, about 75 percent of cancers result mainly from external influences, according to a 1996 report from the Harvard Center for Cancer Prevention. Therefore, although many unknowns still exist, medical experts agree wholeheartedly on the guidelines for lowering your risk of cancer.

Smoking and Tobacco Use

The most important step you can take to prevent cancer is to quit smoking—or never start. Tobacco is the culprit in one-third of all cancer deaths in the United States. Forty-three different cancer-causing substances have been identified in tobacco smoke. Reports by the U.S. Public Health Service and international scientific organizations have documented that smoking is a major cause of cancers of the lung, larynx, mouth, and esophagus. Studies suggest that smoking may also be related to cancers of the breast, bladder, kidney, pancreas, cervix, stomach, liver, colon, and rectum.

Cigarettes are not the only problem: pipes, cigars, and smokeless tobacco are all linked to cancer as well. Women who are tempted to jump into the recent cigar trend should keep in mind that cigar smokers have an even higher risk for cancers of the oral cavity, larynx, pharynx, and esophagus than do cigarette smokers.

Each year, 66,000 American women are diagnosed with lung cancer and 53,000 women die from it. It has been estimated that at least 85 percent of lung cancer deaths are caused by smoking. What that means is at least 45,000 of the women who die annually from lung cancer may have avoided the disease in the first place simply by not smoking. Some studies suggest that women might be more susceptible to the carcinogens in tobacco smoke than men, making smoking even more dangerous for women.

Secondhand smoke, either exhaled or given off by cigarettes, pipes, and cigars, is estimated to be responsible for 3,000 lung cancer deaths in the United States each year. If you do not smoke but live with someone who does, your risk of developing lung cancer increases by about 30 percent. Likewise, if you smoke, that inflates the chances that nonsmokers you live with will develop cancer.

The younger you are when you start smoking, the harder it is to quit. The more you smoke each day, and the longer you have been smoking, the greater your risk of developing cancer and dying from it. Quitting rapidly improves your health (see Figure 1.2 in Chapter 1) and gradually reduces your cancer risk. After 10 to 15 years without cigarettes, your cancer risk and overall health status is likely to be about the same as that of women who never smoked. (For tips on quitting, see Chapter 13.)

A Healthy Diet

Experts estimate that poor diet accounts for one-third of cancer deaths, which means that its influence is equal to that of smoking. Even if you do not use tobacco, your dietary choices may be contributing greatly to your cancer risk.

There are many dietary components to the cancer risk equation, but since cancer develops very slowly, it is hard to know exactly what is safe and what puts you at increased risk. Some general principles seem clear, however, since both the American Cancer Society and the National Cancer Institute have issued nutrition recommendations for preventing cancer that emphasize cutting down on fats and increasing your intake of fiber, fruits, and vegetables.

Fats. Diets high in fat have been linked to an increased risk of breast, colon, and prostate cancers, and may also contribute to cancers of the pancreas, ovary, and uterus. Studies in countries where the population consumes a high percentage of fat consistently have shown a higher incidence of—and more people dying

Anticancer Eating Habits

Here are some dietary tips for reducing your cancer risk:

- **Lower your intake of dietary fat to 20 percent of your total daily calories. Limit consumption of meats, especially high-fat meats.**

- **Increase your intake of dietary fiber to at least 25 grams per day.**

- **Choose most of the foods you eat from plant sources. Eat five to nine servings of fruits and vegetables each day.**

- **Eat foods rich in vitamins A, C, and E.**

- **Cut down on foods that are smoked, salt-cured, or nitrate-cured, such as hot-dogs, ham, and bacon.**

- **Limit your consumption of alcohol to no more than one drink a day.**

- **Avoid overeating, and get plenty of exercise to help maintain your ideal weight.**

Antioxidants Help Prevent Cancer

Foods containing antioxidants may help protect people from cancer by fighting free radicals—unstable molecules that can damage cells.

Researchers have identified the following antioxidants: beta-carotene, which is converted to vitamin A by the body; vitamin C; vitamin E; and selenium, a trace element found in grains, meats, and fish. Many experts believe that eating five to nine servings per day of fruits and vegetables is sufficient for getting the antioxidants you need. Because plant foods are thought to contain hundreds of other potent anticancer compounds that have not been identified yet, dietary supplements should never be relied upon in place of a healthy, balanced diet.

from—breast, colon, and prostate cancers. Saturated fat, the kind most strongly associated with cancer, is found mainly in animal products, specifically beef, pork, poultry skin, whole milk, cheese, and butter.

The average person in the United States gets up to 40 percent of daily calories from fat, far more than is needed to meet the body's needs for energy and essential fatty acids. Experts generally agree that it is best to limit fat intake to no more than 20 percent of your total daily calories.

Fiber. While reducing the amount of fat you eat, you should increase your consumption of fruits, vegetables, grains, and dried beans. Each of these foods contains a substantial amount of fiber, which helps rid the body of toxins. Fiber, also known as "roughage," is especially important for sweeping carcinogens through the intestines, minimizing their contact with the colon's delicate lining. The National Cancer Institute estimates that if every American ate 20 to 30 grams of fiber each day, the incidence of colon cancer could drop by 50 percent.

Fruits and Vegetables. Populations that eat diets high in fruits and vegetables tend to have a lower cancer risk, not only because fruits and vegetables are a good source of fiber, but also because of the vitamins and nutrients they contain. Scientists do not yet know for sure which substances in fruits and vegetables protect against cancer, but they have increasing evidence that the following (from food sources) may be beneficial:

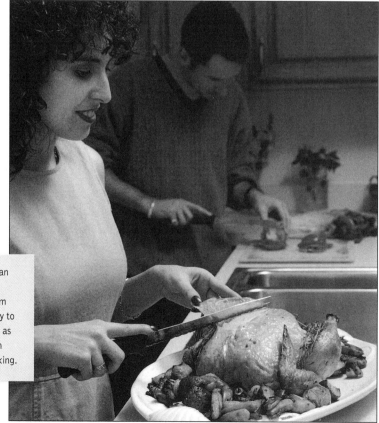

Reducing your intake of saturated fat is an important step in reducing your risk for cancer. For example, remove the skin from chicken before serving. It is not necessary to remove the skin before cooking, however, as studies have shown that fat from the skin does not migrate to the meat during cooking.

- **Vitamin A, beta-carotene, and other carotenoids.** These substances are found in dark yellow and orange vegetables and fruits (such as carrots, sweet potatoes, and cantaloupe) and also in dark green, leafy vegetables (such as broccoli, spinach, and collard greens).
- **Vitamin C.** Found mainly in fruits—especially citrus fruits and juices—and green vegetables, vitamin C is thought to protect against cancers of the esophagus, mouth, and stomach.
- **Vitamin E.** Considered one of the most effective antioxidants for ridding the body of free radicals, vitamin E is found in grains, meat and fish, nuts and seeds, and many vegetables. Studies suggest that vitamin E helps protect against cancers of the lung, breast, cervix, stomach, pancreas, and urinary tract. It also may help build up the immune system so the body can better fight cancer in its earliest stages.
- **Phytochemicals.** These compounds, produced by plants to keep them healthy, seem to help protect people, as well. Although phytochemical research is in its infancy, scientists have identified a number of these compounds that may be beneficial in preventing or fighting cancer. Dietary sources of phytochemicals include fruits, cruciferous vegetables (such as broccoli and cauliflower), garlic and onions, grains, and soy products (such as tofu, soymilk, or soybeans).

Cooking Methods. Research suggests that some cooking methods, especially grilling or frying meats at very high temperatures, create chemicals that might increase cancer risk. When fat burns during open-flame cooking, it forms polycyclic aromatic hydrocarbons (PAHs), which are known to be carcinogenic. The smoke from the burnt fat contains PAHs that settle on the meat. In 1996, scientists from the National Cancer Institute reported finding a higher rate of stomach cancer among people who generally ate their beef barbecued, as opposed to baked or roasted. High consumption of meats cooked at high temperatures has also been linked to colorectal cancer.

Little is known about how often you have to eat grilled or fried meats for it to be harmful. An occasional barbecue is probably fine, but as a rule it is better to use lower-temperature cooking methods for meats, such as steaming, baking, poaching, braising, microwaving, or stewing.

Preservatives. Nitrates and nitrites are chemicals added to some cured foods to keep them from spoiling. Nitrates are commonly found in salt-cured meats, such as ham, bacon, bologna, hot dogs, and sausage; smoked foods, including turkey and salmon; and salt-pickled meats and vegetables.

The bacteria in your mouth convert the nitrates to nitrites. Nitrates also spontaneously turn into nitrites at room temperature. When nitrites combine with other nitrogen-containing compounds in your stomach they form nitrosamines, a known carcinogen thought to contribute to stomach and esophageal cancers.

Alcohol. An occasional vodka tonic or glass of Chardonnay probably will not give you cancer, but some experts believe that too much alcohol may increase your cancer risk. The Harvard School of Public Health estimates that two drinks a day raises a woman's odds of getting cancer by 25 percent, and some epidemiologists think the risk increases by as much as 40 percent. Women who drink more than two drinks a day have an increased incidence of breast cancer.

Anticancer Cooking Habits

How you prepare food can reduce cancer risk:

- **Trim all visible fat from meats before and after cooking.**
- **Before or after cooking chicken, remove the skin.**
- **Instead of grilling or frying, cook meats with lower-temperature methods, such as roasting, baking, steaming, poaching, stewing, or microwaving. Drain the fat from the pan after cooking. When broiling meats, place them at a distance from the heat source.**
- **Use small amounts of cooking spray instead of oils, butter, or grease, and use nonstick cookware to avoid extra fat.**
- **Season meats, fish, and vegetables with herbs, spices, and lemon juice rather than sauces containing fat.**

Researchers have also reported a link between excessive alcohol consumption and colorectal cancer. Furthermore, the combination of alcohol and tobacco markedly increases a smoker's risk of developing cancers in the mouth, pharynx, esophagus, and larynx.

Hazards at Work

Occupational hazards are estimated to account for at least four percent of cancer deaths. Workers in a wide range of occupations are exposed to carcinogens, from metal and ceramics workers who come in contact with arsenic, to waitresses who constantly breathe secondhand smoke. If you work with chemicals or other dangerous substances, be sure you learn all you can about their possible harmful effects and take all possible safety precautions.

Exercise

The Centers for Disease Control and Prevention estimates that 60 percent of Americans lead sedentary lives. Given that exercise can help ward off many illnesses, including the nation's number one killer, heart disease, it is unfortunate that so many shun even moderate exercise. Exercise may reduce the risk of cancer by increasing the numbers of "natural killer cells," a type of immune-system cell that attacks infections and abnormal cells. One study found that exercise increased the level of natural killer cells in the blood threefold.

Exercise also promotes contraction of the bowel, helping it to rid the body more quickly of harmful wastes and carcinogens. Exercise may also reduce the risk of gynecological cancers by lowering levels of hormones that can stimulate abnormal cell growth. Since obesity is a risk factor for many cancers, weight control is another good reason to exercise as a way of preventing disease.

The Mind-Body Link

The roles that stress, depression, emotions, and coping styles play in cancer risk is an area of controversy. Psychological theories of cancer have been proposed since the second century, when the Greek physician Galen observed that melancholy women developed breast cancer more often than other women.

In 1959, research psychologist Lawrence LeShan interviewed more than 250 cancer patients and compared them with 150 healthy people to determine the role of personality and emotions in cancer. His study found that 77 percent of the cancer patients had lost a significant person in their lives (spouse, child, or parent) before being diagnosed with cancer, compared with only 14 percent of the healthy people in the control group. He also found that 64 percent were unable to express hostility, twice the number in the control group. Seventy-nine percent had feelings of self-dislike and self-distrust, compared with 34 percent in the control group. Thirty-eight percent felt tension in their relationship with one or both parents, compared with 12 percent in the control group. This led to theories about a so-called "cancer personality," characterized by bottled-up anger and frustration.

Even experts who discount the existence of a "cancer personality" speculate that factors related to stress can promote cancer and other diseases. For example, extreme emotions might suppress the immune system, giving cancer cells a better environment in which to take root. Studies have shown that stressful events and depression can reduce levels of the cells that activate the immune system. It is an established fact that people with more social ties and a strong support network have a lower death rate from cancer—and other diseases. Another theory is that people under stress engage in more unhealthy behaviors, such as smoking and drinking, which promote cancer in other ways.

Research is still inconclusive about how to use the mind-body connection to prevent cancer. No concrete evidence has been collected to show that feeling good about yourself and keeping stress levels low will prevent you from getting cancer. But there is no question that learning to handle stress more effectively can improve the overall quality of your life—a benefit in itself.

Assessing Hereditary Risk

In some cancers, heredity plays a strong role. For example, if you have immediate family members—a mother, sister, or daughter—with ovarian cancer, you are at greater risk than a woman whose family members have not had ovarian cancer, and your risk is higher if multiple relatives have ovarian cancer. But having a family history of cancer does not mean you are certain to inherit the disease. Knowing that you may be at risk for developing a certain cancer should make you more vigilant about leading a lifestyle that promotes good health and adhering more closely to screening recommendations for that type of cancer.

Only a handful of genes have actually been identified as causing a predisposition to cancer. Those that have been most highly publicized are mutations of tumor suppressor genes—genes that normally restrain cell growth, but when lost or altered by mutation, allow cells to grow uncontrolled. Mutations of the gene BRCA1 or BRCA2 have been linked with higher rates of breast cancer. Studies of families with a very high incidence of breast cancer and a BRCA1 gene mutation suggest that the lifetime risk may reach 85 percent for the development of breast cancer.

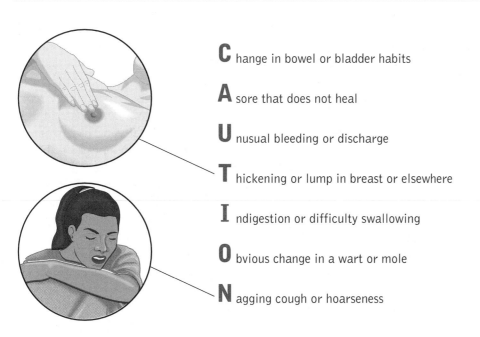

C hange in bowel or bladder habits

A sore that does not heal

U nusual bleeding or discharge

T hickening or lump in breast or elsewhere

I ndigestion or difficulty swallowing

O bvious change in a wart or mole

N agging cough or hoarseness

FIGURE 21.1
The Warning Signs of Cancer
The American Cancer Society identifies these seven warning signs of cancer. If you experience any of these symptoms, see your doctor immediately.

Right now, very few tests are available to pinpoint whether a person carries a mutation that predisposes her to a specific cancer. However, scientists are closing in on the genes for many cancers and are making new discoveries all the time. If your family history suggests a very high risk of breast, ovarian, or colon cancer, there are tests to assess your risk. It is important to keep in mind that these tests deal in probabilities, not certainties.

A negative test can be reassuring and can eliminate the need for frequent tests given to very high-risk people, such as annual colonoscopy to look for colon cancer. A positive test, on the other hand, gives you the opportunity to receive expert counseling and to make decisions that reduce your risk. Genetic counselors play a vital role in predictive testing, making sure that you have balanced information and are psychologically prepared to deal with a positive result. As gene research progresses, scientists hope to develop better tools for diagnosis and treatment.

Genetic screening for mutations associated with high cancer risk is not routinely offered to patients at this time. The decision to have genetic screening should be made with careful consideration of all options. This kind of testing is mainly available at large research centers, although a few commercial laboratories offer testing. If you have a very strong family history—a number of close relatives who have had cancer, especially at a young age and in more than one generation—talk with your doctor. For information about genetic testing and counseling and a listing of centers in your area, call the Cancer Information Service (800-4-CANCER) sponsored by the National Cancer Institute.

Major Types of *Cancer* That *Affect* Women

Although over 150 types of cancer have been identified, the seven most common types of cancer in American women are: breast cancer, lung cancer, colorectal cancer, uterine and cervical cancers, ovarian cancer, and skin cancer. These common cancers are discussed in detail below. For information on other types of cancer, contact the American Cancer Society, or discuss your concerns with your doctor.

Breast Cancer

The thought of breast cancer terrifies most women. Many are more afraid of it than of heart disease, which is actually the top killer of American women. Thanks to better awareness and screening methods, many more cases of breast cancer are being caught at an early, treatable stage. In fact, more than 80 percent of women who find breast cancer in its earliest stage will be cured. Still, there is good reason to be anxious about breast cancer. Its incidence keeps rising, and no one is sure why. Current estimates are that it will strike one out of every nine women who live to age 85.

Researchers have learned a great deal about breast cancer detection and treatment, but much remains unknown, especially about its causes. Genetics, hormones, and diet all appear to play a role. The risk of breast cancer also increases with age, with most cases occurring in women over the age of 50.

Women's breasts are made up primarily of glandular tissue and fat. Inside are clusters of milk-producing glands and a system of ducts for storing milk and channeling it to the nipple. The breasts change continually throughout life and are affected by hormones, pregnancy, menopause, and age. Many women detect worrisome lumps or changes at one time or another, but most do not indicate cancer. Glandular breast tissue tends to be "lumpy" by nature. The reason that doctors promote monthly breast self-examinations is that, if you are familiar with your breasts' normal landscape, it will be easier for you to detect changes that warrant investigation.

The main symptom of breast cancer is a lump or thickening in or near the breast or in the underarm area. It also may show itself as a change in the size or shape of the breast, a discharge from the nipple, or a change in the color or texture of the skin of the breast, areola, or nipple. Some part of the breast may appear dimpled, puckered, or scaly. If you find something that worries you, keep in mind that most breast lumps and changes are not cancer. However, it is essential to make an appointment with your doctor right away so you can be evaluated quickly.

Risk Factors. The following are the common risk factors associated with breast cancer:

- **Increasing age.** Increasing age is the single most important risk factor for developing breast cancer—after female gender. (Breast cancer can strike men but is rare.) It is considered unusual in women under the age of 40. A woman's chance of developing breast cancer before age 40 is 1 in 50, while half of breast cancer cases occur in women 65 years and older.
- **Family history of breast cancer.** If any member of your extended family is diagnosed with breast cancer, you may be at increased risk. But if a first-degree relative (mother, sister, or daughter) has been diagnosed with breast cancer, you are definitely at increased risk, especially if the relative was diagnosed before she reached menopause. Up to 30 percent of breast cancer patients have a history of or close relative with the disease. A woman—Joan, for example—with no family history of breast cancer has a relative risk (called RR) of 1.0, which means her risk is equal to the risk of the general population. Joan's RR is increased to 1.8 if her mother has breast cancer, meaning her risk is 1.8 times the risk of someone in the general population whose mother did not have breast cancer. Her RR is 2.3 if her sister has breast cancer, 2.1 if her mother has breast cancer before age 40, and 2.5 if both her mother and sister have breast cancer.

  About 5 to 10 percent of breast cancers are believed to be inherited. Hereditary breast cancer tends to strike at younger ages, is more likely to strike both breasts, and often appears in multiple family members over three or more generations. It can be passed down through either the mother's or the father's side of the family. Researchers have determined that abnormalities in either of two genes—BRCA1 and BRCA2—are estimated to account for 40 to 50 percent of all hereditary breast cancers. If a woman is found to have an abnormality in one of these genes, detectable by genetic screening tests, her risk is very high. Whether she will actually develop breast cancer, however, is impossible to predict.

wellness **tip**

Read as much as you can about breast changes and breast care so you know which questions to ask your doctor when you go for an examination.

- **A personal history of breast cancer.** If a woman has had invasive or *in situ* (localized, noninvasive) breast cancer, her risk of developing a new breast cancer in any remaining breast tissue in either breast increases by as much as one percent per year.

- **History of benign or fibrocystic breast disease** (also known as "lumpy breasts"). There are many kinds of benign breast changes, including cysts. These changes are *not* associated with an increased risk of cancer, unless a biopsy shows atypical hyperplasia, a condition marked by excessive cell growth.

- **Natural hormonal factors.** Some scientists believe that since hormones promote cell division in breast tissue, they increase the potential for mutations and eventual cancer. Having your first menstrual period before age 12 or having a late menopause theoretically increases your lifetime hormone exposure and could increase your breast cancer risk. Whether this is because of the actual level of hormones present or the actual number of menstrual cycles in a woman's lifetime is unclear. Pregnancy and the timing of pregnancy may also play a role. For example, women who have never been pregnant or have not carried a pregnancy to term before the age of 30 have statistically higher breast cancer rates, for reasons that are unclear at this time.

- **Taking the oral contraceptive pill.** Concerns about whether birth control pills increase a woman's risk of breast cancer have been raised since the pill was introduced in 1961. Several long-term studies with large numbers of participants have been inconclusive. At this point in time, physicians generally agree that the benefits of oral contraception outweigh any possible increase in risk— especially with today's birth control pills, which contain much lower doses of hormone than previous pills contained.

- **Hormone replacement therapy.** Few topics have generated more controversy in breast cancer research than the area of postmenopausal hormone replacement therapy (HRT). At this time, there are not many clear-cut answers for women considering taking estrogen; it is not known what dose or duration of therapy is associated with optimal benefit and lowest risk. Numerous long-term studies are in progress that should shed some light on current practice. Until that data can be examined, the following generalizations can be used for guidance:

  ➤ If you already have breast cancer, estrogen may cause your cancer to grow. On the other hand, some long-term breast cancer survivors with significant cardiac risk or disease are now considering the risks and alternatives of estrogen therapy because of the cardiovascular protection it provides.

  ➤ If you have a strong family history of breast cancer, you may incur some additional risk by using estrogen therapy.

  ➤ High-dose estrogen therapy appears to increase risk more than low-dose estrogen therapy.

  ➤ Long-term use may be associated with greater risk, but experts do not presently have recommendations for how long estrogen therapy should be used to maximize cardiovascular and other protective effects while limiting breast cancer risk. Virtually all studies show no increased risk with less that five years of use.

  ➤ Women who use estrogen therapy live longer. Increased age is associated with increased risk for developing breast cancer.

➤ Quality-of-life issues need to be part of this important debate—especially since there is a rapid accumulation of data about the role of estrogen in the prevention of Alzheimer's disease, coronary heart disease, and other conditions, such as osteoporosis, that affect women's later years. For example, a woman's chances of dying from complications of hip fracture (one woman in five breaks a hip) are the same as her risk of dying from breast cancer.

- **Radiation therapy.** Any medical condition that requires large doses of radiation to the chest increases breast cancer risk.
- **Dense breast tissue in women age 45 or older.** Women in this age group who have at least 75 percent dense breast tissue on a mammogram appear to have increased risk, perhaps because usual screening techniques are less helpful in this group. Women on hormone replacement have denser breasts, which may be related to higher hormone levels.
- **Severe obesity and high-fat diet.** Being more than 40 percent over your ideal weight and eating high-fat foods are thought to promote the development of breast cancer. A 1991 study by researchers at the University of Toronto found that women whose fat intake represented 47 percent of their daily calories were 50 percent more likely to develop breast cancer than women whose fat intake was limited to 30 percent of their daily calories. Ongoing research on low-fat diets limited to less than 15 percent of calories per day may reveal whether low-fat diets reduce breast cancer risk.
- **Excessive alcohol use.** A number of studies suggest there is a link between alcohol consumption and breast cancer. Scientists speculate that alcohol may promote breast cancer by elevating levels of estrogen in the body or by causing certain mammary gland cells to proliferate.

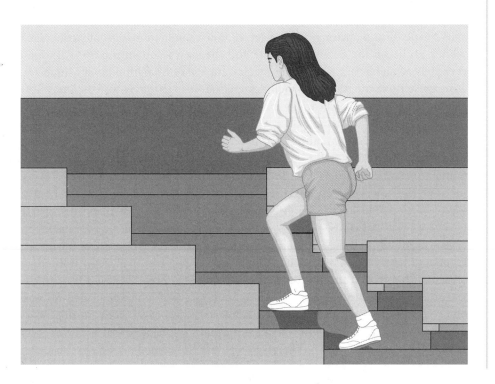

FIGURE 21.2

Lower Your Breast Cancer Risk
A recent study found that women who exercised more than four hours each week had a 37% lower breast cancer risk than women who did not exercise.

Breast Cancer Screening Guidelines

The following recommendations are for women who have an average risk of breast cancer:

Aged 20 to 39
- **Monthly breast self-examination**
- **Clinical breast examination by a doctor or nurse every three years**

Aged 40 and Above
- **Monthly breast self-examination**
- **Annual mammogram**
- **Annual clinical breast examination by a doctor or nurse, conducted close to the time of the mammogram**

Source: American Cancer Society.

Prevention Tips. Given the conflicting results from breast cancer research over the past ten years, it is difficult to provide clear-cut prevention tips. The following suggestions are healthful guides that *may* decrease your risk and promote your overall health:

- Eat a low-fat diet that derives no more than 20 percent of your daily calories from fat.
- Limit alcohol intake to three drinks or fewer per week.
- Get regular exercise.
- Maintain a lean body.
- Conduct monthly breast self-examinations and seek prompt medical attention for abnormalities.
- Talk to your doctor about what combination of clinical breast examination and screening mammograms is best for you.

Screening. With new treatment techniques, almost 90 percent of women who discover their breast cancer while it is still in its earliest stages can be cured of the disease. Screening for early breast cancer, therefore, is crucial. For breast cancer to be detected in its earliest stages, it is important to make use of all three screening methods.

Self-Examinations. All women aged 20 and over should perform breast self-examinations every month. Checking your breasts regularly helps you become familiar with their natural feel and shape, and you can more easily identify changes that may be of concern. If you notice a lump or change in your breast, call your doctor immediately.

Clinical Breast Examinations. Unless you are at high risk, you should have a clinical breast examination by your doctor every three years if you are between ages 20 and 40 and once a year after age 40. The examination is usually conducted while you lie on the examining table and then with you sitting up. Although every physician has her own technique, the clinical examination is very similar to a breast self-examination and includes a visual inspection as well as a physical examination of the breasts and adjacent lymph nodes.

Mammograms. A mammogram can detect many breast tumors when they are very small, often years before tumors are big enough to feel. During a mammogram, a technician flattens each breast between two plastic plates, one an x-ray tube and the other an x-ray cassette. Two views are usually taken of each breast: top to bottom and side to side. Mammograms should be performed by properly trained x-ray technicians on high-quality, low-dose equipment. Be sure the facility is accredited by the American College of Radiology. To learn of approved mammography centers near you, call either the American College of Radiology at 800-ACR-LINE or the National Cancer Institute at 800-4-CANCER.

Studies have shown that regular mammograms for women aged 50 and older identify the greatest number of breast cancer cases because this postmenopausal group is where the most cases occur. Postmenopausal breast cancers tend to be slow-growing, and therefore regularly scheduled mammograms catch these tumors in their early stages.

Conducting a Breast Self-Examination

Inspecting your breasts monthly for possible signs of cancer is an important screening technique. Most breast lumps are found by women themselves, not their doctors. Alert your doctor to any changes you detect. Follow these steps when conducting a breast self-examination:

- Each month, examine your breasts five to seven days after your menstrual period starts; this is when they are likely to be less tender or swollen. If you have already reached menopause or are pregnant or lactating, pick a day of the month and stick to it. If you have undergone a hysterectomy but still have functioning ovaries, avoid times when your breasts are bloated or tender.
- Stand in front of a mirror and look at both breasts. Make sure the contour of the skin is normal, that there is no dimpling or puckering, and that there has been no change in nipple appearance or direction. Stretch your arms over your head and check to see if this brings out any changes.
- With hands on hips, lean your shoulders forward toward the mirror and look for the same signs.
- Now examine the feel of your breasts while showering or bathing. Your fingers glide more easily over wet, soapy skin, making it easier to detect small lumps or changes. Rotate your three middle fingers slowly around each breast, starting at the 12 o'clock position and moving in ever-increasing concentric circles outward. Move your fingers from side to side and top to bottom, carefully feeling every part of each breast and well up into your armpits. A cancerous tumor may be a single, hard lump or a thickening. It is usually painless, but not always.
- Lie flat on your back with a pillow under one shoulder and that arm raised over your head. This flattens the breast and allows easier examination. Rotate your fingers as in the previous step, and repeat on the other breast.
- For an illustration of a breast self-examination, turn to Figure 2.3 on page 29.

Premenopausal breast cancer screening is also very important. Tumors in younger women tend to show faster growth, so the interval between when these tumors can first be detected with a mammogram and when they have spread to the lymph nodes is shorter. For this reason, annual screening for high risk women in their forties has been shown to reduce cancer deaths by 16 percent.

Remember that up to 15 percent of breast cancers do not show up on mammograms until they are far advanced, so breast self-examination and clinical breast examinations are essential in identifying all breast tumors as early as possible.

Lung Cancer

From 1950 to 1988, the death rate from lung cancer jumped fivefold in women—a trend clearly linked to an increase in the number of woman smokers since the 1940s. Today, nearly one-quarter of adult women in the United States smoke. Lung cancer accounts for about 11 percent of all cancer cases among women in the United States, and because of its low cure rate, it is responsible for

wellness **tip**

If you need help to quit smoking, call your local chapter of the American Cancer Society for materials and referrals to smoking cessation programs and support groups. Products such as the nicotine patch and chewing gum are available to help you wean yourself from smoking, and medications can help you handle nicotine withdrawal. See Chapter 13 for more information on how to quit smoking.

21 percent of all cancer deaths in women. The overall five-year survival rate is only 13 percent.

Cigarette smoking is the major cause of lung cancer. The risk of dying from lung cancer is 12 times higher among woman smokers than among those who have never smoked. Other causes include pipe and cigar smoking, secondhand smoke, and exposure to industrial compounds such as asbestos. Keep in mind that brief periods of contact with pollutants is unlikely to lead to lung cancer—the problem is prolonged exposure, or the combination of smoking and industrial exposure.

Common symptoms of lung cancer include a persistent cough, unexplained shortness of breath, and chronic chest pain. You may also develop hoarseness and an increase in mucous secretions from the lungs. Bloody sputum, difficulty swallowing, and recurrent lung infections are other possible signs. Sometimes the face, neck, or upper extremities swell from pressure on blood vessels caused by the cancer.

Risk Factors. The following risk factors have been closely associated with lung cancer:

- **Smoking.** Cigarettes, pipes, and cigars have all been implicated in lung cancer. A history of heavy smoking puts you at especially high risk.
- **Exposure to industrial agents.** Some substances known to be harmful are asbestos, nickel, chromium compounds, chloromethyl ether, beryllium, and arsenic.
- **Having asbestos fibers in your home or workplace.** Asbestos was widely used for insulation in walls, around pipes, and in shingles, siding, and tiles between 1920 and 1970. Asbestos is only a danger when it crumbles or is damaged and the tiny fibers escape into the air. Once you inhale them, they can become lodged in lung tissue. Smokers who are exposed to asbestos are 50 times more likely to develop lung cancer than nonsmokers who are exposed to asbestos.
- **Radon.** An odorless, colorless gas produced by the radioactive decay of radium and uranium in the earth's crust, radon has also been implicated in about ten percent of lung cancer deaths. Radon seeps into some homes through cracks in the foundation, holes for sump pumps, or floor drains.
- **Secondhand smoke.** If you are a nonsmoker, your exposure to tobacco smoke from living with a smoker or chronic exposure to smokers in your workplace is estimated to raise your lung cancer risk by one-third.
- **Radiation.** High levels of radiation exposure, including from treatment of any disease that requires large doses of radiation to the chest, increases lung cancer risk.
- **Health history.** A family history of lung cancer puts you at increased risk, as does a personal history of emphysema, chronic bronchitis, or chronic obstructive pulmonary disease.

Prevention Tips. It is believed that most lung cancer is caused by environmental factors, making it, in many cases, a preventable form of cancer. Follow these tips to reduce your risk of lung cancer:

- **Avoid all forms of tobacco.** If you quit smoking, after ten years your risk of developing lung cancer drops to about half that of people who continue to smoke, and continues to fall the longer you remain a nonsmoker.
- **If anyone in your household smokes, ask them to smoke outdoors or near an open window or in an enclosed space with full ventilation.** Remove ashtrays to deter visitors from smoking. If smoking is allowed in your workplace, ask to change to a nonsmoking area or as far away from smokers as possible. If you are around smoke, keep air circulating with fans and open windows. Many employers—including the federal government—are cracking down on smoking in the workplace. Try giving your employer reports on the harmful effects of secondhand smoke; if that fails, consider changing jobs.
- **Have your home tested for radon.** If high levels are found, steps you can take include increasing the amount of ventilation, covering exposed earth in the basement and other areas, sealing cracks and openings, depressurization, and suctioning radon away from the house. If you want to hire a professional, you can call your state radon agency for recommendations.
- **Check for asbestos in your home, especially tears, flaking, and dislodged chunks.** If you suspect a problem, call an expert for assistance. Do not touch it or try to remove it on your own.

Screening. Lung cancer is difficult to detect at an early stage. Tests, such as examining sputum for malignant cells and regular chest x-rays, have not proved beneficial for people with no symptoms or clear-cut risks. If you are a smoker or have other risk factors for lung cancer, most experts recommend an annual chest x-ray. Some doctors use sputum tests, as well, in which you cough up mucous that is then studied under a microscope for abnormal cells. It is inexpensive and painless but picks up less than half of lung cancer cases. Accuracy of the sputum test increases when done in conjunction with chest x-rays.

Colorectal Cancer

Although the incidence of cancer of the colon and rectum has increased since 1973, insights into the nature of colorectal cancer and how to prevent it have also increased. A growing body of evidence points to the key role of diet in lowering your risk for colorectal cancer.

The colon, also called the bowel or large intestine, is about six feet long and consists of five main sections that curve around the lower abdomen. The rectum is the final five inches of the colon, just above the anus. Digestion begins in the stomach, but is completed in the small intestine. The small intestine empties indigestible waste into the colon. As the waste and digestive fluid are propelled through the colon by muscular contractions, much of the water and mineral content is reabsorbed, leaving behind semi-solid fecal material, containing billions of bacteria, which will be passed at the next bowel movement.

The colon's inner lining, or mucosa, forms new cells and sloughs off cells injured in the process of digestion every four to five days. When the mechanisms that regulate mucosal cell repair become unbalanced, new cells grow faster than old cells can be discarded, producing small growths called polyps. Researchers believe that up to 50 percent of the American population over the age of 40 has polyps. Most are benign, but at least one type, adenomatous polyps, has 1

wellness
warning

A study of more than 88,000 American nurses (called the Nurses Health Study) found that the more red meat consumed — beef, lamb, and pork — the higher the risk of colon cancer. Women who ate red meat daily were found to be two to three times more likely to develop colon cancer than women who ate it less than once a month.

chance in 20 of developing into cancer. Adenomatous polyps generally occur in clusters and take from five to ten years to turn into cancer. Ninety-nine percent of all colorectal cancers evolve from polyps.

Common symptoms of colorectal cancer include cramping, gas pains, bloating, and chronic, unexplained fatigue. You may notice a sudden change in your elimination patterns, such as constipation, diarrhea, or unusually narrow stools. Dark red or bright red blood in your stool is also a possible sign. Another common symptom is having a "full" feeling, even after bowel movements.

Risk Factors. If you recognize any of the following risk factors as pertaining to you, it is recommended that you speak to your physician about screening for colorectal cancer:

- **Hereditary cancer syndromes.** Certain syndromes that run in families increase the risk of adult colon cancer, such as hereditary nonpolyposis colorectal cancer (HNPCC), also known as Lynch syndrome I or II. Another rare, inherited disorder, familial adenomatous polyposis, causes thousands of potentially cancerous polyps to arise, usually around puberty. Other hereditary problems that increase risk are Gardner's syndrome, Turcot's syndrome, and Oldfield's syndrome. Ask your doctor about these syndromes.
- **Ethnic origin.** About six percent of Ashkenazi Jews (Jews of eastern European descent) carry a gene that increases the risk of developing colon cancer.
- **Personal history.** Any of the following can increase the chance of developing colorectal cancer: inflammatory bowel diseases (such as ulcerative colitis or Crohn's disease); breast cancer; ovarian cancer; uterine cancer; or adenomatous polyps.
- **A high-fat, low-fiber diet.** Colorectal cancer is rare in societies where people typically eat little fat and many fruits, vegetables, and grains. Experts theorize that the chemicals in fat can harm the mucosa, increase the level of harsh bile salts in the colon, and may foster the growth of cancer-promoting bacteria. Fiber may guard against colon cancer by neutralizing cancer-promoting materials, breaking down bacteria, and producing a soft stool that moves through the bowel quickly, thus reducing exposure to cancer-causing agents.
- **Obesity and sedentary lifestyle.** More than a dozen studies have shown that low physical activity and obesity are clearly associated with colon cancer.
- **Smoking.** In 1994, a report from the Nurses Health Study showed an increased risk of colorectal cancer among women who smoked. Among women who smoked a pack a day for more than ten years, the risk more than doubled.
- **Excessive alcohol use.** A study reported in 1990 found that just one drink a day raises a person's risk of colorectal cancer by five percent.

Prevention Tips. Although some colorectal cancer is hereditary, there are many steps that women with an average risk can take to prevent the disease:

- Commit to a low-fat, high-fiber diet rich in fruits and vegetables.
- Do not smoke.
- Drink alcohol in moderation, or do not drink at all.

- Consume at least 800 milligrams of calcium per day, which is believed to protect the mucosa from harmful compounds in the stool.
- Get plenty of exercise, which helps food pass through the intestines faster, limiting exposure to potential carcinogens in digestive waste.
- Consider postmenopausal hormone replacement therapy (HRT). Researchers do not understand why, but the incidence of colon and rectal cancers is lower in women on HRT.
- Consider low dose aspirin use. Several studies have shown that women who use aspirin products several times a week have a lower incidence of colon cancer. Check with your doctor regarding this and other medication options.

Screening. In the absence of hereditary risk factors, colorectal cancer is uncommon in women under the age of 40. Beginning about age 40, women are advised to begin regular screening:

- **Digital rectal examination.** A digital rectal examination is recommended starting at age 40. This examination, in which your doctor inserts a gloved, lubricated finger into the rectum to feel for nodules or masses, detects about ten percent of colorectal cancers before symptoms arise.
- **Stool blood tests.** By age 50 you should start having annual stool blood tests, also called the fecal occult blood test. For this test, you are given a set of three cards to take home with you, on which you place a smear of fecal material on three successive days. You close up the cards and mail or return them to your physician, who has them analyzed. Signs of blood in the samples may indicate conditions other than cancer. The sensitivity of this test is sometimes unpredictable: various studies have shown the accuracy to be as low as 26 percent and as high as 99 percent. Also, the test can miss some polyps and cancers that do not always produce bleeding. Still, it can be a useful, easy tool for early detection.
- **Sigmoidoscopy.** This ten-minute procedure, which allows your physician to see inside part of the colon, is recommended every three to five years after age 50. A flexible lighted instrument called a sigmoidoscope is inserted into the rectum and the end of the colon, where up to 45 percent of colorectal cancers and polyps form. As you lie on your side on an examining table, the instrument transmits images from inside the colon to a screen. Although it may produce mild cramping, the procedure is not painful and requires no anesthesia.
- **Colonoscopy.** People at high risk for colon cancer because of personal or family history may be screened with colonoscopy every year or two. For this examination, you are sedated and the physician inserts into your colon a longer fiber-optic viewing instrument, capable of examining the entire colon. Many experts feel that colonoscopy may have a place in routine screening. However, consensus on recommending this technique has not been reached.
- **Barium enema.** Also for high-risk people, this is an x-ray examination in which barium is pumped into the colon to highlight suspicious areas.

Uterine and Cervical Cancers

The uterus is made up of a muscular outer layer called the myometrium and an inner layer called the endometrium. At the lower end of the uterus is the cervix, a cylindrical segment of tissue that opens into the vagina. Cancer of the uterus,

wellness **tip**

Be sure to see your doc-
tor about any abnormal
vaginal bleeding. It is
usually not anything serious, but having irregularities checked out can reassure you that nothing is
wrong, or can ensure
early detection of cancers
while they are highly
curable.

also known as endometrial cancer, is the most common gynecological cancer in the United States, affecting about 31,000 women each year. Both uterine and cervical cancers are highly curable when caught early.

Several conditions of the uterus cause disturbing symptoms. Many women develop fibroid tumors in the uterus, which are not associated with an increase in cancer risk. Fibroid tumors are benign, but they often cause heavy menstrual bleeding or a feeling of pelvic fullness, which are disturbing symptoms for women.

Endometrial hyperplasia is another benign condition of the uterus, but it can progress to endometrial cancer if left untreated. The most common symptom associated with both endometrial hyperplasia and endometrial cancer is abnormal bleeding. Bleeding between menstrual periods or any postmenopausal bleeding should be reported to your doctor.

If the doctor suspects that you have endometrial hyperplasia, she may use a pelvic ultrasound to detect uterine fibroids or to measure the thickness of the endometrium. The definitive test for hyperplasia, however, is done by a pathologist, who examines endometrial cells under a microscope for signs of abnormalities. A sampling of endometrial cells is obtained either by endometrial biopsy or by dilation and curettage (D and C).

The endometrial biopsy is a simple office procedure associated with minimal menstrual-like cramps. The cervix is cleansed, then minimally dilated to allow passage of a tiny suction or scraping instrument that dislodges and collects cells from the lining of the uterus. In some postmenopausal women, the cervix is too atrophied to permit this simple office procedure, so a minor surgical procedure (D and C) must be done to allow endometrial sampling. D and C may also be done in women who have suspicious-looking endometrial biopsies and a more thorough endometrial sampling is needed.

Common conditions that affect the cervix range from infections to benign growths, called cervical polyps, to cervical dyplasia, now called cervical intraepithelial neoplasia (CIN). CIN can be ranked as mild, moderate, or severe; severe dysplasia will progress to cervical cancer if left untreated. It is thought that exposure to viruses or bacteria may contribute to CIN and the development of cervical cancer. Women infected with human papillomavirus (HPV), which causes genital warts, are 15 times more likely to develop cervical cancer than woman without HPV, and the risk increases by 40 times in women who are infected before the age of 21.

Risk Factors. Although the Pap test is recommended every one to three years for all sexually active women over the age of 18 (or anytime a woman has symptoms), a pelvic examination is recommended every year. Women with any of the risk factors listed below will want to be especially vigilant. Risk factors for cervical cancer include the following:

- **Sexual history.** Women who have sexual intercourse before age 16 or have had multiple sex partners over the years are at a higher risk for cervical cancer. Risk also escalates if you have ever had a sexually transmitted disease (STD), including HPV, herpes, gonorrhea, syphilis, and human immunodeficiency virus (HIV). A pregnancy before age 16, or multiple pregnancies, also appears to increase the risk.

- **Tobacco use.** Smoking increases your chances of getting cervical cancer fourfold.

Risk factors for uterine cancer include the following:

- **Increased age.** Women over age 50 and postmenopausal women are at increased risk.
- **Hormonal factors.** "Unopposed" estrogen is believed to play a key role in the development of endometrial cancer. Specific risks include: being markedly overweight, going for long periods of time without ovulating (anovulatory), having your first period before age 12 (early menarche), having your last menses after the age of 55 (late menopause), or never giving birth. Taking just estrogen also increases the incidence of endometrial cancer, and so post-menopausal women who have not had a hysterectomy should take estrogen plus progesterone unless there is a compelling medical reason for not using the progesterone (or artificial progesterone called progestin), as this completely reduces your risk of endometrial cancer.
- **Family history.** Evidence links uterine cancer to a family history of Lynch syndrome II, a disorder that often leads to colorectal cancer, as well.
- **Personal health history.** Atypical endometrial hyperplasia, an excessive cell growth in the lining of the uterus, is the antecedent of endometrial cancer. Increased rates of uterine cancer are also seen in women with colorectal, ovarian, and breast cancers.
- **Severe obesity and sedentary lifestyle.** Women who are obese have higher estrogen than women who are near normal weight, mostly through the production of estrone, an estrogen, by their fat tissue. They are also more likely to go long periods without ovulating, which increases their risk for developing uterine cancer. Hypertension and diabetes, conditions associated with obesity, also appear to increase uterine cancer risk.

Prevention Tips. The following suggestions are believed to reduce your risk of developing cancers of the uterus and cervix:

- **Avoid unprotected sex with multiple partners.** If you are not in a monogamous relationship, be sure to use condoms during sex to limit exposure to viruses and organisms that could increase your risk of cervical cancer.
- **Do not smoke.** Scientists do not understand how smoking promotes cervical cancer, but they have found that cervical cancer risk increases significantly with the number of cigarettes smoked each day and the years of smoking.
- **Eat a healthy diet.** The National Cancer Institute has noted that both vitamin C and folic acid appear useful in reducing the risk of cervical cancer. Folic acid, a member of the B-complex family, is found in dark green, leafy vegetables, such as kale and spinach, as well as in dried beans and peas, wheat germ, asparagus, corn, parsnips, and beets.
- **Maintain a healthy weight and get enough exercise.** Fatty tissue produces an estrogen compound called estrone, which promotes cell growth in the uterus. An obese woman is twice as likely to develop endometrial cancer as a woman of normal weight.

• **Combine estrogen replacement with progesterone.** If you have a uterus and take hormone replacement therapy, be sure to include the hormone progesterone to prevent a buildup of endometrial tissue. This combination actually decreases your risk of uterine cancer to a level that is lower than that of the general population.

Screening. No screening test is currently available for detecting uterine cancer. However, pelvic ultrasound will show increased growth of the uterine lining and lead your doctor to request or perform an endometrial biopsy. The Pap smear is a highly effective test for screening for cervical cancer. With this simple test, your doctor scrapes a thin layer of cells from your cervix and upper vagina and places them on a slide for examination under a microscope.

The Pap test should be performed along with your routine pelvic examination. The pelvic examination itself is an excellent screening opportunity because the doctor asks about symptoms and problems that may warrant further evaluation, such as abnormal bleeding. She also examines the genitals for precancerous changes and feels your pelvic organs for masses or abnormalities. When problems are suspected, additional tests are available that allow doctors to examine samples of tissue. These tests are not used routinely for women with no symptoms or special risk factors.

Asymptomatic women with frequent sexual partners should have the Pap test done annually. Women in mutually monogamous relationships, who have never had STDs or an abnormal Pap test and who have three or more consecutive normal yearly Pap tests can safely extend the time of screening to every two or three years because they are at lower risk of cervical cancer.

Ovarian Cancer

The ovaries are a pair of small, almond-shaped organs with two major functions: they produce and release eggs, and they secrete hormones. Ovarian cancer is the most fatal of the cancers of the reproductive system, largely because it rarely produces symptoms in its early stages. Two out of three cases are detected in advanced stages, after the cancer has infiltrated other parts of the body, such as the lymph nodes and intestine. Although cancer can arise in any of the many types of ovarian cells, the most common form, epithelial carcinoma, develops from the cells covering the ovary's surface.

Scientists believe that the risk of ovarian cancer is related to the number of ovulations, or menstrual cycles, a woman has in her lifetime. Researchers have found that a high number of ovulations can increase by nine times the chances of producing cells with a specific genetic mutation. Late puberty, early menopause, multiple pregnancies, and the use of birth control pills help decrease the risk of ovarian cancer because they decrease the number of ovulations a woman undergoes in her lifetime.

Symptoms of ovarian cancer include feelings of indigestion, appetite loss, gas, nausea, vague discomfort in the lower abdomen, bleeding that is not part of a normal menstrual period, and abdominal swelling, which may be accompanied by constipation and frequent urination.

Risk Factors. The following factors put a woman at an increased risk of ovarian cancer:

- **Hereditary cancer syndromes.** Women in families with a history of Lynch syndrome II, breast-ovarian cancer syndrome, or site-specific ovarian cancer syndromes are prone to malignancies of the ovaries and breast, usually at an early age.
- **Lifetime number of ovulations.** Specific factors related to a high number of ovulations are: no pregnancies, a first pregnancy after age 30, a first menstrual period before age 12, and menopause after age 50.
- **High-fat diet.** In studies from all over the world, a diet high in saturated fats may be linked to the development of ovarian cancer.

Prevention Tips. Experts have no specific prevention tips for ovarian cancer other than following the same healthful lifestyle that helps reduce the risk of many forms of cancer. When selecting a method of birth control, keep in mind the protective effects of the birth control pill as you weigh pros and cons. However, choose the form of contraception that is right for you considering your lifestyle, health factors, and risks. (See Chapter 17 for more information on family planning.)

If you have a strong family history of ovarian cancer, it is critical to discuss your options with a knowledgeable physician. Some women who know their risk is extremely high choose to have their ovaries surgically removed—in a procedure is called prophylactic oophorectomy—once they are absolutely certain that they no longer want to be pregnant.

Screening. There are no screening tests for ovarian cancer that are accurate enough to use routinely in women without symptoms. A blood test is available that checks for an antigen, CA-1,25, that is present in many ovarian tumors. Studies have shown that CA-1,25 is elevated in 80 percent of women with epithelial cell ovarian cancer. About 2 percent of healthy women will have an elevated CA-1,25, which can lead to unnecessary and expensive testing or surgery. Because of that, the test is not used for screening but may be used in women with symptoms suggestive of ovarian cancer, a personal history of ovarian cancer, or a strong family history of ovarian cancer.

The CA-1,25 test is often used in conjunction with transvaginal ultrasound. In this procedure, a probe that pulses ultrasonic beams is inserted into the vagina to provide a picture of the uterus, fallopian tubes, ovaries, and their blood flow. Pelvic ultrasound, in which the probe is moved back and forth across your abdomen, may also be used.

If you have no symptoms and no history that put you at high risk, the best method of screening is an annual pelvic examination, during which your doctor feels your abdomen for masses or abnormalities.

Skin Cancer

Skin cancer is the most common form of cancer, and it is growing at an alarming rate. One in five Americans will be diagnosed with skin cancer over a lifetime. Overexposure to the sun's ultraviolet rays is mainly to blame. Not only have Americans greatly increased the amount of time they spend in the sun since the turn of the twentieth century, but, at the same time, the protective ozone layer in the atmos-

wellness **tip**

Regular use of sun-
screens with sun protec-
tion factor (SPF) of 15
during the first 18 years
of life can reduce the lifetime risk of skin cancer
by as much as 78 percent.

FIGURE 21.3
Warning Signs of Melanoma
Use the "ABCDs" of melanoma to
spot this potentially dangerous
skin cancer.

phere is thinning, which lets through harmful rays. The deadliest type of skin cancer, malignant melanoma, skyrocketed to a 500 percent increase between 1950 and 1985.

Basal cell carcinoma is the most common skin cancer and is also the least dangerous. It has a cure rate of 99 percent if detected early. Basal cell carcinoma develops in the outermost layer of the skin and usually looks like a small, pearly bump—cream-colored to pinkish—most often on the face, neck, or hands.

Squamous cell carcinoma arises from the cells that make up the protective keratin layer of the epidermis. Like basal cell carcinoma, it typically appears on parts of the body exposed to the sun. It looks like a raised red or pink scaly nodule or a wart-like growth and may develop an ulcerated center that is slow to heal.

Actinic keratosis, a benign skin lesion, is a slightly raised, waxy patch of skin one-quarter to one-half inch in diameter that is tan, red, brownish, or grayish. Only rarely do these growths turns into squamous cell carcinoma.

Melanoma arises in pigment-producing cells called melanocytes. It is an aggressive cancer that can spread quickly to any organ or tissue within the body and is one of the most common tumors to spread to the brain and spinal cord. Some melanomas emerge as new growths, while others occur in a preexisting mole—which is simply a cluster of melanocytes. Melanoma is found in people exposed to excessive sun, especially with frequent sunburns. It also can appear in areas of the body not exposed to sun at all.

Most moles and blemishes on the body are benign and no threat to your health. By adulthood the average person has about 25 moles, and new ones can form at any time. To be safe, it is best to have any change or any mole that seems out of the ordinary checked by your doctor. Any spot that suddenly changes in size, shape, or color; any spot that starts hurting, itching, or bleeding; or any spot that first appears after age 20 should be pointed out to your doctor or dermatologist and observed carefully over time.

Risk Factors. Most women will have one or more of the following risk factors associated with skin cancer, and all women are advised to consider themselves at risk for the disease:

- **Sun exposure.** Three or more blistering sunburns before age 20; decades of exposure to the sun, sunlamps, or tanning booths; and living in the South and Southwest, where the sun is strongest, increase the risk of skin cancer.

Total Body Skin Examination: What to Look For

- A mole that is asymmetrical or has irregular borders, is uneven in color, or is wider than the end of a pencil eraser
- Scaly or crusty patches
- A small nodule that progresses into a wartlike bump
- A translucent, flesh-colored, pearly, or red nodule
- A scaly, off-white or yellow patch that looks like scar tissue
- A lesion that is blue, brown, or black
- A wound that does not heal

A=Asymmetry: one half of the mole does not match the other half

B=Border: the edges of the mole are ragged, blurred, or irregular

C=Color: the color of the mole is not uniform throughout or contains shades of tan, brown, black, red, white, or blue

D=Diameter: the diameter of the mole is larger than a pencil eraser

- **Physical traits.** Characteristics associated with higher skin cancer risk include a fair complexion; many freckles; blond or red hair; blue, green, or gray eyes; a higher than average number of moles; atypical moles; or a large congenital mole.
- **Family history.** Conditions that increase your skin cancer risk include any family history of melanoma or certain genetic skin disorders:
  - ➤ *Xeroderma pigmentosum*—a condition that leaves the skin and eyes very sensitive to light
  - ➤ *Albinism*—a lack of protective melanin
  - ➤ *Basal cell nevus syndrome*—a genetic tendency to grow malignancies in areas not usually affected, such as the soles of the feet and palms of the hands
  - ➤ *Dysplastic nevus syndrome*—a susceptibility to melanoma
  - ➤ *Familial atypical multiple mole melanoma syndrome*—puts family members at risk for melanoma, cancers of the eye, breast, respiratory tract, gastrointestinal tract, and lymphatic system

Prevention Tips. The fact that the incidence of skin cancer has grown dramatically over the past 25 years indicates that people's behavior has changed, putting them more at risk. Given the weakening of the protective ozone layer, it is clear that people must, again, change their behavior to reduce the risk:

- **Avoid sun exposure.** Ultraviolet (UV) rays are strongest during the hours 10 AM to 2 PM (or 11 AM to 3 PM during daylight savings time), and these are the times when you are advised to avoid the sun altogether.
- **Wear protective clothing.** When you must be in the sun, use barriers, such as long sleeves, long pants, and a hat with a brim to help reflect UV rays. Remember when wearing a hat that sunlight is often reflected upward from surfaces, such as sand, roads, and water. Sunscreen is always recommended in addition to a hat.
- **Apply sunscreen to unprotected skin.** Many experts recommend using sun screen every day—especially on the face, neck, ears, and hands—whether you expect to be in direct sunlight for any length of time or not. Use it on cloudy days, too. Make sure the sunscreen blocks both UVA and UVB rays.
- **Avoid tanning salons.** Experts emphasize that there is no safe level of tanning from any source, natural or artificial. A suntan is actually a visible sign of injury to the skin.
- **Stay completely out of the sun when using certain medications.** Tetracycline, sulfa drugs, Retin-A, thiazide diuretics, and indo-

> To reduce your risk of skin cancer, be sure to use sunscreen especially on the face, neck, ears, and hands whenever you plan to be outside for any length of time, even on cloudy days.

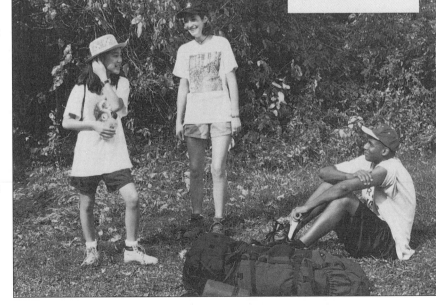

Defining Cancer Cures

There are several definitions of "cure" with respect to cancer:

- **Statistical cure**—when the treated woman has the same mortality as women who did not have the cancer
- **Personal cure**—when the woman with a cancer diagnosis lives a full life and dies of another cause
- **Societal cure**—when options are available to prevent the disease in the first place

When discussing the concept of curing cancer, it is important to differentiate which "cure" we mean, because the cure means different things to the patient, the family, and society as a whole.

methacin all increase sun sensitivity and lead to sunburn even in situations where you would not normally burn.

Screening. Total body skin examinations are the best way to catch skin cancers early. Once a month, check yourself in a brightly lit room, using a full-length mirror and a handheld mirror. Get to know every inch of your skin so you can spot changes when they occur. Do not forget your back, elbows, soles of the feet, between the toes, neck, scalp, buttocks, and vulva.

After age 40, have your skin examined once a year by a physician. Dermatologists are especially trained to identify diseases of the skin. During your annual skin examination the doctor will ask you to remove all your clothing and will look at each part of your body, from head to toe. This takes five to ten minutes. If she finds anything suspicious, she can take a sample of tissue and send it to a laboratory to be examined for signs of cancer.

Approaches *to* Cancer Treatment

Cancer treatment has one of three goals: to cure the disease, to control the disease in an effort to extend the patient's life, or to palliate—which means to relieve or reduce symptoms while the disease runs its course. Many people with cancer live for years after they are diagnosed with the illness. One aspect of wellness that many women will at some point in their lives have to grasp (either for themselves, a friend, or family member) is the idea of staying well while living with a life-threatening disease. If you develop cancer, it is important to learn all you can about your disease so you feel in control, are better armed to make decisions, and can get the best treatment possible. Following is an overview of the avenues doctors typically pursue in treating cancer.

Surgery

The primary treatment for many cancers is to remove the abnormal cells (tumor) through surgery. New high-tech imaging devices are available today that allow surgeons to pinpoint and remove cancerous growths with more accuracy than ever. There are also new surgical tools including cryosurgery, which uses liquid nitrogen to freeze tumors—particularly useful for skin cancers—and laser surgery, which destroys diseased cells using a high-intensity light beam while avoiding damaging nearby crucial tissue.

Radiation

Radiation therapy is a powerful means of shrinking and destroying cancerous tumors. Radiation may be used as the main therapy or it may be used after surgery to kill any stray cancer cells that may have been left behind. Treatment consists of regular exposure (usually every day or every few days) to a radiation beam over a period of several weeks. Sometimes radiation is used before surgery to treat tumors that are very large or difficult to get to surgically.

Although radiation therapy is most often delivered from a machine outside the body, sometimes an internal radiation source is implanted in the body.

Chemotherapy

Chemotherapy is the use of drugs to kill cancer cells throughout the body. There are many different drugs, combinations, and ways of receiving them, from oral pills to injections. A course of chemotherapy usually consists of a cycle of drugs followed by a break, which gives the body a chance to recover from the side effects of the treatment. The course may last 2 to 12 months, depending on the type of cancer. Damage to the body's cells, especially to sensitive blood cells, usually limits the amount of chemotherapy that can be used in a given time period. Newer techniques that accelerate the growth of infection-fighting cells or return a woman's own healthy blood cells allow more aggressive chemotherapy to be given with a higher cure rate.

Immunotherapy

With this new cancer-fighting strategy, the body is encouraged to launch its own form of chemotherapy. In very simple terms, it involves injecting drugs, antibodies, or the patient's own killed tumor cells into the body to zero in on the tumor cells.

Alternative Therapies

Many alternatives therapies, so called because they do not use surgery or drugs, are being tried in conjunction with primary cancer treatments. Some are more widely accepted than others, but these treatments are generally gaining in popularity. Most physicians agree that they certainly do no harm unless they are used instead of conventional medical and surgical treatment. Support groups, help from family and friends, self-help guides on diet and guided imagery, herbal healing, and alternative forms of pain relief abound. Be sure to consult with your oncologist to guarantee that any alternative method of treatment you use is compatible with your conventional treatment regimen.

What *You* Can Do

Cancer is certainly among the most feared diseases. Many women feel that there is nothing they can do to avoid exposure to outside influences that cause cancer. The wellness approach to health empowers women to take a proactive stance to reduce their risk of cancer:

- Commit to a life-sustaining lifestyle. A healthy immune system that is strengthened by a low-fat, high-fiber, nutritious diet and regular exercise, is believed to help keep cell growth within normal bounds.
- Avoid known cancer-causing agents. Tobacco products are the single most dangerous substances that must be avoided. Do not start smoking. If you do smoke, quit. In addition, familiarize yourself with workplace hazards and toxic substances that might be present in your home, and take steps to eliminate your exposure to them.
- Identify personal risk factors and family medical history information that apply to you and discuss them with your physician. Also discuss appropriate screening tests.
- If cancer does strike, be aware that you may live many years with the presence of the disease. Educate yourself about your illness, and continue to practice the principles of wellness.

Protecting *Against* Infection

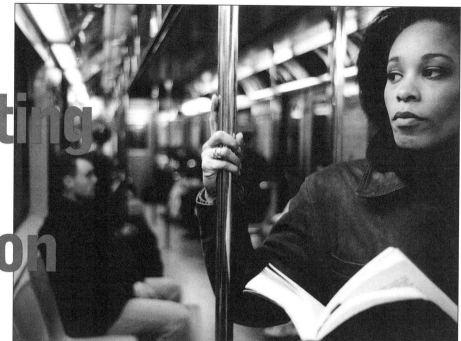

I n medieval times, people explained infections in such elusive terms as "the imbalance of humors," vital fluids that were believed to exist in the body and be responsible for health and illness. Or, they said, infections were caused by "stars in the atmosphere" that carried poisons. By the late 1600s, scientists knew of the existence of microorganisms—tiny organisms visible only through a microscope. But it was not until 200 years later that the medical community began to realize that some of these microorganisms caused disease.

Today, doctors and scientists know a great deal about infections and the microorganisms that cause them. Some infections that once were deadly can now be tamed with the help of drugs. Some are still dangerous and incurable. To stay healthy, it is important that you learn about the most common types of infections and how they are spread, and use that information to avoid infection or reduce its impact.

How Infections Happen

Thousands of species of microorganisms surround us and live within our bodies. Certain microorganisms, when they remain in balance, help keep our bodies healthy. However, when one or more of these organisms get out of balance and invade the tissues of the body, infections develop. These infections can damage and destroy healthy cells.

The Body's Defense System

To understand how infection occurs, it is useful first to see how the body normally protects itself against disease. A number of ingenious natural defenses are set up to keep harmful organisms out or, if they manage to invade, to control or destroy them.

The First Line of Defense. The body produces several defenses that act as natural barriers against disease:

- **Stomach acid** helps the body break down and digest food and can also kill harmful organisms.
- **"Friendly" bacteria** in the lower digestive tract aid the process of digestion while helping keep foreign invaders in check.
- **Skin** forms a protective layer over the entire body, serving as a natural barrier against infection. The oil and perspiration secreted by the skin to keep it from drying out and to keep it cool contain substances that help destroy bacteria on the skin's surface.
- **Mucus** produced by the nose and respiratory tract moistens the airways while also keeping harmful organisms from entering the throat and lungs.
- **Vaginal secretions,** which help keep the vagina lubricated, also contain a substance that kills foreign bacteria.
- **Urine** carries waste products away from the body but is also highly acidic, which tends to discourage bacterial growth.

The Immune System. The body's second line of defense against infection is the immune system. This is a complex system that employs an army of methods to fight invading organisms.

When a foreign organism invades the body, the immune system engages in a battle that may take hours, days, or weeks to resolve. The length of time it takes for the body to rid itself of the attacker depends on several factors, including a woman's overall health, the strength of her immune system, and the potency of the invading organism.

It is during this battle that you experience the symptoms of infection. A fever, for example, is caused by the intense activity taking place in your body's tissues as immune-system cells try to kill attacking microorganisms. A cough, runny nose, pus from a wound or sore, and other discharges are ways in which the body rids itself of harmful bacteria and dead cells.

The immune system has two main methods of operation. It uses patrolling cells to guard continuously against invading organisms, a process called cell-mediated immunity, and it creates special proteins called antibodies to attack specific kinds of foreign cells.

Cell-Mediated Immunity. In a cell-mediated immune response, certain cells seek out and destroy foreign organisms when they invade the body. These cells are called phagocytes. Circulating throughout the bloodstream, these killer cells are constantly on the alert for foreign invaders. This type of immune response is sometimes called nonspecific immunity because these cells are programmed to respond to any attacker.

When invading organisms, such as bacteria, get into the bloodstream, several types of phagocytes are dispatched to the site of the intrusion. A phagocyte destroys an invader by forming a pouchlike structure that surrounds and engulfs it. Once inside the cell, the bacterium is killed by enzymes that break it down and digest it.

Often, cell-mediated immunity is successful in getting rid of an infection. When additional help is needed, however, the body puts specialized defenses into action.

Antibodies. Antibodies are proteins that are produced when a foreign substance (called an antigen) enters and stimulates the body. Antibodies are specifically designed to fit onto the surface of that antigen, somewhat like two jigsaw puzzle pieces. Once attached to the antigen, the antibodies destroy the antigen or render it harmless. This type of immune mechanism is sometimes called antigen specific immunity because each type of antibody is tailor-made to attack the specific antigen that triggered its creation.

Once antibodies have been formed against a specific antigen, they remain in the blood, constantly on guard against future attacks. That is why many of the diseases of childhood, such as mumps and chickenpox, can be contracted only once. Antibodies "stand guard" so that if a person is exposed to these diseases again, the organism will be promptly destroyed, preventing recurrent disease.

The Agents of Infection

Most microorganisms that cause disease fall into two main categories: bacteria and viruses. There are important distinctions between the two that will help you understand the best way to prevent infection.

Bacteria. Bacteria are among the oldest living organisms on earth. They have cleverly evolved over millions of years to live in an impressive number of environments, and, as you might expect, they are everywhere. They live in the soil, inside and on the bodies of animals, in water, and in some types of plants. They can also live on nearly every type of human-made surface.

Many types of bacteria contribute to the good health of the environment and the creatures living there. Some help plants grow by adding important nutrients to the soil. Others help maintain a delicate balance in the ocean, keeping marine life healthy. Bacteria even live inside our bodies, where they help digest food, break down waste products, and keep other, potentially harmful, bacteria in check.

Other types of bacteria, however, can cause illness, disease, and death in plants and animals. In general, these bacteria affect humans in one of two ways. Some invade healthy tissue and attach to cells where they multiply and spread throughout the body. Others produce chemicals called toxins that damage or destroy healthy cells. Such harmful bacteria disrupt the normal functioning of cells—and hence can throw the entire body off kilter.

Viruses. Unlike bacteria, viruses do not have a life of their own. They depend on a living animal's cells to survive. A virus is a tiny structure that consists mainly of a strand of DNA (deoxyribonucleic acid), the molecule that contains the genetic "blueprint" in every living thing. Wrapped around the DNA is a coat of protein that is designed to hook up with cells inside the body. A virus attaches itself to a healthy cell, called a host cell, and then takes over its DNA—its "control center."

Once inside the host cell, the virus orders the cell to make more copies of the virus. These copies spread throughout the body, attaching to more host cells and repeating the process.

Because a virus depends on a host cell, it tends to be very fragile and easy to kill outside of the body. But viruses have "learned" to make up for their fragile nature by acquiring the ability to mutate, or change. One of the reasons that viral diseases are so hard to identify and treat is because they are constantly changing in subtle ways to avoid early destruction by the immune system.

That is why some viral diseases, such as the flu and the common cold, can be contracted many times in a lifetime. Each time you get a cold or the flu, you have actually been infected by a strain of virus that is slightly different from all those that have infected you in the past. Your immune system proceeds to make antibodies to the new virus strain, which it eventually is able to fight off. You are then immune to that particular strain of virus, but another, closely related strain can cause another cold, or in some cases, serious viral illness. Other viruses do not mutate as often but still are difficult to prevent, such as the human immunodeficiency virus (HIV), the virus that causes acquired immunodeficiency syndrome (AIDS).

How Infections Are Spread

Diseases are spread from person to person through contact with the infecting organism. Someone with a cold, for example, can spread the illness by coughing and sneezing. This expels tiny droplets, called fomites, into the air, where they are easily breathed in by someone else. Other organisms are spread on the hands, entering the body when the eye or other body opening is touched. Sharing drinking glasses and eating utensils with a sick person can also result in the rapid spread of infection.

Not all infections are spread this easily, though. Some, like those spread through sexual contact, are passed from one person to another only through contact with infected blood, saliva, semen, or vaginal secretions.

Curing Infections

Most of the infections described in this chapter can be treated with antimicrobial drugs. These drugs attack the organism causing the infection, either killing it outright or slowing down its growth enough so that the body's immune system can finish it off. Antimicrobial drugs can be divided into two groups: antibiotics, which act against bacteria, and antiviral drugs, which attack viruses.

How Antibiotics Work. Well over a century ago, scientists first observed that some microorganisms produced substances that could slow down the growth of or kill other microorganisms. It was not until 50 years ago, though, that the specific chemicals responsible for this activity were identified. In 1948, the famous experiment of Alexander Fleming showed that a species of bread mold could kill bacterial colonies. Fleming was not the first to observe this effect, but he was the first to isolate the agent responsible for it. The substance he discovered came to be known as penicillin, the first antibiotic to be used in medicine.

The discovery of penicillin and of the many antibiotics that followed represented a turning point in the practice of medicine. Many once-fatal diseases, such as syphilis and wound infections, could now be cured with the use of these new drugs.

Food Poisoning

Food poisoning is an infection of the gastrointestinal tract caused by bacteria-contaminated food. Beef, poultry, and eggs are common culprits, but disease-causing bacteria can also be found on raw vegetables and in milk products.

A few simple precautions can lower the risk of these infections:

- Wash your hands after handling raw meats and eggs and before touching other food products.
- Wash dishes, utensils, and cutting boards in hot, soapy water after using them.
- Thoroughly rinse all fresh produce.
- Use one cutting board to prepare raw meat and one for other kitchen tasks. After use, wash all surfaces and utensils thoroughly with hot, soapy water and rinse well.
- Cook chicken, hamburgers, and other meats thoroughly, until there are no pink areas.
- Keep hot foods hot and cold foods cold. If you are not eating foods within the next few hours, refrigerate them; then reheat before serving.
- Avoid eating uncooked eggs or undercooked eggs.

Antibiotics and Bacterial Resistance

Antibiotics can be very good at curing bacterial infections. But scientists and doctors are beginning to realize that too much of a good thing can be bad. Antibiotics have often been prescribed in the absence of infection, or against viruses and other organisms that can't be killed by them.

The result of this practice has been the emergence of new, resistant strains of bacteria. Misuse of antibiotics tends to "weed out" the weaker organisms, leaving stronger ones to reproduce. With their competition gone, these resistant strains are free to grow at an even faster rate—and to cause even more severe infections.

Doctors have begun to be much more cautious in their use of antibiotics. Nowadays, when you see your doctor for a cold, you may be advised to get plenty of rest and drink lots of fluids, rather than getting a prescription for a drug you don't need and that won't work. As more doctors recognize the danger of overprescribing antibiotics, the problem of bacterial resistance will decrease.

More than 100 kinds of antibiotics that are active against infectious organisms have been discovered and synthesized since Fleming's experiment. Most work by interfering with a bacterium's normal functioning. They may break down the organism's cell wall or inhibit its ability to make the proteins it needs to survive.

The type of antibiotic with which a doctor chooses to treat an infection depends on what organism is causing the illness, how widespread and severe the infection is, which drugs are known to be the most effective against it, and which ones the ill person can tolerate. You will hear some antibiotics referred to as "broad spectrum," meaning they are effective against many diverse types of organisms. Often doctors choose broad-spectrum antibiotics as an initial therapy because they are most likely to be effective when the specific cause of infection is not easily identifiable.

If a broad-spectrum drug does not clear up an infection promptly, most doctors will take steps to identify the specific organism causing it. An antibiotic that is targeted specifically to that organism can then be used to cure the infection.

Many people develop allergies or reactions to antibiotics on repeated use. This occurs when your body's immune system attacks the foreign drug. Allergies to drugs limit the body's ability to fight infections and complicate treatment of the disease. Therefore, doctors try to limit the use of antibiotics to infections that truly require them, to reduce the likelihood of developing allergies.

Antiviral Agents. In contrast to the large number of antibiotics that can be used to fight bacterial infections, antiviral drugs are very few in number. Since viruses can quickly mutate and form new strains, most antiviral drugs become obsolete over time. In addition, viruses integrate with the inner workings of host cells, making it difficult to destroy the virus chemically without damaging healthy cells.

Most antiviral drugs—the influenza A antiviral drugs are a good example—work by interfering with the processes by which a virus invades a host cell, takes over its DNA, and orders it to make more copies of itself. Unlike antibiotics, there are no broad-spectrum antiviral drugs. Rather, each antiviral drug is designed to work against a specific type of virus and is usually not effective against other types.

The effectiveness of antiviral drugs varies depending on the types of virus they are meant to attack. Some viral infections can be only controlled, not cured, with antiviral drugs. Others can be slowed down to the point where the body's immune system is able to take over and eliminate the virus.

Preventing *the* Common Cold *and* Flu

Any one of a large number of viruses can cause colds. The so-called "common" cold is most often caused by a group of viruses called the rhinoviruses. Cold symptoms are familiar to everyone: sneezing, runny nose, nasal stuffiness, and sometimes a cough.

"Flu" is a short name for influenza, another viral infection. It is caused by one of three types of influenza viruses. (Many other types of cold- and flu-like illnesses that are not influenza are also commonly referred to as "the flu," which can cause confusion.) The symptoms of influenza come on suddenly and include fever, sore throat, muscle aches, fatigue, weakness, and nasal congestion.

How Colds and Flu Spread

Colds and flu are spread through the respiratory secretions from an infected person. Sneezing and coughing send tiny droplets into the air, where they can easily be inhaled or land on surfaces touched by others. Studies have shown that the most common way in which colds and flu are spread is through physical contact. Typically, the ill person blows her nose and then hands an object to, or shakes hands with, another person. The second person then touches the mucous membranes of her nose, mouth, or eyes, where the virus enters the bloodstream. The symptoms of colds and flu appear within a few days after exposure to the virus.

If you are in contact with people who are sneezing or coughing, one of the best ways to protect yourself is by washing your hands frequently. Also, keep your hands away from your face. Do not touch your eyes after coming into contact with someone who has a cold or the flu; that is the fastest way people become infected.

Treating the Common Cold and Flu

Both colds and flu are caused by viruses; *antibiotics do not help get rid of these infections.* The body's natural defenses are the usual cure, so patience is the key. However, there are things you can do to make yourself more comfortable and to help your body fight the infection.

"Drink plenty of fluids" is common advice, and it is true that drinking water helps your body overcome a virus. Fluids help get rid of waste products and can actually help clear a stuffy nose by keeping the mucus watery instead of thick. Rest is also important. Your body is working hard while it battles a cold or flu, and you need to rest to renew the energy it needs in order to get better quickly.

There is an overwhelming array of over-the-counter products designed to relieve cold and flu symptoms. Aspirin is commonly used for fever and body or headaches, but should be avoided by people with stomach ulcers or those under the age of 25 because of the increased risk of Reye's syndrome. Acetaminophen will relieve symptoms and not cause stomach problems but may worsen the rare occurrence of liver damage from a virus. Nonsteroidal anti-inflammatory drugs, like ibuprofen, may be safer to use, especially for young adults with the flu, but should also be avoided by people with stomach ulcers.

Many of these medications can be helpful in reducing symptoms enough so that you can function during the day and get enough sleep at night. Be aware, though, that if certain products are overused, they can actually extend the life of a cold by working against your body's natural defenses. Antihistamines, for

Should You Get a Flu Shot?

The Centers for Disease Control and Prevention recommends a flu shot each year to prevent influenza. The makeup of this vaccine changes each year because the strain of the virus that is most widespread is usually different each year. Flu shots are especially advised for people with the following conditions:

- Asthma and other chronic respiratory conditions
- Chronic heart, kidney, or lung disease
- Heavy cigarette smoking
- Cystic fibrosis
- Sickle cell anemia
- Diabetes

Flu shots are also recommended for health care workers, teachers and others who work with children, and people who cannot afford to miss several days of work.

Flu shots are generally offered in the early fall. The vaccine is given as a single intramuscular injection (a shot into a muscle), usually in the upper arm. A very small percentage of people have a reaction to the vaccine, though slight fever and muscle aches for about a day following the injection are not uncommon.

Getting a flu vaccine does not absolutely guarantee that you will not get the flu if you are exposed to it. If you do, however, you are more likely to have only a mild case. Because the influenza virus mutates so rapidly, a new flu shot is required each season.

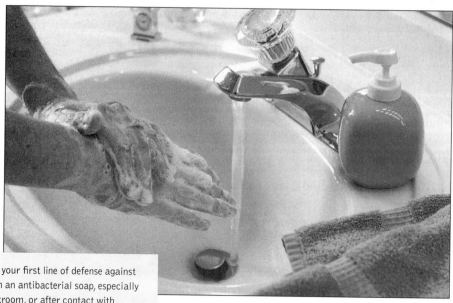

Washing your hands as often as possible is your first line of defense against infection. Wash your hands thoroughly with an antibacterial soap, especially before and after eating, after using the restroom, or after contact with commonly used objects, such as grocery carts and pay phones.

example, which help dry up a runny nose and watery eyes, can also make you tired and drowsy, robbing your body of energy. They also prevent you from getting rid of the viruses through your secretions. Nasal sprays can make stuffiness worse after they wear off. The best policy when you have a cold or flu is to use as few of these drugs as possible to feel reasonably comfortable.

Luckily, colds and flu do not pose serious health risks for the majority of people. Symptoms usually subside after one or two weeks. However, sometimes a secondary bacterial infection develops in the chest, nasal sinuses, throat, or ears as a result of a weakening of the defenses by a particularly stubborn cold or flu. If the viral infection descends into the lower respiratory tract, it can cause viral pneumonia, or lead to bacterial pneumonia, which may require a stay in the hospital. Bronchitis, an inflammation of the upper airway, or sinusitis, an infection of the nasal sinuses, can also develop from a secondary bacterial infection. If symptoms persist for more than two weeks, see your doctor. Antibiotics usually clear up secondary bacterial infections resulting from a cold or the flu.

Preventing *Infections* **of** *Special* **Concern** to **Women**

Many common infections occur only in women. Others, such as urinary tract infections, can occur in either sex but are much more common in women. Some infections are of special concern to women during pregnancy. (See Chapter 18 for infections to be wary of if you are pregnant.)

Of the infections discussed below, many can have serious long-term consequences if they are not treated promptly. As a woman, you need to understand how these infections develop—and what you can do to decrease the likelihood of developing these infections, recognize the signs if you do get them, and promptly get good medical care to prevent complications.

Mononucleosis

"The kissing disease" is so nicknamed because the virus that causes mononucleosis is transmitted primarily through saliva. Women most at risk for the infection are adolescent and young adult students. These women usually live close to a large number of people, often get less sleep than they need, and tend to eat poorly, thus compromising their immune systems.

Symptoms of mononucleosis include fever, sore throat, swollen lymph glands in the neck, underarms, and/or groin, and chronic fatigue. Thirty to forty percent of patients have an enlarged liver or spleen. Symptoms are rarely dangerous, and the infection does not, as some believe, cause miscarriage or birth defects.

Mononucleosis is famous for its long recovery period. Since the infection is caused by a virus, rest—lots of it—and a healthy diet to build up the immune system are the only remedies. Most people need bed rest for two to three weeks. Glands may stay swollen for four weeks, and fatigue may last for six weeks or more. Sometimes medication is given to alleviate symptoms, such as Prednisone for a severe sore throat.

Almost everyone is exposed to mononucleosis at some point, but not everyone contracts the disease. The best way to avoid becoming ill is to keep your immune system healthy. Eat well; get plenty of sleep; don't get "run down." If you know someone who is ill, avoid intimacy, and do not share straws, drinking glasses, or utensils.

Vaginal Infections

The inside of the vagina normally harbors a variety of bacteria and other microorganisms that help to break down substances in vaginal secretions. The acidic environment that is produced as a result allows these organisms to live in balance, keeping the vagina healthy. A vaginal infection can occur when the balance is disrupted, and one type of organism multiplies much faster than the others. Other types of vaginal infections can be caused by organisms not normally found in the vagina that are introduced from outside. Although some vaginal infections may be transmitted sexually, most vaginal infections are not sexually transmitted diseases (STDs), which will be discussed later in this chapter.

An overgrowth of bacteria or yeast in the vagina often results when a woman takes antibiotics to treat another type of infection. These drugs may kill or weaken some of the organisms normally present in the vagina, allowing overgrowth of other species. Frequent use of a vaginal douche can also lead to vaginal infections by allowing overgrowth of other species. A tampon that is left in too long or that is too absorbent for the amount of menstrual flow can irritate the vaginal walls, causing a local inflammation that leads to infection. The use of oral contraceptives changes the vaginal environment and makes overgrowth of yeast more common.

Most vaginal infections do not pose risks to your health, but they can be annoying and extremely uncomfortable. A few can lead to serious health problems if not treated. Symptoms of vaginal infections are generally obvious:

- Itching, burning, and redness of the vulva (the folds of skin that surround the vaginal opening)
- An increased amount of vaginal discharge, which may be yellow and thick and often has an unusual odor

Some vaginal infections can be prevented with good hygiene. Care must be taken, for example, to keep from wiping bacteria from the rectum into the vagina. You can help to prevent this cause of vaginal infections by always wiping from front to back after a bowel movement and generally keeping your vaginal and anal areas

Lyme Disease

In the summer of 1975, several children in the small town of Lyme, Connecticut, began coming down with a bizarre illness. Flu-like symptoms of fatigue, chills, fever, headache, and muscle pain progressed to sore throat, backache, nausea, and vomiting, and then to coordination problems, heart trouble, and arthritis affecting many different joints. Eventually the culprit was found to be a newly discovered bacterium, *Borrelia burgdorferi*, carried by a common species of deer tick.

Since it was first identified, Lyme disease has spread to other parts of New England, as far south as Maryland, and as far west as Oregon and California.

Deer ticks are tiny—about half as big as the common wood tick. Their bite may go unnoticed as they pass bacteria into the host's bloodstream. Anywhere from three days to a month later, a distinctive "bull's eye" rash, with a white center surrounded by a red ring, develops. Weeks or months later, the symptoms of Lyme disease appear.

Lyme disease is best treated in its early stages, when antibiotics can completely eliminate it. Cases that are not caught until later can cause serious problems in the joints, heart, and brain.

The tick that carries Lyme disease is common in woodlands and forests from May through October. To avoid tick bites of any kind, wear long pants tucked into closed shoes, long sleeves, and a hat whenever you are in wooded areas. Check your pets and your own body (and your children's bodies) carefully, especially where hair grows, as soon as you go inside. If you find a tick, pull it out steadily and slowly with a pair of tweezers and drown it in soapy water. Save it in a glass or plastic container for laboratory examination. Seek prompt medical attention at the first sign of illness and make sure your physician is aware of your tick exposure.

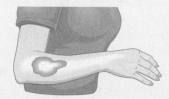

FIGURE 22.1
Spotting Lyme Disease
The typical "bull's eye" rash of Lyme disease has a light center surrounded by clearly defined red areas.

clean. In addition, anything inserted into the rectum, whether it is a penis, a sex aid, or your own or your partner's fingers, should be thoroughly washed with hot soapy water before being placed in the vagina. Changing the condom between anal and vaginal intercourse will prevent the spread of harmful bacteria.

If you are prone to repeated vaginal infections, you may want to consider whether your wardrobe is part of the problem. Tight jeans, slacks, panty hose, or panties, especially if they are made of nonbreathable material, allow the organisms that cause vaginal infections to prosper and multiply. White cotton underpants, loose-fitting slacks or shorts, and pantyhose with a breathable cotton crotch are better choices if you get recurrent infections.

Stress, fatigue, and illness can also contribute to vaginal infection. Sometimes the symptoms of a vaginal infection are a sign that you need to take better care of your whole self.

Following is more advice for preventing vaginal infection:

- Do not use harsh or irritating soaps and douches. Avoid scented tampons, sanitary pads, and toilet paper. Feminine hygiene sprays can also irritate the tissues in and around the vagina.
- Change tampons often during your period—they should not be left in for more than eight hours. Alternate tampons with sanitary pads when menstrual flow is light.
- Avoid daily use of sanitary products to control vaginal secretions.

- Thoroughly clean barrier-type contraceptive devices, such as diaphragms, cervical caps, and spermicide applicators, after each use.
- Do not douche more often than your doctor advises.
- Be careful about using home remedies for vaginal infections. Talk to your doctor about these remedies before using them. Many do not clear up the infection but only mask the symptoms, making the problem worse in the long run.
- If you are taking antibiotics, eating plenty of yogurt and drinking acidophilus milk may help prevent a yeast infection.

Candidiasis. Sometimes called "yeast infection" or "monilia," candidiasis is caused by overgrowth of Candida, a yeastlike organism normally present in small numbers in the vagina. When the yeast organism increases in numbers, it causes a white, thick, cheesy discharge. Candidiasis is usually hard to ignore because it causes intense itching, burning, and redness of the vulva and the vagina.

Candidiasis can usually be cleared up quickly with an antifungal cream inserted into the vagina. Some of these preparations are now available without a prescription, but first-time infections should be seen by your doctor. If this is a recurrent infection that does not respond to treatment, or if the diagnosis is in doubt, check with your doctor.

Oral antiyeast medications are now available by prescription for treating vaginal yeast infections. Only one dose is taken, usually clearing up the infection within two to four days. If the infection persists, contact your doctor.

Bacterial Vaginosis. Previously called nonspecific vaginitis, then Gardnerella vaginitis, bacterial vaginosis is probably caused by several kinds of organisms, including Gardnerella, Mycoplasma, and Mobiluncus species. The most common symptom is an increased volume of watery vaginal discharge with an unusual, fishy odor. Bacterial vaginosis rarely causes redness or itching. Because it can exist along with other types of vaginal infections, your doctor must make this diagnosis before it can be successfully treated.

Bacterial vaginosis can be cured with oral or vaginal antibiotics. Your doctor may recommend simultaneous use of an antiyeast medication, since the antibiotics may cause yeast overgrowth.

Trichomoniasis. Unlike candidiasis and bacterial vaginosis, trichomoniasis is caused by an organism not normally present in the vagina. *Trichomonas vaginalis* is not a bacterium, a virus, or a fungus, but a protozoan—a one-celled organism *(T. vaginalis)* that is much larger than a bacterium. This type of vaginal infection is most often sexually transmitted.

Trichomoniasis often produces an irritating, yellow-greenish discharge from the vagina. The discharge may be bubbly or frothy and may have a bitter or foul odor. Itching and burning often occur with urination because the organism also affects a woman's lower urinary tract. Men can have trichomoniasis, but there are usually no symptoms. A man usually finds out that he has the infection only when it is diagnosed in his sexual partner.

Since trichomoniasis can infect both women and men, both partners must be treated in order to get rid of it. If only the woman is treated, her partner can reinfect her the next time they have unprotected intercourse.

Toxic Shock Syndrome

In 1980, a large number of women began to develop a mysterious illness causing nausea, vomiting, diarrhea, mental confusion, and skin rash. In some cases the symptoms progressed to severe shock—depression of the cardiovascular system that can result in death.

The mysterious illness, called toxic shock syndrome (TSS), was eventually found to be caused by a toxin produced by the bacterium *Staphylococcus aureus.* The cases were traced to the use of a new type of highly absorbent tampon during the women's menstrual period. Since the withdrawal of that tampon in 1981, TSS associated with tampon use has not been reported. Still, it is wise to avoid using tampons with more absorbency than you need. You should change tampons every few hours during your menstrual period, leaving a tampon in place for no more than eight hours. Boxes of tampons now carry a leaflet warning about the dangers of this infection and how to avoid it.

wellness **tip**

After you finish urinating, stand for a few moments. Then sit again and lean forward to allow the last few drops to leave your bladder. This is known as double emptying, and it helps prevent the growth of bacteria from urine that remains in the bladder.

Urinary Tract Infections

The urinary tract is a complex system that regulates the body's balance of fluids and filters out waste products. Women are far more likely than men to develop urinary tract infections. About one of every five women develops at least one urinary tract infection (UTI) at some point during her life, most commonly at the onset of sexual activity and between ages 20 and 50.

A UTI seldom poses a serious health threat, but it must be treated. Otherwise, what starts as a relatively minor infection can progress to affect the kidneys, possibly causing permanent kidney damage. Keeping your urinary system healthy begins with understanding how these infections occur, as well as how they can damage your health if they are not treated promptly.

The urinary tract is made up of four major components: the kidneys, ureters, bladder, and urethra. The kidneys, located in your back just under your ribs, filter out toxins from the blood and produce urine, which is then carried through the tubelike ureters to the bladder, where it is stored. Finally, the urethra carries urine from the bladder to the outside of the body.

Most UTIs are caused by bacteria that enter the urinary tract through the urethra. Normally, these bacteria are flushed away when you urinate, keeping the inside of the urethra sterile. Under some circumstances, however, bacteria begin to grow inside the urethra, causing urethritis (inflammation or infection of the urethra). If the bacteria ascend into the bladder, cystitis (bladder infection) may result. Further movement of the infection upward into the ureters and eventually to the kidneys results in pyelonephritis (kidney infection) or even a systemic blood infection. If pyelonephritis is not treated, permanent kidney damage can result.

Most UTIs are treated long before they reach this point. In women, the infection is usually confined to the lower urinary tract—the urethra and bladder. Ascending infection usually occurs only in people with abnormalities in their organs, people with weakened immune systems, or people in whom infection persists for a long period of time (from a resistant strain of bacteria or inadequate treatment).

Why Is It So Common for Women to Get UTIs? As is true of many types of infection, UTIs are more common in women partly because of the female anatomy. The urethral opening lies very close to the entrance to the vagina, giving organisms from the vagina easy access to the lower urinary tract. Also, a woman's urethra is only a few inches long—about one-quarter the length of a man's. In men, bacteria have to travel about four times as far to reach the bladder. It is thus much easier for bacteria to get to a woman's bladder before they can be flushed out of the body during urination.

It is not uncommon for women to develop urinary tract infections after having sexual intercourse. During foreplay or intercourse, the thrusting motions of the hands or penis can spread bacteria from the vagina into the urethra. The penis can irritate the bladder and make it more susceptible to bacterial infection. Use of the diaphragm can also predispose a woman to UTIs. The rim of the diaphragm fits snugly behind the pubic bone, pushing against the thin front wall of the vagina. On the other side of this wall is the urethra, which can become irritated and infected as a result. If you use a diaphragm and get recurrent UTIs, have your doctor check to make sure it fits you properly.

Symptoms. The symptoms of a urinary tract infection are hard to ignore. The normal urge to urinate becomes a pressing need to find a bathroom. You may rush there several times an hour, only to find that you can pass only a few drops of urine. The urine that does pass may be blood-tinged and followed by intense burning and stinging. You may be awakened several times a night by the feeling that you have to urinate.

You may also have some of the following symptoms:

- An aching feeling, pain, or pressure in the lower abdomen
- Cloudy or bloody urine
- Strong odor in your urine
- Nausea and vomiting, fever and chills, or fatigue (produced by a more severe infection)

Prevention and Treatment. Drinking plenty of water—at least eight glasses a day—is especially important if you have, or are prone to getting, a UTI. Water helps your bladder flush out the bacteria causing the infection. Urinate as often as you feel the urge and empty your bladder completely since holding in urine promotes the growth of bacteria.

Cranberry juice (or cranberry extract) has been used as a home remedy to prevent UTIs or to ward off mild symptoms. Research shows that this practice is helpful. The juices of both cranberries and blueberries contain compounds that keep bacteria from sticking to the inner walls of the bladder. These juices, as well as vitamin C, increase the acidity of urine, which discourages the growth of bacteria. Talk to your doctor about these options, especially before taking high doses of any vitamin.

Sexually Transmitted Diseases

Every sexually active woman should know about STDs—how they are spread, her risk for getting them, and how to prevent them. These infections affect individuals of all ages, races, and backgrounds.

STDs occur in both men and women, but their consequences can be more serious in women. Left untreated, some can lead to pelvic inflammatory disease (PID), infertility, problems during pregnancy, health problems in newborns, an increased risk of cancer, and even death. Since the early stages of STD infection produce few or no symptoms in women, STDs may not be recognized until they are more advanced and more dangerous.

Prevention is the best way to avoid STDs. However, if you do contract an STD, early treatment can prevent complications. The best way to protect yourself is to learn about the most common STDs and how to recognize their symptoms.

Chlamydia. The most common STD in American women, chlamydia is caused by the bacteria *Chlamydia trachomatis*. The organism usually infects the cervix, but it can spread upward into the uterus and fallopian tubes. Chlamydia is one of the most common causes of PID, a potentially life-threatening infection of the upper genital tract (see the section "Pelvic Inflammatory Disease" later in this chapter). About 20 to 40 percent of women with untreated chlamydia develop PID.

wellness **tip**

If you tend to get a urinary tract infection after sex, try drinking a full glass of water both before and after you have intercourse. Urinate before having sex and again after intercourse to help flush out the urethra and prevent bacteria from entering your bladder.

Chlamydia infects an estimated 4 million people in the United States each year—including men who usually have no symptoms but act as carriers. Most are adolescents and young adults. It is estimated that 1 in every 10 teenage girls and 1 in every 20 adult women will get chlamydia at some point in their lives.

In as many as three-fourths of women who are infected with a chlamydial virus, symptoms are few or absent. When they do occur, symptoms can take as long as three weeks to appear after contact with an infected sexual partner. In women, the most common symptoms of chlamydia include the following:

- A yellowish discharge from the vagina
- Itching or burning of the vulva
- Pain, stinging, or burning sensation during urination
- Pain in the lower pelvis during intercourse

In men, the most common symptom is pain, stinging, or a burning sensation during urination. It also causes a thick, yellow discharge from the penis.

A simple test can determine whether you have chlamydia. A technician or doctor will collect a sample of cells from your cervix, which will be viewed under a microscope, grown in a culture medium, or checked by a DNA probe to confirm the presence of chlamydia. Chlamydia is treated with oral antibiotics.

Because chlamydia is often passed back and forth between partners, your sexual partner should be treated at the same time that you are taking antibiotics, even if he has no symptoms. You should refrain from having sex while you and your partner are being treated.

Gonorrhea. Records dating as far back as the 1300s show that gonorrhea has long been a serious health threat. Today gonorrhea is one of the most commonly occurring STDs in the United States. About 1 million cases are reported each year, and researchers estimate that the actual number of cases may be twice as high.

Gonorrhea is caused by *Neisseria gonorrhoeae*, bacteria that grow in warm, moist places of the body. The infection occurs most often in girls ages 15 to 19.

FIGURE 22.2

Pap Smear

A Pap smear is the best screening method to detect certain sexually transmitted diseases. During this procedure, the doctor inserts a device called a speculum into the vagina to examine it. The doctor then uses a small brush or swab to collect a sample of cells from the cervix.

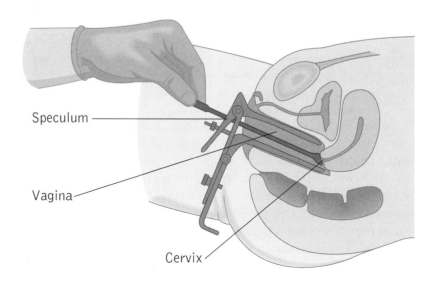

Although the overall incidence of gonorrhea has declined over the past several years, the rate of infected young women has risen as more people in this age group are not practicing safe sex.

Gonorrhea very often occurs with chlamydia. The symptoms—and the consequences if left untreated—of the two infections are similar. About half of women with gonorrhea have no symptoms of the infection. When symptoms do occur, it may be weeks after exposure to the organism.

The symptoms of gonorrhea are nearly identical to those of chlamydia: a yellowish vaginal discharge, painful urination, and sometimes pain in the lower abdomen.

Gonorrhea can also occur in the rectum or the throat after anal or oral sex. Rectal discharge and pain and itching around the anal area can be signs of rectal gonorrhea; soreness and redness in the throat and difficulty swallowing may be symptoms of infection of the throat. Serious gonococcal infections can affect the whole body—causing joint pain and swelling.

A tissue culture is usually needed to diagnose gonorrhea. A sample of cells from the cervix and surrounding areas is examined under a microscope, grown in a culture medium, or checked by a DNA probe test. Results are usually available 48 hours later. Gonorrhea and chlamydia occur together so often that an antibiotic treatment is usually chosen that will be effective against both infections. Recently, however, there have emerged strains of gonorrhea that are resistant to the antibiotics usually used against them. Newer drugs have been developed to combat these resistant strains.

Syphilis. The disease we now know as syphilis is another STD that has plagued people for hundreds of years. Before the advent of antibiotics, the disease was often fatal. Today, it is easily cured if it is caught in time.

An epidemic of syphilis occurred in the United States from 1986 to 1990. The rate of the disease is falling, but tens of thousands of people still become infected each year.

Syphilis is caused by the spiral-shaped bacteria *Treponema pallidum,* which enter the body through the mucous membranes or skin. It can be detected from a culture of the chancre (a small, painless sore) that appears during the primary stage of the infection. Because the chancre can easily go unnoticed, however, the infection may not be detected until the second stage when a rash appears. Blood tests are often used to detect syphilis. Penicillin cures the infection in 98 percent of cases that are diagnosed early. If left untreated, syphilis can spread to the central nervous system, causing tertiary syphilis, which takes years to develop but causes irreversible nerve damage.

Genital Herpes. The virus that causes genital herpes belongs to the same family of viruses (herpes) that cause chickenpox and shingles (herpes zoster). Almost a quarter of a million new cases of infection with herpes simplex virus (HSV) are diagnosed each year in the United States. HSV causes sores in and around the mucous membranes, such as the lips and the genital area. In most infected people, the sores appear (often under stress or during illness), subside, and then recur again and again—with weeks, months, or years between recurrences. The virus cannot be eliminated completely. Once it is in the bloodstream it remains "hidden" in cells at the base of the spine, emerging now and then to cause the sores.

wellness **tip**

Examining your genital area on a regular basis is a good way to catch early signs of many kinds of infections, including STDs. Using a handheld mirror and a bright light, look for redness, swelling, or any type of lump, bump, discoloration, or sore around the vaginal opening, the lips of the vulva, the perineum (area between the vagina and anus), and the anus. See your doctor promptly if you notice anything unusual.

HSV exists in two forms—type 1 and type 2 (HSV-1 and HSV-2). Either of these types can cause herpes sores. HSV-1 is more often responsible for the common "cold sores" around the lips and mouth and is not usually sexually transmitted. HSV-2 is usually (but not always) the cause of herpes sores in the genital area. The herpes sores caused by type 2 seem to be more painful and harder to get rid of than those caused by type 1.

How Herpes Spreads. The most common way that herpes is passed from one person to another is through mucus membrane contact with an open sore—whether a cold sore or a genital sore. Herpes can also be passed from an infected sexual partner even if no sores are apparent at the time. Some people with herpes infections "shed" the virus, even when no sore is visible. In rare cases, a person with herpes never becomes aware that she has the infection because the virus never causes sores. Nevertheless, she can still pass the virus to others.

The sores caused by herpes are small, yellowish lesions that look like blisters. A single sore may erupt by itself, or many small ones may appear in clusters. The sores tend to reappear in the same places on the body, but they can also spread to new areas if you rub or touch them.

The appearance of a herpes sore is usually preceded by a prodromal stage, which signals the onset of a new sore. The area where the sore will appear feels tingly, numb, or more sensitive than usual. Within hours of this tingly sensation, the herpes sore begins to emerge. The very first herpes sore that appears after a person is first infected with the virus is often very painful—more so than subsequent ones. After several days or, in some cases, a few weeks, the sore begins to crust over, dry up, and subside.

Some people never have another herpes sore after the first episode. In others, sores recur within weeks or months. There is no set pattern to the frequency with which the sores erupt. A person may get two or three in a row within a month or two, and then not get any more for months or even years.

Diagnosing Herpes. Herpes is best diagnosed when a lesion is present. Your doctor will examine the sore and can collect a sample to view under a microscope. A blood test is also available but is usually not needed. Antiviral drugs, when started at the first sign of an outbreak, can reduce the severity and duration of the herpes outbreak. Medication can also be taken on a daily basis to prevent or reduce the recurrence of the herpes infection. If you have frequent infections, speak with your doctor about suppressant medication. However, there is currently no way to eliminate the virus from the body.

Genital Warts. Also called condyloma, genital warts are caused by human papillomavirus (HPV). This infection occurs most often in women aged 20 to 24 who have multiple sexual partners.

The virus that causes genital warts belongs to the same family of viruses that causes common warts on fingers and toes. The warts caused by HPV, however, are much more dangerous: some have been linked to cervical cancer.

Genital warts are small growths that appear on or near the cervix, vaginal opening, vulva, anus, or inner and upper thighs. The warts may be raised or flat; flesh-colored, whitish, pinkish, or gray. They may be painless or they may cause

Tips for Preventing Sexually Transmitted Diseases

There is a lot you can do to lower your risk of contracting sexually transmitted diseases (STDs). Follow these simple but important guidelines:

- **Know your sex partner.** Your partner's sexual history is as important as your own. Many STDs can take years to produce symptoms or illness. By having sexual intercourse with someone, you are indirectly exposing yourself to all of his past partners.
- **Use condoms each and every time you have sex.** Aside from abstinence, latex condoms provide the best known protection against STDs, including the virus that causes acquired immunodeficiency syndrome (AIDS). Other forms of birth control that you may be using, such as the diaphragm or the pill, prevent pregnancy but do nothing to stop the spread of disease. Latex condoms should be used in addition to these methods.
- **Avoid high-risk sex.** Any sexual practice that results in damage or microscopic tearing of the mucous membranes can make you vulnerable to STDs. High-risk sexual behaviors, such as anal intercourse, result in a high incidence of STDs.
- **Be alert to the symptoms of STDs.** Any vaginal discharge that is unusual in color, odor, or amount could be a sign of an infection. Pain, itching, burning, or stinging in the genital area are also warning signs. In addition, watch for symptoms in your partner, such as penile discharge, that may mean he is infected.
- **Get regular pelvic examinations.** Your doctor should offer to test you for gonorrhea and chlamydia, two common STDs, at each visit, if she knows you are at risk for STDs. Regular pelvic examinations and Pap smears can also detect possible signs of infection in its early stages, when treatment has a better chance of success.

itching, pain, and bleeding. Often they are clustered in cauliflower-like groups, but they can also appear singly.

A woman with genital warts may not notice any symptoms, especially if the warts are on the cervix. In men, the warts are usually under the foreskin or inside the opening at the end of the penis. HPV can be passed from someone without visible warts. It can take anywhere from a few weeks to several months for warts to appear after a person has been exposed to the virus.

Detecting and Treating HPV. HPV cannot be grown in a culture medium, and there is as yet no blood test that can detect it. For this reason, most cases are diagnosed on the basis of what the doctor can see.

Apart from visual observation, a mildly acidic solution (acetic acid) can be brushed over the cervix and the inside of the vagina. If the mucus membrane turns whitish, a biopsy can confirm the diagnosis of HPV infection.

Getting rid of genital warts is possible but seldom easy. There are many treatments to get rid of visible warts, ranging from topical applications of anti-wart medications to surgical procedures (including laser surgery) to injecting them with interferon. In some cases, the warts go away on their own without treatment, but the virus remains in the affected area and additional outbreaks are common.

HPV and Cervical Cancer. The greatest concern for women with HPV is that some strains of the virus have been linked to cervical cancer. For this reason, it is important to have regular pelvic examinations—usually every six months—if you have ever had genital warts. These regular examinations are important to ensure that the wart virus has not caused any precancerous changes on the cervix or in the vagina.

Pelvic Inflammatory Disease. A potentially dangerous complication of untreated STDs, PID affects more than 1 million U.S. women every year. Almost 100,000 women were hospitalized for PID in 1993 alone. Three-fourths of all cases of PID occur in women under the age of 25. Some research suggests that very young women may be at higher risk for PID because the cells of the cervix are more vulnerable to infection at younger ages.

PID is sometimes called salpingitis, a term that refers to an infection of the fallopian tubes. It almost always develops from an untreated infection of the lower genital tract—usually the cervix. Chlamydia and gonorrhea, two STDs that often occur together, are the most common causes, but other bacterial species are usually present as well in PID.

If not treated properly, an infection in the lower genital tract can move upward into the uterus, fallopian tubes, and ovaries. These structures can then become inflamed and swollen, producing pus and other infected fluid that spreads the infection further inside the abdomen.

The delicate lining of the fallopian tubes is especially susceptible to damage by PID. These narrow passageways can become scarred by the inflammatory process, which results in obstructing the path taken by a fertilized egg on its way to the uterus. In severe cases, the scarring is so severe that sperm cannot reach the egg and a woman becomes infertile. In some cases, the sperm can still get through, but the developing egg cannot, so a woman is at risk for a tubal, or ectopic, pregnancy.

Ectopic pregnancy carries its own risks. The narrow fallopian tubes are not designed to contain a growing embryo, so a fertilized egg that lodges there can eventually grow to the point where the tube bursts, causing bleeding into the abdomen. A ruptured ectopic pregnancy is a serious threat to the woman's life, resulting in shock and even death if surgical treatment is not rapidly available.

Any woman who is sexually active can be at risk for PID. The factors that place you at risk are generally the same ones that increase your risk of acquiring an STD.

Diagnosing PID. Many women do not discover that they have PID until they begin having abdominal pain—dull at first, then increasingly severe. It occurs more commonly after a menstrual period. Some women may first experience painful symptoms with intercourse, while others may experience severe abdominal pain with a routine pelvic examination. The doctor may note that there is pus coming out of the cervical opening and that movement of the cervix causes extreme discomfort. Microscopic examination of the cervical secretions and cultures from the cervix may help to diagnose this serious condition. Other tests can be used to diagnose PID:

- **Ultrasound.** A handheld device is moved over the surface of the abdomen or inside the vagina, creating sound waves that are then transformed into images of the internal structures and organs. An ultrasound will show enlarged, swollen fallopian tubes or signs of abcess formation in the lower abdomen.
- **Culdocentesis.** A needle is inserted through the vaginal wall into the lowest part of the abdomen to collect cells and fluid. If pus is collected, it usually means PID. If blood is collected, it may indicate a ruptured cyst or an ectopic pregnancy.

- **Laparoscopy.** In this minor surgical procedure, a slender, telescope-like tube is inserted through a tiny incision in the abdomen to view the internal organs and collect samples of fluid or tissue if needed to help make a diagnosis.
- **Complete blood count.** White blood cells increase in number with any kind of infection. The white cell count can indicate the severity of the infection and help your doctor determine which treatment to use. Red blood cells decrease with significant bleeding, and severe anemia may indicate bleeding into the abdomen from a ruptured ectopic pregnancy or tubal abcess.

Treating PID. PID must be treated aggressively with antibiotics. Because the infection is almost always caused by a variety of bacterial species, two or more broad-spectrum antibiotics are usually chosen. Often one antibiotic is given as an intramuscular injection and another is taken by mouth over an extended period of time. In severe or life-threatening cases—such as when a woman with PID must be admitted to a hospital—antibiotics are given intravenously. Follow-up examinations by the doctor and follow-up ultrasound or laboratory studies will help to ensure that the infection has been cleared.

Preventing *Viral* Hepatitis

The word hepatitis means "inflammation of the liver." The liver, the largest internal organ in the body, is located in the upper right side of the abdomen. It has the vital function of filtering out wastes from the blood and processing nutrients from the digestive tract. Sometimes the liver and its functions are referred to as the "portal" system because it acts as a gateway through which all elements added to and removed from the blood must pass.

Hepatitis can be caused by liver damage due to certain medications, exposure to toxins, or heavy alcohol use. These cases are more rare, however, than viral hepatitis.

Viral hepatitis can be either acute (short term) or chronic (long term). Acute disease causes symptoms that resolve within several weeks. In chronic hepatitis, the virus is present in a person's body without symptoms (this can sometimes occur after acute hepatitis has cleared up). People with chronic hepatitis are said to be carriers and can infect others, even though they do not appear to be sick.

There are five identified types of viral hepatitis. The most common—hepatitis A, B, and C—are discussed below.

The various types of viral hepatitis have similar symptoms, though some symptoms of B and C tend to be more severe than others. Symptoms usually do not show up until weeks after a person has been infected. Once they do appear, they can include the following:

- Nausea and vomiting
- Diarrhea
- Low-grade fever
- Fatigue
- Jaundice—a yellowing of the whites of the eyes and the skin
- Darkened urine

wellness **tip**

Because contaminated drinking water and food are sources of hepatitis A, people traveling to developing countries where water treatment and food handling are less than optimum are advised to receive the hepatitis A vaccine before traveling, if they are not already immune.

The last two of these symptoms develop because the infected liver cannot clear bile from the blood fast enough.

Although hepatitis A, B, and C produce similar symptoms, their consequences differ widely. Depending on which type of the hepatitis virus is causing the disease, it may be only a mild health problem, or it may have more serious, even fatal consequences.

Hepatitis A

Hepatitis A virus causes almost half of all cases of viral hepatitis and is highly contagious. The virus is spread through contaminated food and water and through the blood and feces of an infected person.

Symptoms of hepatitis A can take as long as two to six weeks to appear after a person is infected. Because of the lag time between infection and the time that symptoms develop, an individual can be infected—and can infect someone else—before being aware that she has hepatitis A.

Most people who develop hepatitis A recover fully within a couple of months, by which time the liver is completely healed. The virus does not remain in the blood, and the person cannot be infected with hepatitis A virus again.

A vaccine is now available that protects against hepatitis A virus. This vaccine can be given to people who are likely to come into contact with the virus. If it is likely that you have been exposed to hepatitis A without the protection of the vaccine, you can receive an injection of an immunoglobulin that can reduce the chances of infection. Immunoglobulin is a protein that can stimulate your immune system to make antibodies against the virus.

The simplest preventative measure against hepatitis A is to avoid poor sanitation, to be sure that your hands are clean when you prepare or eat food, and to wash foods that will not be cooked.

Hepatitis B

Hepatitis B virus (HBV) is mainly transmitted through contact with the blood, semen, or vaginal fluid of an infected person. The symptoms of HBV tend to be more severe than those of hepatitis A. However, up to 90 percent of people who get HBV infection recover fully in three to four months if there is no permanent damage to the liver.

HBV is most commonly transmitted through sex. Other ways in which the infection is spread include the following:

- Sharing of contaminated needles used to inject intravenous drugs
- Contact of a newborn's mucous membranes with the blood of an infected mother at birth
- In a small number of cases, tattooing, body piercing, acupuncture, and injuries from contaminated needles or other medical instruments

Up to ten percent of adults who are exposed to HBV develop a chronic infection and become carriers of the virus, whether or not they ever have symptoms of illness. An HBV carrier can transmit the virus to others and, over time, runs the risk of having permanent liver damage. Early death from cirrhosis (scarring of the liver) or liver cancer occurs in 15 to 25 percent of people with chronic HBV infection.

A vaccine exists to prevent HBV infection and is recommended for anyone who is at increased risk for exposure to the virus. (See Chapter 2 for risk factors associated with HBV infection.) Unlike hepatitis A, there is no vaccine that can prevent infection after exposure to HBV.

The best prevention against hepatitis B is to practice safe sex: limit your sexual partners to those whose sexual history you know, avoid sex with bisexual men or intravenous drug users, and do not share needles used to inject intravenous drugs. Condoms can help prevent the spread of HBV as well as other sexually transmitted infections.

Hepatitis C

The symptoms of hepatitis C may take as long as six to seven weeks to appear after a person has been exposed to the virus. In most people, symptoms are either absent or consist only of very mild fatigue without jaundice. For this reason, hepatitis C infection is often diagnosed not because of symptoms, but because a liver test was done for some other reason.

Hepatitis C is most often transmitted when intravenous drug users share needles. Less often, people who receive blood transfusions or organ transplants contract hepatitis C. Donor blood has been screened for hepatitis C virus since 1990, so this is now a rare cause of infection.

Infection with hepatitis C virus leads to chronic liver disease in about 70 percent of people who are infected. Nearly everyone infected with the virus becomes a carrier and is at increased risk of cirrhosis and liver cancer.

Avoiding sexual contact with known carriers of hepatitis C can prevent this infection. No vaccines or immunoglobulin injections have yet been developed that can prevent infection with the hepatitis C virus. As with HBV, practicing safe sex is the best preventative measure against the infection.

Preventing Tuberculosis

Tuberculosis (TB), a lung infection caused by the bacterium *Mycobacterium tuberculosis,* was common throughout Europe, England, and the United States in the 1700s and 1800s. In fact, it was called "the poet's disease" because it had caused the deaths of so many famous writers, including John Keats and D. H. Lawrence.

Today, people rarely die from TB, but the number of cases diagnosed each year has been growing since the 1980s. This increase is thought to be linked with the decreased immunity caused by AIDS. Many of the same risk factors—in particular, sharing needles among intravenous drug users—are common to both diseases, so people at risk for AIDS are also susceptible to TB.

However, *M. tuberculosis* most often enters the lungs through airborne droplets. From the lungs, it is carried by the blood and lymph systems throughout the rest of the body. The symptoms of TB usually occur within weeks of exposure to the bacterium. In some cases, however, the organism lies dormant for years before TB develops. Symptoms of TB include the following:

- Coughing up blood or discolored sputum
- Pain with breathing and coughing

- Pain in the spine and joints
- Decreased appetite and weight loss
- Fatigue
- Slight fever
- Night sweats

Whether symptoms take weeks or years to appear, the disease is usually well advanced by the time that they are noticeable. TB is still fatal in cases where people do not get the proper diagnosis and treatment.

TB may be diagnosed if your doctor notices a spot on a chest x-ray. If she suspects TB based on your risk factors, a skin test will be ordered to determine whether you have been exposed. It consists of a substance called tuberculin purified protein derivative (PPD). This is a microscopic portion of the TB bacterium that is injected just beneath the surface of the skin. The PPD does not cause disease, but it does have the ability to trigger an immune reaction in the form of raised bumps on the skin's surface. This reaction takes one to three days to develop, so you must return within two to three days to have the results interpreted by a health professional.

TB now can nearly always be cured with antibiotics. However, new strains of TB—often resistant to the commonly used antibiotics—are emerging, especially in patients with AIDS. The antibiotic-resistant form is most common in people who got the disease through intravenous drug use and those who also have AIDS. In these cases, multiple antibiotics are used to combat the infection, but proper diagnosis and identification of the bacterial strain are important.

If you have any reason to suspect that you may have been exposed to TB, contact your doctor right away. The PPD skin test is easy to obtain, and with early treatment you have excellent chances of recovering fully from this disease.

Preventing HIV *and* AIDS

HIV, the virus that causes AIDS, first identified in the early 1980s, has caused the deaths of many thousands of women. More new AIDS cases are diagnosed among women each year in the United States than among men. Younger women are at higher risk for this life-threatening disease than older women. While treatment is available, there is no known cure for AIDS, and so the first line of defense is knowing how to prevent HIV infection.

To become infected with HIV, the virus must get into your bloodstream. Since the virus is present in blood and semen, the most common way women become infected is through sex with an infected partner. Small amounts of the virus reside in vaginal fluid and saliva of affected women, but it is much more easily passed from a man to a woman during sex than from a woman to a man.

Intranvenous drug use is another common source of infection because needles are so often shared among users. Before 1985, when screening of donor blood began, transfusions were a source of HIV infection, as were in vitro fertilization procedures conducted before semen-donor screening began in 1990.

To prevent infection by HIV, women must avoid risky sexual behaviors. The same risk factors apply to HIV infection that apply for other STDs (see previous section in this chapter). The use of a latex condom with partners with uncertain sexual histories is currently the best form of prevention, though it is not considered 100 percent effective.

After HIV enters the bloodstream, the symptoms of AIDS can take months or years to develop. The first signs may be weakness, fatigue, weight loss, night sweats, swollen lymph glands, and low-grade fever. Eventually, any one of a number of opportunistic infections—so called because they "take the opportunity" to attack when defenses are down—may then gain a foothold. Eventually, the AIDS victim becomes seriously weakened and dies.

By the time a person develops "full-blown" AIDS, HIV infection has advanced to a life-threatening point. HIV infection and AIDS ultimately lead to death in 100 percent of the people who become infected. On average, death occurs within five years of the diagnosis of full-blown AIDS. For this reason, more and more doctors are not waiting for AIDS to manifest in their HIV-positive patients. Rather, they are beginning to battle the disease long before any signs or symptoms of illness are present. Doctors are now starting to look at HIV infection not as a necessarily fatal illness, but as a long-term condition that can be managed in order to extend the patient's quality of life.

Research on HIV and AIDS is yielding new treatments. The drug zidovudine (once called azidothymidine, or AZT) has been used for years to treat people with AIDS. The drug seems to slow the rate at which the virus multiplies. Today, AZT is being used with good results in HIV-positive patients who have not yet developed any symptoms of AIDS. Many other antiviral drugs are used, alone or in combination, to reduce the viral load in the body and to raise the level of CD4, a protein on the surface of cells that helps the immune system combat disease. With these treatments, many HIV patients are stabilizing their disease and living long and productive lives.

If you have any of the risk factors for HIV, it is a good idea to get tested. You may be reassured to find you are not infected, or, if you are infected, you can get the best care as

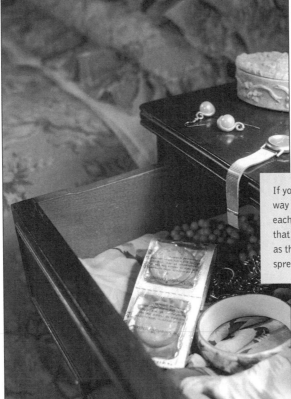

If you are sexually active, the most effective way to prevent HIV is to use a latex condom, each and every time you have sex. Remember that nonbarrier methods of birth control, such as the pill and IUD, do not protect against the spread of infection.

Myths About HIV and AIDS

Numerous misconceptions have sprung up about the ways in which human immunodeficiency virus (HIV) can be spread, causing unnecessary fear and scorn of people infected with HIV. Despite what you may have heard, HIV has *never* been shown to be spread in any of the following ways.

HIV is *not* spread through:

- **Casual contact (touching, hugging, light kissing)**
- **Insect bites**
- **Sneezing or coughing**
- **Toilet seats, doorknobs, or other objects**

Should You Get an HIV Test?

Human immunodeficiency virus (HIV) is now recognized as a health threat to women and men in all walks of life, and of all ages, races, and backgrounds. You can not assume that you are immune to HIV infection because you are in a sexually exclusive relationship and do not use drugs. Your partner's history is as important as your own. Consider getting tested for HIV if any of the following apply to you:

- You have had more than one sex partner.
- You have had sex with an intravenous drug user.
- You use intravenous drugs now, or have used them in the past.
- You had a blood transfusion before 1985.
- You have a sexually transmitted disease (STD) now, or have had one in the past.
- You had artificial insemination with donor semen before 1990.
- You work in a health care setting where you are exposed to blood and other body fluids.
- You have had sex with someone who has any of the above risk factors.

If you have doubts, ask your doctor about your level of risk for HIV and whether you should be tested. Many cities have free or inexpensive clinics that offer anonymous testing, and home kits are available. Remember that these tests do not become positive until you have had the virus in your body for a few weeks or months. If there is any question, you should be rechecked in three to six months.

early as possible. It would also be beneficial (even lifesaving) to change your lifestyle if you have risk factors for HIV, because a negative test now does not mean you will not get the disease in the future. Home and doctor's office tests are available to check for the antibody to HIV, but these tests do not become positive until you have had the virus in your body for a few weeks or months. If there is any question, you should be rechecked in three to six months.

What *You* Can Do

Prevention is the key to keeping your immune system free of infection and boosting your body's own natural defenses:

- Eat well, exercise, and rest. Your immune system can keep you healthy most of the time—if you take care of it. As you care for your overall health by eating well, exercising, and getting enough rest, you strengthen your immune system.
- Reduce stress. Stress and fatigue have a negative effect on the effectiveness of the immune system. How many times have you gotten a cold after a particularly harrowing week at work? After any stressful period—whether it is an important meeting at work or just your normal, activity-filled week—be sure to take some time to relax and renew your energy, even if only for an hour or two. Make time for exercise, a favorite hobby, or relaxation exercises.

- Prevent immune diseases by eliminating your risk of getting AIDS and other sexually transmitted diseases. All STDs weaken your immune system, leaving you open to other infections. There is currently no cure for AIDS, only treatments.
- Make use of screening tests. Whenever you think you might have been exposed to a serious infection, such as tuberculosis or hepatitis, have yourself tested immediately. Early detection is the surest way to a cure.
- Are you at risk for complications from influenza? Discuss with your doctor the advisability of receiving a flu shot.
- If you have any of the risk factors for hepatitis, get vaccinated to prevent this life-threatening infection.

Protecting *Against* Metabolic Disease

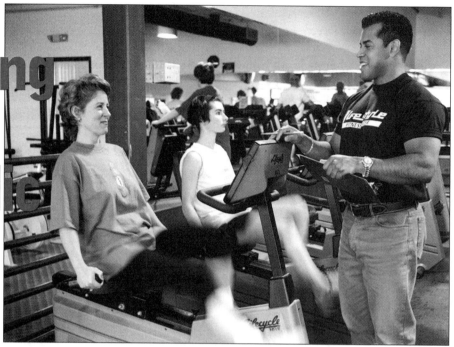

Whether you are exercising hard, sitting and relaxing, or even fast asleep, your metabolism keeps all systems going within your body. It is like the automatic pilot on an aircraft. Another way to think of your metabolism is as your body's furnace. It converts the nutrients you consume into the energy you need to breathe, walk, talk, act, and think. It also provides energy for more basic functions, such as pumping blood, healing cuts, and mending broken bones. If you make sure it is well maintained through proper diet and exercise, you can count on your metabolism to generate the physical and chemical processes necessary to sustain your life.

You have probably heard that people have different metabolic rates. Some people are said to have a slow metabolism, others to have a quick, or fast, metabolism. The speed of your metabolism depends primarily on your age, your weight, your hormonal status, your fitness, and your lifestyle. The younger and the more active you are, the faster your metabolism. An overweight woman usually has a slower metabolism, primarily because more of her body is fat, and she may be less active. Metabolic rate is also influenced by genetic factors. You are born with a faster or slower metabolism. However, the metabolic rate is not fixed in any one individual. It is possible—though not easy—to increase it by becoming more active through regular exercise.

When you go through menopause, the drop in estrogen levels causes a reduction in your metabolic rate. This can be reversed with hormone replacement or an increase in physical activity.

The process of metabolism occurs at the most basic level in your body—in the cell. To prevent your body from processing nutrients too quickly or too slowly, hormones are constantly released by glands in the body's endocrine system, and these hormones, or chemical messengers, regulate cell metabolism. When this process functions smoothly, your body operates at its most efficient level. You maintain an appropriate weight for your age and bone structure, you have the energy you need, and your mental powers are healthy and responsive. The first step in keeping your metabolism functioning at its best is to become familiar with your body's normal metabolic processes. These are handled by the endocrine system.

The **Endocrine** System

A woman's endocrine system is made up of a network of ductless glands—the pituitary gland, the thyroid, the parathyroid, the adrenal glands, and the pancreas—that control a variety of processes:

- Height
- Weight
- Growth
- Sexual development
- Menstruation
- Hair and bone growth
- Fertility
- Pregnancy and breast milk production
- Some aspects of personality and behavior

In addition, the glands manage the body's responses to changes in the internal and external environment, such as illness and stress. The different glands in the endocrine system work interdependently so that the action (or inaction) of one will likely affect the others.

The Pituitary Gland

A small gland located at the base of your brain, the pituitary regulates your body's growth, daily functioning, and reproductive abilities. It is probably the most important of all your endocrine glands because the pituitary acts as the control center for all other endocrine glands, producing hormones that stimulate other glands to do their work. The pituitary gland's production is regulated by your hypothalamus, also located in your brain.

The Thyroid

Your thyroid can be found at the base of your neck, in front of your windpipe. This butterfly-shaped gland secretes the hormones thyroxine and triiodothyronine, which control the metabolic rate. When the thyroid is producing excessive amounts of hormone, your bodily functions, including heart rate, speed up tremendously. If the thyroid does not produce enough hormone, your body slows down, making it difficult to function normally.

The Parathyroid

Your parathyroid includes four glands, also in your neck, located behind or near the thyroid. These glands secrete the parathyroid hormone (PTH), which regulates

Is My Weight Problem Related to My Metabolism?

It is a popular belief among dieters that if you can speed up your metabolism, the pounds will just melt away. Is it true, or is it simply wishful thinking?

It is true that a faster metabolism burns more calories than a slow one. However, it is much harder to alter your natural metabolism than you think. You can temporarily speed it up through exercise, but that is about it.

Interestingly enough, many people with slow metabolisms tend to eat less than those with fast metabolisms, and vice versa. Under normal circumstances people consume the appropriate amount of food for their energy needs. However, if you have a weight problem and you are not eating excessively, your metabolism may be at fault. Studies have shown that some people's bodies inefficiently burn the fuel that comes from food. Their bodies store food as fat instead of burning it for energy.

If your body is a fat-storer, then reducing or eliminating fat from your diet and exercising regularly are the best ways to avoid gaining weight.

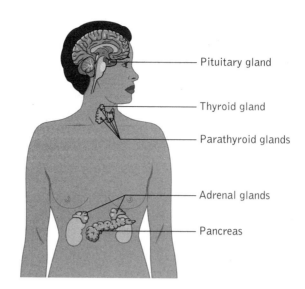

Pituitary gland

Thyroid gland

Parathyroid glands

Adrenal glands

Pancreas

FIGURE 23.1
Your Endocrine System
The glands of the endocrine system effect virtually every part of the body and control a variety of processes, ranging from hair and bone growth to your reaction to stressful situations.

calcium in your bloodstream. PTH regulates the absorption and release of calcium by your bones whenever needed. It also facilitates calcium absorption in the intestines and stimulates the kidneys to make a form of vitamin D.

The Adrenal Glands

Located on the top of each kidney, your adrenal glands are triangular glands about the size of the top sections of your thumbs. They produce a variety of hormones that affect almost every system in your body. These include the hormone adrenaline, which helps you respond to stress by increasing your heart rate, blood pressure, and speed of other body functions. When the adrenal glands fail to function, autoimmune disease or other serious disorders might result. Overproduction of these hormones is also very dangerous.

The Pancreas

Your pancreas is a long, thin gland—about the length of your hand—located behind your stomach. This gland produces the enzymes needed to digest food. It also produces the hormones that allow your body to metabolize the food you eat. The three hormones it produces—insulin, glucagon, and somatostatin—control your body's use of sugar, fats, and proteins. When the pancreas malfunctions, the body cannot efficiently use food as energy.

Metabolism, the Endocrine System, and Wellness

You have already learned that metabolism is like your body's furnace, processing nutrients and producing energy. You also know that the endocrine system controls your body's metabolism. Using the same analogy, imagine what happens if you turn the furnace in your home up too high. Obviously it will burn more fuel and produce more heat than you need. In a similar way, if for any reason the endocrine system "turns up" your metabolism, many of your bodily functions will speed up. Your glands might produce too many hormones, causing dramatic changes ranging from hair growth to a racing heartbeat. Some of these changes are permanent, and some are even life-threatening.

Your Body's Hormones

To keep your metabolism working properly and efficiently, the endocrine system uses hormones. Following is a list of hormones and their functions:

- **Adrenocorticotropin (ACTH)** is released in response to any kind of stress. ACTH controls the adrenal glands' production of the corticosteroid hormones.
  Produced by: pituitary gland
- **Catecholamines** also are secreted in response to stress. These include adrenaline (epinephrine) and norepinephrine.
  Produced by: adrenal glands
- **Follicle-stimulating hormone (FSH)** stimulates the production of estrogen in the first half of the menstrual cycle, which causes egg maturation in the ovary.
  Produced by: pituitary gland
- **Glucocorticoids** help your body deal with stress, reduce inflammation, and increase the level of sugar in the blood. Synthetic forms of these hormones are also available and include prednisone, dexamethasone, and hydrocortisone (cortisol). Synthetic glucocorticoids are used to treat a variety of disorders, such as severe arthritis and asthma.
  Produced by: adrenal glands
- **Insulin** makes it possible for cells to absorb glucose (blood sugar), the fuel necessary for energy. When cells are unable to absorb glucose, blood glucose levels rise (diabetes).
  Produced by: pancreas
- **Luteinizing hormone (LH)** stimulates ovulation and the production of progesterone by the ovaries in the second half of the menstrual cycle.
  Produced by: pituitary gland
- **Mineralocorticoids** keep blood volume normal. Too much of these hormones results in fluid retention, high blood pressure, loss of potassium, and a slight increase of salt in the body. Too little results in low blood pressure, excess potassium, heavy salt loss, and a collapse of blood vessels.
  Produced by: adrenal glands
- **Adrenal sex steroids** stimulate normal sexual development through puberty. These hormones include small amounts of estrogen, testosterone, progesterone, DHEA, DHEA-S, and androstenedione. After puberty, the sex hormones are found in the ovaries in women (and in the testes in men).
  Produced by: adrenal glands
- **Thyroxin** controls the speed of chemical activity in your body. It helps determine how fast you burn up calories.
  Produced by: thyroid gland

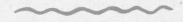

Conversely, sometimes the endocrine system fails to "fire up" your metabolism. (This happens naturally as you age.) A slowing metabolism means the glands do not release enough hormones, which can result in weight gain and extreme fatigue. Again, these changes can also be permanent and life-threatening.

Medically diagnosing a slow-down or an acceleration in metabolic function is the best way to become aware of a disease of this sort. Symptoms vary—severe drowsiness or thirst to sudden weight loss or frequent urination (see box on page 515)—so bring any change to the attention of your physician. Since many endocrine disorders are genetic—that is, they run in families—your doctor can help you determine if you are at risk.

Could *You* Be *at* Risk
for Diabetes *or* Thyroid Disease?

When your body maintains a precise hormonal balance, it functions efficiently and you feel healthy. But because a healthy metabolism requires so many finely tuned interactions among many glands, even small changes can result in problems. Malfunctions sometimes develop into metabolic disease. Women especially are at risk for metabolic disorders, such as diabetes and thyroid dysfunction. These disorders often go undiagnosed for many years, and since half of the 16 million people who are affected by diabetes are unaware that they have the disease, it is wise to be aware of your risk factors and to know what symptoms require further investigation.

What Happens When You Have Diabetes?

Diabetes mellitus, usually called just diabetes, occurs when the body is unable to produce and/or respond to insulin. Insulin, made by the pancreas, is the hormone that enables blood sugar to cross from the bloodstream into the cells where it is used for energy. There are two types of diabetes: Type 1, previously called insulin-dependent, or juvenile, diabetes; and Type 2, previously called non–insulin-dependent, or adult-onset, diabetes.

Type 1 diabetes occurs when the body does not produce any insulin. Experts believe it to be an autoimmune disease caused by a virus or some other "trigger" in the environment. The trigger stimulates the body to destroy pancreatic cells, eventually stopping insulin production. This type of diabetes typically strikes children and young adults.

Type 2 diabetes occurs when the body produces insulin but cannot use it efficiently. The pancreas puts out more and more insulin until it starts to be depleted. This type of diabetes is more common and accounts for 90 to 95 percent of all diabetes cases. It usually does not develop until after age 40.

Symptoms for both types of diabetes are similar. They include frequent urination, extreme hunger, blurred vision, and tingling or numbing sensations in the hands or feet. In addition, female diabetics may experience recurrent skin and vaginal infections. Many of the symptoms of Type 2 diabetes develop so gradually that they are often overlooked or attributed to other causes, such as aging. In Type 2 diabetes, there may be no symptoms at all for the first few years, causing it to go undiagnosed.

Risk Factors. Are you at risk for diabetes? You are if you have a family history of the disease, but experts say that only a quarter of those who contract diabetes are genetically predisposed. Therefore, you can get diabetes if you have no family history—and you may not get it even if you do. If you have any of these additional risk factors, let your doctor know so you can be properly screened for diabetes:

- Delivered a baby weighing more than 9 pounds or had gestational (pregnancy-induced) diabetes
- Had a previous test showing impaired glucose metabolism (borderline diabetes)
- Obesity (more than 20 percent above healthy body weight)
- Ethnic background (African Americans and Hispanics are one and a half to two times more likely to develop diabetes than whites; Native Americans are at even higher risk)
- High blood pressure (140/90 or higher)
- HDL ("good") cholesterol level of 35 or below and/or a blood triglyceride level of 250 or higher
- Impaired glucose metabolism (a fasting blood glucose between 110 and 125 mg/dL or a glucose tolerance test result between 140 and 199 mg/dL)

In addition, women and smokers should be aware of the greater impact that diabetes has on their bodies.

Complications. Both Type 1 and Type 2 diabetes can cause serious health complications. These are usually more severe with the former. For example, Type 1 diabetes can lead to a diabetic coma caused by very high glucose levels. An insulin reaction caused by low levels of glucose is also potentially life-threatening.

Long-term, debilitating complications for both types of diabetes include blindness, kidney failure, nerve damage, heart disease, high blood pressure, cholesterol abnormalities, and damage to blood vessels and nerves. Though not immediately life-threatening, such damage can lead to premature death. In addition, unless carefully monitored, diabetes sometimes causes complications during pregnancy, which can result in miscarriage or fetal death.

Screening. The American Diabetes Association (ADA) strongly recommends routine screening (once every three years) for all Americans starting at age 45, and earlier and more frequently if you are at high risk. There are several methods of screening for diabetes. In addition to evaluating symptoms, your doctor is likely to recommend one or more of the following tests:

- **Fasting Blood Glucose Measurement.** This test measures your glucose level after you have not eaten for 10 to 16 hours. A blood sample is tested for levels of glucose. A blood glucose measurement of 126 milligrams per deciliter (mg/dL) is now considered diagnostic of diabetes if confirmed with a repeat test on a different day, in combination with symptoms of diabetes.
- **Nonfasting Blood Glucose Measurement.** This test measures your glucose level at any time, without regard to when you last ate. A nonfasting blood glucose reading greater than 200 mg/dL is now considered diagnostic of

---

The Warning Signs of Diabetes

Diabetes was once a leading cause of death in the United States. Now, with proper treatment, diabetics can live long, active lives. Early diagnosis is essential; ask your physician for a screening if the following symptoms are present:

Type 1: drowsiness
fruity breath
severe thirst
sudden weight loss
increased passing of urine/bedwetting

Type 2: increased weight gain
frequent urination
itchy skin
frequent infections (e.g., vaginitis)
slow healing of cuts and sores
numbness in extremities

Both: extreme fatigue
blurred vision
increase in hunger

diabetes if confirmed with a repeat test on a different day, in combination with symptoms of diabetes.

- **Glucose Tolerance Test.** This test is often done in conjunction with a fasting test but after the first blood sample is drawn. For the glucose tolerance test, you are asked to drink an extremely sweet glucose drink. Your blood will be tested every 30 minutes for two hours, and then every hour for four hours, in order to examine how your body processes sugar. A glucose level higher than 200 mg/dL may mean you have diabetes. If the result is confirmed by a test on a second day, you have diabetes. (A two-hour version of this test is standard during pregnancy to check for gestational, or temporary, diabetes, caused by the pregnancy.)
- **Urine Test.** This test analyzes a urine sample to detect ketones, a by-product caused by diabetes. Without insulin, the body burns fat instead of glucose. Ketones are the waste product. They build up in the blood and are discharged in urine.

Lifestyle Choices to Prevent or Control Diabetes. Even if you are predisposed to diabetes because of a family history, you can reduce your risk by choosing a healthy lifestyle. If you already have diabetes, changing your lifestyle will help you control it. A healthy diet and plenty of exercise are the keys to preventing and controlling diabetes.

Diet. A diet naturally low in fat and reasonably low in calories helps make insulin receptors more sensitive to insulin. It also helps your body use glucose more efficiently. In addition, a diet low in cholesterol helps to protect against heart disease, a major concern for women with diabetes.

The ADA recommends a diet in which 50 to 60 percent of calories come from complex carbohydrates. This includes breads, fruits, and vegetables. Protein should make up from 12 to 20 percent of the diet, and fats limited to no more than 30 percent. The ADA also recommends small meals eaten throughout the day, rather than two or three large meals.

Diabetes and Cardiovascular Disease

Having diabetes doubles your risk for heart disease and peripheral vascular disease. If you have a heart attack, it is more likely to go undiagnosed, which may increase the damage from that heart attack.

Diabetics also are at increased risk for developing strokes. To help reduce these risks, it is essential that diabetics maintain good control of blood glucose. Because they are already at risk, it is especially important that they avoid high blood pressure, high cholesterol, and smoking.

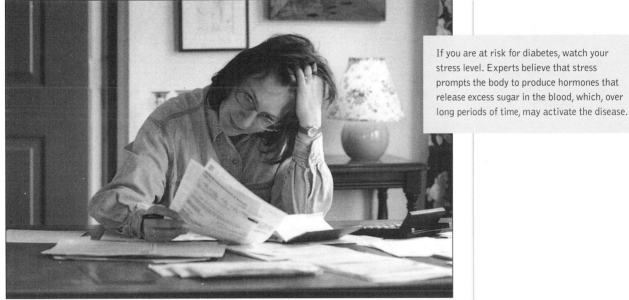

If you are at risk for diabetes, watch your stress level. Experts believe that stress prompts the body to produce hormones that release excess sugar in the blood, which, over long periods of time, may activate the disease.

Weight Loss. If you are overweight, you may need to lose weight in order to protect against or manage diabetes. Obesity is a major risk factor; about 90 percent of all diabetics are overweight. If diabetes runs in your family and you are overweight, you are four times as likely to develop the disease as someone with neither risk factor.

Yet not all overweight people are at increased risk for diabetes. It seems that where a woman carries excess body fat is is important. Women who gain weight around the middle of the body are more at risk than those who gain weight around the buttocks and thighs. In addition, women who gain weight during their adult life are more susceptible than those who gain during childhood or the teen years.

Exercise. Exercise not only helps you reduce your weight, it offers natural protection against diabetes. Physical activity lowers your blood sugar and lowers your blood pressure. In addition, exercise enhances your body's response to insulin, making it easier to process. In fact, studies have shown that doing vigorous exercise—even only once a week—may offer protection against diabetes, while more regular exercise has a stronger effect.

What Happens When You Have a Thyroid Disorder?

The thyroid produces thyroxin (thyroid hormone), which regulates the speed of many bodily functions, including heart rate, cholesterol level, body weight, energy level, muscle strength, skin condition, vision, menstrual regularity, mental state, and many other conditions. Clearly, the effects of thyroid malfunction can be widespread.

While men and women can both get thyroid disease, women are five to eight times more likely to do so. About one woman in eight will develop a thyroid disorder sometime during her lifetime. Between five and eight percent of women develop a thyroid disorder after giving birth.

The following two types of thyroid disorder typically affect women:

- Hypothyroidism, which occurs when an underactive thyroid produces too little hormone
- Hyperthyroidism, which occurs when an overactive thyroid produces too much hormone

Hypothyroidism. The most common of the thyroid disorders, hypothyroidism affects about 11 million Americans and is more common in women than in men. It often is caused by a condition called Hashimoto's disease. Hashimoto's disease is an autoimmune disorder in which the body's white blood cells mistakenly attack thyroid cells, shutting down their function. The thyroid gland can then produce only a limited supply of hormone—not enough for the body to operate efficiently. The resulting increased demand on the gland can cause it to enlarge.

Aside from Hashimoto's disease, hypothyroidism can also result from treatments for an overactive thyroid. This includes medication, surgery, or radioactive iodine treatments.

The chances of your developing hypothyroidism increases with age. In addition, the disease is not limited to adults. One in every 4,000 babies is born with hypothyroidism.

Hypothyroidism often clusters in families, though you can have the disorder even if none of your relatives have it.

Symptoms and Warning Signs. There is a variety of symptoms associated with hypothyroidism. You may experience only some of these. Three or more of the following symptoms indicate a possible problem:

- Goiter (an enlarged thyroid gland that looks like a swelling in the neck)
- Weight gain (even with a loss of appetite)
- Unusually heavy, light, or irregular periods
- Sensitivity to cold
- Slowed heart rate
- Fatigue
- Constipation
- Dry skin and brittle fingernails
- Anemia
- Swollen ankles
- High cholesterol level
- Stiff or weak muscles and/or muscle cramps
- Depression and/or mood swings
- Hoarse voice and/or difficulty swallowing
- Forgetfulness

The symptoms of hypothyroidism are subtle in the beginning. Over time, they become more pronounced. Often, they are mistaken for signs of overwork, stress, or aging.

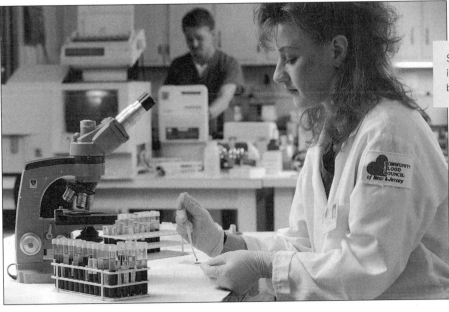

Screening for thyroid disease usually includes both a physical examination and blood tests.

Screening and Treatment. Hypothyroidism is diagnosed by its symptoms, a physical examination, and blood tests. The blood tests measure the levels of thyroid-stimulating hormone (produced by the pituitary gland) and thyroid hormone. If the level of thyroid-stimulating hormone is high and the level of thyroid hormone is low, you have hypothyroidism.

If you do have hypothyroidism, chances are it is a condition that will remain with you through life. Usually, the condition is treated with a synthetic form of thyroid hormone in pill form. Then, to make sure the level of hormone in your blood is not too low or too high, your doctor will monitor your blood and adjust the dose periodically. A dose that is too high can damage your heart, weaken your bones, and cause mood swings and/or indigestion. A dose that is too low will not have the full beneficial effect of the correct dose.

Hyperthyroidism. Hyperthyroidism affects about 1 million Americans—mostly women in their thirties and forties. The most common cause of the condition is Graves' disease. In Graves' disease, your body produces antibodies that mimic thyroid-stimulating hormone, causing your thyroid to produce more hormone. Like hypothyroidism, this condition may cluster in families.

Symptoms and Warning Signs. Below are the symptoms that indicate possible hyperthyroidism. Some symptoms listed here are not exclusive to hyperthyroidism, but three or more of the following symptoms indicate a possible problem:

- Goiter (see hypothyroidism)
- Weight loss (with possible increased appetite)
- Rapid or irregular heart rate
- Trembling of the hands
- Increased sweating and/or sweaty palms
- Difficulty sleeping

- Muscle weakness
- Heat intolerance
- Mood swings, anxiety, and nervousness/irritability
- Light or irregular menstrual periods
- Indigestion
- Diarrhea
- Swelling of the ankles
- Faster-than-usual nail growth or cracking and breaking of the nails
- Hair loss
- Protruding eyes
- High blood pressure

Like hypothyroidism, symptoms of hyperthyroidism develop gradually and often are misdiagnosed for overwork, stress, or aging. Over the long term, if not treated, hyperthyroidism can cause more serious problems. These include heart damage and related problems, and loss of calcium from the bones, which can lead to osteoporosis.

Screening and Treatment. Hyperthyroidism is diagnosed by its symptoms, a physical examination, and blood tests. The blood tests measure the levels of thyroid-stimulating hormone and thyroid hormone. If the level of thyroid-stimulating hormone is low and the level of thyroid hormone is high, you have hyperthyroidism.

Treatment for this disease depends on its cause, how severe it is, and your age and health. Typically, an antithyroid medication is prescribed for three months to one year and is effective in controlling the disease. In conjunction with this medication, a medication called a beta-blocker might be prescribed to reduce a racing heartbeat.

If medication alone does not clear up the condition, your doctor probably will recommend a single treatment with radioactive iodine. In this type of treatment, you take the dose in liquid or pill form. The iodine accumulates in the thy-

The Difficulty in Diagnosing Thyroid Disorders

Exhaustion, lack of concentration, weight gain, depression—the symptoms of the most common type of thyroid disease mimic those of many other conditions. No wonder half of the estimated 13 million cases of thyroid disorders in America remain undiagnosed. In many cases, both women and physicians may attribute symptoms to stress or advancing age.

Studies reveal that many women do not discuss symptoms with their doctors, especially vague symptoms of fatigue or mood disorders. It is best to be direct with your physician. If you have three or more symptoms of thyroid disorder, make a point to describe them and ask, "Should I be tested for thy-

roid disease?" The doctor may be able to tell you definitively that your symptoms do not add up. If she is unsure, then you can ask for a screening test. This is especially important after childbirth and after menopause, when your risk is highest.

For more information on thyroid disease, contact the Thyroid Foundation of America at 800-832-8321.

roid, where the radiation destroys tissue. This reduces the gland's ability to produce thyroid hormone. While one treatment is effective for most people, some need a second or third treatment.

If only part of your thyroid gland is enlarged and overproductive, your doctor might recommend surgery to remove just the damaged portion. Surgery is also recommended for women who wish to get pregnant after treatment. Virtually all women who have been treated for hyperthyroidism will require lifelong thyroid supplements to replace their lost thyroid function.

Subclinical Thyroid Dysfunction. It is possible to have thyroid disease but show few, if any, symptoms. Such a disorder is called subclinical thyroid dysfunction. Subclinical thyroid dysfunction can occur both with an overactive and an underactive thyroid. Many women with subclinical thyroid disease have emotional symptoms, such as depression or anxiety, that are not appreciated because other thyroid symptoms are missing.

Only a blood test can detect when the thyroid hormones are close to, but not at, normal levels. Often subclinical thyroid dysfunction progresses into full-blown thyroid disease, though it may take months or years. Early detection and treatment help prevent the onset of symptoms and curb potentially damaging effects on your body's organs and on your emotional state.

Other **Endocrine** Disorders

The glands in the endocrine system are especially sensitive to hormone malfunctions and tumors. A disruption in the delicate balance of this system can cause serious problems. Knowing your risk factors and being aware of early warning signs enhance your ability to protect against such disorders.

Disorders of the Adrenal Glands

The adrenal glands produce hormones that affect almost every function in the body. Several potentially debilitating diseases can be attributed to dysfunction in the adrenals.

Addison's Disease. This condition occurs when the adrenal glands stop production of steroid-based hormones, such as cortisol. Often considered an autoimmune disease, Addison's disease usually occurs as a result of the body mistakenly attacking the adrenal glands. The attack may be triggered by such disorders as Graves' disease, Hashimoto's thyroiditis, rheumatoid arthritis, and pernicious anemia. Addison's disease can also be caused by tuberculosis, acquired immunodeficiency syndrome (AIDS), or certain fungal disorders, drugs, and congenital defects.

Symptoms of Addison's disease include the following:

- Low blood pressure
- Darkening of the skin
- Weakness and fatigue

- Abdominal pain accompanied by nausea, indigestion, diarrhea, and vomiting
- Low sodium and high potassium levels in the blood

Addison's disease can be diagnosed through a series of tests. The primary test is the cosyntropin stimulation test. First, a blood sample is taken to evaluate the patient's normal hormone levels. Then, the patient is injected with cosyntropin to stimulate the adrenal glands. A second blood sample is taken 30 to 60 minutes later to evaluate whether the adrenal glands are functioning. In some cases, a longer test is necessary, requiring a 48-hour continuous infusion of cosyntropin, for more informative results.

Treatment for the disease includes an oral replacement of the deficient hormones and possibly a second medication to maintain blood pressure or sodium levels. If you do not take these medications regularly, you may experience acute adrenal failure: severe diarrhea, vomiting, dehydration, shock, and loss of consciousness.

Congenital Adrenal Hyperplasia. This disease occurs when the process for converting cholesterol to cortisol is blocked. The pituitary gland senses the low level of cortisol, so it produces more adrenocorticotropin (ACTH) to stimulate the adrenal glands. However, increased stimulation causes an excess of other hormones—typically male hormones such as androstenedione, DHEA, and DHEA-S.

Symptoms of the disease include the following:

- Growth of hair in areas typically associated with males, such as the upper lip, the chin, the breast, and below the navel
- Acne
- Irregular menstruation
- Infertility

Congenital adrenal hyperplasia is usually diagnosed in infancy or childhood because of the telltale growth of hair. However, if the blockage is only partial and hormone levels are only slightly elevated, symptoms may not appear.

A medical history and physical examination help make an initial diagnosis. Blood tests confirm it. These tests detect the presence of male hormones. Sometimes, a cosyntropin stimulation test is used to confirm the diagnosis.

Treatment depends on the severity of the disease. If the disease does not affect menstruation or fertility, there may be no treatment given. If symptoms are more severe, patients may take small oral doses of steroid hormones to reduce the overall hormone level in the body. If congenital adrenal hyperplasia is diagnosed in infancy or childhood, usually it is more severe, and lifetime treatment with supplements to replace missing hormones is necessary.

Cushing's Syndrome. Cushing's syndrome is the opposite of Addison's disease. While a woman with Addison's disease does not produce enough hormone, a woman with Cushing's syndrome produces too much—specifically cortisol and other glucocorticoid hormones. The elevated hormone levels cause protein to break down and fat to be deposited in the tissues.

DHEA Dietary Supplementation

Recent interest in the use of DHEA as a dietary supplement has been based on its reported anti-aging properties. Research has noted that DHEA levels are high during your teens and twenties, and they progressively diminish after that. Taking DHEA as a dietary supplement has made some people claim to feel young again.

Scientists are exploring the effects of hormones like DHEA. So far, DHEA studies have shown that laboratory rodents stay slimmer and live longer. Even animals bred for cancer have an easier time resisting the disease. Older mice taking DHEA can fight off disease as well as those half their age. They also look younger.

Results have not yet been proven with humans. Small studies of fewer than 50 people have shown some effects—but nothing that can be extrapolated to the general population.

There may be risks as well. Excessive amounts of DHEA may cause liver cancer or other side effects. Most people are limiting replacement to 25 milligrams a day. Women generally need less than men and may find that as little as 15 milligrams a day is useful. In the case of DHEA, more is not better.

Cushing's syndrome has a number of causes. An adrenal-stimulating tumor in the pituitary gland or the lung might trigger the excess cortisol. Benign (non-cancerous) tumors called adrenal adenomas can produce the extra hormone, as can adrenal carcinomas. Certain medications—such as those which contain glucocorticoid hormones—can cause the disease.

Symptoms of the disease include the following:

- Unexplained weight gain, especially in the abdomen, above the collar bone, or behind the neck
- Rounded face, ruddy complexion, and/or increased facial hair
- Wide, dark purple stripes on the abdomen, buttocks, or near the armpits
- Weakness
- Thinning of the skin, resulting in easy bruising and poor wound healing
- Change in menstrual periods
- Decrease in sexual drive

Cushing's syndrome is often initially diagnosed through a medical history and a physical examination. The diagnosis is confirmed through tests. One such test is the dexamethasone suppression test, where a dose of this substance is given to the patient to turn off the production of cortisol. Nine hours later, cortisol levels are measured in the blood. Urine specimens are collected over the next 24 hours to determine the amount of cortisol eliminated from the body. If necessary, the test is continued with a small amount of another glucocortoid hormone administered every six hours for two days with blood cortisol levels measured during this time.

Not only does a test like dexamethasone suppression confirm a diagnosis of Cushing's syndrome, it helps doctors determine the possible causes. A CAT scan or MRI might then be needed to locate the source of the problem. A CAT, or CT, (computed axial tomography) scan combines the use of a computer and x-rays to reveal cross-sectional images of tissues. MRI (magnetic resonance imaging) uses a powerful electromagnet to make your cells resonate, producing waves that scan a plane, or cross-section of the body, and reveal abnormalities.

Treatment depends on the cause of the disease. Surgery is routinely used to remove adrenal or pituitary tumors. If medication is the culprit, doses are usually decreased to eliminate problems.

Hirsutism. This disease creates male-patterned hair growth in women, including hair on the face, chest, and abdomen. It occurs when an excess of testosterone stimulates hair follicles producing thick, coarse hair usually associated with men. Although all women have testosterone in their systems, levels are usually not high enough to stimulate hair growth of this type. Not every case of excess hair is related to a glandular disorder. Some women's bodies are simply hypersensitive to normal amounts of testosterone, and the hair they find is only cosmetically annoying. Hirsutism, though, occurs when the adrenal glands produce an excess of male hormone and can also be caused by certain tumors and other disorders of the adrenal glands.

Symptoms of the disease include the following:

- Coarse hair on the upper lip, chin, chest, or abdomen
- Menstrual irregularities
- Infertility
- Acne

Hirsutism is diagnosed through a medical history, a physical examination, and blood tests. The blood tests measure the amount of male hormones in the body.

Treatment depends on the cause of the disease. Tumors may be removed by surgery. Hormonal supplements may control a hormonal imbalance. Medications may also be used to block testosterone's effect on the hair follicles.

Pheochromocytoma. These are tumors that typically develop in the central portion of the adrenal glands. Pheochromocytomas affect the production of the hormones adrenaline and norepinephrine. Usually, they develop in one or the other gland, but occasionally can be found in both. Only five percent of pheochromocytomas tend to be hereditary, while the rest occur spontaneously.

Symptoms of pheochromocytomas include the following:

- Palpitations and/or fainting
- Severe headaches
- Blood pressure that is erratically high and/or difficult to control
- Anxiety attacks
- Increased sweating
- Tremors
- Weight loss

Diagnosis of the disease includes a medical history and physical examination. Paroxysmal (sudden) attacks of symptoms are common, and the examination and tests are most accurate immediately after an attack. Technicians measure the patient's pulse and blood pressure while she is lying down and standing up. The physical examination usually is followed by a blood test and a 24-hour urine specimen collection, where levels of adrenal medulla hormones are measured. If levels are high, the patient will undergo an MRI to pinpoint the tumor.

Most tumors are found in the adrenal glands. Only ten percent are found in the abdomen. Surgery is required to remove the tumors.

Disorders of the Parathyroid

When the parathyroid glands are not working properly, calcium levels in the blood may be decreased, or they may be elevated. Decreased calcium absorption can lead to osteoporosis, or brittle bone disease. Elevated calcium absorption can lead to hypercalcemia, with symptoms ranging from nausea and lethargy to extreme fatigue and muscle weakness.

Hyperparathyroidism. This condition occurs when the parathyroid glands produce too much PTH, the hormone that increases the amount of calcium and decreases the amount of phosphorus in your blood. In most cases, hyperparathyroidism is caused by a benign parathyroid tumor. Occasionally, it is triggered by enlargement of the parathyroid glands or other causes.

Hyperparathyroidism primarily affects women over 50. Its symptoms include the following:

- Mild fatigue, lethargy, and/or apathy
- Nausea and indigestion
- Muscle weakness
- Abdominal pain
- Increased urination and thirst
- Constipation

In mild cases, there are no symptoms at all. In severe cases, the condition can cause vomiting, kidney stones, kidney failure, peptic ulcers, pancreatitis, stupor, and comas.

This disease is diagnosed by elevated levels of calcium in the bloodstream. Specific tests include blood samples to measure serum calcium, phosphorous, total proteins, PTH, and urine specimens to test for calcium.

Treatment usually involves surgery to remove the benign tumors. If surgery is not possible, treatments include increased water intake, diuretics, estrogen, and increased physical activity.

Hypoparathyroidism. This is the opposite of hyperparathyroidism and far less common. In this case, the parathyroid produces too little PTH, preventing the body from making proper use of calcium. Typically, hypoparathyroidism is triggered by damage to the parathyroids during neck surgery. Symptoms of the disease include the following:

- Numbness and tingling of the hands, feet, and mouth
- Muscle cramps and/or spasms
- Cataracts

Diagnosis is made through a medical history, physical examination, and blood tests. Treatment includes calcium and vitamin D supplements.

Disorders of the Pituitary Gland

If the pituitary gland is not functioning properly, your body's growth, functioning, and reproductive capabilities are affected, leading to a variety of potentially serious diseases.

Cushing's Syndrome. Cushing's syndrome can be caused by either a dysfunction of the adrenal glands or of the pituitary. For a summary of the disease, see the description under "Disorders of the Adrenal Glands."

Diabetes Insipidus. Sometimes the pituitary gland produces too little antidiuretic hormone (ADH), the hormone that controls the balance of water in the body. This results in diabetes insipidus, a condition unrelated to diabetes mellitus (commonly known as diabetes) where the body holds too much salt. Usually caused by a pituitary tumor, the condition also may result from a head injury or pituitary tumor surgery or because of a kidney defect in responding to ADH.

Symptoms of the disease include the following:

- Excessive urination
- Severe thirst

FIGURE 23.2

A Healthy Metabolism

Maintaining a healthy weight is an important step toward keeping your metabolic system healthy. If you need to lose weight, aim for a gradual loss of about a pound each week to allow your body to adjust.

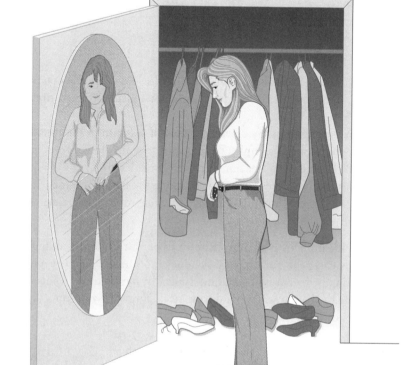

A combination of a water deprivation test and blood tests will determine the salt and water balance in the patient's body. If the balance is off, increased fluid intake and a salt-restricted diet can help. In addition, an antidiuretic hormone in the form of a nasal spray or injection is given. Tumors, if present, are removed by surgery.

SIADH. Syndrome of inappropriate antidiuretic hormone (SIADH) occurs when the pituitary produces too much ADH. This condition is usually caused by a pituitary tumor, stroke, or head trauma. Symptoms include body swelling and edema, and scant urine. SIADH is screened for using tests similar to those used to diagnose diabetes insipidus. Treatment consists of medications that suppress the production of ADH or removal of tumor.

Hypopituitarism. When the pituitary gland produces insufficient quantities of one or more of its hormones, hypopituitarism results. Usually, the cause is a tumor on the pituitary gland, but it can also develop after a serious head injury. Symptoms of the disease include the following:

- Cessation of menstruation
- Infertility
- Inability to lactate following childbirth
- Fatigue
- Depression
- Loss of pubic hair
- Decreased appetite

A medical history, physical examination, and blood tests to measure hormone levels confirm the diagnosis. The disease is treated by taking a synthetic version of the deficient hormones.

Prolactinoma. This disease is characterized by an overproduction of the hormone prolactin, necessary for stimulating milk production after childbirth. Typically, it is caused by a benign tumor, but it can be triggered by certain oral contraceptives, tranquilizers, and hypothyroidism.

Symptoms of the disease include the following:

- Irregular or lack of menstrual periods
- Infertility
- Appearance of breast milk unrelated to pregnancy

Prolactinoma can be diagnosed with blood tests that detect prolactin and thyroid hormone levels. If your prolactin levels are high while your thyroid hormone levels are normal, you may have the disease. The presence of a tumor can be confirmed with CAT or MRI of your pituitary.

The disease is treated with drugs and/or surgery. Drugs can decrease prolactin levels to a more normal range. Surgery is used to remove tumors, especially those causing visual problems.

Sheehan's Syndrome. This syndrome is a form of hypopituitarism that occurs after childbirth. Normally, the pituitary gland grows during pregnancy. When it grows too much, the body is unable to supply it with enough oxygen and nutrients. Some or all of the gland dies as a result.

Symptoms of the disease include the following:

- No production of breast milk following birth
- No menstrual periods
- Loss of body hair in the underarm and pubic areas
- Depression

Sheehan's syndrome is diagnosed and treated in the same manner as hypopituitarism.

What *You* Can Do

Since many metabolic diseases and endocrine disorders are hereditary, knowing your family history will help keep you alert for symptoms. Knowing the specific risk factors—and reducing or eliminating them—is a good first step toward preventing the onset of disease. In addition, if you know you have or are at risk for an endocrine disorder, initiate the practical lifestyle changes listed below:

- Maintain a healthy weight within a normal range. A slow, steady gain or loss is preferable. Avoid fad diets or quick weight loss programs. If you need to lose weight, a sensible loss of about a pound a week will allow your body to adjust.
- Eat a nutritious, balanced diet. Some endocrine disorders are especially sensitive to diet. Increase your consumption of complex carbohydrates (fruits, beans, and breads) and fresh vegetables. Keep fat and cholesterol at a minimum.
- Get enough calcium. If you are not getting enough in your diet, consider calcium supplements. Check with your doctor to determine the appropriate dosage.
- Exercise regularly. Exercise protects against most diseases.
- Schedule routine physical examinations with your doctor even if you are feeling well. Alert her to the endocrine disorders that run in your family. Ask to be screened for them to ensure early detection of any problems. Make sure postpregnancy checkups include tests of thyroid function.

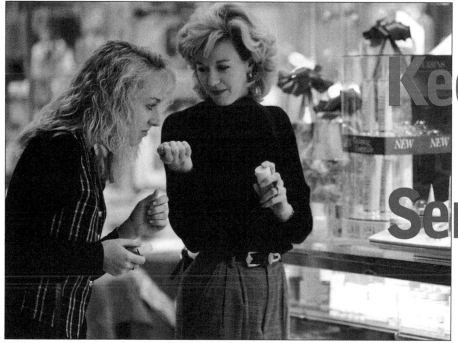

Chapter 24

Keeping *the* Senses Sharp

You depend on your senses to interpret the world around you. Without a complex sequence of events occurring within your central nervous system at every moment of your life, you could not perceive that a kitten is soft, a rose is sweet-smelling, and soup is hot or spicy. Changes in the ability to see, hear, smell, and taste usually begin gradually in middle age, so that, for example, even a woman who has never needed glasses may find "suddenly" that the small print in the newspaper is blurry. A lifelong commitment to caring for your eyes, ears, nose, and mouth—the primary agents through which you perceive the world—enhances your ability to enjoy life by keeping your senses sharp. Taking measures to care for the senses also helps prevent premature loss of function due to illness or injury.

How *Do* **Your Senses**
Interpret Your *Environment?*

Sensory receptors provide information about your environment to your central nervous system. This complex system helps you interpret and react to information from outside and inside your body. Each sensory receptor is responsive to a particular stimulus, such as texture, heat, sound, or light.

Sensory receptors convert various forms of energy to signals in order to send distinct messages to your brain and central nervous system. For example, sensory receptors are involved in converting mechanical energy (to transmit touch and sound), thermal energy (to relate temperature), electromagnetic energy (to detect light), and chemical energy (to transmit smells and taste).

The Information Network of the Brain

How does a sensory message, such as the odor of lemons, get to your brain? When you inhale the scent of a lemon, an impulse or "message" is initiated. Chemicals called neurotransmitters carry that message to specialized cells called sensory neurons, or nerves, in the brain. These brain, or cranial, nerves then interpret the message as "lemon" smell.

Research has demonstrated that exercise, which increases the amount of oxygen supplied to the brain, can improve the neurotransmitter system of the brain. Research also confirms that parents and caregivers of young children from birth to age five can foster children's neurotransmitter systems by reading to them, talking to them, singing or playing music, and engaging them in a rich variety of activities and experiences.

Perceiving Information from the External Environment

When you "sense" someone is behind you or hear your child crying, your body is perceiving sensory information from the outside. Several elements of the central nervous system are involved in picking up and interpreting these signals. The rods and cones in your eyes, for example, are sensitive to light. The hair cells in your ears are especially sensitive to sound waves. The olfactory neurons in your nose specialize in picking up scents. Receptor cells on your tongue primarily sense taste, and sensory nerves in your skin detect texture, pain, and temperature.

All of your senses are interrelated and often work together. Sensors in your nose work not only to pick up smells, but also to help provide information about taste. Your skin functions not only to protect your body and signal pain, but also to transmit information about textures and temperature.

Interpreting Messages from Inside Your Body

Visceral senses help you perceive information about your "internal environment," what your body feels like inside. When you "feel" your lungs expanding, tension in your neck, hunger, a sore throat, or nausea, for example, your visceral senses are at work. Sudden and excessive dilation and/or contraction of the blood vessels in your head, for example, can create pressure that alerts you and makes you "feel" a headache.

The Pain Response

Pain is transmitted by nerve endings throughout your body in response to electrical, mechanical, and chemical energy. There are two pathways for pain—one slow and one fast—and, therefore, two major types of pain: sharp and localized (such as that from a puncture wound or a paper cut); and dull and diffused (such as pain from some types of headache or toothache).

Your Eyes

The eye is a complex sense organ that is made up of layers of sense receptors: the outer layer (sclera and cornea), the middle layer (choroid and iris), and the inner layer (retina). The outer layer serves as protection. The sclera is situated at the front of the eye, where it forms the cornea, a transparent layer that allows light rays to enter the eye. The middle layer, the choroid, provides nutrients to the retina, where the receptor cells are located. The lens allows incoming light to focus on the retina. The iris—the colored portion of your eye—is a continuation of the choroid. It contains muscle fibers that automatically dilate the pupils to allow variable amounts of light to enter your retina. The retina contains the rods and cones (visual receptors), a network of blood vessels, and connecting fibers. Rods are especially sensitive to light and provide us with night vision, but not details or color. Cones provide bright light, color distinctions, and greater detail than do rods.

How Do the Eyes Perceive Light?

We actually do not see objects, but only light reflected off objects. That is why if you enter a room that is completely dark, you will not be able to see at all. Light enters the eye through the cornea and rests on the lens and the retina. Once the light reaches the retina, the rods and cones converge their signals into a network of nerve fibers that make up the optic nerve. The retina receives images upside down; the brain must reinterpret them and restore them right side up. Images from both eyes are merged by the brain to produce three-dimensional vision.

The optic nerve transmits data to the brain, where signals are relayed to other parts of the brain as necessary to process information. If someone throws a ball to you, your eyes will signal your brain that the ball is coming, and your brain will send signals that will help you decide either to catch the ball or duck to avoid being hit.

How Do the Eyes Move?

Eye movement is accomplished with the help of six ocular muscles. Four muscles move the eye up and down; two muscles control rotary movement. There are four types of eye movements: jerky movements, smooth movements, vestibular movements (which occur in response to stimuli), and convergence movements (which help you focus on objects nearby).

Protecting and Caring for Your Eyes

Just like the rest of your body, your eyes must be protected, rested, and well fed. A balanced diet that includes fresh fruits and vegetables helps you maintain healthy eyes. Be sure to eat foods high in beta-carotene, vitamin B complex, vitamins C and E, and the minerals selenium and zinc (see Table 24.1). Adequate amounts of vitamin A are necessary, but excess amounts are toxic.

Working with Computer Terminals. Women who hold office jobs that require sitting for hours in front of a computer may be concerned about whether such work is safe for their eyes. It is true that poor lighting in work areas, poor

---

More Than Five Senses

Although you may have learned that there are only 5 senses (sight, sound, smell, taste, and touch), there are actually at least 11 conscious senses that convey information to your central nervous system without your full awareness. Different sensory receptors allow you to experience the following conscious sensations, in addition to the basic 5:

- Warmth
- Cold
- Pain
- Joint position and movement
- Awareness of the position of parts of your body in space, such as whether you are lying down, standing up, sitting down, or bent over, or if your arm is up or down
- Acceleration, the sense of slowing down or speeding up, even when you are not physically causing the change

TABLE 24.1

Eating for Healthy Eyes

VITAMIN / MINERAL (SOURCE)	HOW IT HELPS
VITAMIN A / BETA-CAROTENE (fish, fruit, eggs, carrots, other "yellow" or "red" vegetables, fortified milk)	Help prevent night blindness; build immunity against viruses that cause conjunctivitis; essential for dry and irritated eyes; helpful against photophobia (light sensitivity); help repair damage to the retina; provide relief from lid infections or styes. Severe vitamin A deficiencies in children may cause corneal deterioration, resulting in blindness.
POTASSIUM (oranges, bananas, dried fruits, meat and poultry, milk, yogurt)	Balances excess sodium. Low potassium levels have been associated with vision problems in some people.
COPPER, MANGANESE, SELENIUM, and ZINC (nuts, legumes shellfish, grains, potatoes, tea, vegetables, brewer's yeast, wheat germ)	Important for healing; retard cataract growth; enhance immune response.
ESSENTIAL FATTY ACIDS (red meat, poultry, fish, butter, soft or squeeze margarine products, cooking oil)	Beneficial for dry eyes.
VITAMIN C (Citrus fruits, red peppers, strawberries, broccoli, cauliflower, cantaloupe)	Helps reduce intraocular pressure in patients with glaucoma; helps heal ulcerated eyes; beneficial for dry eyes if taken with vitamin B_6.
VITAMIN B complex (whole grains, legumes, wheat germ, nuts, fish, brewer's yeast, leafy greens, milk, eggs, bananas, lean meats)	Improves intraocular cellular metabolism; prevents loss of eyelashes; B_{12} helps prevent nerve damage to the eyes.
CALCIUM (milk, salmon, sardines, dark green, leafy vegetables, shellfish); **MAGNESIUM** (whole grains, nuts, bananas, apricots, soybeans)	Improve circulation in blood vessels of the eyes.

machine design and setup, poor blinking habits, or not resting the eyes periodically throughout the day can cause problems, such as dry eye, eyestrain, and headaches.

To minimize damage to your eyes from a video display terminal do the following:

- Use an antiglare screen (sized to fit over your regular screen) to diminish glare.
- Reduce the brightness of the screen to soften the contrast between the words and the screen background.
- Be sure that your work area is adequately lit from sources other than the screen itself.

- Work at least one arm's length from the screen.
- Take frequent breaks from the computer and allow your eyes to rest and focus on objects at a greater distance. (A brief walk around the office is also good to stretch your back and legs and loosen your shoulders.) Post a favorite picture on the wall beyond the monitor to focus on and rest your eyes.
- Blink often to keep your eyes moist, such as at the end of every line of type. If the office air is dry, apply rewetting drops to your eyes to prevent redness. Over-the-counter rewetting drops, most often made from plain saline (salt) water that is specially sterilized for use in the eye, are very helpful.

Preventing Eye Injury. Eye injuries can impair your vision or deprive you of sight entirely. Many injuries are avoidable if the proper precautions are taken. It has been estimated that 90 percent of all eye injuries can be prevented by following safety guidelines and using protective eyewear on the job or while participating in sports.

Be aware of and recognize potential hazards, such as dust from wood or metal, sparks from welding, and fumes from chemicals. Harm can also come from light rays, such as those generated from electrical welding or acetylene equipment. These can cause painful eye burns unless your eyes are adequately protected.

Follow these precautions:

- Wear appropriate protective eyewear (glasses, goggles, face shields, or helmets) for any activity that might lead to eye damage.
- For low-risk sports, such as track and field, it is sufficient to use protective eyewear with lenses made of plastic.
- For high-risk sports, such as racquetball and squash, wear lenses made of polycarbonate, a material stronger than plastic.
- Eyeglasses do not qualify as protective eyewear. If you wear corrective lenses, protective eyewear should be worn over them.
- Protective eyewear must meet standards of the American National Standards Institute.
- In order to provide adequate protection, your eyewear must fit properly, be clean, and be in good condition. Do not wear faulty eyewear.
- Learn basic first aid for eye injuries.
- Know the location of emergency stations, such as eye wash stations in a laboratory, school, or gas station.
- Get medical attention immediately if your eyes become injured.

Exercising Your Eyes

Like the rest of your body, your eyes need exercise to maintain flexibility and strength. The following exercises can help you maintain healthier eyes and flexible eye muscles:

- Sit in a comfortable position. With your head facing forward, locate an object in the farthest upper left-hand corner of the room. Allow your eyes to focus on the object for a minute or two.
- Next, bring your index finger within six inches of your nose. Allow your eyes to focus on your finger for a minute or two.
- Now focus on an object in the upper right-hand corner of the room for a minute or two.
- Once again, focus on your index finger, keeping it six inches from your nose.
- Now focus on an object in the lower left-hand corner of the room.
- Focus on your stationary finger.
- Focus on an object in the lower right-hand corner of the room.

You may also wish to try focusing on your finger as it moves slowly near and far. First bring your index finger within six inches of your nose and focus. Then move your finger six inches farther away from you and focus. Keeping your head stationary and your finger within your field of vision, move your finger as far to the right as you can, then as far to the left as you can.

Preventing Damage from Ultraviolet Rays. Ultraviolet (UV) light is the damaging component of sunlight. UV rays reflected from sand, snow, pavement, or water can burn the surface of the eye just as direct light rays can. Sunburn on the eye surface will burn just as sunburn on the skin does. Although painful, the pain is temporary. The concern lies in cumulative damage created by repeated exposure to UV rays. Long-term exposure to UV rays affects not only the surface of the eye, but also the internal structures, the lens and retina. UV exposure is also a risk factor for pterygium (a growth that invades the cornea of the eye), macular degeneration (breakdown of the macula, which controls central vision), and cataracts (clouding of the lens).

People who spend a significant amount of time in the sun, or who live at high elevations or near the equator, are at greatest risk for eye damage from UV rays. Some drugs, such as psoralens, tetracycline, doxycycline, allopurinol, and phothiazine, also can cause light sensitivity. Women who take these "photosensitizing" drugs must be extra careful to shield their eyes (and skin) from harmful rays.

Experts recommend protecting your eyes from the sun with wide-brimmed hats and sunglasses that screen out 99 to 100 percent of UV light, including both UVA and UVB rays. Although you can purchase sunglasses off-the-rack, it is safer to buy a pair from your ophthalmologist or optometrist, even if you do not require prescription sunglasses. Then you will be assured that the lenses are properly ground and that they will provide adequate protection from harmful rays.

Avoiding Damage from Cosmetics. One of the most common ways women damage their eyes is through poor makeup habits. Here are several simple rules regarding the correct use and application of eye makeup:

- Purchase only small amounts of eye makeup when you shop.
- Discard and replace cosmetics after six to eight weeks to minimize bacterial buildup.
- If you suspect that a product has been contaminated, throw it out.
- No product is totally allergy proof. Ask for a free sample to test new products before you make a purchase. If you have a reaction to a makeup product, return it promptly to the store you purchased it from with your receipt. Most stores allow refunds or exchanges for makeup.
- While at the store, only test eye shadow color on the inside of your arm or wrist. The color of your skin there is similar to the color of your eyelids. Use a new cotton swab or tissue to apply a new color. Applying tester shades to your eyelid may transmit infection.
- Apply mascara only to the tips of your lashes, not down to the base of your lashes, to avoid getting particles in your eye or risk having the mascara wand brush across your cornea.
- Never apply eye makeup while in a moving vehicle. You may poke yourself in the eye or, worse, cause an accident.
- Never borrow someone else's makeup. Infections can be easily transmitted this way, or you may be allergic to the brand.

Choosing Sunglasses for Maximal Protection

When you buy sunglasses, check the label to be sure that they will block 99 to 100 percent of UVA and UVB light. Choose a wraparound, close-fitting pair that will prevent light from hitting your eyes from the sides. Ignore ads that suggest that certain color lenses offer greater protection than others. Lens color and darkness are fashion concerns. UV protection is actually provided by a chemical coating applied to the surface of the lens.

Removing Foreign Particles. Specks of dust or dirt can sometimes blow into your eyes. Your tears usually wash them out, but occasionally particles are more stubborn to remove. Do not rub your eye or attempt to remove a foreign particle with your fingers. Use the flat surface of a clean, lint-free cloth, such as a handkerchief, and very gently dab the particle so that it sticks to the cloth. Otherwise, try flushing the object out with an eye cup, using a sterile saline eye wash solution. If you succeed in removing the particle, but experience persistent pain, see your ophthalmologist as soon as possible. If the particle is embedded in your eye, go to the hospital emergency room. Do not attempt to remove it, or you may seriously injure your eye.

Correcting Your Vision

Vision correction services should only be provided by licensed, trained specialists. Following are the three main categories of specialists you should know about:

- **Ophthalmologists** are physicians who are specially trained to care for eyes. They are medical doctors with a minimum of four years of additional training in diagnosing and treating eye problems. These doctors not only prescribe glasses and contact lenses, but also treat injuries to the eye and perform surgery when necessary.
- **Optometrists** mainly diagnose poor vision and prescribe corrective lenses. They are also trained to identify eye diseases through retinal examinations and can conduct simple tests to confirm their findings. Some states allow optometrists to treat certain eye diseases.
- **Opticians** fill prescriptions (for glasses and contact lenses) written by ophthalmologists and optometrists. They are not qualified to examine eyes, to treat diseases of the eye, or to correct faulty vision.

What Causes Poor Vision? Nearsightedness (myopia), farsightedness (hyperopia), inability to focus on nearby objects (presbyopia), and astigmatism (asymmetrical cornea) are among the most common eye correction problems. All of these problems result from refraction errors of the lens or cornea.

Refraction refers to what happens when light enters the eye. When light hits the eye, the cornea and lens refract or "bend" the light to allow the rays to converge at the retina. Nearsightedness occurs when the shape of the eye is too long, causing the rays to converge at a point in front of the retina. As a result, objects will appear blurry. Farsightedness occurs when the shape of the eye is shortened, causing the point of convergence to occur behind the retina. Objects will then appear out of focus. Nearsightedness or farsightedness may occur as a result of heredity. Presbyopia occurs, however, with aging and a gradual hardening of the lens, making it difficult to focus at close range.

FIGURE 24.1
What Causes Poor Vision
The nearsighted eye is elongated in shape, causing light rays to converge at a point (the focal point) in front of the retina. The farsighted eye is compacted in shape, causing light rays to converge behind the retina.

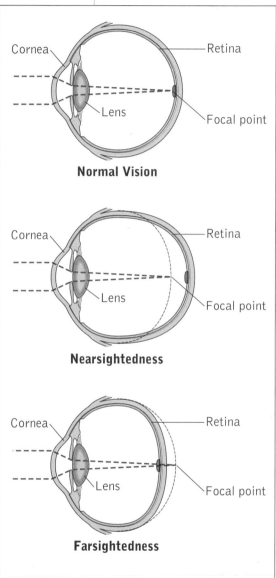

Normal Vision

Nearsightedness

Farsightedness

wellness **tip**

Use a soft cloth to keep your glasses clean and to avoid scratching them. Always carry a lined case in your purse or keep one in your car. When you travel, pack an extra pair of glasses or take your prescription with you as a precaution in case you break or lose your glasses.

Astigmatism occurs from a refraction error related to the uneven surface of the cornea. In a normal eye, the cornea is symmetrical. In an astigmatic eye, areas of the cornea are steeper or flatter than normal. If you have been diagnosed with astigmatism, portions of your field of vision will be blurred. Astigmatism does not worsen with age. It may occur with either nearsightedness or farsightedness, and can be treated with either corrective glasses or contact lenses.

Options for Correcting Poor Vision. There are several options available to correct eyesight. Women can choose from eyeglasses, contact lenses, and even surgery.

Eyeglasses. Nearsightedness and farsightedness are easily corrected with eyeglasses. After a thorough examination, your eyecare specialist will prescribe concave lenses to correct nearsightedness or convex lenses to correct farsightedness. Bifocal lenses are designed to provide correction for both close-up and distance vision.

If you decide to wear eyeglasses, you may choose between plastic or glass for your lenses. Plastic lenses are lighter, less breakable, and provide better protection than glass. They do, however, scratch more easily. Glass lenses, although resistant to scratches, are heavier and breakable. Glass lenses and newer plastic lenses are available with a photochromatic coating, which darkens to protect your eyes from bright light. Your eyecare specialist can help you choose a lens suited to your needs.

If your glasses become loose or uncomfortable, see your optician immediately. If you find that they no longer adequately correct your vision, see your optometrist or ophthalmologist immediately. The problem may be solved with a new prescription.

Hard Contact Lenses. These lenses are easy to care for and provide good vision correction; however, they may require a longer adjustment period and may cause problems if foreign particles become lodged between the contact and cornea. One type of hard contact lens, the gas-permeable lens, contains pores that allow oxygen to reach the cornea. They are made of thin, rigid plastic that move with each blink of the eye and allow tears to circulate across the cornea. This type is generally more comfortable than regular hard lenses. They are also more expensive. However, they are easier to clean and more durable than soft lenses, and provide excellent vision correction.

Use fresh solution every time you clean your contact lenses, to prevent contamination of the eye and lenses and to rid the lenses of protein buildup.

Soft Contact Lenses. Although more comfortable and more easily adapted to than hard lenses, soft lenses are more expensive to buy and to maintain. Soft lenses are also not as durable as hard lenses. A daily cleaning routine must be strictly followed to avoid contamination of the eye and lenses and to rid the lenses of protein buildup. Although they correct vision well, contact lenses may become dry in windy weather, when the humidity is low, or when the lenses are worn for more than 12 hours a day. Special soft contact lens rewetting drops can be applied when this occurs.

Soft lenses are available in daily-wear, extended-wear, and disposable models. Daily-wear lenses are designed to be worn during waking hours and generally need to be replaced at least once a year. Extended-wear lenses are designed to allow oxygen to reach the cornea and can be worn around the clock, even as you sleep, owing to the high water content in the lens itself. Some types can be worn for up to two weeks. Although less handling is involved, the risk of eye infection is greater. Extended-wear lenses are more expensive, thinner, and more fragile than other types of lenses, and they require more frequent monitoring by your doctor.

Disposable lenses are similar to the extended-wear variety, but are usually discarded after two weeks of constant use and consequently do not require cleaning or maintenance. Some disposable lenses are designed to be disposed of and

wellness **warning**

While wearing contact lenses, avoid exposure to tobacco smoke or aerosols. The porous lens of the contact can absorb these chemicals, eventually leaking them onto the surface of your eye.

Cleaning Your Contact Lenses

Keeping your lenses clean and disinfected will ensure comfort and help prevent medical complications. Several kinds of contact lens disinfection are available. The two most popular are heat and chemical disinfection.

The eye itself maintains a relatively germfree environment, owing to the antibacterial quality of your tears. The most common eye contaminates come from your own hands, from tap water used to clean lenses, and from airborne mold spores that are often found in bathrooms, storage cases, and uncapped lens solution bottles.

Inadequate disinfection of contact lenses can result in corneal inflammation from *Acanthamoeba* (commonly found in tap water and swimming pools) or *Pseudomonas aeruginosa* (a bacterium frequently bound to a component of your tears). *Acanthamoeba* infections can result in severe ulcerative infections of the cornea and permanent decreases in vision. *P. aeruginosa* problems arise when you rub your eyes or roughly reposition your contacts, causing a microtear in the cornea. The microtear allows the cornea to become "inoculated" with the bacterial agent.

Follow these care tips:

- If your eyes become red or irritated, immediately remove your contact lenses. If pain persists, see your eye care specialist as soon as possible.
- Avoid rubbing your eyes while you wear contact lenses.
- Shield your eyes from dust and debris on windy days.
- Always wear high-quality sunglasses outdoors, even on cloudy days.

- Avoid wearing contacts while you swim, unless you have been fitted with watertight goggles.
- Avoid using a hair dryer while wearing contacts. This can cause your contacts and your eyes to dry out.
- Avoid using chemicals that emit fumes. These can cause irritation and/or dryness. Protect your eyes when using household cleaning products, glues, and paints.
- Do not substitute one cleaning solution for another. This switch may cause your contacts to become cloudy or may cause the surface of the lens to deteriorate. Not all brands are compatible. Check with your eye care specialist before switching to another brand.
- If you experience an allergic reaction to your contact lens cleaning agent, see your doctor to confirm the presence of an allergy, to make sure infection or other problems are not present, and to get help deciding on another preparation.
- If you wear makeup, use water-soluble cosmetics.
- Apply makeup after you have inserted your contact lenses. Make sure that your hands are clean to avoid contaminating the lenses. Avoid getting makeup particles in your eyes.
- Do not remove makeup until you have removed your contact lenses. This will help avoid getting potentially irritating particles on your lenses.
- Use fresh solution in your lens case when disinfecting your lenses.
- Avoid contaminating your lenses or your eyes with lotions, creams, or sprays.
- Never use saliva to rewet or clean your contacts.

replaced daily. However, they are generally more expensive than other varieties of contact lenses.

Bifocal Contact Lenses. As with bifocal glasses, bifocal contact lenses provide correction for both close-up and distance vision. The lenses are usually weighted to ensure that close-up correction remains at the bottom of the lens. This type of lens may require a period of adjustment.

Radial Keratotomy. Most refraction problems can be treated with corrective glasses or contact lenses. However, people with mild nearsightedness may choose a more permanent surgical solution, such as radial keratotomy. The procedure requires making precise surgical incisions in the cornea of each eye in a radial pattern. This causes the center of the cornea to flatten, which allows the light rays to focus more correctly on the retina. Radial keratotomy is performed as an outpatient procedure, requiring only a local anesthetic. Following the procedure, patients will be instructed to wear a patch or dark glasses for several days. However, recovery can take up to several months and results are not guaranteed. Almost half of patients will have fully corrected vision; others will still require glasses or contact lenses, and others may become farsighted or experience serious complications, including infections and corneal rupture.

Photorefractive Keratotomy. Photorefractive keratotomy is also known as laser vision correction. Following the procedure, more than 80 percent of patients maintain 20/20 vision; 98 percent will see 20/40 or better. Laser vision correction is used to treat mild to moderate myopia (nearsightedness) with low astigmatism. A computer-controlled excimer laser is used to achieve precise changes in the shape of the cornea, and it is far less variable in results than radial keratotomy. With the aid of a cold beam of ultraviolet light, the excimer laser reshapes a microscopically thin layer of superficial corneal tissue. Unlike radial keratotomy, this procedure does not weaken the cornea.

This treatment can be used to correct nearsightedness, farsightedness, and astigmatism. The excimer laser is not used to treat presbyopia. However, clinical trials are in progress to determine if this laser can be used to induce nearsightedness in one or both eyes to correct presbyopia. Since presbyopia is a continuing degenerative disease associated with aging, any treatment will correct only current problems. If laser surgery becomes an option, people with presbyopia will more than likely require several procedures over their lifetimes.

Eye Disorders

Of course, it is troubling when any change occurs in your eyes, especially when the change seems symptomatic of disease rather than of poor vision. While certain symptoms do suggest the possibility of a serious underlying disease that could threaten your eyesight if not treated, others are caused by more common eye disorders that may or may not need extensive treatment. It is important to know the difference.

Less Serious Eye Disorders. Almost everyone develops a common eye disorder at some point in her life. Most of these problems can be treated with a home remedy or over-the-counter medication. The only exception is conjunctivitis, which is highly contagious and must be treated immediately by your physician.

Flashes and Floaters. Flashes are caused when the vitreous—the gelatinous material that fills the space between the lens and the retina—shrinks and tugs on the retina, creating a sensation of flashing lights. This sensation can occur repeatedly over a period of several months and occurs more frequently with aging. If light flashes develop frequently, see your ophthalmologist. It may mean that you have a torn retina, requiring immediate treatment to save your vision.

Flashes of light may also occur as part of a migraine. These flashes are caused by spasms occurring in blood vessels in the brain. Sometimes headache follows the flashes. When the flashes occur in lines or waves without a headache, the condition is called an ophthalmic migraine.

Floaters are small specks or clouds that occur in your field of vision. The floaters are actually inside your eye and cast a shadow on the retina. They may take several shapes, including dots or lines.

Floaters are more likely to occur in people who are nearsighted, who have undergone cataract operations, laser surgery of the eye, or who have had inflammation inside the eye. If floaters develop suddenly, see your ophthalmologist immediately.

Sometimes floaters are a sign of a torn retina. When the retina tears, a small amount of bleeding can occur. The blood in the eye may appear as floaters. If a new floater appears or if you see sudden flashes of light, see your ophthalmologist immediately.

A few floaters may not cause a serious disturbance in your vision. However, if a large number of floaters are apparent (or a very large blind spot, called a scotoma) then your eyes need immediate attention. Many floaters may indicate a hemorrhage into the back of the eye.

Dry Eyes. Dry eyes occur from a lack of natural tears. This condition sometimes accompanies rheumatoid arthritis or other connective tissue disorders. Such a disorder is called Sjögren's syndrome. Sjögren's syndrome usually affects middle-aged women. Eye drops or lubricant ointment may relieve dryness. In some cases, corticosteroids may be prescribed.

Styes. A stye is an infection occurring near the root of the eyelash. It appears as a reddish, painful, and pus-filled lump. Although styes are not harmful to your sight, you may need to see your ophthalmologist if they recur frequently or interfere with your sight. Styes can be treated with warm compresses several times a day. Allow the pus sac to burst on its own. Do not attempt to squeeze it out or increased infection can occur. Your physician may prescribe a topical antibiotic cream for your eyelid.

Conjunctivitis. Conjunctivitis is an inflammation of the conjunctiva, the transparent membrane of the eye. Commonly known as "pinkeye," it may be caused by viral or bacterial infection, or by an allergic reaction. It can also occur in newborns if a tear duct is not completely opened. In the case of newborns, eyesight can be threatened if conjunctivitis is not treated immediately.

Viral conjunctivitis is distinguished by a watery discharge. Bacterial conjunc-

wellness **tip**

It is recommended that women under the age of 40 have their eyes examined every two to three years. Between 40 and 60 years of age, an eye examination is recommended at least every two years, or more often if vision changes or a family history of glaucoma is present. By age 60, yearly eye examinations are recommended.

tivitis produces thickened discharge. Any symptoms of conjunctivitis (redness, itching, discharge, blurred vision, sensitivity to light, and a gritty feeling in the eye) should be examined by your doctor or ophthalmologist as soon as possible.

Although it does not usually harm vision, conjunctivitis is highly contagious. It may be associated with corneal complications in adults, accompanied by severe pain in the eye and swollen eyelids.

More Serious Eye Disorders. See your doctor at once if you have symptoms of the more serious eye disorders. Immediate treatment may be necessary to prevent further complications or even loss of sight.

Ptosis. Ptosis (drooping eyelid) is caused by a weakness in the muscles that raise your eyelids. It may run in families, but is more often caused by aging and injury or by diseases, such as a viral infection, diabetes, stroke, myasthenia gravis, brain tumor, or cancers occurring at the base of the neck or top of the lung. Drooping eyelids may be relieved when an underlying disease is treated. If a child is born with ptosis, surgery may be necessary.

Glaucoma. Glaucoma is caused by pressure building up within the eyeball, which eventually damages the optic nerve causing blurred vision and even blindness. The disorder is often a product of aging; up to three percent of the population over the age of 65 develops glaucoma. Also prone to the disease are diabetics, African Americans, those who take cortisone or medication to reduce blood pressure, and those who are nearsighted.

The most common form of glaucoma is called open-angle glaucoma, which develops gradually over several years and may cause no symptoms until the optic nerve is actually damaged. The second type, called closed-angle glaucoma, develops rapidly and causes sudden blurring of vision, nausea and vomiting, and redness in the affected eye. Persons suffering from closed-angle glaucoma might also notice a halo around lights when they look directly at them. These symptoms require immediate medical attention.

Glaucoma can be treated with surgery, but it must be caught early. Since open-angle glaucoma does not usually produce symptoms, regular eye examinations that include a test for glaucoma are essential for all women. When you schedule your eye examinations (every two or three years for women under 40; every two years for women over 40), be sure to ask your eyecare specialist if she routinely tests for glaucoma, and ask what kinds of tests she performs. The most reliable way to detect glaucoma is to combine three simple procedures. One measures for loss of peripheral vision, which is a subtle symptom of early glaucoma. Another, called tonometry, measures the pressure within the eyes. A third test is a thorough examination inside the eyes while the pupils are dilated.

Cataracts. There is growing evidence that cataracts, unlike glaucoma, are preventable when certain health habits are followed. Cataracts occur when the normally clear lens of your eye becomes clouded, impairing the ability of the lens to focus images on the retina. The condition is associated with aging, but recent research, though not conclusive, strongly indicates that cigarette smoke, strong sunlight, and a diet weak in certain vitamins all contribute to the formation of cataracts. Vitamins C and E along with beta-carotene seem to guard against the environmental factors (cigarette smoke and ultraviolet light) that are now believed to be the cause of cataracts in some people.

The existence of a cataract need not be debilitating. Unless it causes limitations in your lifestyle, such as the inability to read or the failure to pass a driver's test, a small cataract can go untreated and may never get worse than when it is first diagnosed. While cataracts are traditionally the leading cause of blindness, they can now be effectively treated with surgery. The ophthalmologist usually removes the affected parts of the lens and then implants an artificial replacement lens. In some cases laser surgery is required to correct a blurring in the artificial lens. Both treatments are usually performed on an outpatient basis and are almost always successful.

Your Ears

The ear is made up of several delicate structures designed to carry sound waves to your brain. Your external ear—called the pinna—is made up of cartilage and bone. The pinna gathers sound and funnels it to your middle ear. The middle ear houses the tympanum, commonly called the eardrum, and three auditory bones, or ossicles (the malleus, the incus, and the stapes, named for its resemblance to stirrups). The movement of the auditory ossicles translates movements of the tympanic membrane (which vibrates when it is hit by sound) into the fluid of the inner ear. Hair cells in the inner ear stimulate the auditory nerve, which then transmits impulses to the brain. Finally, the brain translates the auditory impulses into sound.

Protecting and Caring for Your Ears

Like your eyesight, whether your hearing remains reasonably sharp throughout your life depends to a degree on the care you take to protect your ears from exposure to environmental hazards, injury, and illness. Many people despair when they notice a gradual loss of hearing because it represents the advancement of the aging process. Fortunately, research reveals that proper care can delay or prevent the onset of hearing loss, and modern science now provides many products to improve hearing for people with hearing problems, even into old age.

Excess Noise and Your Ears. One preventative measure against hearing loss is almost completely within your control: protecting your ears from excess noise. Noise is measured in units called decibels (dB). Exposure to a decibel level higher than 85 that is sustained for an 8-hour period constitutes excess noise.

The effect of excess noise that you experience in the course of a day is cumulative. For example, if you encounter 80 dB of noise at work for only a 4-hour period, but return home and listen to music at very high volume or operate power tools without hearing protection, you could exceed your noise exposure limit and risk gradual and permanent hearing loss. Even everyday tasks and activities, such as using vacuum cleaners and driving on busy roads, can expose you to excess noise.

wellness
warning

If you suspect you have a cataract, contact your eye care specialist to determine the seriousness of the problem. Typical symptoms include double vision, poor night vision, difficulty driving at night because of extreme glare from oncoming headlights, blurring of vision, and colors appearing faded or yellowed.

wellness **warning**

Hair cells in your ears can become damaged by prolonged exposure to loud noise. When hair cells become damaged, they cannot be replaced or rejuvenated. The result is permanent hearing loss.

Follow these tips to prevent hearing loss due to excess noise:

- After exposure to inordinate noise levels, allow your ears to rest for 24 hours by avoiding all increased noises.
- Wear earplugs, special protectors, or canal caps when using noisy tools, firearms, or equipment, or when riding in noisy vehicles or airplanes. Be sure they fit properly and can reduce the noise rating by at least 15 dB.
- Employees who are exposed to potentially damaging noise should wear protective earplugs in the ear canal or earmuffs that cover the entire external ear. For optimal protection, both devices should be worn simultaneously.
- Avoid plugging your ears with cotton. Cotton can become stuck in your ear canal, and it will not offer adequate protection against noise.
- Have your hearing tested annually.
- If you are in a room where you must shout to be heard, leave the area for a period of time. If you cannot hear a conversation that is less than two feet away, or you must raise your own voice to be heard, assume that noise levels are excessive.
- Avoid loud recreational noises. Many adults today have reduced hearing from listening to loud music at home or at concerts, or from using headphones.
- Watch the volume of your stereo headphones, cellular phones, and earphones. If you can hear the sound produced by your headphones or cellular phone when you hold them an arm's length away, the noise level is too high and can damage your hearing. Lower the volume!

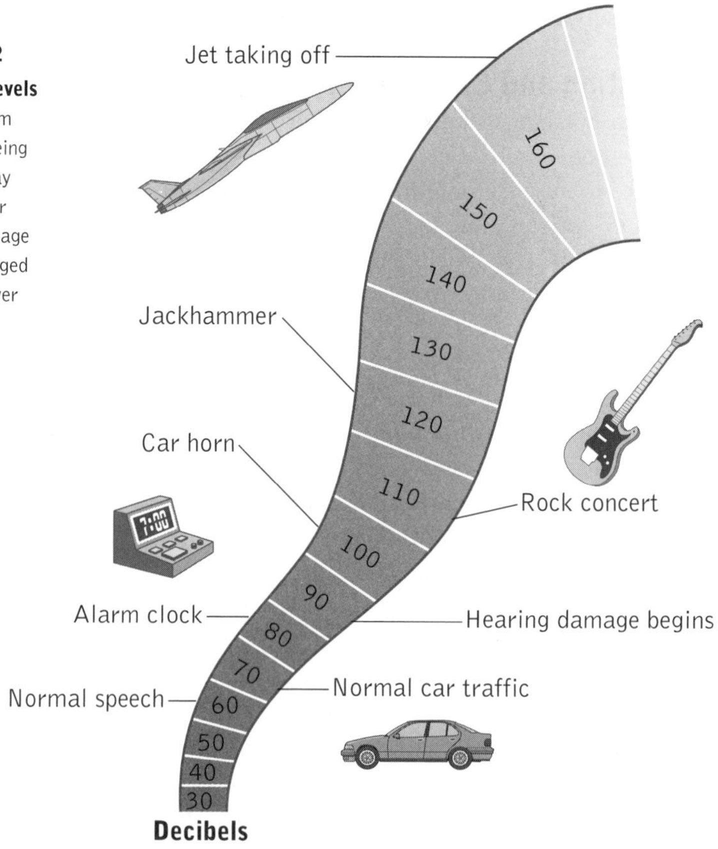

FIGURE 24.2
Everyday Decibel Levels
Protect your ears from hearing damage by being aware of how everyday sounds can effect your hearing. Hearing damage can begin with prolonged exposure to sounds over 85 decibels.

Jet taking off — 160
150
140
Jackhammer — 130
120
Car horn — 110
100
90 — Hearing damage begins
Alarm clock — 80
70 — Normal car traffic
Normal speech — 60
50
40
30

Rock concert

Decibels

Ear Protection Devices. You can purchase earplugs at most drugstores, sporting goods, or music stores. They come in a variety of materials, including foam, rubber, silicone, or wax. Most earplugs are disposable and provide moderate protection against excess levels of noise. Earplugs are also recommended for swimming, especially for people prone to ear infections.

Musician's plugs are also available to help filter out dangerous levels of noise generated by electric instruments commonly used by rock bands. Musician's plugs help filter out noise without sacrificing the sound of voices.

Cleaning Your Ears Safely. Your outer ear contains glands that produce ear wax. Ear wax traps dirt and prevents it from reaching your eardrums. The wax often dries out by itself and causes no problems. Sometimes, however, the wax accumulates to such a degree that it interferes with your hearing or causes a bothersome clicking sound when you swallow. A large buildup of wax can be removed by a physician who has the proper tools to avoid the danger of puncturing or perforating the eardrum. If you have a small wax buildup, if your ear is otherwise healthy, and if you do not have a perforated eardrum or have not had mastoid surgery, follow these safety tips to remove the wax on your own:

- Loosen the wax by placing a few drops of baby oil or mineral oil in each ear canal. Be sure that the oil is at room temperature.
- Fill a 3-ounce rubber bulb syringe with water that is body temperature.
- Tilt your head to the right side if you are cleaning your right ear (and vice versa), and pull your outer ear up and back to straighten your ear. Gently squirt water into the canal. If this causes pain, stop immediately.
- If there is no pain, repeat this process until the wax falls out.
- When the wax has fallen out, dry your ear canal with a soft, lint-free cloth, and insert six to ten drops of drying solution, such as ear drops with alcohol or rubbing alcohol. This will help destroy fungal and bacterial growth.
- Tip your head to one side to drain excess alcohol.
- Over-the-counter ear wax removal kits are also available. If these attempts do not work and if the wax exerts uncomfortable pressure on your ear, see your physician right away.

Overcoming Problems During Air Travel. Ear problems can occur during flight because there is an air pocket in the middle ear that is vulnerable to rapid changes in air pressure.(Air pressure changes can also occur when driving on mountain roads, diving in deep water, or riding in elevators in tall buildings.) Follow these suggestions to prevent or minimize blocking of your ears or to unblock your ears when the air pressure changes rapidly:

- Take a decongestant pill (over-the-counter pseudoephedrine, 30 milligrams) or use a nasal decongestant spray one hour before ascent or descent to shrink membranes and allow your ears to "pop" more naturally. Avoid decongestants if you are pregnant or take other medications, unless you have checked with your doctor first.
- If you have allergies, take an antihistamine at the beginning of the flight. However, avoid antihistamines if you are pregnant, have high blood pressure or a

heart condition, or take other medications, unless you have checked with your doctor first.

- Swallowing and yawning often help. Yawning helps activate the muscle that opens the eustachian tube. Try chewing gum or sucking on hard candy to encourage the swallowing reflex.
- If yawning or swallowing does not work, pinch your nostrils; take in a mouthful of air; using your cheeks and throat muscles, force air out by blowing it forcefully out of your nose. You should hear a "pop" from the reduced air pressure.
- Do not sleep during descent. Have the flight attendant awaken you before descent. (It is also wise to wake infants and toddlers during ascent and descent, and to nurse the child or offer a bottle or pacifier.)
- If pain persists following the flight, repeat the dose of decongestant and see your physician.

Ear Disorders

Most illnesses that affect the ear, while not always preventable, are treatable and may not cause hearing loss if they are caught early. The longer ear problems are left untreated, however, the harder they are to remedy.

Ear Infections. Infection of the outer and middle ear can occur as a result of bacterial, viral, or fungal infection. Middle ear infections may be triggered by high altitudes, cold climates, and decompression experienced during air travel. The most common type of ear infection is *otitis externa,* also known as swimmer's ear.

Swimmer's ear is also called "fungus" of the ear and "jungle" ear (so called by soldiers who fought in the South Pacific during World War II). The infection is often caused by bacteria. It is caused when water becomes trapped in the ear canal following swimming or showering. The canal extending from the eardrum to the outside may become swollen and reddened. Patients may have fever, discharge from the ear, and sensitivity upon touch. Temporary hearing loss may result from the inflammation. Ear infections of this type usually require treatment with antibiotics.

Choosing an Ear Doctor

A variety of health care specialists have been trained to treat disorders of the ear. If you see your primary care physician first for problems related to your ears, you may be directed to see a specialist.

- **Otolaryngologist.** These specialists diagnose and treat disorders of the ear, nose, and throat, including hearing loss and disorders related to sinuses, larynx, and throat. They are trained to perform head and neck surgery and cosmetic reconstruction.

- **Otologist.** These physicians specialize in treatments listed above, but related only to the anatomy, pathology, and physiology of the ear.

- **Audiologist.** These specialists are licensed and trained to perform tests related to hearing and hearing assessment. Those with the letters CCC-A (Clinical Certification of Competence-Audiology) after their names have been certified by the American Speech-Language-Hearing Association.

If you experience dizziness, ringing, bleeding, sudden pain, or hearing loss, see your physician immediately, as it might indicate a punctured eardrum. Punctured eardrums can result from a severe middle ear infection, sudden loud noises, or sudden inward pressure to the ear.

If you have an ear infection, keep the ear canal dry and warm. If you must blow your nose, do so very gently. Avoid getting water in your ear. Do not swim. A course of antibiotics or even surgical draining of the affected area may be necessary.

Tinnitus. Tinnitus refers to ringing in the ears. This common ailment may be intermittent or persistent. Temporary tinnitus may be caused by a small plug of ear wax. However, tinnitus is often associated with hearing loss as a result of exposure to loud noises, infection, perforation of the eardrum, fluid in the middle ear, or rigidity of the bones in the middle ear. Tinnitus may also signal the presence of other diseases or disorders, such as cardiovascular disease, anemia, or aspirin excess.

Your physician can make the diagnosis and may conduct tests for otosclerosis, Ménière's disease, acoustic trauma, hereditary hearing loss, occupational hearing loss, or other ear conditions.

Otosclerosis. Otosclerosis is a disorder that results in a gradual hearing loss. It often runs in families, afflicting more women than men. Otosclerosis occurs most frequently during childbearing years. During pregnancy, hearing loss often becomes more pronounced. Calcium growths at the entrance to the inner ear and stiffening of the stapes may occur. Once the stapes no longer vibrates, sound waves cannot be passed on to the inner ear. Otosclerosis can be surgically corrected.

Ménière's Disease. Ménière's disease is characterized by episodes of dizziness (vertigo), ringing in the ears (tinnitus), pressure in the ears, and distorted hearing. It can be caused by excess fluid in the cochlea (the hearing organ) or the semicircular canal (the balance organ). Most patients have a combination of the two.

Attacks may last from hours to days. Sometimes, they are severe enough to cause nausea and vomiting and impair your ability to walk. Episodes may become increasingly more serious and can result in hearing loss.

If you experience these symptoms, see your physician immediately. Your physician may have you undergo a test called electronystagmography. This involves flooding your ear with water, which, for reasons uncertain even to medical professionals, causes your eyes to flicker. Your physician will study the flicker and may repeat the test with water of varying temperatures. Your response to each will be noted to determine the ability of your inner ear to help you maintain balance. While Ménière's is rarely curable, vitamin supplement treatments may reduce the frequency and severity of the episodes.

Cholesteatoma. This is a middle ear disorder caused by a blockage of the eustachian tube, resulting in an inward bend of the eardrum. Sometimes skin from a tumor or a cyst grows through a hole in the eardrum. The growth is called a cholesteatoma. The cholesteatoma can damage the small structures of the middle ear, causing hearing damage or loss. However, it is a benign condition and will not spread to other areas. Surgery is required for removal. Unfortunately, since

wellness **tip**

Swimmer's ear can be prevented by shaking the water out of your ear following swimming. Apply a drying solution, such as ear drops with alcohol or rubbing alcohol, to the canal. This will help dry up excess water and retard the growth of fungus and bacteria. If you are prone to swimmer's ear, wear earplugs while swimming or showering.

the condition is chronic, it can return. In serious cases, surgery may also be required to create a cavity from which periodic cleaning can be conducted.

Hearing Aids

Improved technology has made hearing aids better than ever. Costs range from $500 to $2,000. Three types of hearing aids are available:

- Those worn behind the ear
- Those worn in the ear
- Those worn in the ear canal

Behind-the-ear models are relatively unobtrusive and quite small. They are powerful and easy to use. Hearing aids worn in the ear are usually custom molded for comfort. This type does not offer sufficient correction for people with severe hearing losses. Hearing aids worn in the canal are the smallest version. Because they are worn closer to the eardrum, they require less power and volume. This variety is also insufficient for people with severe hearing loss.

Cochlear implants are also available for persons with profound hearing loss. The implants restore auditory sensation via electrical stimulation of the auditory nerve. An electrode is implanted into the inner ear. Sound enters a microphone, where a speech processor encodes the sounds and transmits them to a coil.

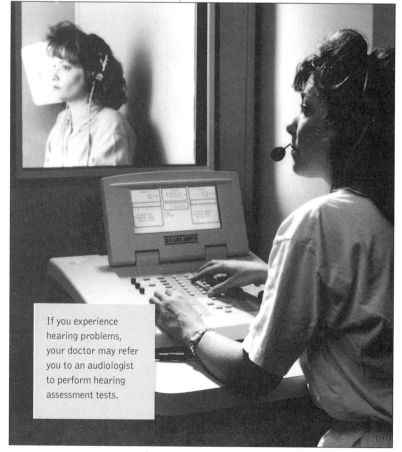

If you experience hearing problems, your doctor may refer you to an audiologist to perform hearing assessment tests.

Deciding Whether You Need a Hearing Aid. Hearing loss due to aging is a gradual process that may go unnoticed for quite some time unless a family member or friend points out that you seem to be having trouble. If you think you are experiencing hearing loss, your first step is to visit your primary physician or to go directly to an otolaryngologist (ear, nose, and throat doctor). These doctors can check for other causes of hearing loss that can be more easily treated or that would not respond to a hearing aid.

If your hearing is so reduced that you cannot function well, your physician may give you an audiogram, or she might refer you directly to an audiologist for testing and recommendations regarding hearing aids.

Choosing an Audiologist. Once you and your doctor have determined that a hearing aid is appropriate, your next step is to choose an audiologist, someone trained to perform tests that determine precisely how much amplification you need in order to hear better.

Just as some optometrists sell eyeglasses, some audiologists dispense hearing aids. However, there are audiologists who are not genuinely qualified to sell you a hearing aid, so it is important that you choose one who is certified by the American Speech-Language-Hearing Association as indicated by the letters CCC-A (Clinical Certification of Competence-Audiology). To be sure you will get satisfaction, take the following steps before you buy:

- Ask your doctor to recommend a qualified audiologist.
- Look for the CCC-A designation after the audiologist's name.
- Be direct in asking the person selling you a hearing aid for her qualifications.
- Check the store with the Better Business Bureau before you buy a hearing aid to be sure there is no record of misleading conduct.
- Ask to see a state license.
- Make sure the salesperson offers a written warranty that will allow you to return an unsatisfactory hearing aid. Some warranties provide for low-cost replacement of lost or damaged products.
- Ask the audiologist to give you another hearing test while you are wearing the device.

Your Sense of **Smell**

Your sense of smell shares a common chemical sensing system with your sense of taste. What affects one usually affects the other. For example, nerve cells in your nose, mouth, and throat work together to alert your brain to the presence of a barbecue by transmitting messages about the molecules that the smoking meat puts out into the environment. If you are unable to smell the barbecue, you will not be able to taste it as well as you do when your sense of smell is sharp. Here are some other fast facts about your sense of smell:

- Humans are capable of recognizing approximately 10,000 odors, although most people can only distinguish 2,000 to 4,000 odors.
- Your sense of smell not only enables you to enjoy pleasant scents and fragrances, but also alerts you to potential danger, such as spoiled foods, smoke or fire, and chemical fumes.
- Women are more sensitive than men to smells. Some women report that their sense of smell sharpens during pregnancy, and it is said that a mother will know her own baby by scent alone a few hours after birth.

Did you ever wonder why certain tastes or smells jar your memory? For example, you might smell a certain brand of hand cream and suddenly, vividly picture your mother getting ready to go out on a Saturday evening from your childhood. When you smell an odor or taste a food, that sensory information is transmitted directly to two specific parts of the brain: the amygdala, which stores memories associated with emotion, and the hippocampus, which stores memories related to spatial information. The combination stimulates the memory and often elicits a particular emotion. Smelling old books, for example, may make you feel sad if your grandfather who has passed away had a wonderful collection of old books

Alternatives to Hearing Aids

Before you seek out hearing aid referrals, check with your doctor to make sure your hearing loss is severe enough to merit a hearing aid. Understand that a hearing aids will not help you in a noisy room or hear people who mumble. If you have decreased hearing, there are ways to improve your ability to understand people without using a hearing aid:

- Tell family members and friends that you have a hearing problem.
- Ask them to face you when they speak, to talk clearly, and not to rush what they are saying.
- Ask people to speak one at a time rather than all at once.
- Reduce background noise, such as television, radio, and stereo.
- Arrive early to meetings and ask to be seated up front where you can see the speaker's mouth and hear better without distraction.

that you used to read together. "Comfort food" is so called because smelling it and eating it can bring back memories of home-cooked meals and childhood treats.

Protecting and Caring for Your Nose and Sinuses

As with your eyesight and your hearing, a gradual loss of your ability to smell and taste accompanies the aging process. Your nose needs to remain moist to be healthy and function properly. However, there are steps you can take throughout your life to protect these senses.

Treating Colds and Allergies Sensibly. We all get colds occasionally. When we have one, we are miserable and we try to cure it, and when it is gone, we forget about it. But it is important to know that the annoying symptoms of a cold can protect you from worse disorders, and that some cold treatments produce a lasting negative effect on the nose and throat and so should be used sparingly.

The mucus produced in reasonable quantities when you are in good health protects your lungs, sinuses, and nose by trapping dust and other impurities. When the nose becomes irritated, as with an allergic reaction or a cold, it alerts the mucus glands to send more help. The increased mucus in your nose and sinuses warms and moistens cold air before it reaches your lungs, and it traps bacteria and viruses before they can take root. Given that your immune system is somewhat depressed during a cold, these are valuable preventative measures your body automatically takes.

This is not to say you should not treat a cold. But you should be aware of the negative side effects of the most common treatments so you can make informed choices. Antihistamines, for example, make it easier for you to breathe by drying up the mucus in your nose, but they may over-dry membranes, causing pain, bleeding, or prolonged congestion. They may make you feel drowsy unless you look for the newer nondrowsy formulas. Decongestant pills temporarily bring relief by opening up nasal passages to allow drainage of swollen membranes. When they wear off, congestion can actually be worse than before (a condition called rebound). Use of decongestant nasal sprays is not recommended unless congestion is severe, because they directly affect a large part of the mucous membrane of the nose and have more significant rebound. Take care not to overuse these products.

Nonprescription nasal drops and sprays that contain decongestants should be used no more than three or four times a day for no longer than a few days. Prolonged use can cause irritation and chronic inflammation of the mucous membrane, called rhinitis medicamentosa. It is not uncommon for the unwary to become addicted to nasal sprays. If this happens, a cycle begins where the spray works for a short time, then the mucous flows more heavily than ever, prompting the sufferer to use even more nasal spray. The rebound cycle is difficult to break. If you think you have become dependent on nasal sprays, see your allergist or your otolaryngologist.

Chemicals and Your Sense of Smell. Another step you can take to preserve your sense of smell is to limit your exposure to industrial agents that might be present in your workplace or in household products. Be especially aware of the potential harm from benzene, carbon disulfide, formaldehyde, paint solvents, methyl bromide, cadmium, and nickel dust. If you work around these or similar agents, encourage your employer to inspect the ventilation system in your workplace to be sure it is working at maximum efficiency. When you use any chemical household product or work with paints and paint thinners at home, open as many windows as possible, or work outside.

Finally, reduce your exposure to cigarette smoke by quitting, if you are a smoker, and by asking family members to smoke outside. The chemicals in cigarettes damage your sense of smell. If they refuse, ask them to smoke only in a certain room, with the door closed and the windows open to keep smoke out of the rest of the home.

Disorders of the Nose

The loss of taste or smell may be caused by illness, disease, trauma, surgery, medication, or

Loss of a Sense of Smell and Your Safety

If you do not have a sense of smell, or if it has been compromised in some way, you are missing an important warning sense. To protect yourself from injury, follow these safety tips:

- Routinely check the sell dates on all foods; discard items that are beyond the recommended dates.
- Install smoke, gas, and carbon monoxide detectors in your home and at work.
- Consider changing your applicances from gas to electric.
- Do not smoke. Encourage family members to quit smoking.
- Avoid using excess salt or sugar to compensate for lack of flavor.
- Seek the aid of a nutritionist for guidance in healthful eating habits to prevent malnutrition or obesity.
- Check to see if you have a zinc deficiency. Zinc supplementation has been demonstrated to improve the sense of smell in patients with zinc deficiencies.
- Consider seeking psychiatric help for support in coping with olfactory dysfunction.
- Eliminate drugs or toxins that may be causing or adding to your problem.
- Explore medical or surgical intervention that may help with obstructive diseases of the sinonasal tract. Medical therapy can include decongestants or a course of nasal or oral steroids taken under supervision.

environmental exposure. The loss of smell is usually described three ways. Anosmia indicates complete loss of the sense of smell. (Many patients with anosmia can usually detect the difference between categories of taste, such as salty, sweet, sour, and bitter, since these are sensed on the tongue; however, more subtle flavors will be lost to them.) Hyposmia indicates a reduced sense of smell; paraosmia indicates a distortion of the sense of smell. A loss of smell may be associated with the following:

- Chronic disease of the sinonasal tract, such as chronic sinusitis
- Allergic rhinitis
- Nasal obstructions and polyps
- Upper respiratory tract infection
- Psychiatric disorders (schizophrenia and depression)
- Neurodegenerative disease (Alzheimer's and Parkinson's diseases, neurosyphilis)
- Immune disorders (Wegener's granulomatosis, sarcoidosis, Sjögren's syndrome—common among postmenopausal women—and multiple sclerosis)
- Aging (half of all people over 65 show a decline in the ability to smell)
- Congenital dysfunction
- Drugs, including opiates, analgesics, cocaine, and antibiotics (aminoglycosides, macrolides, tetracycline, ampicillin, amphotericin B, griseofulvin)
- Zinc deficiency
- Trauma to the head or nose

As you can see, reduction or loss of the ability to smell can be minor, temporary, and easily treated, or it may indicate a serious condition. If your physician cannot identify a treatable nasal condition, she may refer you to a neurologist to determine if the problem is associated with brain function.

Environmental *Problems* *and* the Senses

Women seem to be more prone than men to environmental illnesses, possibly because many chemicals mimic estrogen when they are absorbed into the body. Principle culprits are benzene, phenol, chlorine, and formaldehyde. Be aware of the materials that surround you and take note of those you suspect may be causing discomfort, especially if you have recently changed jobs, cosmetics, or household products. If you have problems with any of your senses, ask yourself whether you have come into contact with any of the following objects or substances, or whether you are experiencing internal changes that might be the cause of the problem:

External Environment
- New paint or synthetic carpets in the home
- New car or office furniture with soft plastic fabrics
- Renovations at the workplace
- Chemical pollutants in the neighborhood or workplace

FIGURE 24.3
Environmental Threats to Your Senses
Many people are unaware that they are allergic to common chemicals or materials in their surroundings. If you think one of these substances may be causing you problems, speak with your doctor.

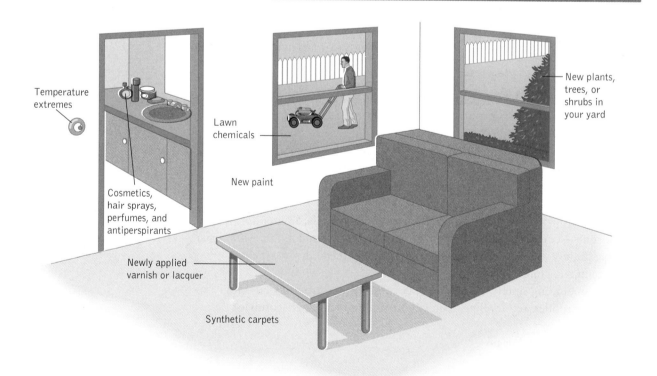

Temperature extremes

Cosmetics, hair sprays, perfumes, and antiperspirants

Lawn chemicals

New paint

New plants, trees, or shrubs in your yard

Newly applied varnish or lacquer

Synthetic carpets

- Toxic incinerators in the neighborhood
- New plants, trees, or shrubs in your yard or the neighbor's yard
- Pesticides or lawn chemicals
- Newly applied varnish, lacquer, or glues
- Extremes in temperature
- Extreme humidity or dryness
- Chemical cleaners
- Cosmetics, hair sprays, perfumes, and antiperspirants

"Internal" Environment
- Medications
- Stress
- Vitamin deficiency or excess
- Hormonal imbalance
- Food or drug allergy
- Implanted medical devices or prostheses
- Excessive consumption of hydrogenated oils
- Contaminated drinking water

What *You* Can Do

Protecting your senses from injury or premature loss of function will enhance your enjoyment of life into old age. Although a certain loss of acuity in eyesight, hearing, smell, and taste is considered normal during the aging process, you need not accept every change as "inevitable." Approach the wellness of your senses as you do every other aspect of your health. Listen to your body but be aware of changes, note whether there is something you can do to improve the situation, and if there is, do it! In particular, you can begin at a young age preparing your senses for a long life if you:

- Shield your eyes from bright sunlight with hats and UVA- and UVB-blocking sunglasses.
- Eat a diet high in beta-carotene and vitamins E and C.
- Have your eyes checked regularly.
- Avoid situations where the noise level is excessive (above 85 dB).
- Rest your ears after exposure to excessive noise.
- Use cold and allergy medications sparingly.
- Limit your exposure to chemical sprays and fumes.
- See your doctor anytime you have problems with your eyes, ears, or nose that last more than a few days.
- Quit smoking.

Strengthening *Your* Bones *and* Muscles

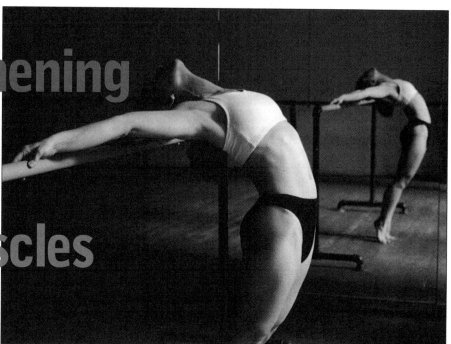

Every time you pick up a pencil, answer the telephone, walk to the store, or take a dance class, your musculoskeletal system is at work. This complex system of bones, joints, and muscles forms a strong frame that supports and protects tissues and organs and enables you to perform all physical activities.

What keeps the musculoskeletal system healthy? Maintaining a sensible lifestyle that includes regular exercise, good nutrition, and injury prevention helps women build and maintain healthy bones, muscles, and joints, as well as improve their cardiovascular fitness and overall energy level.

Women are prone to a number of conditions affecting their joints, muscles, and bones, many of which can be painful and debilitating. A strong musculoskeletal system helps prevent these conditions or lessen their symptoms and can help women function independently well into their elder years.

The Building Blocks *of the* Musculoskeletal System

The term musculoskeletal system describes the many components that work together to give the body its structure, strength, and ability to move. In addition to the muscles and skeleton, there are two types of fibrous connective tissues: ligaments, which connect bones at the joints; and tendons, which attach muscles to bones.

By gaining a basic understanding of the building blocks of the musculoskeletal system, you will not only become familiar with how the system works, but you will also be able to recognize the warning signs of a malfunction. This knowledge also helps you identify the steps necessary to keep your bones, joints, and muscles in healthy, working order.

Anatomy Lesson: Bones, Joints, and Muscles

The skeleton contains 206 bones. Some bones are large and quite visible to the eye, especially those at the elbows, wrists, knees, and ankles. Others (those deep within the hands and feet) are tiny, and you may not be aware of them until you feel pain or strain in a particular spot. Bones are connected by joints. More than 600 muscles enable the bones and joints to move.

Bones. Bones are living tissue, much like the skin, heart, and lungs. Composed of calcium and protein, bones have a solid, hard casing on the outside; spongy bone is located inside. As its name suggests, spongy bone is full of small holes, which keep the skeleton relatively lightweight. The interlacing, honeycomb structure that forms these holes is highly intricate and lends bones their strength by providing a barely perceivable, but very important, degree of flexibility. Inside the spongy bone is marrow, which produces blood cells for the body. In healthy, young adults, the bones retain an optimal amount of minerals that give bones strength.

Remodeling. Like all the cells in the body, bone is constantly being renewed. Through a process called "remodeling," old bone is broken down and new bone is created. In healthy young adults, this is a balanced process, so bone mass, also referred to as bone density, and bone strength remain constant. After age 35, however, a gradual loss of bone mass begins, with more bone being broken down than produced. This process is called resorption. If resorption accelerates, bone mass and strength are greatly reduced and can lead to osteoporosis, a condition in which low bone density leaves the bones vulnerable to fracture.

Improving Bone Strength. You can enhance your bone mass by working and conditioning your bones, through weight lifting or weight-bearing exercises that bear the body's own weight, such as walking, running, and aerobic exercises in which one or both feet leave the floor.

Main Bones of the Arms. The long bone running from the shoulder to the elbow is the humerus. In the forearm are two parallel bones, the ulna (which runs up the outside of the arm and forms the knob of the elbow) and the radius. The wrist and hand have many smaller bones in three basic groups: the carpals (the bones of the wrist), the metacarpals (forming the trunk of the hand), and the phalanges (finger bones).

Main Bones of the Legs. The leg is fairly similar to the arm, having a single long bone in the thigh (the femur) and two parallel bones in the lower leg: the tibia (the larger bone comprising the shin) and fibula. At the bottom of the leg are the smaller, more agile bone configurations of the ankle (tarsals) and foot (metatarsals).

Skull and Ribs. There are two areas where bones work to encase and protect vital organs. The skull, which is actually made up of several bones, encases the

wellness **tip**

Think of bone strength as a bank account. Up until sometime in your thirties, you make more "deposits" to the account than "withdrawals." During the middle adult years, deposits and withdrawals are about even. After menopause, withdrawals far outweigh deposits.

brain. The rib cage protects the heart and lungs. The ribs wrap around each side of the torso and are joined by cartilage to the sternum (breastbone) in the front and to the spine in the back. The rib cage is capped by the clavicle (collar bone), which runs from the top of the sternum out both sides to the scapula (shoulder bone).

The Spine. Perhaps the most important part of the skeleton, the spine, or backbone, runs from the base of the skull, down the back, and through the pelvis. This flexible yet strong structure of interlocking bones (called vertebrae) is the foundation of the entire body. Like the main beam of a roof, the spine supports and links all other sections of the skeleton. It also encases the spinal column, the bundle of nerves that carries signals from the brain down to the nervous system. Layered in between the spine's 24 vertebrae are discs, gel-filled pads of cartilage, that act as shock absorbers and enable the spine to flex and sustain weight. There are very few motions or positions that do not in some way involve the spine and the many back muscles and ligaments that support it. For this reason, the back is highly prone to strain and injury.

Joints. Without joints, your skeleton would function as little more than a shoe tree or mannequin. Deftly constructed of muscles, tendons, and ligaments, as well as the bones they join together, joints are the spots where your frame bends at the knee, wrist, hip, neck, ankle, elbow, jaw, hand, and foot. Every physical action you perform—from keyboarding a computer and turning the car keys in the ignition, to shoveling snow and dancing—involves the fluid, coordinated movement of one or more joints.

FIGURE 25.1

Your Joints

The joints in your body function in a manner very similar to mechanical joints. These illustrations show the three main types of joints in your body.

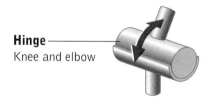
Gliding
Wrist and ankle

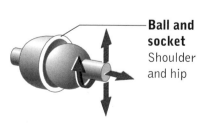
Hinge
Knee and elbow

Ball and socket
Shoulder and hip

There are three major types of joints— gliding (which includes the wrist and ankle), hinge (knee and elbow), and ball and socket (shoulder and hip)—each of which provides a different range of motion. Cartilage at the end of each joint bone (both in the ligaments that hold the bones together and on the facing surfaces of the bones) allows the joints to flex and move. In the small cavity between the two bones, a highly slippery substance called synovial fluid flows around and lubricates the bones, ligaments, and membranes. Made up of water and mucus, this fluid thickens when pressure is exerted on the joint. Small sacs called bursae further ease movement by protecting muscles and tendons when they rub against the harder bones and ligaments. The intricate design of the joint's component parts, combined with the synovial fluid and bursae, give the healthy joint an incredible smoothness of motion.

Muscles. Muscles are made up of fibers that contract and release in response to electronic impulses transmitted through nerves from the brain. Muscles are powered by glycogen, a natural body sugar produced in the liver.

Muscles are generally organized in groups that provide opposing, push-pull forces, defined as extension (pushing) and flexion (pulling). When you pull open a door, for instance, you flex one set of muscles in your upper arm; when you close it, you extend another, opposing set. Muscles also mediate the amount and force of movements, creating, for example, the difference between walking and running.

In addition to propelling your limbs and helping you lift and exercise, muscles do the important work of supporting your body. Your stomach muscles, for example, help keep you erect, hold your back in position, and also hold the digestive organs in place. Your leg muscles do not just move your legs, they also help you keep erect by subtly flexing or extending as you walk down a bumpy sidewalk, lean into a strong wind, or carry a heavy package or small, wriggling child. The leg muscles help compensate for any factor that could throw you off balance.

Muscles work best when they are used regularly. During everyday use and during exercise, muscles are flexed or extended against resistance, building mass, tone, and strength. Lifting weights or performing isometric, or resistance, exercises that target specific muscle groups helps keep your muscles toned and strong. Weak muscles are more prone to sprains and strains.

Physiology Lesson: How You Move

By learning about the musculoskeletal system and the intricate ways in which different parts work together to give you mobility and dexterity, you can see that it is a marvel of design and engineering. Take, as an example, the versatility of the arm. When you reach to pick up the phone, electrical impulses from your brain, delivered through your nerves, stimulate the muscles in your upper arm and forearm. When these muscles contract, the tendons attaching them to the bones transfer the force of these contractions to the bones, which causes the arm to move. This chain reaction of impulse, contraction, force transfer, and motion occurs at lightning speed in all the required muscles, in a highly coordinated fashion. The result is a smooth reach. When your hand gets close enough to the receiver, it executes a similar coordinated chain reaction (powered by other muscles and tendons in your forearm plus those in the hand) in each of your fingers, and the receiver is grasped. Similar processes occur as other muscles in your arm are stimulated to bring the receiver up to your ear.

This simple action would not be possible without the joints—shoulder, elbow, wrist, and finger joints. By going through their ranges of motion, also in a highly coordinated fashion, joints make the movement of arm and hand possible. They do it smoothly and silently, thanks to the lubricating power of the synovial fluid, which "greases the gears" of the joints. The ligaments and other joint tissues are specially engineered to facilitate the movement of the bones. As the hand reaches out for the receiver, the forearm twists as its two bones, the ulna and radius, rotate at both the wrist and elbow and cross over one another. As the hand comes up to the ear, these two bones cross back to a side-by-side position. All this, just to pick up the telephone. Similarly orchestrated impulses and movements occur throughout your body countless times each day.

Unfortunately, there are a number of conditions that threaten the smooth functioning of the musculoskeletal system. Some arise with age, some from disease, and many from lifestyle factors. Most, however, can be avoided or curbed if you work to keep your bones, muscles, and joints healthy.

Musculoskeletal Problems
Most Affecting Women

Everyone suffers various aches and pains, especially as they get older. Three conditions—low back pain, osteoporosis, and osteoarthritis—are quite common in women. These conditions illustrate most dramatically the impact of aging, menopause, general inactivity, and everyday stresses and strains on the musculoskeletal system.

Low Back Pain

Low back pain is among the most common of all physical complaints. It is, however, one of the most preventable and treatable. The back works hard every day, bearing a great deal of weight, helping you carry out hundreds of movements and activities, such as lifting, running, and walking. It also works to keep you upright when standing or sitting. The back's complex network of muscles, ligaments, bones, joints, and nerves is highly vulnerable to strain and injury—especially in the lower (lumbar) portion of the spine, where the greatest pressure is felt.

Low back pain affects 80 to 90 percent of adult Americans at some point in their lifetime. In more than 90 percent of these cases, however, low back pain is not a serious condition. Back pain typically develops over time. Although many back pain sufferers can trace their condition to a specific incident of lifting or twisting, it seems that just as many cannot pinpoint the cause. They just know that it hurts—often so much that they cannot perform their normal activities. In fact, low back pain is the leading cause of disability for those under age 45.

Most cases of low back pain stem from a long-term lack of care—poor posture, improper lifting technique, and weak and underused stomach and back muscles, as well as from stress and obesity. These factors combine to render the

FIGURE 25.2
Classic Back Stretch
Try this basic back stretch first thing in the morning or during the day to relieve stiffness or tightness.

STEP 1 Lay on your back. Pull left knee to chest, hold to a count of five, then return to starting position. Repeat on right.

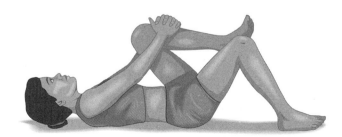

STEP 2 Bring both knees up toward chest, separating slightly so they point toward your shoulders. Hold to a count of five, then return to starting position. Repeat whole sequence 5 times. Do not use your arms or hands to help raise knees.

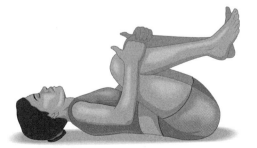

back vulnerable to injury, even an activity as simple as leaning over the sink to brush your teeth or sneezing.

What Causes Low Back Pain? Low back pain is usually caused by a pulled muscle, an inflamed tendon, or an injured ligament. Sometimes it may involve strain in one of the discs nestled between the vertebrae. Such problems usually take care of themselves, resolving in four to six weeks without the use of medication or surgery. (Treatments for low back pain are discussed later in this chapter.)

Ruptured Disc. A ruptured disc is a fairly serious condition. When a spinal disc tears, tissue from its soft center often leaks out, exerting pressure against nerves running along the spine. Symptoms often include pain shooting down through the buttock and leg, as well as numbness and limited leg function. In the past, surgery was considered the only option for treating this condition, but advances in knowledge about back pain, diagnosis, and treatment make it only a last resort.

Sciatica. One fairly common low back condition is sciatica, a form of pain that shoots down from the lower back through the buttock and into the leg. Sciatica is often caused by a ruptured or inflamed disc pressing against the sciatic nerve. The nerve may be irritated in other ways, however, and sciatica is often resolved with simple treatment.

Who Is at Risk? According to the American College of Orthopedic Surgeons, you face an increased risk for back pain if:

- Your job requires frequent bending and lifting.
- You keep your knees stiff and bend your back when you lift objects.
- You stretch, reach, or twist your body when moving or lifting objects.
- You are overweight.
- You slouch when standing or sitting.
- You do not regularly stretch and exercise or do not engage in recreational activities.
- You smoke.

Other factors known to contribute to low back pain include depression, anxiety, and work stress. Various forms of arthritis (especially osteoarthritis) are known to affect the lower back. Pregnancy can also cause low backache.

Preventive Measures. The great majority of low back disorders are preventable. Following are some tips to help you strengthen your back.

Maintain Good Posture. The inward curve of you lower spine is designed to help the back sustain the weight of the upper body. Slouching pushes back on that

---

Warning Signs of a Serious Back Condition

Although most back problems heal without treatment, there are four serious conditions that have symptoms of low back pain: fracture of the spine; spinal tumor; infection; and cauda equina syndrome (a compression of nerves running down from the lower portion of the spinal cord into the lower extremities). Call your doctor immediately if your back pain is accompanied by any of these symptoms:

- Loss of bladder or bowel control; difficulty in starting or stopping urination, especially of sudden onset
- Numbness in the genital or rectal area
- New leg numbness or weakness not due just to pain
- Unexplained fever and/or painful urination
- Severe pain that keeps you from standing or walking
- No improvement for 10 to 14 days

wellness **tip**

A firm mattress is essential for people who are prone to low back pain. It prevents you from staying in one position all night and getting stiff. If your mattress is too soft and you are not able to buy a new one, use a bedboard (sold in stores, or make your own with 3/4-inch plywood) under the mattress.

curve, thereby straining the lower back's muscles, bones, and other tissues. Stand and walk with your back straight and your shoulders back but relaxed. Your lower back should not arch, and your upper back should not stoop. Keep your shoulders and head erect and your stomach in at all times.

When working at a desk for long periods, sit close to the work surface to avoid leaning forward. Also, make sure that your desk is the proper height, allowing your arms to rest in a way that flexes your elbows at a 90-degree angle. (There are more workspace suggestions later in the chapter.)

You can even have good posture in bed. Avoid lying flat on your back or sleeping on your stomach; this can worsen swayback. If you want to sleep on your back, make sure to put a pillow under your knees to support them. Avoid high pillows under your head, which can strain neck, arms, and shoulders. The best sleeping position is lying on your side with knees bent. This position rests your lumbar spine altogether. If you put a pillow between your knees, it will ease the natural pressure of your upper thigh pulling down on the hip. A flat pillow under your head is acceptable to support the neck, especially if you have broad shoulders.

Standing Tall

To find the best standing position for you, stand with your back toward the wall one foot away, then lower your knees until you are in a sitting position. Tighten your abdominal and buttock muscles, which will tilt your pelvis back and flatten your spine against the wall. Hold this position while inching up the wall to a standing position. Practice walking while maintaining this same posture.

Rest Your Back. If your job requires you to sit for long periods, get up every hour to stretch your back. If possible, walk around for a few minutes to loosen back muscles and ligaments. On long car trips, pull over every hour or so to get out and rest your back. When driving with someone else, switch drivers regularly, especially if you are feeling back strain.

Alleviate Stress. Emotional stress can have a direct impact on your back. For some, an aching back accompanies pressure on the job or personal distress. Try to relieve stress in healthy ways, such as through meditation, deep breathing, or listening to music. If stress is unavoidable, find ways to keep it from "going straight to your back." Sit properly at work. Maintain good posture. Exercise to stretch and strengthen your back while helping alleviate stress.

Exercise. Regular exercise helps tone muscles responsible for back stability—the rectus abdominus and oblique muscles in the abdomen, and the back's erector spineae and latissimus dorsi muscles. Exercise slowly, and do not perform any exercises that cause you pain. If you are prone to low back pain, it is recommended you do exercises to strengthen the abdomen several times a week, especially upon rising in the morning.

Secret Exercises

Try these tension relievers and muscle-toning exercises during the day while at your desk, stopped at a red light, or in the elevator:

- Rotate shoulders forward and backward.
- Turn head slowly side to side.
- Very slowly, touch left ear to left shoulder; right ear to right shoulder. Raise both shoulders to touch ears; drop them as far down as possible.
- Pull in abdominals, tighten, and hold for a count of eight. Relax slowly. Gradually increase the count.

wellness **tip**

Bend your knees whenever you bend down (for example, to pick up an object, even one as light as a pencil) or bend over (for example, to turn on the bath faucet).

Proper Lifting Technique. Improper lifting is a common source of low back strain and injury. By taking a few very simple precautions, you can lift and carry almost any reasonable weight with minimal strain:

- Get close to the object you are going to lift and face it squarely. Do not twist your back as you lift.
- Bend your knees and squat down gently to grab the object and tense your stomach muscles.
- Lift using your thigh muscles. Keep your back straight. Do not use your back muscles to lift.
- As you lift the object, keep it close to your body. Keep your back straight.
- If you must change directions, do not twist your torso, but turn your whole body with your feet and legs.
- When setting the object down, bend your legs again and keep your back straight.

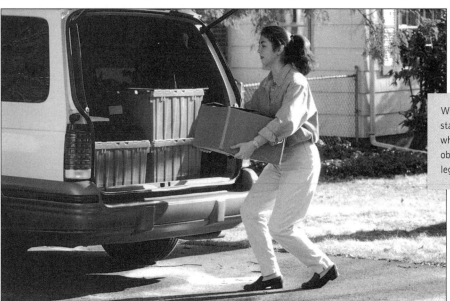

When lifting a heavy object, be sure to stand close to the object, bend your knees while keeping your back straight, grasp the object firmly, breathe in, and lift with your legs, not your back.

Lifetime Habits to Prevent Low Back Pain

- Never bend from the waist only. Always bend the hips and knees.
- Always turn and face the object you wish to lift. Never lift a heavy object higher than your waist. Hold heavy objects close to your body.
- Never lift or move heavy furniture. Leave it to professionals.
- Never sit on soft chairs or couches. When sitting for long periods of time, cross and recross your legs occasionally, to rest your back.
- When exercising, avoid any movements that arch or overstrain the lower back, backward or forward bends, or touching the toes with knees straight.
- Wear shoes with moderate heels, one inch or lower.
- Put a footrest under your desk.
- Buy or borrow a rocking chair. Rocking rests the back by changing the muscle groups used.
- Concentrate on developing good posture and strong abdominal muscles.

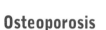

Osteoporosis

Osteoporosis, sometimes referred to as brittle bone disease, is a condition that causes bones to become porous and weakened. As you age, the balanced process of remodeling (old bone being replaced with new bone) slows down. Bones slowly begin to lose their mass, or bone density, as bone is broken down faster than it is made. The holes in the inner, spongy bone become larger as important minerals are depleted, causing the honeycomb structure to thin out. The outer compact bone also begins to thin, and the bone loses its ability to absorb the strains of bodily motion—and even to bear weight.

This disease affects the entire skeleton. People with osteoporosis often develop stooped shoulders (also called a hunchback or dowager's hump), as the weakened vertebrae compress under the weight of the upper body. Other bones also become brittle, greatly increasing the likelihood of fracture, primarily in the spine, hip, and forearm (radius).

Every year, at least 1.2 million fractures related to osteoporosis occur in the United States. Some of these fractures, especially those in the hip, can be disabling and require treatment in a long-term care facility. Hip fractures have been associated with more deaths, disability, and expense than all other types of osteoporotic fractures combined. Osteoporosis has also been linked to tooth loss and to painful compression fractures of the spine. The health care costs associated with osteoporosis have been estimated at a staggering $10 billion annually, including $6 billion a year to treat hip fractures alone.

Who Is at Risk? Just being female puts you at risk for osteoporosis. By and large, osteoporosis is a disease of aging women. Of the more than 25 million Americans suffering from osteoporosis, 80 percent are women. According to the National Osteoporosis Foundation, one in every two women over the age of 50 will suffer an osteoporotic fracture in her lifetime.

Why do women suffer from this disease in such high numbers? To begin with, a woman's bones are smaller and lighter than a man's, so that when bone loss occurs, the effects are more pronounced. Secondly, menopause places women at risk for developing osteoporosis. The female hormone estrogen appears to protect against bone loss. During and after menopause, the amount of estrogen produced by a woman's ovaries drops to very low levels. As a result, her rate of bone loss, already under way due to her age, increases dramatically.

Still other factors can increase a woman's risk of osteoporosis. Race is one important factor, with white and Asian women suffering at a rate much greater than African American women. Some scientists believe this disparity is due to differences in body size, structure, and bone metabolism associated with ethnicity. Some women are genetically predisposed to the condition: the female blood relatives (daughters, sisters, and nieces) of women with osteoporosis often develop the disease.

Those women who have their ovaries surgically removed (as during hysterectomy), also run a high risk of osteoporosis—especially if that surgery occurs before the natural time of menopause and the woman does not take hormone supplements to maintain the protective effects of estrogen. Risk is also increased for those women who stop menstruating early because of eating disorders, such as anorexia or bulimia. Some athletes who train at the professional level, such as gymnasts, runners, and some skaters, are also at risk because excessive exercise and training disrupts their menstrual cycles.

Certain medications have been linked with osteoporosis. Women who take glucosteroids for certain diseases and conditions, such as arthritis, severe asthma, and inflammatory bowel disease, have an increased incidence of osteoporosis. Other medications that can put women at risk are anticonvulsant medications (for epileptics), heparin, methotrexate, and lithium. Some medical conditions can also make a woman more vulnerable to osteoporosis. These include thyroid disorders, kidney or liver disease, celiac disease, Cushing's disease, diabetes mellitus, prolactinoma, hypercalciuria, and rheumatoid arthritis.

Poor nutrition and lack of exercise can lead to the development of osteoporosis. Calcium is essential for strong, healthy bones and must be stored in a woman's body to stave off the effects of natural bone resorption, which begins at age 35. By not consuming adequate amounts of calcium, a woman risks an early depletion of bone mass, and therefore, osteoporosis. Women who take the "yo-yo" approach to weight loss—repeatedly dieting and fasting—are at greater risk of developing osteoporosis. Because exercise, especially weight-bearing exercise, is important in developing strong bones, inactive women are more likely to develop osteoporosis. Conversely, women who exercise excessively over may years can wear down bone mass, and their risk of osteoporosis rises.

Researchers point to three lifestyle behaviors—cigarette smoking, coffee consumption, and excessive alcohol consumption—as actively raising one's risk of developing osteoporosis. Smoking is perhaps the worst of the three, simply because of its detrimental impact on a woman's overall health (increasing the risk of developing lung cancer and heart disease). But smoking also appears to have a specific impact on a woman's bones. A study conducted in Australia in the early 1980s compared the levels of bone mass in pairs of identical twin sisters whose risk for osteoporosis was also identical—except for the amount that each sister smoked. The researchers determined that the sisters who smoked more (a

wellness
warning

In postmenopausal women who have developed osteoporosis, hip fractures can be fatal. It has been estimated that a woman's risk of sustaining a potentially life-threatening hip fracture is equal to her combined risk of developing breast, uterine, and ovarian cancers.

pack of cigarettes a day during their adult lives) experienced a five to ten percent greater deficiency in bone mass by the time they reached menopause. Alcohol contributes to bone loss by increasing the amount of calcium lost through urine and stools. Research shows that drinking five or more caffeinated beverages a day reduces bone density.

Detecting Bone Density. There are tests, similar to x-ray imaging, available to assess a woman's bone density and determine her risk for osteoporosis. These tests are not yet used routinely but may be helpful for monitoring the condition of women who are at significant risk for osteoporosis. The National Osteoporosis Foundation recommends testing for all women approximately six months after menopause; early detection can signal the need for preventive measures. In women with some of the risk factors mentioned earlier, screening for osteoporosis even before menopause is critical to diagnosis and instituting treatment.

Preventive Measures. Osteoporosis is by no means inevitable. There are a number of highly effective steps women can take to lower their risk of osteoporosis, or at least curb its negative effects.

Diet. Make sure to consume enough calcium. According to the National Institutes of Health (NIH), a large percentage of Americans fail to get adequate amounts of this important mineral. The NIH recommends that women consume the following amounts of calcium, according to age and reproductive status:

- 1,200 to 1,500 milligrams a day for females aged 11 through 25, and pregnant and breastfeeding women
- 1,000 milligrams a day for women aged 25 to 50, and postmenopausal women taking estrogen replacement therapy
- 1,500 milligrams a day for postmenopausal women not taking estrogen replacement therapy

A number of foods contain calcium, especially milk, cheese, and other dairy products. Eating low-fat cheeses and skim milk provides calcium without excessive fat. You may wish to consider calcium supplements, which are available over-the-counter in any drugstore. These supplements are especially good for women who must avoid dairy products because of lactose intolerance. Supplements may cause difficulty for some women, however, especially those who have experienced kidney trouble; it is best to check with your doctor before taking them. For people who have difficulty tolerating calcium because of stomach upset, a form of calcium called calcium citrate may be easier to take than calcium carbonate, which is found in most supplements.

To absorb calcium efficiently, however, your body also needs sufficient amounts of another nutrient, vitamin D, which is also found in many common foods and vitamin supplements. The recommended daily amount of vitamin D is 400 IU (International Units) for adult women and 800 IU for elderly women.

Exercise. Exercise, such as walking, helps you avoid osteoporosis by building bone mass and strength. Even if you have already begun to lose bone mass, exercise can be helpful in slowing that process. Exercise also helps keep joints agile and strengthens your muscles, which provide your bones with much-needed support.

Hormone Replacement Therapy. Estrogen provides an important benefit for a woman's bones, helping them retain minerals and mass. This benefit is greatly reduced when women reach menopause and estrogen production falls to a very low level. Estrogen's protective effect can be maintained, however, through hormone replacement therapy (HRT). (HRT has other benefits and risks; for a full discussion of HRT, see Chapter 19.)

A number of experts have recommended HRT for women at high risk for osteoporosis. It may be especially helpful for women whose ovaries were removed before age 50, and those who have experienced natural menopause and have multiple osteoporosis risk factors, including early menopause, a close relative with osteoporosis, or less-than-normal bone mass for one's age.

Alternatives to HRT. Women who choose not to take HRT, or who do not tolerate it well, have several alternatives to consider beyond calcium and exercise: calcitonin, alendronate sodium, and selective estrogen receptor modulators (SERMs). Calcitonin is a synthetic version of a hormone made in the parathyroid gland that has been shown to alleviate severe back pain, slow bone loss, and increase bone density. It is intended only for short-term use and does not provide the protection against heart disease and Alzheimer's disease that is offered by estrogen. Alendronate sodium, approved by the Food and Drug Administration (FDA) for the treatment of osteoporosis and prevention of fractures, has also been shown to slow bone loss and actually increase bone density, though it also does not provide the benefits of estrogen. Alendronate must be taken on an empty stomach with at least eight ounces of water to ensure proper absorption and to reduce the side effects of nausea, heartburn, or abdominal discomfort. The FDA has recently approved a low dose of alendronate for women at high risk of developing osteoporosis in order to prevent osteoporosis from developing. Raloxifene hydrochloride, a SERM, was approved by the FDA in 1997 for the prevention of osteoporosis. This medication has positive estrogen-like effects on bone but lacks the negative effects on breast and uterine tissue. It lowers "bad" cholesterol (LDL) but does not improve "good" cholesterol (HDL). Further clinical trials with this and other SERMs will show whether this class of medication will have benefits for those women who cannot take estrogen.

Osteoarthritis

The word arthritis simply means pain and swelling in the joints. Osteoarthritis (OA) is the most common form of this complaint: the simple wearing out of a joint due to common, lifelong use. Unlike rheumatoid arthritis, a more rare, systemic, and chronic inflammatory disease (discussed later in this chapter), OA is largely related to age and thus is largely not preventable, although overuse of joints can play a role in its onset.

As people age, the natural lubrication in their knees, hips, knuckles, and other joints dries up. As OA sets in, a joint's surfaces rub together and break down, causing friction between bones. This friction and subsequent breakdown

wellness
warning

Swimming and bicycling are very good forms of aerobic exercise, but they are not weight-bearing and need to be supplemented with other forms of exercise to build strong bones.

of bone tissue prompts the bones to regenerate, yielding spurs (osteophytes). Spurs are painful and limit motion in the joint.

Where Osteoarthritis Strikes. OA usually occurs in the weight-bearing joints (hips and knees), as well as in the hands, feet, back, and neck. OA of the hip is widely considered the most painful and crippling form of this disease. With the growth of bony changes, this ball-and-socket joint loses much of its range of motion, hampering the leg's ability to move from side to side. The pain and debilitation caused by hip arthritis have been cited as one of the primary reasons elderly people are confined to a nursing home or continuous care facility. In the hands, OA causes the knuckles to become knobby (with the growth of bone spurs) and the fingers misaligned. OA rarely affects the elbows, shoulders, or ankles.

Who Is at Risk? According to the National Institute of Arthritis and Musculoskeletal and Skin Diseases, some 16 million Americans suffer from OA. OA affects 11.7 million women, which represents 74 percent of all cases. The condition strikes both men and women and affects virtually everyone to some degree in their middle-to-late years. Because it is caused largely by everyday wear and tear on the joints, progressing age is a major risk factor.

OA is also prompted by other factors, such as diabetes or Lyme disease, injury to the joint, surgery, or constant and extreme stress (caused by being overweight, poor posture, or constant, repetitive strain from use of the joint in the workplace or in recreational activities).

Those who are overweight appear to suffer at much higher numbers because their excess body weight exerts undue pressure on weight-bearing joints. Those who perform certain physical movements repeatedly over many years, such as manual laborers, factory workers, or athletes, also experience the disease more commonly. There are other, less controllable factors that can increase the risk of OA. One is the presence of a congenital deformity that causes a joint to function improperly and hasten its degeneration. Another has to do with genetics. Women in certain families seem predisposed to develop osteoarthritis. Researchers have

Living with Arthritis

Important factors in the treatment of all forms of arthritis are a positive attitude and active participation in your treatment. To help cope with your disease and pursue normal activities, the following proactive steps are suggested:

- Learn about your form of arthritis. Read professional and lay articles on the topic. If you have access to a computer, investigate a support group on-line. As you do your research, write down questions to ask your doctor. Staying well informed will help you feel in control and build your confidence in discussing issues with your doctor.
- Find a type and level of exercise that is comfortable for

you. Some arthritis pain comes from swelling and stiffness due to swelling; this restricts mobility that, in turn, promotes further stiffness and pain. Simple, moderate exercise can help break this cycle, and it need not be strenuous to be effective. Be sure, however, to discuss exercise with your physician first.

- Set goals. Having a specific goal to accomplish can help reduce pain because it absorbs your attention and provides a surge of positive feelings when you reach the goal.

Source: The Arthritis Foundation.

demonstrated, for instance, that, in the case of identical female twins, osteoarthritis is often suffered by both sisters, regardless of any other contributing factors.

Rheumatoid Arthritis

Rheumatoid arthritis (RA) does not strike just at different joints, but rather involves the entire body. Synovial tissues become inflamed, with joint pain, swelling, and stiffness. During late-stage RA, other parts of the body become affected, such as the skin and blood vessels (often creating leg ulcers), the eyes (triggering such disorders as conjunctivitis), the lungs, and the nerves. Anemia (lack of iron) is another common manifestation of RA. People suffering from this disease often feel fatigued and weak in general. Still, joint swelling and degeneration are the most common and troubling aspects of RA.

According to the Arthritis Foundation, this disease afflicts approximately three percent of all Americans, mostly women. It usually strikes adults between the ages of 30 and 40 and becomes most serious for those aged 40 to 60 years. RA is an extremely disabling disease. Even with appropriate drug therapy, up to seven percent of patients are disabled to some extent five years after they contract RA, and 50 percent are too disabled to work ten years after disease onset. Some sufferers experience periodic attacks (called flares), and others experience steady progression of symptoms over time.

The exact cause of RA is not known. It is an autoimmune disorder—one in which the body reacts to some foreign bacteria or virus. Because its cause is unknown, risk for RA is difficult to determine. The condition affects 2.5 million Americans of all ethnic backgrounds and ages. Women represent some 71 percent of all cases, but no one knows for sure why that is. There appears to be a genetic predisposition to developing the disease, but RA is not consistently passed from sufferers to their children.

Repetitive Stress Injuries

There are several types of repetitive stress injuries, all caused by the repetitive use of one part of the body over long periods of time during athletic or work activi-

Avoiding Repetitive Stress Injuries

Repetitive stress injuries can often be avoided, primarily by resting your hands frequently and stretching your wrist joint. If your job requires you to work on a keyboard or to perform some other manual activities (such as machine work or sewing) for long periods of time, make sure you have good positioning and wrist support. Take a break every 10 or 15 minutes to stretch and give your hard-working nerves and tendons a rest. One good stretch is to place your hands together with your finger tips up, as though you were praying, with your elbows out to your side. Slowly rotate your finger tips toward your chest. You will feel the stretch in your wrists as you do this. Hold for a count of five and then release.

Workstation Tips

If you work at a desk for long periods of time, you may need to rethink how your work area is arranged. The simple act of sitting exerts stress on your body, especially when the arrangement of your desk and chair restricts your circulation or places undue pressure on your muscles and joints. Computers pose an additional hazard if the monitor and keyboard are not placed appropriately in relation to your body.

By making the following adjustments to your work space, you can work with minimal bodily restriction and stress and can greatly reduce your risk of carpal tunnel syndrome, neck tension, and low back pain:

- **Proper seating.** Make sure that your chair provides ample support in the lower back and that its height and backrest are adjustable. The chair should have wheels so that you can move it easily. Arm rests are recommended.

- **Waist, knee, and elbow angle.** When sitting at your desk or workstation, your waist, knees, and elbows should each be arranged at 90-degree angles. Adjust your chair and arm rest heights accordingly. Make sure you sit so that your feet are flat on the floor. If the height of your chair does not permit you to sit with your feet squarely on the floor, use a foot rest. When your hands are placed on the desk, your elbows should also form a right angle.

- **Monitor placement.** Your computer monitor should be adjusted so that the top sits at, or just below, eye level.

Placement any higher can cause neck strain. Position the screen at a comfortable viewing distance, about two feet away from your eyes.

- **Wrist angle.** If your keyboard is positioned properly, your wrists should be able to rest comfortably on the table in front of it. If the thickness of the keyboard requires you to bend your wrists upward, use a wrist-rest pad. This will prevent your wrists from contorting upward, which is a major cause of carpal tunnel syndrome among computer users. Also, position your mouse so that it is level with your keyboard. Allow enough space so that you can use it without stretching or leaning over. Consider one of the new "natural" ergonomically designed keyboards that automatically places your hands and wrist in the least stressful position.

- **Elbow placement.** When keyboarding, try to hold your elbows in, close to your sides. This will help minimize "ulnar displacement," the sideways bending of the wrist caused by many keystrokes.

- **Keyboarding.** When you use the keyboard, relax your upper arms. Use a light touch, keeping your hands and fingers relaxed.

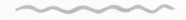

ties. Two repetitive stress injuries that are common in women are carpal tunnel syndrome and deQuervain's tenosynovitis. Sports injuries related to overuse are discussed later in this chapter.

Carpal Tunnel Syndrome. Carpal tunnel syndrome (CTS) is a painful condition that affects the wrists and hands. The carpal tunnel is the space through which the median nerve and flexor tendons extend from the forearm into the hand. When you move your hands and fingers, the flexor tendons rub against the walls of the tunnel. If this action is done repeatedly, it can cause irritation and swelling. When the inflamed tendons press against the median nerve, it causes tingling, numbness, pain, and weakness in the thumb, index finger, and middle finger.

Carpal tunnel syndrome affects people who perform activities that require the repetitive movement of the hands and wrist. The condition often strikes drafts-people, musicians, assembly-line workers, and those who work at a computer.

De Quervain's Tenosynovitis. This condition is caused by inflamed tendon sheaths in the thumb muscles. Women often experience it in the last three months of pregnancy or in the months following delivery. Others may contract this disorder performing jobs or activities requiring repetitive wrist and hand use. This condition is characterized by pain in the hand and a catching or "triggering" sensation when the thumb is moved toward the pinky finger.

Foot *and* Ankle Care

Your feet are made up of 28 bones, ligaments, muscles, and tendons, and provide you with balance and stability, whether you are walking on city streets or climbing up a rocky trail. Feet serve as your flippers when you swim and shock absorbers when you jump. Nevertheless, women often neglect foot care, cramming their feet into poorly fitting shoes, cleaning and drying them improperly, leaving them vulnerable to fungus, or walking barefoot without protection against tacks and splinters. There are a number of foot disorders. Some are unavoidable, while others can be treated or prevented altogether with proper foot care.

Corns and Calluses

These protective layers of dead skin form as a result of repeated pressure and friction on the skin. Corns develop on toes; calluses are found on the soles of the feet. Both result most often from ill-fitting shoes. Wear proper-fitting shoes and look for shoes in wide widths if your feet need the extra space.

Cutting out corns and calluses with a knife or razor is clearly dangerous and can cause serious damage and infection. Over-the-counter corn and callus removers have strong chemicals, so be careful when using them. In many cases, it is best to seek the advice of a podiatrist (foot doctor).

Metatarsalgia

If it hurts to walk or put pressure on the ball of your foot, your metatarsal bones may be inflamed. Metatarsalgia can be caused by being overweight, by pounding the foot down when walking or running, or by foot deformities that flatten the front of the foot.

You may find relief by using padded shoe inserts or by switching to more comfortable footwear altogether. If pain is severe or persistent, see a podiatrist.

Bunions

This painful, bony lump on the inside joint linking the big toe to the foot is a form of bursitis that develops when the toe is forced inward, causing pressure on the joint. A genetic predisposition appears to cause bunions in some people, and they often occur in women with flat feet. Often, however, the culprit is a constricting shoe. Women who wear narrow-toed high heels are especially prone to developing bunions.

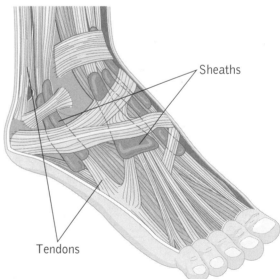

Sheaths

Tendons

FIGURE 25.3
Foot Pain
Most foot pain is caused by injury to or inflammation of tendons or the protective sheaths that surround them.

Bunions cannot always be avoided, even with the right shoe, but the right shoe can make you more comfortable. If you feel pressure on the big toe joint, try switching to shoes with plenty of room for your toes. If you wear high heels, switch to flats; a raised heel exerts undue pressure on the toes and joints. If the pain is severe or is not eased by changing shoes, see your doctor. You may need orthopedic inserts and pads to correct toe alignment. If the toe will not bend back on its own, surgery may be required.

Hammer Toes

This deformity of the second through fourth toes is almost always caused by a combination of heredity and footwear. Constant constriction forces the toe bones to bend, resulting in a "scrunched" appearance. Treatment of hammer toes includes use of proper footwear, corrective pads, and in some cases, surgery to shave down protruding bone.

Heel Pain

The sole of the foot is padded by a piece of fibrous, fatty tissue called the plantar fascia. Because the heel often takes the greatest pounding, sustaining the initial impact in running and walking, the heel portion of the plantar fascia can become tender and inflamed. Heel pain is often exacerbated by a number of contributing factors, including age, improper footwear, excessive stress from running and other physical activities, being overweight, and foot deformities that inhibit proper weight distribution throughout the foot. Other conditions, including arthritis, gout, and spurs on the heel bone, also cause discomfort in the rear of the foot.

Heel pain can be relieved, and often avoided, by ensuring that your shoes have proper padding, by moderating participation in such sports as running and tennis (which exert great force on the heel) and by watching your weight. If you experience pain, cut back on those activities that aggravate it, and try taking aspirin or other nonsteroidal anti-inflammatory medications (NSAIDs), like ibuprofen and naproxen. You can also try using shoe inserts specially designed to absorb pressure on the heel.

Sprained Ankles

The ankle is a complex joint central to all activities involving the leg. Every time you stop, turn, or jump, a good deal of force is concentrated in the ankle joint. The ankle is highly prone to injuries involving its bones and ligaments.

Preventing Ankle Sprains

To help prevent ankle sprains in activities that involve jumping or quick stops and starts, such as basketball, tennis, or aerobics, wear good-quality athletic shoes that provide adequate ankle support and are designed for that particular sport. High-top athletic shoes are especially effective for ankle support. If you have weak ankles, or if your ankles feel tired or achy, you might also consider taping your ankles or wearing braces.

A sprain is the irritation or tearing of a ligament. Ankle sprains can occur any time you twist the ankle, be it tripping over a child's toy, stumbling on steps, or landing on the side of the foot after a jump in aerobics class. Sprains are characterized by swelling and immediate pain, especially when flexing the ankle or trying to put weight on it.

Seek medical help promptly if you feel a snapping sensation or hear a pop while sustaining an ankle injury, if the pain and swelling are severe, or if the foot is misaligned. These could be signs of a severe sprain (a torn ligament) or a broken bone. If you are able to put some weight on your foot, you can try to treat the sprain yourself with the following steps, known as RICE: rest, ice, compression, and elevation. Ice the ankle promptly for up to 60 minutes every 2 hours and elevate it to reduce swelling. Then apply compression with an ankle brace or bandage. Try NSAIDs for pain and avoid putting weight on the ankle for 48 to 72 hours. Then, keeping the ankle wrapped, try walking on it lightly. You may need to use crutches or a brace for support. As the pain and swelling decrease, begin a slow return to normal activity, but keep the ankle wrapped and use care until all symptoms have gone away completely. Avoid wearing high heels until your sprain has healed completely. Let pain be your guide as to how much to do. Some time after the second week, when you are able to walk free of pain, you will want to start gentle exercises to regain ankle flexibility and to strengthen the supporting muscles. You can test whether or not you are able to return to regular activity by seeing if you can stand on your toes for 20 seconds and hop on your toes 10 times. If you are able to do this, you may begin jogging slowly until you get stronger and increase activity. Always stop immediately if you feel any pain.

Neck Pain

Neck pain often strikes with little warning and for no apparent reason. It is often severe and can make it virtually impossible to find a comfortable position in which to sit or sleep. Stiffness makes it difficult to turn your head.

Neck pain is often the result of some general life aggravation or stress. Many women "carry" stress in their neck and shoulders, and muscles and ligaments tense up. The condition is worsened by poor posture and work habits. Sometimes just sleeping with the window open, which can cause a draft, or making an usual movement of the head can result in neck strain or pain.

While some neck pain can signal serious conditions, such as meningitis and shingles, and is a common symptom of osteoporosis, osteoarthritis, and rheumatoid arthritis, most neck disorders are mild and resolve themselves with time and care. Following are some specific types of neck pain, as well as guidelines for prevention and treatment.

Neck Arthritis

With aging, natural wear and tear can cause the discs of the cervical spine to degrade. As the discs begin to shrink and bone spurs form, the spine's range of motion is greatly restricted, causing a stiff neck. Apart from achiness and limited movement of the head and neck, this does not generally lead to great pain or dis-

wellness **tip**

Airplane travel is a notorious source of neck stiffness. When flying for long periods, nestle a small pillow into the curve of your neck. You can also try creating a bolster with a rolled up airplane blanket or a towel. Special inflatable neck supports have been designed for this purpose. They are often sold in airport shops and some catalogs.

ability. As with other forms of osteoarthritis, this type of neck pain can be treated with a mixture of pain relief (NSAIDs) and regular exercises to ease flexibility.

Whiplash

Whiplash injuries are caused by a sudden, violent movement of the head. A common source of whiplash is rear-end car collisions. When a car is hit from behind, the force of the impact pushes the driver or passenger's body forward and the head back, thereby hyperextending the neck. As the car stops, the head flips forward, causing hyperflexion, the opposite and equally violent snapping motion. Whiplash can result in a simple strain of the neck muscles and ligaments, a sprain (the actual stretching or tearing of ligaments), dislocation or hairline fractures of the vertebrae, inflammation or rupture of a cervical disc, and damage to the spinal column or to the different nerves running along the spine.

Whiplash causes symptoms in other areas as well, including sore shoulders, pain in the jaw, and headaches and dizziness. Most whiplash injuries cause pain that gradually increases over the week after the injury. It is important to seek medical attention as soon after a whiplash incident as possible to reduce the intensity of symptoms. Treatment includes use of a soft cervical collar, applying ice to the area, taking NSAIDs (such as aspirin and ibuprofen), and, later, physical therapy.

Ruptured Disc

As discussed earlier, this condition can result from severe trauma, such as whiplash, or from other, milder events. When a spinal disc in the neck tears, tissue from its soft center often leaks out, exerting pressure against nerves running along the spine. A ruptured disk causes severe pain and limited motion. Symptoms may also include tingling or numbness in the neck, arms, and scalp. Treatment includes the use of a cervical collar, applying ice, traction, NSAIDs, and physical therapy or careful manipulation. Surgery may be required in some cases.

Sprain

Neck sprain typically causes pain at the injury site and sometimes in the surrounding muscles, as well as inflammation and limited range of motion. There are a number of treatment options, including collars, heat and cold treatments, massage, physical therapy or careful manipulation, and use of anti-inflammatory agents.

General Neck Strain (Cervical Fibrositis)

This mild condition can result from a night sleeping on a too-soft hotel pillow or with the window open, which can cause a draft. Many people develop neck aches after long periods of reading or working with their heads down and their necks hyperflexed. Cases are usually mild and respond to simple therapies, including heat, and use of anti-inflammatory agents.

Preventing Neck Pain and Strain

Bad posture, inadequate support, and stressful contortions can all lead to neck injury. Here are some tips for avoiding neck strain and subsequent stiffness or injury:

- Try to be conscious of the posture in your upper spine. When reading, do not slump in your chair. Hold the item you are reading at eye level so that you do not bend (hyperflex) your neck. At work, make sure that your computer screen is adjusted so that the top of the monitor is at or just below eye level. When writing, do not slump over your desk. Sit up straight and close to the writing surface. Look down at your work without tilting your head forward. Make sure your chair provides adequate low back support, which will help your neck posture. (For more information on adjusting your workstation, see the box on page 566.)

- Always make sure that your neck is properly supported, whether lying in bed or sitting up. When reading in bed, arrange the pillows so that you can sit up and read comfortably without flexing your neck. When lying down or sleeping, lie on your side or back, and adjust your pillow to support your neck without tilting your head. You can also try a bolster or cervical support pillow, a cylindrical piece of foam designed to fit right into the back curve of the neck. A rolled up towel will serve this same purpose.

- At the movies, do not sit too close to the screen. When bird watching or star gazing, try to cup one or both hands around the back of the neck.

- Be careful in the shower. If you are too tall to fit under the shower head, bend your knees to rinse your hair, or support your neck when tilting your head back.

- Avoid lying on your stomach. Whether you are on the floor or on the bed, watching TV or sleeping, this position puts strain on your neck muscles and ligaments.

Neck Exercises

Here are three basic exercises to ease stiffness and aid healing in your neck:

- **Basic relaxation.** Try the following exercise each morning, shortly after waking up. Lie on your back with your knees drawn up and your neck supported by a bolster. Take a deep breath, expanding your lungs as far as possible. Exhale slowly. Repeat five times.

- **Head turn.** Using the same position as above, turn your head to the left, and then return it to a normal position. Do the same on the right side. Repeat three to five times.

- **Stress relief.** The following exercise helps ease tension, especially after long periods spent working at a desk or driving a car. Draw your head back and tuck your chin in toward your chest. Take a deep breath. Then raise both shoulders up as close to the ears as possible and hold, counting to five. Relax and let your shoulders drop. Then draw your shoulders backward as far as possible, counting to five. Relax. Repeat these two motions in succession three times.

Source: Adapted from *The Whiplash Handbook* by Monique Harriton. Charles C. Thomas Publishers, 1989.

Neck Stretches

Here are three basic stretches to limber up your neck and help avoid injury:

- **Side neck stretch.** Tilt your head to the left, keeping your shoulders down. Place your left hand on the right top side of your head. Gently pull your head toward your left shoulder for 20 seconds. Reverse position and stretch to the right.

- **Neck pull-down.** Clasp your hands behind your head and let it lean forward. Hold for 15 seconds. Then pull down gently on your head for another 15 seconds. Breathe and relax in this position, keeping your back straight. Rest briefly and repeat.

- **Isometric exercise.** To strengthen neck muscles, place your left hand against the side of your head. Without moving your head or arm, push your head against your hand for 10 seconds. Repeat three times. Then reverse and use your right hand.

- Never cradle the telephone between your head and shoulder, as this can strain your vertebra, muscles, and ligaments. Instead, hold the receiver in your hand and put off that task requiring both hands until after you are through on the telephone. If you simply must use your hands while on the telephone, use a neck cradle support device or speaker phone.
- If it is chilly or drafty, make sure your neck is covered. Cold weather can cause a stiff neck. In cold weather, always wear a scarf to cover up your neck, even if you are only going out to get the mail.

Knee *Problems*

The knee is often a source of pain, especially in women who are physically active. This joint bends in one direction and is stabilized by two sets of ligaments, the tough connective tissue which connects bone to bone. Two ligaments, called the anterior and posterior cruciate ligaments, keep the knee from over-rotating and hyperextending. The co-lateral ligaments keep the knee from moving side to side and attach the lower leg bone, the tibia, to the upper leg bone, the femur. Cartilage lines the joint and acts as a shock absorber. The patella, or kneecap, sits on top of the joint.

Some of the largest and strongest muscle groups of the body work the knee—the quadriceps, or front thigh muscle, and the hamstrings, or back thigh muscles. These help support and protect the knee joint, but can also be a cause of some problems, especially when the quadriceps pulls excessively on the knee joint. Women are susceptible to more knee problems than men are because their wider hips cause the femur to meet the knee at a greater angle. This causes the quadriceps muscle to pull at a slight angle on the knee joint, rather than straight up and down as in most men. This angle means the kneecap pulls a little to one side.

Common Knee Conditions. The most common complaint is pain in the kneecap or patella. This is often a roughening of the joint, caused by minor arthritis changes in the kneecap, or inflammation, often caused by overuse of the joint or overdeveloped quadriceps. Patellofemoral syndrome (PFS), common in women, is the pain in the front of the kneecap that worsens with activity, such as sitting or walking up stairs. Often clicking or other noises are heard when the knee is bent. This is caused by the uneven pull of the quadriceps muscle that causes excessive damage to the underside of the patella. It is often treated with special exercises to strengthen the quadriceps and muscles on the inside of the knee and stretching the tight muscles on the outside of the knee. Treatments that help the patella move in the proper direction and avoiding aggravating activities are also helpful.

Athletic women will often suffer a tear of their knee ligaments. The anterior cruciate ligament (ACL) tear is most common, especially in soccer and basketball players. It occurs when the athlete overdevelops her quadriceps without adequately developing her hamstring muscles. Uneven pressure on the knee with sudden movements will cause the pop and pain of an ACL tear.

Preventing Knee Injuries. To help prevent knee injuries in activities, wear good-quality athletic shoes that are designed for the sport to give you sure footing.

Regular muscle stretching and balancing the development of the leg muscles and making sure that the inner knee muscle is strengthened will reduce PFS and ACL tears. If you have knee pain, wraps may help, but get assistance from a trainer or specialist to make sure you are using them properly.

Headaches

It is the rare individual who can claim she never gets headaches. The cause of most headaches is easily traced when the sufferer thinks back a few hours and realizes that she stayed in the sun too long, ate or drank too much, has not eaten in several hours, or read for a long period of time with inadequate lighting. The garden-variety headache usually disappears without medical treatment, or can be taken care of with mild, over-the-counter medications. Migraines and cluster headaches, which strike relatively few individuals, sometimes require more aggressive treatment. And certain unexplained headaches may be a signal of a serious underlying condition.

Tension Headaches

Muscle tension is the most common cause of the relatively mild, transitory headaches almost all women experience from time to time. Stress, which causes you to tense the muscles of your head and neck for long periods of time, is the prime suspect in such headaches. Lack of sleep, depression, and general fatigue also contribute to stress, and therefore to headaches. Tension headaches rarely indicate serious illness.

Most tension headaches respond to over-the-counter pain medication, such as ibuprofin, acetaminophen, and aspirin. Some women find that aspirin upsets the stomach, in which case one of the other medications is recommended. If you have frequent tension headaches and none of these over-the-counter medications work for you, talk to your physician to determine the probable source of your headaches and to decide on the appropriate pain reliever.

Regular exercise, especially flexibility training, helps some women prevent tension headaches. Strength training improves posture and prevents muscle strain. If your work involves sitting in front of a computer throughout the day, for example, you are likely to develop tension headaches. Practicing relaxation techniques, which make you aware of the difference between tense and relaxed muscles, reduces the frequency of tension headaches, as does getting up and walking around or stretching every half hour or so.

Preventing Tension Headaches in the Workplace

If you sit or stand in one position through most of your workday, take a few minutes during each hour to relax your neck muscles. When you become conscious of them, you may notice that they are pulling your shoulders up toward your ears. Breathe slowly and deeply, and consciously let your shoulders fall back and down. As you notice the difference between tight and relaxed neck muscles, work toward keeping them relaxed most of the time.

Headaches to Take Seriously

Although headaches are a common affliction, most are not caused by life-threatening conditions. However, some headaches may be a sign of serious disease and should not be underestimated. If a headache is accompanied by any of the following symptoms, see your physician immediately or go to the emergency room:

- **Frequent sleeplessness caused by headache**
- **Confusion or changes in awareness**
- **Seizures**
- **Failed or irregular muscle coordination**
- **Difficulty tilting the head forward; stiff neck**
- **Unusually severe facial pain**
- **Headache with exercise or sexual intercourse**
- **Spread of head pain to the neck or as far as the lower back**
- **Sustained double vision**
- **Local swelling and tenderness anywhere on the head or face**
- **Acute neck pain on one side that radiates to the face, eye, or ear**
- **Rash**

Cluster Headaches

Cluster headaches are characterized by sharp pain usually localized in one temple or behind one eye. They usually strike at night or in the morning, and may be linked to smoking and drinking. It is not clear why some people get cluster headaches, but it is known that they are more likely to occur in men and they begin in early adulthood, usually continuing throughout a person's life.

Migraines

Classic migraines occur four times as frequently in women as they do in men. Symptoms include distorted vision and debilitating pain, sometimes occurring on one side of the head only. A migraine sufferer may become sensitive to touch and experience coldness in her extremities. She may sense phantom smells before the onset of an attack or see flashing lights and other "hallucinatory" optical disturbances, sometimes called an aura.

Susceptibility to migraines appears to be inherited. Researchers theorize that the pain stems from the sudden narrowing and then widening of the blood vessels near the brain. Most people report that their migraines are usually "triggered" externally by changes in altitude, barometric pressure, humidity, or temperature; smog; bright lights; sunshine; flickering lights; computer monitors; loud noises; perfumes; or chemical odors. Others report internal triggers that are probably the body's reaction to stimulants, such as alcohol, monosodium glutamate, sulfites, tyramines, nitrites, red wine, salt, and caffeine.

If you suffer from migraines and do not know what triggers them, keep a diary, speak to your physician about the likeliest causes, and see if you can narrow down the possibilities to one or two. Once you know the cause, you and your doctor can identify the most appropriate and effective therapy for your specific situation. Recognizing the signs at the onset of a migraine and beginning treatment immediately sometimes shortens the duration significantly.

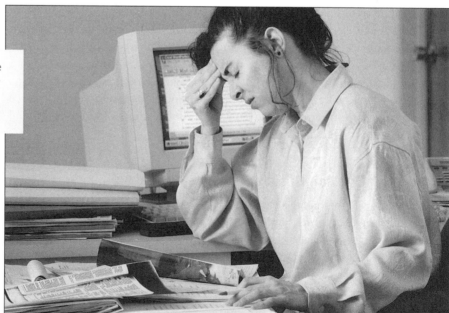

Stress, which causes tension in the muscles of your head and neck for long periods of time, is a common cause of tension headaches.

The Benefits of Massage

Massage not only feels good, it can also aid healing. The gentle but firm manipulation of the muscles during massage increases blood flow to ease stiff muscles and reduce spasm. If you have sustained a serious injury, your massage should be performed by a trained physical therapist or massage therapist. If your injury is minor, however, or your muscles just feel a little stiff, see a professional masseur/masseuse, or ask your spouse or a friend to gently rub the muscles in your back, shoulder blades, neck, arms, and legs. Do not let them try "cracking" your spine or apply too much pressure to tender areas: this could cause damage.

Hormonal changes may influence migraines. Some women are more likely to have an attack during menstruation. Some find birth control pills to be a trigger. To the extent that hormones play a role in a woman's experience with migraines, she may find that the frequency of attacks decreases during pregnancy and after menopause.

Avoiding Soft Tissue *Joint* Disorders

The soft tissues of your joints are susceptible to a number of different strains and disorders, described generally as rheumatism. When joint pain occurs throughout the body, that "achiness all over" may be a signal of rheumatoid arthritis (described earlier) or fibromyalgia. Localized pain or discomfort in only one or two joints may fall into one of the following categories: tendinitis, bursitis, or myofascial pain. These soft tissue problems in particular joints are most commonly caused by overuse of unconditioned joints in work and sports activities (including manual labor, taking up a new sport, or "do-it-yourself" weekend marathons of home repair or home improvement tasks). They can also be caused by congenital deformities and by other illnesses or conditions, such as pregnancy, during which hormones are secreted to relax ligaments and tendons. Preventive measures, discussed later in the chapter, can help lower your risk of such conditions.

Fibromyalgia

Fibromyalgia is a syndrome that is poorly understood and often misdiagnosed. It is not damaging to the body but is characterized by general body aches that can range from mild to incapacitating. In women, it is strongly associated with other symptoms, including chronic muscle pain, aching, irritable bowel syndrome, chronic headaches, PMS, depression, and sleep disorders (including difficulty sleeping and chronic fatigue syndrome).

The American College of Rheumatology's criteria for this diagnosis includes widespread pain affecting both sides of the body for at least three months with tenderness in at least 11 of 18 "tender points" in areas of the upper neck, back, shoulder, and hip. Fibromyalgia is not a joint pain or musculoskeletal disorder, but seems to be a pain modulation condition. Many factors can contribute to

wellness
warning

Seek medical help promptly if you feel a snapping sensation or hear a pop while sustaining an injury in the workplace or during sports or recreational activities, if the pain and swelling are severe, or if there is bruising at the wound site. These could be signs of a severe sprain, a torn muscle, joint dislocation, or a fractured bone.

fibromyalgia, including decreased circulation, minor injury, fitness, smoking, inappropriate exercise, emotional trauma, and lack of sleep.

Treatments consist of reducing contributing factors to the extent possible and trying to improve sleep, which is often impaired. Low-impact aerobic exercises, such as swimming or stationary bicycling, should be started at a very low level and only gradually increased. Limiting caffeine and alcohol, which can interfere with sleep, also helps. Low doses of medications that raise your body's serotonin, a neurotransmitter that modulates sleep and pain, and pain medications, such as NSAID, are also used. Trigger point injections, massage and physical therapy, relaxation, and acupuncture or acupressure can be beneficial.

Tendinitis

Tendinitis is a fairly common complaint that involves inflammation or irritation in one or more tendons. These tissues attach muscles to bone and play an important role in creating limb movement. Most cases of tendinitis are caused by sports injury. Common forms of tendinitis are Achilles tendinitis, affecting the heel and ankle, elbow tendinitis (or "tennis elbow"), and rotator cuff tendinitis in the shoulder.

Bursitis

The inflammation of one or more of the bursae, the small buffering tissues that ease limb movement by protecting muscles and tendons when they rub up against bones and ligaments, is called bursitis. It is most commonly experienced in the shoulder but also occurs in the knee, elbow, hip, heel, and foot. Bursitis tends to occur after the age of 40 and is often found after overuse of joints, especially the shoulder.

Myofascial Pain

Myofascial pain is a type of muscular pain that strikes specific areas of the shoulder and upper back and the lower back and buttocks. Set off by pressure on tender areas (called "trigger points"), myofascial pain is sharp and often shoots through the muscle area into the adjacent limb.

Who Is at Risk?

Soft tissue joint disorders can strike anyone. Still there are some whose risk is higher. Those who are overweight, for instance, put undue pressure on their weight-bearing joints, thereby leaving them open to strain or injury. In addition, those who perform certain physical movements repeatedly over many years also experience these disorders more often. For example, manual laborers or people who are heavily involved in sports, either recreationally or professionally, often develop soft tissue joint disorders.

Preventive Measures

The best way to reduce your risk of soft tissue injury is to avoid strain. Key recommendations include knowing your limits, warming up and stretching, and avoiding overuse.

Know Your Limits. Do not engage in strenuous activity unless you are physically up to the task. If you have been sedentary for a long time and want to begin exercising, do not go out and run three miles. Take a short walk. Then work up to a more demanding routine. If you want to learn a new sport, learn it gradually. For example, you might start off your tennis career by gently knocking a few balls around. Don't try to "murder" the ball, or lunge for difficult shots, until you have been playing regularly for several weeks. A good way to make sure you pace yourself is to take a class. A good instructor will teach you how to warm up, practice good technique, and build stamina—all of which help avoid injury in any sport.

Warm Up and Stretch. You can prevent many activity-related injuries by adequately warming up your body and stretching for five to ten minutes. Once your muscles have warmed up, stretch them thoroughly. Work your major muscle groups first, then concentrate on those muscles you will be using. See Figure 9.2 on page 178 for examples of basic warm-up stretches. Also, take time to cool down after exercising or engaging in a sports activity. Keep moving for a few minutes. Then stretch for five minutes more.

Avoid Overuse. It may sound like plain common sense, but avoiding overuse, or "listening to your body," is an important guideline for reducing your risk of injury. A tired body is more prone to injury. If your joints or limbs start to ache during an activity, rest immediately. Consider cutting back on your activities to give your joints and muscles a rest. If your body is sending you signals to slow down in the form of aches or twinges, you may need to leave a day or two in between tennis games or aerobics classes.

What *You* Can Do

A healthy musculoskeletal system is your primary means to an independent, active life. Many of the disorders that cause pain and disability—threatening your physical independence as you age and your ability to enjoy physical activity at any life stage—can be prevented or curbed if maintaining healthy muscles and bones is a priority in your wellness program:

- Choose and stick with a regular, moderate exercise program to maintain strength and agility and avoid injury.
- Choose a healthy diet that contains recommended amounts of calcium, protein, and vitamin D. Try to get these nutrients from food sources and not supplements.
- Watch your weight to avoid unnecessary strain on your muscles, joints, and bones.
- Avoid unhealthy behaviors, such as smoking and excess alcohol consumption, that pose risks to your musculoskeletal system (and jeopardize your overall health).
- Avoid injury by following simple safety precautions and by using good judgment in sports and other physical activities, such as pacing yourself and wearing proper footwear.

Resources

CHAPTER 1
A Dynamic Approach for a Longer, Healthier Life

The American College of Obstetricians and Gynecologists (ACOG)
409 12th Street, SW
PO Box 96920
Washington, DC 20090-6920
202-863-2518
www.acog.com

American Medical Women's Association (AMWA)
801 N. Fairfax Street
Suite 400
Alexandria, Virginia 22314
703-838-0500
www.amwa.org

Centers for Disease Control and Prevention
Office of Women's Health
1600 Clifton Road, NE
Atlanta, GA 30333
404-639-3311
www.cdc.gov/od/owh/whhome.htm

CHAPTER 2
Family History and Lifestyle Assessment

National Society of Genetic Counselors
233 Canterbury Drive
Wallingford, PA 19086
610-872-7608
www.members.aol.com/nsgcweb/nstchome.htm

CHAPTER 3
Making Informed Health Care Decisions

American Association of Retired Persons
601 E Street, N.W.
Washington, DC 20049
800-424-3410
www.aarp.org

American Board of Medical Specialties
1007 Church Street, Suite 404
Evanston, IL 60201-5913
800-776-2378
847-491-9091

Health Insurance Association of America
555 13th Street NW
Washington, DC 20004
202-824-1600
www.hiaa.org

National MEDICARE Issues Hotline
Health Care Financing Administration
200 Independence Avenue SW
Washington, DC 20201
800-638-6833

CHAPTER 4
Childhood: Birth to Ten Years

American Academy of Pediatrics
141 Northwest Point Blvd.
P.O. Box 927
Elk Grove Village, IL 60009-0927
847-981-7084
www.aap.org

U.S. Consumer Product Safety Commission
4330 East-West Highway
Bethesda, MD
800-638-2772
www.cpsc.gov

Vaccine Adverse Event Reporting System
P. O. Box 1100
Rockville, MD 20849-1100
800-822-7967
www.vaers@cais.com

CHAPTER 5
Adolescence/Early Reproductive Years: Ages 11 to 24

Al-Anon/Alateen
Al-Anon Family Group Headquarters, Inc.
1600 Corporate Landing Parkway
Virginia Beach, VA 23454-5617
800-344-2666
www.Al-Anon-Alateen.org

American Academy of Family Physicians
8880 Ward Parkway
Kansas City, MO 64114
800-274-2237
www.aafp.org

Vaccine Adverse Event Reporting System
P. O. Box 1100
Rockville, MD 20849-1100
800-822-7967
www.vaers@cais.com

CHAPTER 6

Later Reproductive/Mature Years: Ages 25 to 45/46 to 64

American College of Obstetricians and Gynecologists (ACOG)
409 12th Street, SW
PO Box 96920
Washington, DC 20090-6920
202-863-2518

American Association of Retired Persons
601 E Street, N.W.
Washington, DC 20049
800-424-3410
www.aarp.org

CHAPTER 7
Older Years: Ages 65 and Over

American Association of Retired Persons
601 E Street, N.W.
Washington, DC 20049
800-424-3410
www.aarp.org

National Osteoporosis Foundation
1150 17th Street NW
Suite 500
Washington, DC 20036-4603
202-223-2226
www.nof.org

CHAPTER 8
Eating for Wellness

American Dietetic Association
216 West Jackson Boulevard
Chicago, IL 60605-6995
312-899-0040
www.eatright.org

U.S. Department of Agriculture (USDA)
Washington, DC 20250
202-720-2791
www.usda.gov

CHAPTER 9
Exercising for Strength and Stamina

Aerobics and Fitness Association of America (AFAA)
15250 Ventura Boulevard
Suite 200
Sherman Oaks, CA 91403
800-446-2322
www.afaa.com

CHAPTER 10
Sleeping Peacefully

National Sleep Foundation
729 15th Street NW
4th Floor
Washington, DC 20005
202-785-2300
www.sleepfoundation.org

SleepNet
www.sleepnet.com

The Sleep Well
www-leland.stanford.edu/~dement

CHAPTER 11
Fostering Good Relationships

American Psychiatric Association
1400 K Street, NW
Suite 501
Washington, DC 20005
202-682-6220
www.psych.org

National Mental Health Association, Inc.
1021 Prince Street
Alexandria, VA 22314-2971
800-969-6642

CHAPTER 12
Maintaining Your Mental and Emotional Health

National Depressive and Manic Depressive Association
730 North Franklin, Suite 501
Chicago, IL 60601
800-826-3632
www.ndmda.org

Anxiety Disorders Association of America
11900 Parklawn Drive, # 100
Rockville, MD 20852
301-231-9350
www.adaa.org

National Mental Health Association, Inc.
1021 Prince Street
Alexandria, VA 22314-2971
800-969-6642

American Psychiatric Association
1400 K Street, NW, Suite 501
Washington, DC 20005
202-682-6220
www.psych.org

CHAPTER 13
Controlling the Use of Harmful Substances

Center for Substance Abuse National Drug Hotline
800-662-4357

National Institute of Alcohol Abuse and Alcoholism
600 Executive Boulevard
Willco Building
Bethesda, MD 20892-7003
301-443-3860
www.niaaa.gov

National Institute on Drug Abuse
Room 10A39 5600 Fishers Lane
Rockville, MD 20857
301-443-1124
www.nida.nih.org

National Clearinghouse for Alcohol and Drug Information (NCADI)
P.O. Box 2345, Rockville, MD 20847-2345
800-729-6686
www.health.org

CHAPTER 14
Identifying and Overcoming Violence

National Domestic Violence Hot Line
800-799-7233

Hot line for reporting suspected child abuse
800-422-4453

National Clearinghouse on Child Abuse and Neglect Information
P.O. Box 1182
Washington, DC 20013-1182
800-394-3366
www.calib.com/nccanch

Administration for Children, Youth, and Families
www.acf.dhhs.gov/programs/acyf

National Center on Elder Abuse (NCEA)
810 First Street, NE
Suite 500
Washington, DC 20002-4267
www.gwjapan.com/NCEA

Rape, Abuse, and Incest National Network (RAINN)
Toll-free number that will route you to a local rape crisis center:
800-656-4673
www.cs.utk.edu/~bartley/other/RAINN.html

CHAPTER 15
Preventing Injury and Accidents

American Academy of Pediatrics
141 Northwest Point Blvd., P.O. Box 927
Elk Grove Village, IL 60009-0927
847-981-7084
www.aap.org

American Red Cross
17th & D Streets, SW
Washington, DC
202-737-8300
www.redcross.org

Educational Fund to End Handgun Violence
100 Maryland Avenue, SE, #303
Washington, DC 20002
202-544-7227

National Safety Council
1121 Spring Lake Drive
Itasca, IL 60143-3201
630-285-1121
www.nsc.org

U.S. Consumer Product Safety Commission
4330 East-West Highway
Bethesda, MD
800-638-2772 Consumer Hotline
301-504-0990 Main Line
www.cpsc.gov

U.S. Department of Labor
Occupational Safety and Health Administration
Washington, DC
800-827-5335
www.ohsa.gov

CHAPTER 16
Nurturing Your Sexuality

American Association of Sex Educators, Counselors, and Therapists (AASECT)
P.O. Box 238
Mount Vernon, IA 52314
319-895-8407
www.aasect.org

Sexuality Information and Education Council of the United States (SIECUS)
130 West 42nd Street, Suite 350
New York, New York 10036-7802
212-819-9770
www.siecus.org

CHAPTER 17
Planning Your Family

American College of Obstetricians and Gynecologists
409 12th Street, SW
PO Box 96920
Washington, DC 20090-6920
202-638-5577

American Society for Reproductive Medicine
1209 Montgomery Highway
Birmingham, AL 35216-2809
205-978-5000

RESOLVE, Inc. (Infertility Support)
1310 Broadway
Somerville, MA 02144
617-623-0744

Natural Family Planning (Couple-to-Couple League)
www.itek.net/~mission/cathlc/ccl

Emergency Contraception Hotline
800-584-9911

CHAPTER 18
Planning a Healthy Pregnancy

Depression After Delivery
P.O. Box 1282, Morrisville, PA 19067
800-944-4773
215-295-3994
www.pleiades-net.com/org/DAD.1.htm

Planned Parenthood (to make appointment for reproductive health care)
800-230-7526

CHAPTER 19
Planning for Menopause

American Association of Retired Persons
601 E Street, NW
Washington, DC 20049
202-434-2277

National Institute on Aging Information Center
PO Box 8057
Gaithersburg, MD 20898-8057
800-222-2225

CHAPTER 20
Lowering Your Risk for Cardiovascular Disease

American Heart Association
7272 Greenville Avenue
Dallas, Texas 75231-4597
214-706-1442
www.amhrt.org

The American Medical Women's Association Education Project on Coronary Heart Disease in Women
801 N. Fairfax Street #400
Alexandria, VA 22314
703-838-0500
www.amwa-doc.org

The National Heart, Lung, and Blood Institute
National Institutes of Health
9000 Rockville Pike
Bethesda, Maryland 20892
301-496-4236
www.nhlbi.nih.gov

CHAPTER 21
Reducing Your Risk for Cancer

National Cancer Institute
  9000 Rockville Pike
  Bethesda, MD 20892
  800-422-6237
  www.nci.nih.gov

American Cancer Society
  1599 Clifton Road NE
  Atlanta, GA 30329
  800-227-2345
  www.cancer.org

CHAPTER 22
Protecting Against Infection

National Sexually Transmitted Disease Hotline
  800-227-8922

Centers for Disease Control and Prevention
  National AIDS Clearinghouse
  P.O. Box 6003
  Rockville, MD 20849-6003
  800-458-5231

Centers for Disease Control and Prevention
  Office of Women's Health
  1600 Clifton Road NE
  Atlanta, GA 30333
  404-639-3311
  www.cdc.gov/od/owh/whhome.htm

CHAPTER 23
Protecting Against Metabolic Disease

American Diabetes Association
  P.O. Box 25757
  1660 Duke Street
  Alexandria, VA 22314
  800-342-2383
  www.diabetes.org

The National Institute of Diabetes and Digestive
Kidney Diseases (NIDDK)
  Division of Diabetes, Endocrinology, and Metabolic
    Diseases
  31 Center Drive
  Building 31 Room 9A04
  Bethesda, MD 20892
  301-496-3583
  www.niddk.nih.org

Thyroid Foundation of America
  Ruth Sleeper Hall, RSL 350
  40 Parkman Street
  Boston, MA 02114-2698
  800-832-8321

CHAPTER 24
Keeping the Senses Sharp

American Academy of Ophthalmology
  655 Beach Street
  San Francisco, CA 94109
  415-561-8500
  www.aao.org

The National Institute on Deafness and Other Communication
Disorders (NIDCD)
  1 Communication Avenue
  Bethesda, MD 20892-3456
  800-241-1044

The National Headache Foundation
  5252 North Western Avenue
  Chicago, IL 60625
  800-843-2256
  www.headaches.org

CHAPTER 25
Strengthening Your Bones and Muscles

American Academy of Orthopedic Surgeons
  222 South Prospect Avenue
  Park Ridge, Illinois 60068
  800-346-2267
  www.aaos.org

Arthritis Foundation
  PO Box 19000
  Atlanta, Georgia 30326
  800-283-7800
  www.arthritis.org

National Osteoporosis Foundation
  1150 17th Street NW, Suite 500
  Washington, DC 20036-4603
  202-223-2226
  www.nof.org

Index

I

P

Pacemaker, 456
Pain response, 530
Painkillers, 269, 399
Pancreas, 512
Panic disorder, 242-243
Pantothenic acid, 151
Pap test, 6, 31, 90-91, 108, 130
Paranoid personality disorder (PPD), 247
Parasomnias, 205-207
Parathyroid, 511-512
    disorders of, 525-526
Passive smoking, 28, 264-265, 454, 463, 474
Patellofemoral Syndrome (PFS), 572
PCP (phencyclidine), 268
Peer pressure, 92-93
Pelvic examination, 91
Pelvic inflammatory disease (PID), 91, 347-348, 497, 502-503
Penicillin, 489
Pericardial disease, 437-438
Pericarditis, 437-438
Perimenopause, 410-412
Periodic health examinations
    adolescence, 87-103
        counseling, 92-101
        immunizations, 101-103
        overview, 87-89
        screening, 89-92
    adulthood, 104-121
        counseling, 110-119
        immunizations, 119-121
        overview, 104-105
        screening, 105-110
    cardiovascular disease and, 446-447
    childhood, 69-84
        counseling, 75-81
        immunizations, 33, 81-84
        overview, 69-70
        screening, 70-74
    hormone replacement therapy and, 421
    importance of, 5
    senior years, 123-140
        counseling, 132-139
        immunizations, 139-140
        overview, 123-126
        screening, 126-132
Periodontal disease, 119
Personality disorders, 246-248
Pertussis, 82

Phenylalanine (PKU) test, 74
Pheochromocytoma, 524-525
Phobias, 241-242
Phosphorus, 152
Photorefractive keratotomy, 538
Physical activity. See Exercise
Physical relationships, 30-32. *See also* Sexuality
Physician
    "board eligible," 58
    communication with, 59-61
    experience, 58
    private practice of, 62
    relationship with patient, 25
    training/certification, 57-58
    visiting, patient checklist for, 61
Phytochemicals, 465
Phytoestrogens, 419
Pinkeye, 539-540
Pituitary gland, 511
    disorders of, 526-528
Placental interruption, 383
Plantar fascia, 568
Plaque, arterial, 173, 433, 440, 443
Plasma, 433
Platelet inhibitors, 457
Platelets, 433
Pneumococcal vaccine, 139
Point-of-service (POS) plans, 45-46
Poisoning, preventing, 76-77, 311
Poliovirus vaccine, 82
Polycyclic aromatic hydrocarbons (PAHs), 465
Polysomnography, 204
Post-abortion syndrome, 369
Postmenopausal Estrogen Progestin Interventions (PEPI) Trial, 418, 420, 446
Postmenopausal years, 168, 425-429, 561
Postovulation method of birth control, 362
Postpartum blues, 404, 406
Postpartum depression (PPD)/psychosis, 239, 404, 406
Posttraumatic stress disorder (PTSD), 243-244, 288, 291
Potassium, 152
Power of attorney, durable, 65-67
Preconception care, 376
Preeclampsia, 383
Preexisting conditions, 40

Preferred provider organizations (PPOs), 44-45
Pregnancy. *See also* Birth control; Childbirth; Infertility
    abortion and, 367-369
    acquired immunodeficiency syndrome and, 507
    in adolescence, 97-98
    in adulthood, 117
    alcohol consumption in, 262, 387
    caring for newborn, 402-403
    diabetes and, 14
    diet in, 385-386
    domestic violence and, 280, 388-389
    due date and, 379
    exercise in, 186-188, 387
    high blood pressure in, 106, 383
    home test kit, 377
    hormonal changes in, 187
    illicit drug use in, 388
    infection in, 389
    intercourse and, 390, 393
    lifestyle and, 385-390
    morning sickness and, 391
    personal responsibilities in, 408
    physical changes/challenges in, 187, 390-393
    post-childbirth, 402
    postpartum blues and, 404, 406
    preconception care, 376
    prenatal care, 379-385
    preparing for childbirth and, 393-396
    prescription drugs in, 388
    questions about, 375-379
    from rape/sexual assaults, 291
    rest in, 390
    rubella in, 92, 110, 121
    sexual fulfillment and, 338
    sleep and, 199, 392
    smoking in, 11, 264, 387-388
    subsequent, 407-408
    travel and, 390
    unintended, 97-98, 117, 326, 337, 369
    weight gain in, 187
    work and, 388-390
Prejaculatory fluid, 361
Premarin, 419
Premature ejaculation, 342
Premenstrual syndrome (PMS), 239
Prenatal care, 379-385

Photo Location Acknowledgments

Broadway Dance Center, New York, NY
Community Blood Council of New Jersey, Trenton, NJ
Helene Fuld Medical Center, Trenton, NJ
HiTOPS—Health Interested Teens' Own Programs on Sexuality, Princeton, NJ
Lawrence Ob-Gyn Associates, Lawrenceville, NJ and Yardley, PA

Lifestyle Fitness Center, Plainsboro, NJ
Offices of Edward Von Der Schmidt, III, M.D., Neurologist, Princeton, NJ
Presbyterian Homes of New Jersey, Princeton, NJ
Princeton Indoor Tennis Center, Princeton, NJ
Princeton YWCA, Princeton, NJ

AP 13 '02

DATE DUE

JUN 0 5 2002		

GAYLORD   #3523PI   Printed in USA